IMMUNOSUPPRESSIVE AND ANTIINFLAMMATORY DRUGS

ANNALS OF THE NEW YORK ACADEMY OF SCIENCES
Volume 696

IMMUNOSUPPRESSIVE AND ANTIINFLAMMATORY DRUGS

Edited by Anthony C. Allison, Kevin J. Lafferty, and Hans Fliri

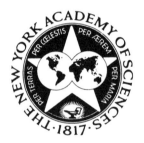

The New York Academy of Sciences
New York, New York
1993

Library of Congress Cataloging-in-Publication Data

Immunosuppressive and antiinflammatory drugs / edited by Anthony C. Allison, Kevin Lafferty, and Hans Fliri.
    p. cm. — (Annals of the New York Academy of Sciences, ISSN 0077-8923 ; v. 696)
    Includes bibliographical references and index.
    ISBN 0-89766-835-9 (cloth : alk. paper). — ISBN 0-89766-836-7 (pbk. : alk. paper)
    1. Immunosuppressive agents—Congresses. 2. Anti-inflammatory agents—Congresses. I. Allison, Anthony C. (Anthony Clifford), 1925-   . II. Lafferty, Kevin. III. Series.
    [DNLM: 1. Anti-Inflammatory Agents—congresses.
2. Immunosuppressive Agents—congresses. W1 AN626YL v. 696 1993 / QV 247 I33 1993]
Q11.N5   vol. 696
[RM373]
500 s—dc20
[615'.7]
DNLM/DLC
for Library of Congress   93-41797
                                                  CIP

SP
Printed in the United States of America
ISBN 0-89766-835-9 (cloth)
ISBN 0-89766-836-7 (paper)
ISSN 0077-8923

ANNALS OF THE NEW YORK ACADEMY OF SCIENCES

Volume 696
November 30, 1993

IMMUNOSUPPRESSIVE AND ANTIINFLAMMATORY DRUGS[a]

Editors and Conference Organizers
ANTHONY C. ALLISON, KEVIN J. LAFFERTY, AND HANS FLIRI

CONTENTS

[a]This volume is the result of a conference entitled Immunosuppressive and Antiinflammatory Drugs held on April 12–15, 1993 in Orlando, Florida and sponsored by the New York Academy of Sciences.

Part III. Novel Antiinflammatory Strategies

Part IV. Immunosuppressive Drugs for Transplantation

Poster Papers

Financial assistance was received from:

Supporters
- DUPONT MERCK PHARMACEUTICAL COMPANY
- NIPPON KAYAKI CO. LTD.
- SANDOZ PHARMACEUTICALS CORPORATION
- SYNTEX (USA) INC.
- SYNTEX LABORATORIES, INC.
- WYETH-AYERST RESEARCH

Contributors
- ABBOTT LABORATORIES
- AFFYMAX RESEARCH INSTITUTE
- BOEHRINGER INGELHEIM PHARMACEUTICALS, INC.
- GLAXO INC. RESEARCH INSTITUTE
- HOECHST-ROUSSEL PHARMACEUTICALS INC.
- HOFFMANN-LA ROCHE INC.
- RW JOHNSON PHARMACEUTICAL RESEARCH INSTITUTE
- MERCK RESEARCH LABORATORIES
- MILES INC.
- MONSANTO COMPANY
- PFIZER CENTRAL RESEARCH
- THE UPJOHN COMPANY
- WARNER-LAMBERT/PARKE-DAVIS

Novel Immunosuppressive and Antiinflammatory Drugs

A 1993 Perspective

ANTHONY C. ALLISON[a]

Dawa Corporation
Belmont, California

IMMUNOSUPPRESSIVE DRUGS

The advantages and limitations of currently used immunosuppressive drugs are well known. Several antimetabolites synthesized for cancer therapy were incidentally found to have immunosuppressive activity. In 1951, 6-mercaptopurine (6-MP) was synthesized as an inhibitor of nucleic acid base metabolism. First used in leukemia, 6-MP was found to suppress antibody formation and allograft rejection; later the prodrug azathioprine was found to a better immunosuppressive *in vivo*.[1] Used with glucocorticoids, azathioprine made human organ transplantation feasible.[2] However, efficacious doses of azathioprine are close to those producing bone marrow suppression and other side effects. Methotrexate, which inhibits synthesis of thymidylate as well as of purines *de novo*,[3] is a nonselective antiproliferative agent active on many cell types. Developed for cancer therapy, methotrexate was later found to have immunosuppressive and antiinflammatory effects that are useful in rheumatoid arthritis and other diseases. However, methotrexate can produce liver damage, pneumonitis, and bone marrow suppression. Coming to drugs now in development, Brequinar was synthesized by the E.I. DuPont de Nemours Company as an antimetabolite for use in solid tumors. The drug was shown to inhibit dihydroorotate dehydrogenase, thereby blocking *de novo* pyrimidine synthesis, and to exert antiproliferative activity on a variety of cell types. Later Brequinar was found to be a potent immunosuppressive, and it is currently being studied in human organ graft recipients.[4]

The second strategy for identifying immunosuppressive drugs has been screening of fermentation products. The prototype is, of course, cyclosporine, shown in 1977 to prevent proliferation of lymphocytes *in vitro* and to exert immunosuppressive activity *in vivo*.[5] Combination therapy with cyclosporine, azathioprine, and a glucocorticoid greatly improved the survival of organ grafts, and cyclosporine has also been approved for treatment of psoriasis. However, side effects of cyclosporine include nephrotoxicity, hypertension, hypercholestrolemia, diabetogenic effects, neurotoxicity, hirsutism, and gingival hyperplasia. Using a nephrotoxic drug to prevent kidney graft rejection is obviously not the final answer. Cyclosporin G is somewhat less nephrotoxic in experimental animals than cyclosporin A, and comparative studies in humans are required.

The clinical and commercial success of cyclosporine led other companies to screen fermentation products for immunosuppressive activity. The most potent is FK-506, which has a mode of action and toxicity profile similar to those of cyclospo-

[a]Correspondence: 2513 Hastings Drive, Belmont, California 94002.

rine. Another potent immunosuppressive identified in a similar way is rapamycin. Although there is a structural resemblance to FK-506, its mode of action is different. The fermentation product spergualin and its derivative, 15-deoxyspergualin, were developed for anticancer use and later found to be immunosuppressive. The search for natural products with immunosuppressive activity continues. In Orlando, Longley reviewed the immunosuppressive effects of discodermolide, a polyhydroxylated lactone derived from a marine sponge.

For a decade, cyclosporine was used clinically without understanding its mode of action at the molecular level. It was known that the drug blocks early events in the activation of T lymphocytes, including IL-2 gene transcription. Identification of cognate intracellular receptors of cyclosporine and FK-506 as proline isomerases, and the binding of calcineurin to the drug-isomerase complexes, with consequent inhibition of its Ca^{2+}-dependent phosphatase activity, was a major advance. The molecular biological studies leading to this conclusion were reviewed by Clipstone and by Weiderrecht in Orlando. Fliri reviewed structure-activity relationships of cyclosporins, which show that the cyclosporin molecule has two functional domains, one mediating cyclophilin binding and the other endowing affinity of the complex to calcineurin, thereby inhibiting its enzyme activity. Cyclophilin-binding cyclosporin analogues that do not inhibit the phosphatase activity of calcineurin are not immunosuppressive. NFAT, a DNA-binding protein complex required for IL-2 gene transcription, contains a 120 kD subunit present in unstimulated T-cells. NFATp is a substrate for calcineurin *in vitro*.[6] Interaction of the lymphocyte-specific factor, NFATp, with the ubiquitous transcription factors Fos and Jun provides a novel mechanism for combinatorial regulation of IL-2 gene transcription, which integrates the calcium-dependent and protein kinase C–dependent pathways of T cell activation.[6] These studies focused attention on proline isomerases, which are found in a wide range of organisms, prokaryotic as well as eukaryotic, as Hemenway and Heitman reminded us during the conference. In principle proline isomerases can facilitate rapid changes in protein conformation, as required for ion channels and other functions; it will be interesting to learn the role of these proteins.

Sehgal, one of the discoverers of the biological effects of rapamycin, pointed out that the mechanism of action on lymphocytes is distinct from that of other immunosuppressive drugs. Cyclosporine and FK-506 block Ca^{2+}-dependent cytokine gene transcription and do not affect IL-2 dependent proliferation. Rapamycin inhibits cytokine-mediated signal transduction pathways late in the response to proliferative signals. Flanagan presented evidence that rapamycin arrests T cells at their entry into the S-phase of the cell cycle and inhibits IL-2-induced expression of p34[cdc2], a serine/threonine kinase that is required for all cells to progress through the cell cycle. This progression is correlated with the synthesis, phosphorylation, dephosphorylation, and disappearance of cell-cycle-dependent proteins termed cyclins. Albers reported the identification of a rapamycin-sensitive, cyclin-dependent kinase activity that correlates with the arrest point in osteosarcoma cells. It would be interesting to learn the mechanism by which rapamycin prevents the association of cyclin D1 with specific cyclin-dependent kinases, and to have comparable information on lymphocytes.

Another strategy is the rational design of immunosuppressive drugs. Observations on children with inherited defects of purine metabolism led Allison and his colleagues to conclude that *de novo* synthesis of guanosine nucleotides is required for proliferative responses of human T and B lymphocytes to antigenic and mitogenic stimulation. The enzyme limiting the rate of *de novo* synthesis of GMP is inosine monophosphate (IMP) dehydrogenase. The fermentation product mycophenolic acid (MPA), a nonnucleoside inhibitor of IMP dehydrogenase, proved to have more potent antiproliferative effects on lymphocytes than on other cell types. Natsumeda pointed out that this selectivity may be explained, at least in part, by the existence of two isoforms of IMP dehydrogenase. Type I IMP dehydrogenase is the housekeeping enzyme expressed in resting cells, including lymphocytes. When T and B lymphocytes respond to proliferative signals, expression of the type I gene is unchanged while that of the type II gene is rapidly induced. The type II enzyme is five times more sensitive to MPA than is the type I enzyme. MPA has other activities, including inhibition of the glycosylation of adhesion molecules. That could decrease recruitment of lymphocytes and monocytes into sites of ongoing organ graft rejection and inflammation, such as the synovia of patients with rheumatoid arthritis. MPA and rapamycin, alone among the immunosuppressive drugs in development, inhibit the proliferation of human arterial smooth muscle cells in clinically attainable doses, which has implications for chronic rejection.

APPLICATIONS OF IMMUNOSUPPRESSIVE DRUGS

The first application of immunosuppressive drugs discussed in Orlando was the prevention of organ graft rejection. Since Japanese investigators introduced FK-506 and 15-deoxyspergualin, their accumulated experience with these drugs was informative. Takahara pointed out that FK-506 is, like cyclosporine, nephrotoxic and produces hyperglycemia; it can also produce hyperkalemia, cardiac symptoms, and abdominal distention. Although the activity of FK-506 in renal allograft recipients is comparable to that of cyclosporine, there is no indication of superiority. However, in a multicenter prospective, randomized trial comparing FK-506 (now termed tacrolimus) to cyclosporine after liver transplantation, the incidence and severity of rejection were significantly lower in the tacrolimus group.[7,8] Similar results were recorded in a European trial. Preliminary findings suggest that tacrolimus has efficacy in some autoimmune diseases (see the useful review—Reference 8, and papers in this volume). The drug is active in psoriasis; as presented by Lemster in Orlando, tacrolimus treatment decreases IFN-γ and adhesion molecule expression in psoriatic skin.

Suzuki described an unusual activity of 15-deoxyspergualin (DSG). In rats with heterotopic heart allografts, delaying the administration of DSG to the time of onset of rejection allowed the development of suppressor cells. In human renal allograft recipients, quadruple induction (cyclosporine, mizoribine, DSG, and methyl prednisolone) has been used with the objective of withdrawing the steroid during the maintenance phase of immunosuppression. Of 19 treated patients, 8 have been maintained steroid free with good graft function.

Cramer described the use of Brequinar (BQR) in transplantation. BQR is an effective primary immunosuppressive for preventing the rejection of vascularized allografts and xenografts. It is better than cyclosporine for inhibiting antibody formation and rejection reactions dependent on humoral responses. BQR is also more effective in the rescue of rejecting allografts. Combination therapy (BQR and cyclosporine) is more effective than monotherapy. Ongoing clinical trials in human renal and liver allograft recipients will establish whether this combination is effective in the principal target species, without limiting side effects.

COMBINATION THERAPIES

Ochiai described effects of various drug combinations on survival of renal allografts in dogs. As found also in other laboratories, most combinations were more effective than single drugs. He concludes that several immunosuppressive drugs developed during the past few years show not only remarkable potency but also side effects. Combination treatment is safer and more efficacious, and it will prevail in the future. The problem is that there are so many possible combinations. Antibodies against lymphocytes, antigen-presenting cells, and adhesion molecules all have activity in allograft recipients, adding to the possible combination regimes. The doses and timing of administration of different modalities can also be varied. It will be impossible to test all the combinations in humans in controlled studies. Combination therapies are routine in cancer therapy, and are likely to be required also for optimal treatment of allograft recipients, patients with rheumatoid arthritis, and those with other diseases. With so many possible combinations, how can one decide which ones to try first? There are two approaches: one is to analyze the mode of action of different immunosuppressive drugs, and the observed effects in experimental animals, and try to assess which combinations are likely to be most effective in man. That requires understanding of the limitations of currently used drug combinations, followed by an attempt to overcome them. The second approach is to start with clinical observations on combination therapies and extrapolate them to the likely effects of new combinations.

Despite the advances in human organ transplantation, the limitations are well known. Doses of immunosuppressives required to prevent allograft rejection are close to those decreasing resistance to infectious agents. The effects of drugs on lymphocytes should be rapidly reversible, so that if herpesvirus or other infections occur, and it is necessary to withdraw the drug, immune function is rapidly restored. Combination therapy with standard regimes (cyclosporine and low-dose steroid, with or without antilymphocyte globulin (ALG), and/or azathioprine) prevents rejection in about one-half of organ graft recipients. Treatment of ongoing rejection with a high-dose steroid and/or ALG can increase susceptibility to infections and late non-Hodgkin's lymphomas, so that rejection should be avoided if possible. The incidence of lymphomas is raised not only in organ graft recipients[9] but also in patients with rheumatoid arthritis treated with azathioprine.[10] The frequency of lymphomas has decreased since doses of cyclosporine were reduced, but it is still much higher than in age-matched controls.[9]

The most obvious need is for a combination therapy that reduces the incidence of rejection crises in organ graft recipients. Mycophenolate mofetil, the prodrug of mycophenolic acid, administered with relatively low doses of steroids and cyclosporine, has reduced the incidence of rejections to 17%. Ongoing trials with Brequinar in combination with cyclosporine should serve as a comparator. The second need is for a better treatment of ongoing rejection. Again mycophenolate mofetil looks promising in humans, and findings in experimental animals suggest that Brequinar may also be effective for this application. Both drugs inhibit the glycosylation of adhesion molecules, which could explain their efficacy even when populations of effector lymphocytes have expanded.

The third need is for a drug combination that avoids the late lymphomas. Two pathogenetic mechanisms have been implicated. One is Epstein-Barr virus (EBV) driven proliferation of B lymphocytes,[9,11] while the other is chromosomal translocations that convert such polyclonal proliferation into frank malignancy. A well-known example is the *c-myc/Ig* locus translocation,[12] but other chromosomal translocations leading to lymphoma development have been identified.[13] In retrospect it is ironic that the cyclosporine/azathioprine combination is an unfortunate combination from this point of view. Cyclosporine does not prevent the proliferation of EBV-transformed B lymphocytes but suppresses T-cell-mediated surveillance against that phenomenon, increasing the population of B cells susceptible to malignancy.[15] Azathioprine is mutagenic[14] and thioguanosine incorporated into DNA[1] can increase chromosome breakage. Of the new immunosuppressives, mizoribine produces a high incidence of chromosome breaks[16] whereas MPA, which is not a nucleoside, does not. It is a reasonable inference which drug is less likely to be a predisposing factor in lymphoma development.

Now that acute rejection can be reasonably well controlled, chronic rejection is the principal limitation of long-term survival of organ grafts. This is a proliferative arteriopathy that narrows coronary vessels three to five years after heart transplantation and can limit survival of renal allografts beyond five years. Both cellular and humoral immune responses, producing many growth factors for smooth muscle cells, are likely to be involved, so the most promising strategy seems to be inhibiting one of the major pathogenetic mechanisms: proliferation of smooth muscle cells in the neointima. Mycophenolic acid (MPA) and rapamycin are the only immunosuppressive drugs currently in development known to have that effect in clinically attainable concentrations. Mycophenolate mofetil inhibits intimal proliferation in rat aortic allografts, whereas cyclosporine and Brequinar do not.[17] The most striking experimental finding so far is in primate heart xenografts by the group of McManus. Cynomolgus monkey hearts were transplanted into baboons, which received various immunosuppressive regimens. A combination therapy of cyclosporine with azathioprine allowed mean survival of 94 days, with severe arteriopathy. Combination therapy of cyclosporine and mycophenolate mofetil increased survival, with coronary arteries remarkably free of intimal proliferation, as discussed in Orlando. Of course there is no certainty that these findings in rats and nonhuman primates can be extrapolated to humans, but they certainly suggest that by choice of an appropriate combination therapy, the limitation imposed by chronic rejection will be lessened.

A major problem in xenografts, as well as in some allografts and other situations, is humoral immune responses. Humans nearly always produce antibodies against mouse and other foreign immunoglobulins, and even humanized antibodies often elicit antiidiotypic responses. Immunotoxins can elicit the formation of antibodies against both the targeting immunoglobulins and the protein toxins. It would be useful if such humoral responses could be prevented. Mycophenolate mofetil, Brequinar, rapamycin, and 15-deoxyspergualin can all suppress humoral responses in experimental animals, and findings in humans are awaited with interest.

An obvious strategy for treatment of asthma, especially in steroid-resistant patients, would be suppression of the formation of immunoglobulin E (IgE). As Chang, de Vries, and colleagues point out, Brequinar and mycophenolate mofetil inhibit IgE formation more efficiently than cyclosporine and apparently by different mechanisms.

Furst discussed the optimization of combination chemotherapy for rheumatoid arthritis. His approach combines knowledge of mechanisms of action, kinetics, and toxicities to look for "nonoverlapping" combinations. Although Furst was considering disease-modifying antirheumatic drugs, the strategy is applicable to combinations of immunosuppressive drugs. For example, cyclosporine and tacrolimus have similar mechanisms of action and toxicities, so they would be expected to be a bad combination: clinical experience shows that to be the case. Following these principles would restrict the number of drug combinations considered suitable for clinical trials.

OTHER CLINICAL APPLICATIONS OF IMMUNOSUPPRESSIVE AND ANTIINFLAMMATORY DRUGS

Analyzing the efficacy of drugs is often limited by end points. For example, in rheumatoid arthritis, traditional measures include functional status, numbers of swollen and tender joints, and rheumatoid factor levels. It would be useful to have accurate measures of cartilage and bone erosion, and to identify subsets of patients with rapidly progressive disease. Jeffcoat described a method, digital subtraction radiography, for measuring small changes in bone density. Developed to follow changes in alveolar bone in periodontal disease, this method also shows promise in rheumatoid arthritis. In some patients joint erosion occurs rapidly, and in that subset it would be relatively easy to establish whether an experimental drug can retard bone erosion. Some cyclooxygenase inhibitors can prevent bone erosion in periodontal disease, a common disorder.

Another disease in which one can literally see what is happening is autoimmune uveitis. Whitcup described the efficacy of several immunosuppressive drugs in experimental autoimmune uveoretinitis and in patients with autoimmune uveitis. Many patients who would previously have become blind can now be treated, but less toxic drugs are needed. Immunosuppressive drugs are also needed for corneal transplants under some circumstances (regrafting following rejection and following herpetic or traumatic keratitis). Regimes currently used for organ transplantation have too many side effects for this application, in which a new drug would be useful.

Immunosuppressive drugs are also needed in chronic liver disease, reviewed by Jones and Bergasa in Orlando. Several chronic liver diseases are thought to have an autoimmune basis, notably idiopathic chronic active hepatitis, primary biliary cirrhosis, primary sclerosing cholangitis, and immunocholangitis. Glucocorticoids and azathioprine, often used in combination, are effective in autoimmune chronic active hepatitis. Methotrexate has shown efficacy in primary biliary cirrhosis. In one trial, prednisolone showed beneficial effects in this disorder, but exacerbated metabolic bone disease. There is scope for use of new immunosuppressive drugs in chronic liver diseases.

A particularly exciting prospect for the new immunosuppressive drugs is for treatment of insulin-dependent (type I) diabetes mellitus. The conference of the New York Academy of Sciences in Orlando preceded the International Diabetes Workshop, so as to allow exchanges of ideas between representatives of the two groups. Maclaren stated that it is now possible to identify humans with type I diabetes before their pancreatic islets are destroyed by an autoimmune and inflammatory reaction. Autoantibodies to an isoform of glutamic acid decarboxylase (GAD) and to insulin are markers of early disease. As he and Stiller emphasized, this is the time when immunosuppressive drugs could inhibit the autoimmune process before the islets are destroyed. Cyclosporine and azathioprine have delayed the onset of diabetes, but not indefinitely. As Bach and Stiller pointed out, the nephrotoxicity of cyclosporine limits is utility for this purpose. Elliott described the use of nicotinamide to prevent type I diabetes in genetically predisposed mice and humans. The mechanism by which nicotinamide exerts this effect is unknown. However, dietary nicotinamide can stimulate NAD synthesis and influence purine and pyrimidine metabolism;[18] for example the level of NAD and the NAD/NADH ratio can change the proportion of adenosine and guanosine nucleotides. Hence administration of nicotinamide could have metabolic effects similar to those of mycophenolic acid.

Hao showed that mycophenolic acid can suppress the development of diabetes in genetically predisposed BB rats. These findings, and those on azathioprine and nicotinamide in humans with type I diabetes, suggest that a prospective, placebo-controlled trial of mycophenolate mofetil in human with antibodies to GAD and to insulin would be worth undertaking. Avoiding the late complications of diabetes (vascular problems, renal failure, blindness) would be a major achievement.

ANTIINFLAMMATORY DRUGS

The most widely used antiinflammatory drugs are glucocorticoids and cyclooxygenase inhibitors. While these have brought many therapeutic benefits, their side effects are serious. Glucocorticoids can increase susceptibility to infections, and they have widespread metabolic effects, e.g., on bone and carbohydrate metabolism. The gastrointestinal erosion produced by cyclooxygenase inhibitors remains a serious limitation. New strategies for antiinflammatory therapy are obviously needed.

This includes better understanding of mechanisms of action, as well as new applications of currently used drugs. For a long time the antiinflammatory effects of glycocorticoids were attributed to induction of lipocortins, inhibitors of phospholipase A_2. When lipocortins were cloned, it became obvious that they are abundant cytosolic proteins, not inducible by glucocorticoids, and they bind phospholipids rather than functioning as phospholipase inhibitors. An alternative to the lipocortin hypothesis is that glucocorticoids inhibit the production and effects of proinflammatory cytokines TNF-α and IL-1β. There is substantial evidence supporting this hypothesis, and the underlying molecular biology has been analyzed. When macrophages are activated by lipopolysaccharide (LPS), expression of the TNF-α gene is induced, but a major effect is to increase the efficiency of translation of TNF-α messenger RNA. Glucocorticoids have little effect on TNF-α gene transcription but decrease the efficiency of specific mRNA translation.[19] LPS induces the expression of the IL-1β gene in monocytes; glucocorticoids have no demonstrable effect on transcription but decrease the stability of IL-1β mRNA, and thereby suppress the synthesis of IL-1β.[20] Glucocorticoids also suppress effects of IL-1, including induced expression of genes for neutral metalloproteinases[21] and of the type II cyclooxygenase discussed below. While it is gratifying to understand better how glucocorticoids exert inflammatory effects, the many metabolic disturbances produced by molecules of this class remain a barrier to future developments. A great deal is now known about glucocorticoid receptors and related molecules, and that may open the way to discriminate between clinical efficacy and side effects.

It has been known for a long time that while cyclooxygenase inhibitors have similar overall effects, they differ in clinical utility. Some have central nervous effects, others do not; some are better analgesics than others. One such difference was presented in Orlando: the remarkable difference in potency of cyclooxygenase inhibitors for preventing IL-1-induced bone erosion. One inhibitor, ketorolac, blocks this effect in the low nanomolar concentration range. This raises the possibility that the drug can be used topically, in a mouthwash formulation, to prevent alveolar bone erosion in periodontal disease. The major current development in this area, as discussed by Hla in Orlando, is the recognition that there are two isoforms of cyclooxygenase, the Cox 1 and Cox 2 isoenzymes, showing about 60% amino acid identity. The Cox 1 enzyme is constitutively expressed in most cell types whereas Cox 2 is rapidly inducible by LPS in monocytes and by IL-1 in fibroblasts. Inflammatory tissues, such as synovia of patients with rheumatoid arthritis, express Cox 2 message and have Cox 2 protein. This raises the possibility that by inhibiting Cox 2 selectively it may be possible to exert antiinflammatory activity without gastrointestinal erosion. Most inhibitors (flurbiprofen, ibuprofen, meclofenamic acid, and docosahexaenoic acid) affect both isoenzymes with near equal potency, whereas piroxicam, indomethacin, and sulindac sulfide are more potent Cox 1 inhibitors. The active metabolite of nabumetone, 6-methoxy-2-naphthyl acetic acid, was reported to be a selective inhibitor of murine Cox 2,[22] but appears to be less active against human Cox 2. Several large pharmaceutical companies are looking for selective inhibitors of Cox 2, and compounds with that activity should soon be identified. It will be interesting to know whether they will have clinically useful antiinflammatory activity in humans without producing gastrointestinal erosion, affecting renal blood flow, or exhibiting other toxicities.

A series of selective inhibitors of mediator production and effects developed during the past few years will likewise be useful reagents for analyzing their role in the pathogenesis of diseases. In Orlando two strategies for inhibiting 5-lipoxygenase were reviewed: the redox inhibitors Zileuton and A-78773 (Bell) and inhibitors of translocation of the 5-lipoxygenase-activating protein (Evans). In several experimental animal models of inflammation and allergy, these inhibitors decrease edema, inflammatory cell influx, and bronchospasm. Preliminary clinical studies suggest that 5-lipoxygenase inhibitors have activity in asthma and ulcerative colitis. It will be interesting to examine the efficacy of these drugs in controlled clinical trials, and analyze how they compare with other drugs such as leukotriene and PAF antagonists.

In Orlando another novel antiinflammatory strategy was discussed: the use of small molecules to inhibit the production of the proinflammatory cytokines TNF-α and IL-1β. There is substantial evidence that these cytokines are major mediators of inflammation and the pathophysiological disturbances in septic shock.[23] Attempts to inhibit the effects of either one, for example, using antibodies to TNF-α or the IL-1 receptor antagonist, have had limited success, suggesting that it will be necessary to inhibit both to treat inflammatory diseases and shock. The only drugs known to inhibit the production of both TNF-α and IL-1β are glucocorticoids, with all their complications. During the past few years, anecdotal reports of the inhibition of either TNF-α or IL-1β have been replaced by systematic studies showing the feasibility of using single drugs to inhibit the production of both cytokines.

Eugui and her colleagues reviewed evidence that when cells of the monocytic-macrophage lineage are stimulated by LPS, reactive oxygen intermediates can activate transcription factors (e.g., NF-κB and AP-1) which are required for the coordinate expression of the TNF-α, IL-1β, and IL-6 genes. Some antioxidant drugs can prevent the activation of transcription factors and the expression of all these genes. These effects are not due to overall inhibition of protein synthesis and are gene selective: antioxidants suppressing cytokine production can actually increase production of the IL-1 receptor antagonist (Waters). The effects are cell-type selective: the antioxidants suppressing IL-6 synthesis in monocytes do not inhibit synthesis of the same cytokine in fibroblasts. Thus, activity in septic shock and inflammatory states may be achievable without limiting side effects. Lee discussed bicyclic imidazoles, which selectively inhibit the translation of TNF-α and IL-1β messenger RNAs in cells of the monocyte-macrophage lineage. Thus the feasibility of using one drug to inhibit the production of both TNF-α and IL-1β is established. Other strategies for inhibiting the production of individual cytokines have been developed. For example, agents elevating cyclic AMP levels in monocytes, such as prostaglandins and type IV cAMP phosphodiesterase inhibitors, suppress the production of TNF-α but not IL-1β.[23] As discussed by Miller in Orlando, the IL-1β converting enzyme is another potential therapeutic target. Cloning and expressing this thiol proteinase, and synthesizing inhibitors, has been elegant science. However, it remains to be seen whether an inhibitor of IL-1β production, without effects on TNF-α, IL-1α, or IL-6, will have clinical utility.

SUMMARY

Research on immunosuppressive and antiinflammatory drugs is progressing rapidly. Several new drugs are in development, and learning how to combine them optimally, for treatment of different diseases and prolonging graft survival, will be a major task for the next few years. Decreasing the incidence of complications following transplantation will reduce patient anxiety and cost, and the shortage of donor organs is an additional reason for wishing to prolong graft acceptance. Many clinical findings with the new drug combinations should be published by the end of the century. We can begin the next millennium with improved immunosuppressive and antiinflammatory drugs discussed at the Orlando conference.

REFERENCES

1. ELION, G. B. 1989. The purine path to chemotherapy. Science **244:** 41.
2. MURRAY, J. E. 1993. Biological spinoff of organ transplantation. Ann. N.Y. Acad. Sci. **685:** 389.
3. JOLIVET, J., K. H. COWAN, G. A. CURT, et al. 1983. The pharmacology and clinical use of methotrexate. N. Engl. J. Med. **309:** 1094.
4. MAKOWKA, I. & D. V. CRAMER, Eds. Brequinar sodium: a new immunosuppressive drug for transplantation. Transplant. Proc. 25(Suppl. 2): 1.
5. BOREL, J. F., C. FEURER, C. MAGNEE & H. STAHELIN. 1977. Effects of the new anti-lymphocytic peptide cyclosporin A in animals. Immunology **32:** 1017.
6. JAIN, J., P. G. McCAFFREY, Z. MINER, et al. 1993. The T-cell transcription factor NFATp is a substrate for calcineurin and interacts with Fos and Jun. Nature **365:** 352.
7. McDIARMID, S., et al. 1993. A multi-center prospective randomized trial comparing FK-506 to cyclosporin A (CyA) after liver transplantation: comparison of efficacy based on incidence, severity and treatment of rejection. American Association of Transplant Surgeons Meeting, Houston, Texas, May 1993.
8. PETERS, D. H., A. FITTON & G. PLEGLER. Tacrolimus: a review of the pharmacology and therapeutic potential in hepatic and renal transplantation. Drugs (In Press.)
9. HANTO, D. W., K. J. GAJL-PECZALSKA, D. C. FRIZZERA, et al. 1983. Epstein-Barr virus (EBV) induced polyclonal and monoclonal B cell lymphoproliferative diseases occurring after renal transplantation. Clinical, pathologic and virologic findings and implications for therapy. Ann. Surg. **198:** 356.
10. MATTESON, E. L., E. Y. HICKEY, L. MAGUIRE, et al. 1991. Occurrence of neoplasia in patients with rheumatoid arthritis enrolled in a DMARD registry. J. Rheumatol. **18:** 809.
11. YOUNG, L., C. ALFIERI, K. HENNESY, et al. 1989. Expression of Epstein-Barr virus transformation-associated genes in tissues of patients with EBV lymphoproliferative disease. N. Engl. J. Med. **321:** 1080.
12. KLEIN, G. & E. KLEIN. 1989. How one thing led to another. Annu. Rev. Immunol. **7:** 1.
13. KORSMEYER, S. S. 1992. Chromosomal translocations in lymphoid malignancies to several novel protoncogenes. Annu. Rev. Immunol. **10:** 785.
14. RICKINSON, A. B., M. ROWE, V. HART, et al. 1984. T-cell-mediated regression of "spontaneous" and Epstein-Bar virus-induced B-cell transformation in vitro: studies with cyclosporin A. Cell. Immunol. **87:** 646.
15. HERLIA, P., L. MURELLI, M. SCOTTI, et al. 1988. Organ specific activation of azathioprine in mice: role of liver metabolism in mutation induction. Carcinogenesis **9:** 1011.
16. SAKAGUCHI, K., M. TSUJINO & M. YOSHIZAWA. 1975. Action of bredinin on mammalian cells. Cancer Res. **35:** 1643.

17. STEELE, D. M., D. A. HULLETT, W. O. BECHSTEIN, *et al.* 1993. Effects of immunosuppressive therapy in the rat aortic allograft model. Transplant. Proc. **25:** 754.
18. MICHELI, V., C. RICCI, S. SESTINI, *et al.* 1991. Pyridine nucleotide metabolism, purine and pyrimidine interconnections. Int. J. Purine Pyrimidine Res. **2**(Suppl. 1): 19.
19. HAN, J., P. THOMPSON & B. BEUTLER. 1990. Dexamethasone and pentoxyphylline inhibit endotoxin-induced cachetin/tumor necrosis factor synthesis at separate points in the signaling pathway. J. Exp. Med. **172:** 391.
20. AMANO, Y., S. W. LEE. & A. C. ALLISON. 1993. Inhibition by glucocorticoids of the formation of interleukin-1α, interleukin-1β and interleukin-6: mediation by decreased mRNA stability. Mol. Pharm. **43:** 176.
21. MATRISIAN, L. M. 1990. Metalloproteinases and their inhibition in matrix remodeling. Trends in Genet. **6:** 121.
22. MEADS, E. A., W. L. SMITH & D. L. DE WITT. 1993. Differential inhibition of prostaglandin endoperoxide synthase (cyclooxygenase) isoenzymes by aspirin and other nonsteroidal antiinflammatory drugs. J. Biol. Chem. **268:** 6610.

Immunosuppressive Profile of Rapamycin

SUREN N. SEHGAL

Wyeth-Ayerst Research
CN 8000
Princeton, New Jersey 08545-8000

INTRODUCTION

Rapamycin (FIGURE 1) is a macrolide antibiotic produced by *Streptomyces hygroscopicus* isolated from a soil sample that was collected from Rapa Nui, commonly known as Easter Island.[1,2] It was originally identified as an antifungal agent with potent anticandida activity. However, subsequent studies demonstrated impressive antitumor and immunosuppressive activities. For example, rapamycin exhibited activity against B16 melanocarcinoma, colon 26 tumor, EM ependymoblastoma, CD8F1 mammary, and colon 38 murine tumors.[3,4] The earliest evidence of rapamycin's immunosuppressive activity was demonstrated by its ability to prevent the development of autoimmune adjuvant arthritis and experimental allergic encephalomyelitis in the rat.[5] The current interest in rapamycin as a potent immunosuppressive agent is a result of its unique mechanism of action and discovery of its superior potency in preventing allograft rejection.[6,7]

IN VITRO IMMUNOSUPPRESSIVE PROPERTIES

Rapamycin belongs to the class of macrocyclic immunosuppressants that block the T cell proliferation between G1 and S phase of the cell cycle. However, its effects are distinct from those of cyclosporin A (CsA) and FK506, the other macrocyclic immunosuppressants in this class. The immunological studies related to these drugs were recently reviewed by Sehgal and Bansbach[8] and Sehgal *et al.*[9] Briefly, rapamycin inhibits murine, porcine, and human T lymphocyte proliferation induced by mitogenic lectins, antigens, cross-linking of cellular receptors with monoclonal antibodies (e.g., CD3, CD28), alloantigens, phorbol esters, and calcium ionophore and lymphokines (IL-2, IL-4, IL-6) with IC_{50} values in the 0.1–300 nM range.[10–13] In contrast, CsA and FK506 block T cell activation induced only by stimuli employing Ca^{2+}-dependent pathways with IC_{50} values for FK506 that are 50- to 100-fold lower than that of CsA.[10,14–17]

Rapamycin inhibits proliferation of activated T cells even when the drug is added up to 12 hours after stimulation, whereas CsA and FK506 lose their effect when added two hours after cell stimulation.[10,18] IL-2-dependent T cell proliferation is inhibited by rapamycin, but not by CsA or FK506.[18] Taken together, these data support the conclusion that, unlike CsA and FK506 which block Ca^{2+}-dependent cytokine transcription early in G1 phase, rapamycin inhibits cytokine-mediated signal transduction pathways later in G1 phase.

Rapamycin inhibits Ca-dependent proliferation of B cells with a potency the same as that of FK506 and about 70-fold higher than that of CsA. However, unlike FK506 and CsA, which inhibit proliferation completely, the inhibition with rapamy-

1

cin plateaus between 70% and 90%.[19] In addition, rapamycin inhibits lipopolysaccha-ride (LPS) induced B cell proliferation, a calcium-independent pathway that is resistent to FK506 and CsA.[18,19] Rapamycin has significant effect on spontaneous and pokeweed mitogen (PWM) induced production of immunoglobulin M (IgM), immunoglobulin G (IgG) and immunoglobulin A (IgA) from human B cells.[20] IL-4-stimulated IgE production by human peripheral blood mononuclear cells and IL-2 plus *Staphylococcus aureus* Cowan I (SAC) stimulated IgG and IgM production by pure tonsillar B cells are also suppressed by rapamycin.[20] These results imply that in addition to affecting T cell function, rapamycin directly affects B cell function.

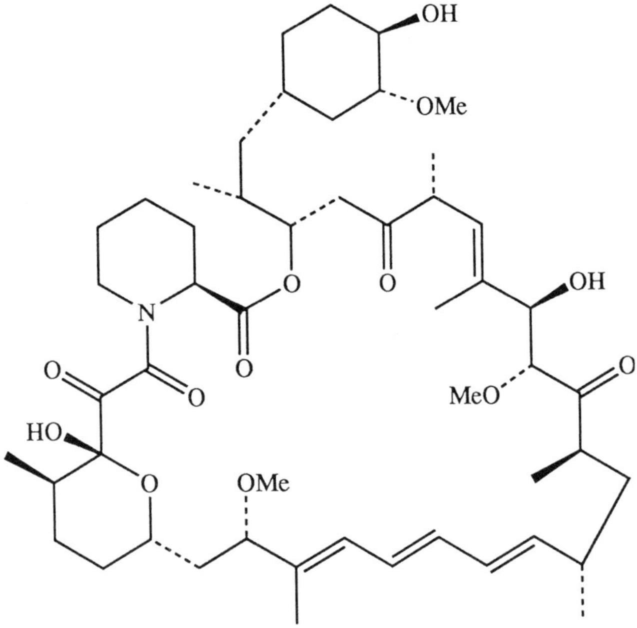

FIGURE 1. Chemical structure of the immunosuppressive macrolide rapamycin.

MECHANISM OF ACTION

Rapamycin and CsA act synergistically in the inhibition of T and B cell prolifera-tion *in vitro*.[13,21,22] Equimolar concentrations of FK506 and rapamycin also inhibit con-A-induced T cell proliferation in an additive manner.[18,23] While no antagonism between CsA and rapamycin can be detected, FK506 and rapamycin in 50- to 1000-fold molar excess are selective reciprocal antagonists for all parameters tested to date.[8] This suggests that a common intracellular receptor may be involved in mediating the inhibition by rapamycin and FK506. Since the effects of FK506 and rapamycin are distinct, it also suggests that different molecular targets mediate the biological activity of these agents. The common cellular receptors of rapamycin and FK506 are the FK506 binding proteins (FKBPs). Like cyclophilins, which are the specific binding proteins of CsA, FKBPs are peptidyl prolyl *cis-trans* isomerases.[24–26] Both rapamycin and FK506 bind to and inhibit the isomerase activity of FKBPs;

however, since they function as reciprocal antagonists, either binding to PPIase or inhibition of PPIase activity is not sufficient to mediate their immunosuppressive effect.

FK506 and CsA are known to mediate their inhibition in the early G1 cell cycle phase during T cell activation, principally via inhibition of cytokine production. They inhibit IL-2 gene transcription induced by a Ca^{2+}-dependent stimulant in T cells. When bound to their respective immunophilins, FK506 and CsA appear to form a ternary complex with calcineurin and inhibit its ability to dephosphorylate peptide substrates.[27-29] Specifically, this results in the inhibition of dephosphorylation of the cytoplasmic subunit of NF-AT, which is required for its translocation to nucleus and subsequent activation of the transcription factor NF-AT.[30,31]

Despite the intensive research activity in this area, the molecular target of rapamycin, homologous to calcineurin, has not yet been identified. However, the following is known about the biochemical targets of rapamycin. (1) Rapamycin at immunosuppressive concentrations inhibits IL-2-stimulated phosphorylation of P70 S 6 kinase (p^{70S6k}) and its subsequent activation.[32-34] (2) The rapamycin:FKBP complex is necessary for the inhibition, since molar excess of FK506 can block rapamycin's effect.[33,34] (3) Rapamycin:FKBP complex has no inhibitory effect on p^{70S6k} activation in a cell-free system, indicating that it may form a ternary complex mediating direct or indirect inhibition of kinases or other phosphatases. In addition to inhibition of p^{70S6k} activation, which takes place during early G1 phase, rapamycin's major inhibitory effects on the proliferation of T cells block progression of the cell cycle at mid to late G1 phase. This is evidenced by the following. First, delayed addition experiments indicated that the critical steps sensitive to rapamycin occurred up to 16 hours post–mitogen stimulation[10,18] and 8–9 hours post–IL-2 induction.[35] Second, rapamycin does not affect gene transcription of early genes including *c-jun, c-myc, c-fos,* but does decrease c-myb production.[35,36] Thirdly, although rapamycin does not decrease cdk2 and cyclin E levels in a D10.G4 T cell clone, the kinase activity of cdk2/cyclin E complex is dramatically diminished in rapamycin-treated cells.[36] Rapamycin treatment blocks the hyperphosphorylation of retinoblastoma protein (pRB) and the subsequent augmented synthesis of cdc2 and cyclin A. The inhibition of hyperphosphorylation of pRB may be a result of the inactivation of kinase activity of cdk2/cyclin E complex, which has been reported to be involved in the phosphorylation of pRB.[37,35,36] Taken together, these data suggest that rapamycin may activate a phosphatase(s) or inhibit a kinase whose substrate pool includes $p70^{S6k}$ and the cdk2/cyclin E complex.

IN VIVO IMMUNOSUPPRESSIVE PROFILE

Rapamycin is currently in phase I clinical trials for inhibition of organ transplant rejection. The rationale for the clinical evaluation is based on demonstrated transplant rejection inhibitory effect of rapamycin in animal models. Early in its investigation, rapamycin was reported to be threefold more potent than FK506 and 50-fold more potent than CsA in a quantal mouse heart allograft model.[38] Rapamycin has subsequently been reported to be very effective in prolonging the survival of both heterotopically and orthotopically transplanted organs in various animal species ranging from mouse to baboon (TABLE 1). Some of the significant recent studies are reviewed here.

Rapamycin was effective in the engraftment of islet cells in streptozotocin-induced diabetic mice with hyperglycemia.[39] Successful transplantation of the islet cell under the kidney capsule restored the normoglycemic state. Graft failure in

TABLE 1. Animal Models Of Transplantation in which Rapamycin Is Effective

Animal Species	Graft	References
Mouse		
BALB/c → C3H	Heterotopic heart	38
BALB/c → C3H	Skin	48
Rat		
BN → LEW	Heterotopic heart	43
DA → PVG	Heterotopic heart	6
BUF → WFu	Heterotopic heart	49
BUF → WFu	Orthotopic kidney	49
	Heterotopic small bowel	49
	Bone marrow (GVHD)	56
Dog		
	Orthotopic kidney	6, 50
Pig		
Mismatch by MLR	Orthotopic kidney	45, 50
Baboon		
Mismatch by MLR	Orthotopic kidney	51
Cynomolgus monkey		
Mismatch by MLR	Heterotopic heart	52

untreated allografts occurred at 22 ± 4.7 days, and vehicle-treated allografts at 16 ± 1.8 days. The groups treated with rapamycin at 0.1 and 0.3 mg/kg per day intraperitoneally (ip) for 7 days gave graft survival of 56 ± 11 and 57 ± 9 days, respectively. However 10- to 50-fold higher doses were not as effective in maintaining normoglycemia, possibly due to rapamycin's effect on transplanted islet grafts at these higher doses, resulting in failure of the graft function. Histopathologic analysis of the kidney, liver, heart, lung, and small intestine demonstrated no abnormalities at any dose.[39] This is the first report of the effectiveness of rapamycin in cellular transplantation.

Allografted rats without immunosuppressive therapy showed acute rejection of transplanted heart, kidney, and pancreas at day 4 posttransplant, as evidenced by histopathological analysis of the biopsied specimens of the grafts. Treatment with rapamycin [0.8 mg/kg delivered intravenously (iv) by continuous infusion from day 4 posttransplant to day 14] reversed or significantly delayed the ongoing acute rejection.[40] The extension of these studies shows[41] that rapamycin reverses the ongoing heart allograft rejection in a dose-dependent manner at doses of 0.02, 0.08, and 0.8 mg/kg for 14 days to 30.8 ± 5.8, 44.7 ± 15.9, and 96.4 ± 35.9 days, respectively (untreated controls rejected grafts on day 7.0 ± 2.5). Under the same experimental conditions, CsA, 2 mg/kg, was able to extend the graft survival to only 10 ± 2 days. However, when CsA was given in combination with rapamycin (0.02 mg/kg per day), the grafts survived for more than 100 days. The synergism between rapamycin and CsA has been previously reported for prophylaxis of rejection.[42,43] This study has demonstrated that CsA and rapamycin synergistically inhibit and reverse the ongoing rejection of heterotopic heart allografts in the rat. These results suggest that rapamycin alone and/or in combination with CsA may be useful in the treatment of ongoing acute allograft rejection.

Yatscoff and coworkers have correlated rapamycin blood levels with its efficacy in prolonging heart allografts in the rabbit.[44] Heterotopic heart transplanted New Zealand white rabbits, treated with rapamycin at doses of 0.05, 0.1, 0.5, and 1.0 mg/kg per day, exhibited excellent allograft survival. Only two animals in the lowest dosage group (0.05 mg/kg per day) rejected their grafts. The rapamycin dose was correlated with trough drug concentrations. The whole blood concentrations of rapamycin resulting in maximal efficacy with minimal toxicity were in the range of 10–60 ng/ml; rabbits having trough whole blood concentrations of <10 ng/ml rejected their grafts and rabbits with levels >60 ng/ml exhibited increased incidence of infections due to overimmunosuppression. These results suggest that therapeutic monitoring of trough blood concentrations of rapamycin, as with CsA and FK506, may be useful in guiding dosage adjustments to maximize the immunosuppressive efficacy while minimizing drug-induced side effects.

The evidence of the efficacy of rapamycin as an antirejection agent in a large animal was first demonstrated in orthotopic kidney allografted pigs.[6] In a recent study, rapamycin was compared with triple therapy (TT) consisting of CsA, azathioprine, and prednisone in a porcine renal transplant model.[45] TT and rapamycin (0.25 mg/kg per day) significantly improved renal transplant survival versus control (from 10 days to 46 days and >59 days, $p = 0.0025$ and 0.001, respectively after 30 days treatment). Serum creatinine was lower in the rapamycin-treated group than in the TT-treated group. These data suggest that rapamycin, besides being a potent immunosuppressant, has a reduced nephrotoxic potential relative to CsA in the pig.

EFFECT IN AUTOIMMUNE DISORDERS

We have reported the effect of rapamycin in several spontaneous and induced autoimmune disorders (TABLE 2).[46] Recently, Roberge *et al.* have reported the effect of rapamycin in experimental autoimmune uveoretinitis,[57] an antigen-induced autoimmune disorder of the eye in rats. Rapamycin administered iv for 14 days via an osmotic pump reduced the incidence of uveoretinitis in a dose-dependent manner. At lower doses of 0.025 and 0.05 mg/kg, rapamycin had no significant effect on the incidence of the disease. However, at 0.1 and 0.5 mg/kg iv, rapamycin prevented the onset of disease in 12 of the 14 rats in each dose group. At the dose of 1 mg/kg, rapamycin completely prevented the onset of disease. CsA at a dose of 2 mg/kg intramuscularly (im) prevented the onset of disease in 3 of 15 total animals from three separate experiments consisting of 5 animals each. However, CsA at 2 mg/kg im, combined with rapamycin (0.01 mg/kg iv) prevented the onset of disease completely.[47] These data clearly demonstrate the synergistic effect of rapamycin and CsA in an antigen-induced autoimmune disorder.

TABLE 2. Animal Models of Autoimmune Diseases in which Rapamycin Is Effective

Model	Disease	Dose Range	References
Mouse			
MRL/1pr	SLE	12.5–25 mg/kg per oral (po) 3 × week	53
NOD	Type 1 diabetes	0.6–6 mg/kg po 3 × week	54
Collagen-induced arthritis	Arthritis	2.5–25 mg/kg po 3 × week	46
Rat			
BB	Diabetes	4 mg/kg po 2 × weeks	55
E.A.E.	M.S.	$ED_{50} = 5.9$ mg/kg po 3 × week	46
Adjuvant arthritis	Arthritis	$ED_{50} = 2.3$–3.7 mg/kg po 3 × week	46

CONCLUSION

In conclusion, rapamycin, a macrolide natural product, is a potent immunosuppressive agent. Unlike FK506 and CsA, which block cytokine gene expression, rapamycin's effects on immune functions are mediated via inhibition of cellular responses to cytokines. Thus, rapamycin's mechanism of action is different from that of FK506 and CsA. Rapamycin's unique immunosuppressive profile and remarkable efficacy in a variety of organ transplantation and autoimmune animal models point to its high clinical potential.

ACKNOWLEDGMENTS

I express my thanks to Ms. Linda Warner, Mr. J. DeJoseph, and Drs. Katherine Molnar-Kimber and Alan Lewis for their critical reading of the manuscript.

REFERENCES

1. VEZINA, C., A. KUDELSKI & S. N. SEHGAL. 1975. J. Antibiot. 28(10): 721–726.
2. SEHGAL, S. N., H. BAKER & C. VEZINA. 1975. J. Antibiot. 28(10): 727–32.
3. DOUROS, J. & M. SUFFNESS. 1981. Cancer Treatment Rev. 8: 63–87.
4. ENG, C. P., S. N. SEHGAL & C. VEZINA. 1984. J. Antibiot. 37(10): 1231–1237.
5. MARTEL, R. R., J. KLICIUS & S. GALET. 1977. Can. J. Physiol. Pharmacol. 55: 48–51.
6. CALNE, R. Y., S. LIM, A. SAMAAN, D. S. J. COLLIER, S. G. POLLARD, D. J. G. WHITE & S. THIRU. 1989. Lancet 1989: 227.
7. MORRIS, R. E. & B. M. MEISER. 1989. Med. Sci. Res. 17(14): 609–610.
8. SEHGAL, S. N. & C. C. BANSBACH. 1993. Ann. N.Y. Acad. Sci. 685: 58–67.
9. SEHGAL, S. N., K. MOLNAR-KIMBER, T. D. OCAIN & B. M. WEICHMAN. Med. Res. Rev. (In press.)
10. DUMONT, F. J., M. J. STARUCH, S. L. KOPRAK, M. R. MELINO & N. H. SIGAL. 1990. J. Immunology 144(1): 251–258.
11. ADAMS, L. M., L. M. WARNER, W. L. BAEDER, S. N. SEHGAL & J. Y. CHANG. 1989. J. Cell Biol. 109(4): Abstr. 163.
12. BANSBACH, C. C., E. CASILIO-LONARDO, L. M. ADAMS, S. N. SEHGAL & J. Y. CHANG. 1990. FASEB J. 4(7): Abstr. 1768.
13. KAHAN, B. D., S. GIBBONS, N. TEJPAL, S. M. STEPKOWSKI & T.-C. CHOU. 1991. Transplantation 51(1): 232–239.
14. SAWADA, S., G. SUZUKI, Y. KAWASE & F. TAKAKU. 1987. J. Immunol. 139: 1797–1803.
15. KAY, J. E., C. R. BENZIE, M. R. GOODIER, C. J. WICK & S. E. DOE. 1989. Immunology 67: 473–477.
16. JUNE, C. H., J. A. LEDBETTER, M. A. GILESPIE, T. LINDSTEN & A. J. THOMPSON. 1987. Mol. Cell. Biol. 7: 4472–4481.
17. LIN, C. S., R. C. BOLTZ, J. J. SIEKERKA & N. H. SIGAL. 1991. Cell. Immunol. 133(2): 269–284.
18. KAY, J. E., L. KROMWEL, S. E. A. DOE & M. DENYER. 1991. Immunology 72: 544–549.
19. WICKER, L. S., R. C. J. BOLTZ, V. MATT, E. A. NICHOLS, L. B. PETERSON & N. H. SIGAL. 1990. Eur. J. Immunol. 20(10): 2277–2283.
20. LUO, H., H. CHEN, P. DALOZE, J. CHANG & J. WU. 1992. Transplantation 53: 1071.
21. KAHAN, B. D., S. GIBBONS, N. TEJPAL, T. C. CHOU & M. STEPKOWSKI. 1991. Transplant. Proc. 23(1,2): 1090–1091.
22. DUMONT, F. J., M. R. MELINO, M. J. STARUCH, S. L. KOPRAK, P. A. FISHER & N. H. SIGAL. 1990. J. Immunol. 144(4): 1418–1424.
23. MORRIS, R. E. 1992. Transplant. Rev. 6(1): 39–87.

24. HARDING, M. W., A. GALAT, D. E. UEHLING & S. L. SCHREIBER. 1989. Nature 341(6244): 758–760.
25. SIEKIERKA, J. J., G. WIEDERRECHT & H. E. A. GREULICH. 1990. J. Biol. Chem. 265: 21011–21015.
26. FRETZ, H., M. W. ALBERS, A. GALAT, R. F. STANDAERT, W. S. LANE, S. J. BURAKOFF, B. E. BIERER & S. L. SCHREIBER. 1991. J. Am. Chem. Soc. 113: 1409–1411.
27. LIU, J., J. D. FARMER, JR, W. S. LANE, J. FRIEDMAN, I. WEISSMAN & S. L. SCHREIBER. 1991. Cell 66: 807.
28. LIU, J., M. W. ALBERS, T. J. WANDLESS, S. LUAN, D. G. ALBERG, P. J. BELSHAW, P. COHEN, C. MACKINTOSH, C. B. KLEE & S. L. SCHREIBER. 1992. Biochemistry 31(16): 3896–3901.
29. FRUMAN, D. A., P. E. MATHER, S. J. BURAKOFF & B. E. BIERER. 1992. Eur. J. Immunol 22(10): 2513–2517.
30. FLANAGAN, W. M., B. CORTHESY, R. J. BRAM & G. R. CRABTREE. 1992. Nature 352(6338): 803–807.
31. MCCAFFREY, P. C., B. A. PERRINO, T. R. SODERLING & A. RAO. 1993. J. Biol. Chem. 268(5): 3747–3752.
32. PRICE, D. J., J. R. GROVE, V. CALVO, J. ARVUCH & B. E. BIERER. 1992. Science 257: 973–977.
33. KUO, C. J., J. CHUNG, D. F. FIORENTINO, W. M. FLANAGAN, J. BLENIS & G. R. CRABTREE. 1992. Nature 358(6381): 70–73.
34. CHUNG, J., C. J. KUO, G. R. CRABTREE & J. BLENIS. 1992. Cell 69(7): 1227–1236.
35. FLANAGAN, W. M., E. FIRPO, J. M. ROBERTS & G. R. CRABTREE. Science. (In press.)
36. TERADA, N., J. J. LUCAS, R. A. FRANKLIN, A. SZEPESI, J. DOMENICO & E. W. GELFAND. 1992. J. Cell Biochem. Suppl. 16B: 180.
37. AKIYAMA, T., T. OHUCHI, S. SUMIDA, K. MATSUMOTO & K. TOYOSHIMA. 1992. Proc. Natl. Acad. Sci. USA 89: 7900–7904.
38. MORRIS, R. E., J. WU & R. SHORTHOUSE. 1990. Transplant. Proc. 22(4): 1638.
39. FABIAN, M. C. & N. M. KNETEMAN. 1992. Diabetes 41(Suppl. 1): 156A.
40. CHEN, H. F., J. P. WU, H. Y. LUO & P. M. DALOZE. 1991. Transplant. Proc. 23: 2241–2242.
41. CHEN, H., J. WU, D. XU, H. LUO & P. M. DALOZE. 1993. Transplant. Proc. 25(1): 719–720.
42. KAHAN, B. D., J. Y. CHANG & S. N. SEHGAL. 1991. Transplantation 52(2): 185–191.
43. MORRIS, R. E., B. M. MEISER, J. WU, R. SHORTHOUSE & J. WANG. 1991. Transplant. Proc. 23(1): 521–524.
44. FRYER, J., R. W. YATSCOFF, E. A. PASCOE & P. J. THLIVERIS. 1993. Transplantation 55(2): 340–345.
45. ALMOND, P., A. MOSS, R. NAKHLEH, M. MELIN, S. CHEN, A. SALAZAR, K. SHIRABE & A. J. MATAS. 1993. Transplant. Proc. 25(1): 716.
46. CARLSON, R. P., W. L. BAEDER, R. G. CACCESE, L. M. WARNER & S. N. SEHGAL. 1993. Ann. N.Y. Acad. Sci. 685: 86–113.
47. MARTIN, D. F., L. R. DEBARGE, R. B. NUSSENBLATT, C. C. CHEN & F. G. ROBERGE. 1993. Invest. Opthalmol. Vis. Sci. 34(Suppl.): 476.
48. ENG, C. P., J. GULLO-BROWN, J. Y. CHANG & S. N. SEHGAL. 1991. Transplant. Proc. 23(1): 868–869.
49. STEPKOWSKI, S. M., H. CHEN, P. DALOZE & B. D. KAHAN. 1991. Transplantation 51(1): 22–26.
50. COLLIER, D. S. J., S. R. CALNE, S. THIIRU, S. LIM, S. G. POLLARD, P. BARRON, M. DACOSTA & D. J. G. WHITE. 1990. Transplant. Proc. 22(4): 1674–1675.
51. COLLIER, D. S., R. Y. CALNE, S. G. POLLARD, P. J. FRIEND & S. THIRU. 1991. Transplant. Proc. 23(4): 2246–2247.
52. MORRIS, R., J. WANG, C. GREGORY & B. ZHENG. 1991. J. Heart Lung Transplant. 10(1 part 2): 182.
53. WARNER, L. M., T. A. CUMMONS, J. Y. CHANG, S. N. SEHGAL & L. M. ADAMS. 1990. FASEB J. 4(3): Abstr. 538.
54. BAEDER, W. L., J. SREDY, S. N. SEHGAL, J. Y. CHANG & L. M. ADANS. 1992. Clin. Exp. Immunol. 89(2): 174–178.

55. BRAYMAN, K. L., S. ALMOND, A. MOSS, S. CHEN, R. NAKHLEH, D. E. R. SUTHERLAND, J. S. NAJARIAN & A. J. MATAS. 1991. Surg. Forum **42**(10): 405–407.
56. BLAZAR, B. R., P. A. TAYLOR, S. N. SEHGAL & D. A. VALLERA. 1993. Ann. N.Y. Acad. Sci. **685:** 73–85.
57. ROBERGE F. G., D. XU, C. CHAN, M. D. DE SMET, R. B. NAUSSENBLATT & H. CHEN. 1993. Curr. Eye Res. **12**(2): 197–203.

The Mechanism of Action of FK-506 and Cyclosporin A

GREG WIEDERRECHT, ELSA LAM, SHIRLEY HUNG,
MARY MARTIN, AND NOLAN SIGAL

Department of Immunology Research
Merck Research Laboratories
Post Office Box 2000
Building R80W-107
Rahway, New Jersey 07065-0900

INTRODUCTION

The T lymphocyte plays a fundamental role in the process of organ transplant rejection as well as in the generation of autoimmune disease. Upon presentation with antigen by the antigen presenting cell (APC), the T cell undergoes a differentiation process that results in lymphokine secretion and its own proliferation.[1] The secreted lymphokines are responsible for a number of subsequent events, including conversion of B cells into antibody-secreting plasma cells, chemotaxis of macrophages and natural killer cells, and conversion of precytotoxic T lymphocytes (pre-CTLs) into CTLs, all of which contribute to the eventual destruction of the targeted tissue. In order to prevent tissue rejection, it is clear then why the prevention of T cell activation is an important pharmacological target.

Cyclosporin A (CsA) was introduced in 1983 as a therapeutic agent for renal allograft rejection and revolutionized the field of clinical transplantation due to the improved organ transplant survival rate.[2] Since that time, its use has expanded to cardiac, liver, heart-lung, and multiple organ transplants as well as to the treatment of certain autoimmune diseases such as psoriasis and insulin-dependent type I diabetes.[3,4] Use of CsA is limited by its side-effect profile, particularly its chronic nephrotoxicity, and so safer immunosuppressive agents have been sought. FK-506, a compound 10- to 100-fold more potent than CsA, began clinical testing in 1989 for the prevention of liver transplant rejection.[5,6] Surprisingly, both FK-506 and CsA have almost identical toxicities when used at equivalent therapeutic doses.

FK-506 AND CsA INHIBIT EARLY EVENTS IN T CELL ACTIVATION

FK-506 and CsA block early events in T lymphocyte activation. Both compounds exert their immunosuppressive effects downstream from the very early membrane-associated events, such as phosphoinositide turnover, that occur upon contact between the antigen presenting cell and the T cell receptor-CD3 complex.[7-9] These early membrane-associated events result in a rise in the levels of intracellular calcium and activation of the protein kinase C family, neither of which is affected by CsA or FK-506. Both drugs act proximally to transcription of a set of early lymphokine genes, IL-2, IL-3, IL-4, TNF-α, GM-CSF, and IFN-γ, which are expressed within two to four hours following the initiation of T cell activation.[10] Administration of either drug after expression of these early lymphokine mRNAs has no effect upon the T

9

cell.[9] The inhibitory effects of both drugs are IL-2 reversible because addition of IL-2 to drug-treated cells rescues the cells from their antiproliferative effects. In addition to their effects upon T cells, FK-506 and CsA block mast cell, neutrophil, basophil, and cytotoxic T lymphocyte degranulation—events that do not require active transcription—at a potency comparable to that observed for inhibition of T cell activation.[11,12] A stringent requirement for drug sensitivity is that the T cell activation or exocytosis pathway utilized by the cell involve an increase in intracellular calcium levels.[13] Pathways not involving a rise in intracellular calcium concentration, such as T cell activation via the CD28 pathway or C5a-induced neutrophil degranulation, are not sensitive to the effects of either FK-506 or CsA.[14-16] These results demonstrate that FK-506 and CsA do not inhibit specific transcriptional or exocytosis events. Rather, the two drugs block a calcium-dependent signal transduction event common to certain calcium-dependent pathways.

To understand the biochemical mechanism of action of FK-506 and CsA, two directions of research have been fruitful—forward from the identification of the intracellular receptors for these drugs, and backward from the inhibition of expression of IL-2.

THE MAJOR INTRACELLULAR RECEPTORS FOR FK-506 AND CsA

Based upon the clear similarities in the mechanisms of action of FK-506 and CsA, it was not surprising when it was found that the intracellular receptors for these chemically dissimilar drugs share at least four interesting properties. First, both of the major receptors are small cytosolic proteins. The molecular weight of the major receptor for FK-506 is 12 kilodaltons (kDa) and is termed FKBP12.[17,18] The major receptor for CsA is a 17-kDa protein and is named CypA.[19] Second, CypA and FKBP12 are among the most abundant proteins within the cell, comprising between 0.2% and 0.4% of the total cytosolic protein. Third, both receptors appear to be ubiquitous and are extraordinarily well conserved throughout phylogeny.[20,21] Not only have they been found in nearly every cell type and tissue examined, but the amino acid sequences within each receptor family are highly similar in organisms ranging from yeast to man.

The fourth, and perhaps the most interesting, characteristic shared by the two receptors is that they share an enzymatic activity. Both proteins catalyze the cis-to-trans isomerization of peptidyl-prolyl bonds and are termed peptidyl-prolyl-isomerases (PPIases).[17,22,23] CypA has little preference for the amino acid preceding the proline residue, while the substrate preferences for FKBP12 can vary over three orders of magnitude with Leu-Pro substrates being preferred.[24] CsA and FK-506 are potent inhibitors of their cognate receptors' PPIase activity. Initially, it seemed possible that inhibition of PPIase activity would be relevant to the immunosuppressive activity of the drugs. However, FK-506 and CsA analogues were soon discovered that were potent PPIase inhibitors but that had no inhibitory effect upon IL-2 transcription. One such compound is rapamycin, which is chemically related to FK-506, but which antagonizes the ability of FK-506 to block IL-2 transcription.[25,26] Rapamycin is at least equipotent to FK-506 in its ability to inhibit the PPIase activity of FKBP12. Another compound is the MeAla[6] derivative of CsA, which has no immunosuppressive activity but which is 70% as active as CsA at inhibiting the PPIase activity of CypA.[27] These observations demonstrate that inhibition of PPIase activity is not sufficient to block T cell activation.

The great abundance of FKBP12 and CypA within cells as well as their high degree of conservation throughout phylogeny suggest that these proteins would have some fundamental and critical role in cellular physiology. Their PPIase activity led to the suggestion that these proteins might be "foldases," required for proper protein folding within the cell. However, disruption of the genes encoding CypA and FKBP12 in *Saccharomyces cerevisiae* demonstrated that, in yeast, neither gene is essential for viability.[28,29] The precise roles for the CypA and FKBP12 proteins within the cell are presently an area of active investigation. FKBP12 is specifically associated with the ryanodine receptor, a calcium channel in the sarcoplasmic reticulum of smooth muscle cells involved in excitation-contraction coupling.[30] The role of FKBP12 in mediating calcium flux through the channel is unknown at present. It is possible that the PPIase activity of FKBP12 functions to help open and close the channel.

The absence of any correlation between inhibition of PPIase activity and immunosuppression showed that loss of function of FKBP12 or CypA was not the underlying mechanism of immunosuppression mediated by FK-506 or CsA, respectively. Further evidence against the loss-of-function model came from cell-loading experiments which indicated that only a fraction of the intracellular pool of FKBP12 or CypA is bound by either of the drugs at immunosuppressive doses. Alternatively, a gain-of-function model suggested that FK-506 and CsA were not active by themselves but were, in fact, prodrugs that became active upon binding to their cognate receptors. This model would help to explain the observations listed above. Lending further support to the gain-of-function model were the observations that CsA and FK-506 undergo radical changes when bound by their receptors and exist in conformations not observed when they are free in solution. The resulting drug-receptor complex is a novel chemical entity that might then be the active immunosuppressive drug.

CALCINEURIN IS A SIGNALING COMPONENT OF IL-2 EXPRESSION

The hunt for targets of the FKBP/FK-506 and the Cyp/CsA drug-receptor complexes led to the isolation of the calcium- and calmodulin-dependent serine-threonine phosphatase calcineurin (CaN), on FKBP12/FK-506 and CypA/CsA affinity columns.[31,32] Calcineurin is a heterotrimer of a 59-kDa catalytic subunit (CaNα), a 19-kDa regulatory subunit (CaNβ), and the 15-kDa calmodulin (CaM).[33] A strong correlation exists between the immunosuppressive activity of the FK-506 or CsA analogues and the ability of the receptor-analogue complex to bind calcineurin *in vitro* and to inhibit its phosphatase activity against an artificial substrate *in vitro*.[25] For example, rapamycin, which does not inhibit IL-2 synthesis, does not bind calcineurin in the presence of FKBP. Likewise, the nonimmunosuppressive CsA analogue MeAla[6]-CsA binds to cyclophilin with an affinity similar to that of CsA, but the Cyp/MeAla[6]-CsA complex does not inhibit CaN phosphatase activity. Careful characterization of the requirements for FKBP/FK-506/CaN complex formation using a high-performance liquid chromatography (HPLC) gel filtration assay demonstrated an absolute requirement for the presence of calmodulin.[34] A requirement for the presence of the CaNβ regulatory subunit was demonstrated in experiments measuring CypA/CsA-mediated inhibition of calcineurin phosphatase activity.[35]

The calcineurin catalytic subunit consists of a catalytic domain in the N-terminal half of the protein, followed by two allosteric control regions in the C-terminal third of the protein, a calmodulin-binding domain and an autoinhibitory domain. It has been proposed that, *in vivo*, calmodulin releases the autoinhibitory domain from the catalytic site of calcineurin, allowing the FKBP/FK-506 complex to bind. This hypothesis would be consistent with the observation that a 43-kDa proteolytic fragment of CaN, which lacks the calmodulin and autoinhibitory domains, is constitutively active and calcium and calmodulin independent.[36,37] The proteolytic subunit is bound by drug-receptor complexes even in the absence of calmodulin. The PPIase activity of FKBP12 has no role in calcineurin complex formation. This was demonstrated using a PPIase-deficient FKBP12 mutant, F37Y, which has FK-506 binding activity but only 0.01% of the wild-type PPIase activity.[34] Titration of wild-type and F37Y proteins into incubation mixtures that contained FK-506 and calcineurin demonstrated that both proteins have equivalent IC_{50}s for inhibiting phosphatase activity.

Some of the first experiments confirming calcineurin as a relevant *in vivo* target for FK-506 and CsA were performed by measuring calcineurin activity in extracts prepared from T cells cultured in the presence of the drugs. By treatment of the extracts with okadaic acid, a potent inhibitor of protein phosphatases 1 and 2A, it was shown that calcineurin activity decreased in a dose-dependent manner when the cells had been incubated with FK-506 or CsA.[38] IL-2 production by the drug-treated cells correlated with the decrease in calcineurin phosphatase activity. Rapamycin had no effect upon calcineurin activity and reversed the effects of FK-506, evidence that it is an FK-506/receptor complex that is the actual inhibitory molecule. That FKBP12 is the receptor relevant to FK-506's effects is suggested by experiments performed in mast cell lines deficient in FKBP12. Treatment of these FKBP12-deficient cells with FK-506 failed to inhibit calcineurin phosphatase activity or lymphokine secretion.[39]

Validation of calcineurin as a physiological component of the TCR signal transduction pathway was confirmed in transfection experiments using a construct, named ΔCaM-AI, encoding the 43-kDa calcium- and calmodulin-independent form of CaN described above and Jurkat cells, a human T-lymphoma cell line.[40] Jurkat cells can be activated to produce IL-2 in response to the mitogens ionomycin and PMA which provide the stimuli needed to increase the intracellular calcium levels and activate the protein kinase C family, respectively. The Jurkat cells were cotransfected with a reporter gene that measured IL-2 promoter activity. In cells transfected with wild-type calcineurin, there was no IL-2 promoter activity when the cells were stimulated with either PMA or ionomycin alone. In cells transfected with ΔCaM-AI, there was no activity of the IL-2 promoter in response to ionomycin alone. However, treatment of the ΔCaM-AI transfected cells with PMA alone bypassed the calcium requirement and resulted in a >150-fold induction of promoter activity that was sensitive to FK-506 and CsA. Thus, ΔCaM-AI acted in synergy with PMA to render the cells independent of calcium signaling. This provided the first *in vivo* demonstration that calcineurin is a component of calcium-dependent transcriptional activation of the IL-2 gene via the TCR signal transduction pathway.

Further corroboration of calcineurin as the drug-sensitive target came from drug titration experiments with CsA and FK-506.[40] Transfection of Jurkat cells containing an IL-2 reporter construct with either wild-type calcineurin or ΔCaM-AI increased the IC_{50} of FK-506 and CsA between four- and sixfold. Rapamycin reversed the inhibitory effects of FK-506. These results confirmed that calcineurin is the FK-506- and CsA-sensitive component of the TCR signal transduction pathway.

THE HUMAN IL-2 PROMOTER

As a mediator of the calcium signaling emanating from the T cell receptor, calcineurin probably dephosphorylates one or more substrates that are either directly or indirectly involved in transcribing the IL-2 gene, as well as other early lymphokine genes. One strategy aimed at identifying the substrates for calcineurin and, hence, identifying novel therapeutic targets for immunosuppression has been to start with the IL-2 promoter and work backward. The human IL-2 promoter has been extensively characterized, and the region required for maximal IL-2 expression extends approximately 300 base pairs (bp) upstream from the transcription initiation site.[41] Deletion and mutational analysis has identified five enhancer sites that have been labeled NFIL-2A through NFIL-2E. These enhancers contain binding sites for several transcription factors. Some of these transcription factors such as octamer/octamer associated protein (Oct/OAP), NF-κB, and AP-1 are relatively well characterized proteins that are required for transcribing genes in other cell types. Other enhancer elements on the IL-2 promoter bind factors that appear to be unique to T cells such as nuclear factor of activated T cells (NF-AT) and a CD28-responsive factor.

To understand the role that each enhancer element plays in the FK-506 and CsA sensitivity of the IL-2 promoter as well as to understand which enhancer elements are responding to signals from calcineurin, each of the enhancer elements has been multimerized, placed upstream of a basal promoter element (containing the IL-2 TATA box), fused to a chloramphenicol acetyl transferase (CAT) reporter gene, and the constructs transfected into Jurkat cells.[42] The IL-2A (Oct/OAP), IL-2E (NF-AT), and NF-κB multimerized elements yield maximal levels of CAT expression when the cells are costimulated with ionomycin and PMA. In all three cases, that activity is inhibited by FK-506 and CsA, indicating the involvement of calcineurin. Further evidence of calcineurin's role in the transcription driven by these factors is that when the cells are cotransfected with ΔCaM-AI, the requirement for ionomycin treatment is bypassed.[42] Interestingly, ionomycin/PMA cotreatment of ΔCaM-AI transfected cells results in hyperactivation of transcription driven by the IL-2A and IL-2E elements, suggesting that additional calcium-dependent signaling pathways may be required for maximal induction through these elements. The ΔCaM-AI/PMA-induced transcriptional activity exhibited by these reporter constructs is, in all cases, inhibited by FK-506 and CsA.

In contrast to the observations made with the IL-2A, IL-2E, and NF-κB elements, transcription driven by multimers of the AP-1 element is maximal when the cells are treated with PMA alone.[42] Ionomycin/PMA cotreatment actually results in less CAT expression driven by the AP-1 elements. Pretreatment of PMA/ionomycin-stimulated cells with FK-506 results in more AP-1-dependent CAT expression. This result suggests that inhibition of calcineurin appears to enhance transcription through the AP-1 element.

The transcriptional results, taken together, make it clear that calcineurin activates the IL-2 promoter via at least three different transcription factors (NF-AT, NF-κB, and Oct/OAP) and that multiple calcium-sensitive signals regulate IL-2 promoter activity. One model for calcineurin's action in the T cell is that it dephosphorylates one or more transcription factors in the cytoplasm that can then be translocated to the nucleus to activate the IL-2 promoter. Precedent for this model is found in *Saccharomyces cerevisiae* where the transcription factor SWI5 is dephosphorylated in the cytoplasm and is then translocated to the nucleus.[43] It has been proposed that, in the T cell, calcineurin dephosphorylates a constitutive cytosolic component of the NF-AT complex (NF-AT$_C$) which is then translocated to the nucleus, combines with a nuclear NF-AT component of the complex (NF-AT$_N$), and the resulting NF-AT$_C$/NF-AT$_N$ heterodimer binds to its regulatory site on the IL-2 promoter contributing to IL-2 expression.[44] Experimental support for this hypothesis has recently been reported.[45] The FK-506 sensitivity of the NF-κB site is particularly intriguing as it participates in the induction of numerous promoters in a variety of cell types and might therefore be associated with some of the toxic effects of FK-506 and CsA. In addition to its effects on these transcription factors, calcineurin almost certainly dephosphorylates other, as yet unidentified, substrates in the T cell and in other cells that are not involved in IL-2 expression. For instance, inhibition of FK-506- and CsA-sensitive exocytosis pathways does not require new transcription. Therefore, the substrates for calcineurin in granulocytic cells are almost certainly different from those in T cells. Other calcineurin substrates relevant to the neuro- and nephrotoxic side effects of FK-506 and CsA will be discussed in a later section.

THE HUMAN FKBP, CYCLOPHILIN, AND CALCINEURIN GENE FAMILIES

The binding activity for FK-506 was first identified in the cytosol of Jurkat cells.[46] Later, a 12-kDa binding activity, FKBP12, was purified to homogeneity by two groups.[17,18] In addition to FKBP12, three more human FKBPs have been identified and are named, according to their mass, FKBP13, FKBP25, and FKBP52.[46-53] We have cloned, expressed in *Escherichia coli,* purified, and characterized each of these

TABLE 1. Characterization of Human FK-506 Binding Proteins[a]

FKBP	Binds FK-506	PPIase Activity Inhibited by FK-506	Drug-FKBP Inhibits Calcineurin
12	+	+	+
13	+	+	−
25	+	+	−
52	+	+	−

[a]Known human FK-506 binding proteins are listed in order of increasing molecular weight in kilodaltons. Binding of FK-506, inhibition of PPIase activity by FK-506, and inhibition of bovine calcineurin phosphatase activity by the FKBP/FK-506 complex are indicated by pluses and minuses.

proteins. Northern analysis has demonstrated that all three are expressed at the message level in Jurkat cells. All of them bind FK-506, and all have PPIase activity that is antagonized by FK-506 and rapamycin. The FKBP12/FK-506 complex is, by far, the most potent at inhibition of bovine calcineurin phosphatase (TABLE 1). At our present level of understanding, FKBP12 is probably the relevant FKBP mediating the immunosuppressive effects of FK-506. However, a formal demonstration of this awaits gene knockout experiments in mice.

The fact that all of the FKBPs are PPIases is the only clue that we have concerning their *in vivo* function. Given their PPIase activity, it is not surprising that two of the FKBPs, FKBP12 and FKBP52, have been found associated with other proteins within the cell. The association of FKBP12 with the ryanodine receptor has already been discussed. Cloning of the cDNA encoding rabbit FKBP52 revealed that it contains three FKBP homologous regions, the most conserved of which is contained N-terminally and which is probably most responsible for its FK-506 binding activity.[54] FKBP52 binds to hsp90 alone as well as when hsp90 is complexed with untransformed steroid receptors.[55] The amino acid sequence of FKBP52 contains consensus elements indicating binding to calmodulin, and FKBP52 has been purified using calmodulin affinity columns.[56] FKBP52's relevance to steroid receptor function as well as FK-506's effects upon steroid function is, as yet, undetermined.

Binding of FKBP13 or FKBP25 to other proteins has not yet been reported, although the two proteins have been characterized to some extent. FKBP13 contains a signal sequence and an endoplasmic reticulum retention sequence.[47] The processed protein is associated with heavy membrane fractions. Interestingly, while FKBP12 is the most abundant FKBP in most cells and tissues, FKBP13 is more abundant than FKBP12 in rat basophilic leukemia cells.[12] However, FKBP13 has not been implicated in the drug sensitivity of serotonin release in these cells. FKBP25 is homologous to FKBP12 in the C-terminal half of the protein.[49,52] The N-terminal half of the protein is unrelated to any protein in the current databases. FKBP25 binds rapamycin with much greater avidity than it binds FK-506. Cloning and sequencing of the FKBP25 cDNA as well as sequencing of the protein have revealed that it has five nuclear localization sequences in the N-terminal half of the protein and one in the C-terminal, FKBP12 homologous, half. Nuclear localization of FKBP25 has recently been confirmed.[57] The *in vivo* function of FKBP25 or whether it mediates the effects of rapamycin on IL-2 dependent T cell proliferation is not known.

Like the FKBPs, the cyclophilins comprise an ever-expanding gene family. Southern analysis of human genomic DNA suggests the presence of at least 20 related genes or pseudogenes.[58] Thus far, in addition to the 165 amino acid major human cytosolic cyclophilin, CypA, three other human cyclophilins have been purified or their cDNAs cloned. CypB, also called Cyp2 or S-cyclophilin, is a 208 amino acid protein having a 32 amino acid hydrophobic leader sequence, an endoplasmic reticulum retention sequence, and has been detected in human milk.[59–61] Cyp3 is a 207 amino acid protein having a 42 amino acid hydrophobic leader sequence.[59] Subcellularly, CypB and Cyp3 are associated with membrane fractions. NK-TR (natural killer-tumor recognition molecule) is a 1403 amino acid protein with a cyclophilin like domain at its *N*-terminus.[62] Like FKBP12, CypA appears to have a ubiquitous tissue and cell distribution. By northern analysis, CypB and Cyp3 appear to have a more restricted tissue distribution relative to CypA, although all three have message expressed in T lymphocytes. However, the message levels of CypB and Cyp3 are 10 to 100 fold lower, respectively, than the message level of CypA in a number of tissues and cell types. CypA, CypB, and Cyp3 all have PPIase activity that is inhibitable by CsA. CypA and CypB have been examined for their ability, in the presence of CsA, to inhibit CaN phosphatase activity. Both CypA/CsA and CypB/CsA drug complexes inhibit CaN phosphatase activity with the CypB/CsA complex being the more potent inhibitor.[35] NK-TR is found only on the surface of natural killer cells. As yet, there have been no reports measuring NK-TR's affinity for CsA or whether it has PPIase activity. In addition to these human cyclophilins, a 40-kDa cyclophilin-related protein that will almost certainly have a human counterpart has been purified from bovine brain and characterized.[63] Cyp40 appears to be ubiquitously expressed, binds CsA, and has PPIase activity that is inhibitable by CsA.

Based upon isoelectric focusing experiments, six isoforms of the catalytic subunit of calcineurin can be discerned in extracts prepared from brain.[64,65] To date, the accumulated data indicate that there are at least three genes encoding the catalytic subunit of mammalian calcineurin.[66–73] These genes, encoding the type 1, type 2, and type 3 isoforms, can undergo alternative splicing events to give additional variants (type 1δ, type 2δ, and type 3δ) in which 10 amino acids in the resulting protein are deleted between the calmodulin binding and autoinhibitory domains. All of the calcineurin catalytic subunits are extremely well conserved. Message for the type 1, type 2, and type 3 variants has been detected in T lymphocytes.[74] Activation of the IL-2 promoter by PMA and either the type 1, type 2, and type 3 isotypes is inhibited by FK-506 suggesting that, in contrast to the FKBPs, at our present level of understanding, there is little to distinguish the calcineurins from one another.[75]

TOXICITY

Although FK-506 appears to have some benefits over CsA, both drugs have significant toxic side effects. Both compounds show acute neurological toxicity, which improves over time, and both drugs exhibit chronic nephrotoxicity. The similar toxicity profiles indicate that toxicity is mechanistically linked to the similar biochemical effects exerted by the two drugs. Support for mechanism-based toxicity came from an analysis of CsA analogues demonstrating that more immunosuppressive compounds had greater nephrotoxic potential.[27] Further support for mechanism-linked toxicity came from an analysis of the effects of L-685,818, an FK-506 antagonist. L-685,818 and FK-506 bind with equal affinity to FKBP12. However, the FKBP12/L-685,818 complex is a much poorer inhibitor of CaN phosphatase activity and, in the cell, it reverses the effects of FK-506. Unlike FK-506, L-685,818 exhibits no toxicity and can, in fact, antagonize the toxic effects of FK-506.[25] These data indicate that binding of FK-506 or CsA by their cognate receptors is not responsible for toxicity but that inhibition of calcineurin by the drug-receptor complex is. As discussed earlier, inhibition of calcineurin-mediated dephosphorylation of substrates in cells other than T cells may be deleterious to the organism. These toxic side effects may be the consequence of perturbations in transcriptional regulation, inhibition of other cellular signaling pathways in which CaN plays a role, or both. Potential mediators of toxicity include calcineurin-regulated Ca^{2+} channels in the brain and the membrane Na^+/K^+ pump in renal tubule cells, which is also regulated by calcineurin and which is sensitive to FK-506 and CsA.[76-78] Long-term disruption of sodium and potassium homeostasis in tubule cells might be responsible for the problems in renal clearance that occur during CsA and FK-506 therapy. While the FKBPs and cyclophilins may not be relevant to toxicity from a mechanistic perspective, it is possible that these receptors act as potential drug sinks in cells and in tissues and that the ability of a particular analogue to penetrate a particular organ may be related to the FKBP or cyclophilin concentration within the cells of that organ.

CONCLUSION

The efforts to understand the mechanistic basis for the immunosuppressive effects of FK-506 and CsA have led to a partial dissection of the signal transduction pathway between the T cell receptor and expression of IL-2. Calcineurin has been identified as a component of the pathway that is activated in response to increases in intracellular calcium. However, the calcineurin substrates relevant to activation of IL-2 synthesis remain to be identified. Identification of the calcineurin substrates and an understanding of the FK-506 and CsA receptors may yield safer and more beneficial immunosuppressive drugs.

SUMMARY

FK-506 and cyclosporin A (CsA) are potent immunosuppressive agents used clinically to prevent tissue rejection. Interest in the development of more effective immunosuppressive drugs has led to an intense effort toward understanding their biochemical mechanism of action with the result that these compounds have now become powerful tools used in deciphering the signal transduction events in T lymphocyte activation. Although chemically unrelated, FK-506 and CsA exert nearly identical biological effects in cells by inhibiting the same subset of early calcium-associated events involved in lymphokine expression, apoptosis, and degranulation. FK-506 binds to a family of intracellular receptors termed the FK-506 binding proteins (FKBPs). CsA binds to another family of intracellular receptors, the cyclophilins (Cyps), distinct from the FKBPs. The similarities between the mechanisms of action of CsA and FK-506 converge upon the calcium- and calmodulin-dependent serine-threonine protein phosphatase calcineurin (CaN). Both the FKBP/FK-506 complex and the Cyp/CsA complex can bind to calcineurin, thereby inhibiting its phosphatase activity. Calcineurin, a component of the signal transduction pathway resulting in IL-2 expression, catalyzes critical dephosphorylation events required for early lymphokine gene transcription.

REFERENCES

1. CRABTREE, G. 1989. Science **243:** 355–361.
2. KAHAN, B. 1989. N. Engl. J. Med. **321:** 1725–1738.
3. BOUGNERES, P., P. LANDAIS, C. BOISSON, J. CAREL, N. FRAMENT, C. BOITARD, J. CHAUSSAIN & J. BACH. 1990. Diabetes **39:** 1264–1271.
4. ELLIS, C., M. FRADIN, J. MESSANA, M. BRAWN, M. SIEGEL, A. HARTLEY, L. ROCHER, S. WHEELER, T. HAMILTON, T. PARISH, M. ELLISMADU, E. DUELL, T. ANNESLEY, K. COOPER & J. VOORHEES. 1991. N. Engl. J. Med. **324:** 277–284.
5. KINO, T., H. HATANAKE, S. MIYATA, N. INAMURA, M. NISHIYAMA, T. YAJIMA, T. GOTO, M. OKUHARA, M. KOHSAKA, H. AOKI & T. OCHAI. 1987. J. Antibiot. **40:** 1256–1265.
6. FUNG, J., S. TODO, A. TZAKIS, M. ALESSIANI, K. ABUELMAGD, A. JAIN, O. BRONSTER, M. MARTIN, R. GORDON & T. STARZL. 1991. Transplant. Proc. **23:** 1902–1905.
7. MIZUSHIMA, Y., H. KOSAKA, S. SAKUMA, K. KANDA, K. ITOH, T. OSUGI, A. MIZUSHIMA, T. HAMAOKA, H. YOSHIDA, K. SOBUE & H. FUKIWARA. 1987. J. Biochem. **102:** 1193–1201.
8. SAWADA, S., G. SUZUKI, Y. KAWASE & G. TAKAKU. 1987. J. Immunol. **139:** 1797–1803.
9. DUMONT, F., M. STARUCH, S. KOPRAK, M. MELINO & N. SIGAL. 1990. J. Immunol. **144:** 251–258.
10. TOCCI, M., D. MATKOVICH, K. COLLIER, P. KWOK, F. DUMONT, S. LIN, S. DEGUDICIBUS, J. SIEKIERKA, J. CHIN & N. HUTCHINSON. 1989. J. Immunol. **143:** 718–726.
11. FORREST, M., M. JEWELL, G. KOO & N. SIGAL. 1991. Biochem. Pharmacol. **42:** 1221–1228.
12. HULTSCH, T., M. ALBERS, S. SCHREIBER & R. HOHMAN. 1991. Proc. Natl. Acad. Sci. USA **88:** 6229–6233.
13. SIGAL, N. & F. DUMONT. 1992. Annu. Rev. Immunol. **10:** 519–560.
14. JUNE, C., J. LEDBETTER, M. GILLESPIE, T. LINDSTEN, C. THOMPSON. 1987. Mol. Cell. Biol. **7:** 4472–4481.
15. KAY, J. & C. BENZIE. 1989. Immunol. Lett. **23:** 439–445.
16. LIN, C., R. BOLTZ, J. SIEKIERKA & N. SIGAL. 1991. Cell. Immun. **133:** 269–284.
17. SIEKIERKA, J., S. HUNG, M. POE, C. LIN & N. SIGAL. 1989. Nature **341:** 755–757.
18. HARDING, M., A. GALAT, D. UEHLING & S. SCHREIBER. 1989. Nature **341:** 758–760.
19. HANDSCHUMACHER, R., M. HARDING, J. RICE, R. DRUGGS & D. SPEICHER. 1984. Science **226:** 544–547.
20. SIEKIERKA, J., G. WIEDERRECHT, H. GREULICH, D. BOULTON, H. HUNG, J. CRYAN, P. HODGES & N. SIGAL. 1990. J. Biol. Chem. **265:** 21011–21015.
21. TRANDINH, C., G. PAO & M. SAIER. 1992. FASEB J. **6:** 3410–3420.
22. TAKAHASHI, N., R. HAYANO & M. SUZUKI. 1989. Nature **337:** 473–475.
23. FISCHER, G., L. WITTMANN, K. LANG, T. KIEFHABER & F. SCHMID. 1989. Nature **337:** 476–478.
24. HARRISON, R. & R. STEIN. 1990. Biochemistry **29:** 3813–3816.
25. DUMONT, F., M. STARUCH, S. KOPRAK, J. SIEKIERKA, C. LIN, R. HARRISON, T. SEWELL, V. KINDT, T. BEATTIE, M. WYVRATT & N. SIGAL. 1992. J. Exp. Med. **176:** 751–760.
26. BIERER, B., P. MATTILA, R. STANDAERT, L. HERZENBERG, S. BURAKOFF, G. CRABTREE & S. SCHREIBER. 1990. Proc. Natl. Acad. Sci. USA **87:** 9231–9235.

27. SIGAL, N., F. DUMONT, P. DURETTE, J. SIEKIERKA, L. PETERSON, D. RICH, B. DUNLAP, M.
    STARUCH, M. MELINO, S. KOPRAK, D. WILLIAMS, B. WITZEL & J. PISANO. 1991. J. Exp.
    Med. 173: 619–628.
28. TROPSCHUG, M., I. BARTHELMESS & W. NEUPERT. 1989. Nature 342: 953–955.
29. WIEDERRECHT, G., L. BRIZUELA, K. ELLISTON, N. SIGAL & J. SIEKIERKA. 1991. Proc. Natl.
    Acad. Sci. USA 88: 1029–1033.
30. JAYARAMAN, T., A.-M. BRILLANTES, A. TIMERMAN, S. FLEISCHER, H. ERDJUMENT-
    BROMAGE, P. TEMPST & A. MARKS. 1992. J. Biol. Chem. 267: 9474–9477.
31. LIU, J., J. FARMER, W. LANE, J. FRIEDMAN, I. WEISSMAN & S. SCHREIBER. 1991. Cell
    66: 807–815.
32. FRIEDMAN, J. & I. WEISSMAN. 1991. Cell 66: 799–806.
33. KINCAID, R., S. HIGUCHI, J. TAMURA, P. GIRI & T. MARTENSEN. 1991. Adv. Prot.
    Phosphatases 6: 73–98.
34. WIEDERRECHT, G., S. HUNG, H. CHAN, A. MARCY, M. MARTIN, J. CALAYCAY, D.
    BOULTON, N. SIGAL, R. KINCAID & J. SIEKIERKA. 1992. J. Biol. Chem. 267: 21753–21760.
35. SWANSON, S., T. BORN, L. ZYDOWSKY, H. CHO, H. CHANG, C. WALSH & F. RUSNAK. 1992.
    Proc. Natl. Acad. Sci. USA 89: 3741–3745.
36. KINCAID, R., T. MARTENSEN & M. VAUGHN. 1986. Biochem. Biophys. Res. Commun.
    140: 320–328.
37. HUBBARD, M. & C. KLEE. 1989. Biochemistry 28: 1868–1874.
38. FRUMAN, D., C. KLEE, B. BIERER & S. BURAKOFF. 1992. Proc. Natl. Acad. Sci. USA
    89: 3686–3690.
39. KAYE, R., D. FRUMAN, B. BIERER, M. ALBERS, L. ZYDOWSKY, S. HO, Y. JIN, M. CASTELLS,
    S. SCHREIBER, C. WALSH, S. BURAKOFF, K. AUSTEN & H. KATZ. 1992. Proc. Natl. Acad.
    Sci. USA 89: 8542–8546.
40. O'KEEFE, S., J. TAMURA, R. KINCAID, M. TOCCI & E. O'NEILL. 1992. Nature 357: 692–694.
41. ULLMAN, K., J. NORTHROP, C. VERWEIJ & G. CRABTREE. 1990. Annu. Rev. Immunol.
    8: 421–452.
42. FRANTZ, B., E. NORDBY, C. PAYA, R. KINCAID, M. TOCCI, S. O'KEEFE & E. O'NEILL.
    EMBO. (Submitted.)
43. MOLL, T., G. TEBB, U. SURANA, H. ROBITSCH & K. NASMYTH. 1991. Cell 66: 743–758.
44. FLANAGAN, W., B. CORTHESY, R. BRAM & G. CRABTREE. 1991. Nature 352: 803–807.
45. MCCAFFREY, P., B. PERRINO, T. SODERLING & A. RAO. 1993. J. Biol. Chem. 268: 3747–
    3752.
46. SIEKIERKA, J., M. STARUCH, S. HUNG & N. SIGAL. 1989. J. Immunol. 143: 1580–1583.
47. JIN, Y., M. ALBERS, W. LANE, B. BIERER, S. SCHREIBER & S. BURAKOFF. 1991. Proc. Natl.
    Acad. Sci. USA 88: 6677–6681.
48. JIN, Y.-J., S. BURAKOFF & B. BIERER. 1992. J. Biol. Chem. 267: 10942–10945.
49. WIEDERRECHT, G., M. MARTIN, N. SIGAL & J. SIEKIERKA. 1992. Biochem. Biophys. Res.
    Commun. 185: 298–303.
50. YEM, A., A. TOMASSELLI, R. HEINRIKSON, H. ZURCHER-NEELY, V. RUFF, R. JOHNSON &
    M. DEIBEL. 1992. J. Biol. Chem. 267: 2868–2871.
51. PEATTIE, D., M. HARDING, M. FLEMING, M. DECENZO, J. LIPPKE, D. LIVINGSTON & M.
    BENASUTTI. 1992. Proc. Natl. Acad. Sci. USA 89: 10974–10978.
52. GALAT, A., W. LANE, R. STANDAERT & S. SCHREIBER. 1992. Biochemistry 31: 2427–2434.
53. FRETZ, H., M. ALBERS, A. GALAT, R. STANDAERT, W. LANE, S. BURAKOFF, B. BIERER & S.
    SCHREIBER. 1991. J. Am. Chem. Soc. 113: 1409–1411.
54. CALLEBAUT, I., J.-M. RENOIR, M.-C. LEBEAU, N. MASSOL, A. BURNY, E.-E. BAULIEU &
    J.-P. MORNON. 1992. Proc. Natl. Acad. Sci. USA 89: 6270–6274.
55. RENOIR, J., D. RADANYI, L. FABER & E. BAULIEU. 1990. J. Biol. Chem. 265: 10740–10745.
56. MASSOL, N., M.-C. LEBEAU, J.-M. RENOIR, L. FABER & E.-E. BAULIEU. 1992. Biochem.
    Biophys. Res. Commun. 187: 1330–1335.
57. RIVIERE, S., A. MENEZ & A. GALAT. 1993. FEBS Lett. 315: 247–251.
58. HAENDLER, B. & E. HOFER. 1990. Eur. J. Biochem. 190: 477–482.
59. BERGSMA, D., C. EDER, M. GROSS, H. KERSTEN, D. SYLVESTER, E. APPELBAUM, D.
    CUSIMANO, G. LIVI, M. MCLAUGHLIN, K. KASYAN, T. PORTER, C. SILVERMAN, D.
    DUNNINGTON, A. HAND, W. PRICHETT, et al. 1991. J. Biol. Chem. 266: 23204–23214.

60. PRICE, E., L. ZYDOWSKY, M. JIN, C. BAKER, F. MCKEON & C. WALSH. 1991. Proc. Natl. Acad. Sci. USA. **88:** 1903–1907.
61. SPIK, G., B. HAENDLER, O. DELMAS, C. MARILLER, M. CHAMOUX, P. MAES, A. TARTAR, J. MONTREUIL, K. STEDMAN, H. KOCHER, R. KELLER, P. HIESTAND & N. MOVVA. 1991. J. Biol. Chem. **266:** 10735–10738.
62. ANDERSON, S., S. GALLINGER, J. RODER, J. FREY, H. YOUNG & J. ORTALDO. 1993. Proc. Natl. Acad. Sci. USA **90:** 542–546.
63. KIEFFER, L., T. THALHAMMER & R. HANDSCHUMACHER. 1992. J. Biol. Chem. **267:** 5503–5507.
64. KLEE, C., T. CROUCH & M. KRINKS. 1979. Proc. Natl. Acad. Sci. USA **79:** 6270–6273.
65. BILLINGSLEY, M., K. PENNYPACKER, C. HOOVER, D. BRIGATI & R. KINCAID. 1985. Proc. Natl. Acad. Sci. USA **82:** 7585–7589.
66. KINCAID, R., M. NIGHTINGALE & B. MARTIN. 1988. Proc. Natl. Acad. Sci. USA **85:** 8983–8987.
67. GUERINI, D. & C. KLEE. 1989. Proc. Natl. Acad. Sci. USA **86:** 9183–9187.
68. ITO, A., T. HASHIMOTO, M. HIRAI, T. TAKEDA, H. SHUNTOH, T. KUNO & C. TANAKA. 1989. Biochem. Biophys. Res. Commun. **163:** 1492–1497.
69. KUNO, T., T. TAKEDA, M. HIRAI, A. ITO, H. MUKAI & C. TANAKA. 1989. Biochem. Biophys. Res. Commun. **165:** 1352–1358.
70. RATHNA GIRI, P., S. HIGUCHI & R. KINCAID. 1991. Biochem. Biophys. Res. Commun. **181:** 252–258.
71. MCPARTLIN, A., H. BAKER & P. COHEN. 1991. Biochim. Biophys. Acta **1088:** 308–310.
72. MURAMATSU, T., P. RATHNA GIRI, S. HIGUCHI & R. KINCAID. 1992. Proc. Natl. Acad. Sci. USA **89:** 529–533.
73. MURAMATSU, T. & R. KINCAID. 1992. Biochem. Biophys. Res. Commun. **188:** 265–271.
74. PARSONS, J. & S. O'KEEFE. Unpublished data.
75. PARSONS, J., T. MURAMATSU, R. KINCAID, M. TOCCI, E. O'NEILL & S. O'KEEFE. (Manuscript in preparation.)
76. ARMSTRONG, D. 1989. Trends Neurosci. **12:** 117–122.
77. APERIA, A., F. IBARRA, L.-B. SVENSSON, C. KLEE & P. GREENGARD. 1992. Proc. Natl. Acad. Sci. USA **89:** 7394–7397.
78. TUMLIN, A. & J. SANDS. 1993. Kidney Int. **43:** 246–251.

Calcineurin Is a Key Signaling Enzyme in T Lymphocyte Activation and the Target of the Immunosuppressive Drugs Cyclosporin A and FK506[a]

NEIL A. CLIPSTONE AND GERALD R. CRABTREE

Howard Hughes Medical Institute
Stanford University School of Medicine
Stanford University
Stanford, California 94305

INTRODUCTION

The immunosuppressive drugs cyclosporin A (CsA) and FK506 have proven to be extremely powerful therapeutic agents both in the prevention of allograft rejection following solid organ engraftment and in the prophylatic treatment of graft-versus-host disease after bone marrow transplantation.[1-3] The immunosuppressive properties of CsA and FK506 can largely be ascribed to their potent inhibition of the T cell activation dependent transcription of the T cell growth factor interleukin 2 and other immunologically important T lymphocyte derived lymphokines.[4-6] In normal T lymphocytes, physiological triggering of the T cell antigen receptor results in the generation of a number of distinct intracellular biochemical signals (e.g., elevated intracellular calcium, activation of protein kinase C, and tyrosine phosphorylation), which together act to initiate the orderly expression of specific T cell genes resulting in T cell activation, cellular proliferation, and ultimately acquisition of immune function.[7,8] Although structurally unrelated, both CsA and FK506 inhibit this complex sequence of events at a similar step. In this regard, CsA and FK506 do not inhibit the initial generation of biochemical second messengers, but rather, act at a subsequent step in the signaling cascade to specifically interfere with a Ca^{2+}-sensitive T cell signal transduction pathway,[9-12] thereby preventing the activation of specific transcription factors (such as NF-AT and NF-IL2A) involved in lymphokine gene expression.[9,13-15]

CsA and FK506 appear to act via interaction with their cognate intracellular receptors,[16-18] cyclophilin and FKBP, respectively (reviewed in Reference 19). Despite the lack of any significant homology between these two receptor families, both possess peptidyl prolyl-*cis-trans* isomerase activity, an enzymatic activity involved in the catalysis of the *cis-trans* isomerization of proline residues in polypeptide substrates.[19-23] The observation that CsA and FK506 specifically inhibit the isomerase activity of their respective receptor[19-23] led initially to the notion that isomerases were directly involved in T cell activation. Arguing against this simple model is the observation that certain nonimmunosuppressive analogues of FK506 can bind to FKBP fully inhibiting its isomerase activity and, moreover, can antagonize the inhibitory effects of FK506.[16,17,19] These and other findings have led to the proposal

[a]This work was supported by the Howard Hughes Medical Institute, the National Institutes of Health, and the Anna Fuller Fund (N.A.C.).

of an alternative model wherein the drug-isomerase complex itself directly interferes with signal transduction events.

The Ca^{2+}/calmodulin regulated serine/threonine phosphatase, calcineurin, was identified by affinity purification as the major target of drug-isomerase complexes in tissue and cell extracts.[24,25] Calcineurin is comprised of two subunits, a calmodulin binding 59-kDa catalytic subunit (CNA) and a Ca^{2+}-binding 19-kDa regulatory subunit (CNB) (reviewed in References 26 and 27). It is ubiquitously expressed, but is most abundant in brain and is highly conserved from mammals to yeast.[26,28] In the present study, we have directly tested whether the interaction of drug-isomerase complexes with calcineurin observed *in vitro* is responsible for the *in vivo* immunosuppressive effects of CsA and FK506.

MATERIALS AND METHODS

Transfections and Reporter Gene Assays

TAg Jurkat cells are a derivative of the human T cell leukemia line Jurkat stably transfected with the SV40 large T antigen.[29] TAg cells (10^7) were transiently transfected as described previously.[9] Two micrograms of the indicated plasmid was used for each transfection; the amount of DNA was kept constant by addition of pBJ5. Twenty-four hours posttransfection, cells were cultured under the appropriate stimulation conditions and reporter gene activity was assessed after a further 20 h incubation. Secreted alkaline phosphatase activity was determined as previously described.[30] Chloramphenicol acetyltransferase activity was determined using standard procedures.[31]

RESULTS

Experimental Rationale

From *in vitro* studies, drug-isomerase complexes have been found to have dichotomous effects on the enzymatic activity of calcineurin. Thus, while FKBP-FK506 complexes completely inhibit calcineurin's enyzmatic activity towards a phosphopeptide substrate derived from the regulatory subunit of cAMP-dependent protein kinase, the activity towards the synthetic substrate *p*-nitrophenyl-phosphate is, in contrast, significantly enhanced.[24,32] It appears therefore that drug-isomerase complexes can potentially mediate either gain or loss of function effects on calcineurin.

Assuming that calcineurin is the relevant *in vivo* target of CsA and FK506; based upon the observed effects of the drug-isomerase complex on the enzymatic activity of calcineurin, two potential models to explain the putative role of calcineurin in the mechanism of action of CsA and FK506 can be proposed. In the first, the loss of function model (FIGURE 1a), calcineurin is assumed to be an integral component of the T cell signal transduction pathway, which mediates the calcium-dependent dephosphorylation and subsequent activation of an important signaling intermediate. In this model, drug-isomerase complexes simply bind to calcineurin and directly inhibit its activity, consequently preventing the dephosphorylation and activation of the signaling intermediate and thereby inhibiting T cell activation. In the second, or gain of function model (FIGURE 1b), calcineurin is not itself a component of the T cell signal transduction pathway per se. Rather the drug-isomerase complex acts in a dominant gain of function fashion to recruit calcineurin, altering its substrate specificity and redirecting it to dephosphorylate an illegitimate substrate that is an important signaling intermediate, thereby rendering it inactive and consequently preventing T cell activation. This latter phenomenon of an enzyme subunit (in this case, the drug-isomerase complex) affecting the substrate specificity of a phosphatase is not wholly without precedent and has been well documented in the case of protein phosphatase 2A (PP2A).[33-35]

In order to distinguish between these two alternative possibilities, we have investigated the consequences of calcineurin overexpression on the sensitivity of T cells to CsA and FK506. We reasoned that if the loss of function model were correct, overexpression of calcineurin should simply overcome the inhibitory effects of CsA or FK506. In contrast, if the gain of function model were correct, overexpression of

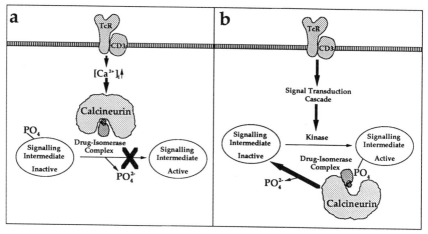

FIGURE 1. Two potential models to explain the putative role of calcineurin in the mechanism of action of CsA and FK506. **a:** Loss of function model. The drug-isomerase complex simply inhibits calcineurins' essential role in T cell signal transduction. **b:** Gain of function model. Calcineurin is not directly involved in T cell signaling, but rather is recruited by the drug-isomerase complex to inactivate a critical signaling molecule. See text for details.

calcineurin would either have no effect, since the concentration of drug should limit calcineurin participation, or, if the cellular concentration of calcineurin were itself very low and therefore limiting, overexpression of calcineurin should render cells more sensitive to the effects of CsA/FK506.

Overexpression of Calcineurin Renders Cells Resistant to the Immunosuppressive Effects of CsA and FK506

The *cis*-acting elements in the promoter of the IL-2 gene that are targets for the action of CsA and FK506 have been identified.[8,9,13,14] The transcription factors that bind to two of these sites, namely, NF-AT and NF-IL2A, are critical for IL-2 gene expression,[8,36] are induced by ionomycin/phorbol myristyl acetate (PMA; 12-*O*-

tetradecanoyl-phorbol-13-acetate), and their function is inhibited by FK506 and CsA in a dose-dependent fashion.[8,9,13] We therefore utilized plasmids containing multiple copies of binding sites for either NF-AT or NF-IL2A located upstream of the minimal IL-2 promoter and the secreted alkaline phosphatase reporter gene (NFAT-SX and NFIL2A-SX respectively), to monitor the effects of CsA and FK506. To determine the consequences of calcineurin overexpression on the sensitivity of T cells to CsA and FK506, TAg Jurkat cells were transiently cotransfected with either expression vectors encoding the murine catalytic CNAα1[28] and regulatory CN-B subunits (pBJ5-CNA and pBJ5-CNB respectively) or control plasmids, together with either the NFAT-SX or NFIL2A-SX reporter genes. Transfected cells were cultured in the presence of various concentrations of CsA and FK506, and after stimulation with ionomycin and PMA, reporter gene activity was assessed. The results of these experiments are shown in FIGURE 2. Transfection of both pBJ5-CNA and pBJ5-CNB resulted in a dramatic shift in the FK506 dose-response curve to the right relative to cells transfected with the control expression vector pBJ5 alone (FIGURE 2a and b), indicating that calcineurin overexpression renders transfected cells resistant to the effects of FK506. Similarly, overexpression of calcineurin also made cells more resistant to the effects of CsA (FIGURE 2c and d). This effect was observed whether cells were stimulated either with ionomycin and PMA (FIGURE 2a–d) or CD3 mAb and PMA (data not shown). Transfection of pBJ5-CNA alone produced a small but reproducible increase in the resistance of TAg Jurkat cells to CsA and FK506 (data not shown). The marked resistance observed in FIGURE 2 however was dependent upon cotransfection of pBJ5-CNB; transfection of pBJ5-CNB alone was without effect. Calcineurin is highly related in its catalytic domain to other serine/threonine phosphatases.[26,28,33,37] We therefore tested whether overexpression of another class of phosphatase could also cause transfected cells to become more resistant to the effects of drug. In this regard, transfection of an expression vector encoding the catalytic domain of human protein phosphatase 2A (PP2A) had no significant effect on the FK506-mediated inhibition of NFAT-SX activity (FIGURE 2a, open squares), indicating that the ability to make cells more resistant to the immunosuppressive effects of CsA and FK506 appears specific to calcineurin.

Overexpression of Calcineurin Enhances NFAT- and NFIL2A-Dependent Transcription

The foregoing data demonstrate that calcineurin overexpression renders TAg Jurkat cells markedly resistant to the effects of the immunosuppressive drugs CsA and FK506. What underlies the molecular basis of this effect? Clearly these data are most consistent with the loss of function model outlined in FIGURE 1a. In this model, calcineurin is assumed to be an essential enzyme in the T cell signaling cascade. Consequently, overexpression of the enzyme should result in an excess of calcineurin relative to the concentration of the inhibitory drug-isomerase complex, therefore overcoming the inhibitory effect of the drug and allowing signaling to proceed normally. Importantly, however, the experiments in FIGURE 2 do not directly address whether calcineurin is an integral component of the T cell signal transduction cascade, an important prerequisite of this model. With that caveat in mind, an equally plausible alternative is that overexpression of calcineurin acts indirectly to make cells resistant to CsA and FK506. In this case, calcineurin may not actually play a role in T cell signaling and may not represent the relevant *in vivo* target of CsA and FK506. Rather, calcineurin may simply bind and sequester the inhibitory drug-isomerase complex and thereby prevent it from interacting with its relevant intracellular target.

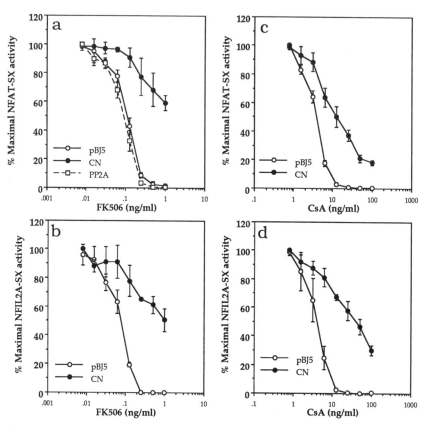

FIGURE 2. Overexpression of murine calcineurin renders TAg Jurkat cells more resistant to CsA and FK506. TAg Jurkat cells were cotransfected either with NFAT-SX (a and c) or NFIL2A-SX (b and d) together with either pBJ5-CNA and pBJ5-CNB (filled circles), pBJ5 alone (open circles), or pBJ5-PP2A (open squares). Transfected cells were stimulated with ionomycin and PMA in the presence of various concentrations of FK506 (a and b) or CsA (c and d) and assayed for secreted alkaline phosphatase activity. The results are expressed as percent of maximal reporter gene activity and represent the mean of values determined from three independent transfections. Error bars represent standard deviations. The data are representative of at least four independent experiments.

In order to distinguish between these two possibilities, it was important to establish the role, if any, of calcineurin in the T cell signal transduction cascade. To this end, the effect of calcineurin overexpression on the signaling requirements for NFAT- and NFIL2A-dependent transcription in transfected TAg Jurkat cells was examined. Optimal expression of both NFAT- and NFIL2A-dependent transcription requires two stimuli,[9] namely, phorbol ester and calcium ionophore, which activate protein kinase C and increase the concentration of intracellular calcium respectively. As calcineurin is a calcium-regulated phosphatase[26,27] and could, therefore, in part, mediate the effects of the calcium signal during T cell activation, we attempted to establish whether overexpression of calcineurin could affect the requirement for an increase in intracellular calcium. Thus, TAg Jurkat cells were cotransfected with pBJ5-CNA and pBJ5-CNB or as a control pBJ5 alone, together with either NFAT-SX or NFIL2A-SX, then stimulated with a constant concentration of the phorbol ester PMA (10 ng ml^{-1}) and various concentrations of the calcium ionophore ionomycin. As shown in FIGURE 3, transfection of pBJ5-CNA and pBJ5-CNB was found to result in a significant shift in the ionomycin dose-response curves for both NFAT-SX (FIGURE 3a, filled circles) and NFIL2A-SX (FIGURE 3b, filled circles) compared to control cells transfected with pBJ5 alone (FIGURE 3a and b, open circles), indicating that overexpression of murine calcineurin augments both NFAT- and NFIL2A-dependent transcription in response to elevated intracellular calcium levels. Note that high levels of ionomycin actually inhibit reporter gene activity. This effect was

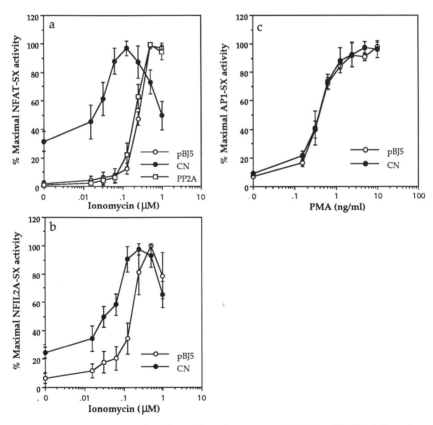

FIGURE 3. Overexpression of murine calcineurin augments NFAT- and NFIL2A-dependent transcription. TAg Jurkat cells were cotransfected with either NFAT-SX (a), NFIL2A-SX (b), or AP1-SX (c) together with either pBJ5-CNA and pBJ5-CNB (filled circles), pBJ5 alone (open circles), or pBJ5-PP2A (open squares). Transfected cells stimulated either with a constant concentration of PMA and various concentrations of ionomycin (a and b) or various concentrations of PMA (c) were assayed for secreted alkaline phosphatase activity. The results are expressed as percent of maximal reporter gene activity and represent the mean of values determined from three independent transfections. Error bars represent standard deviations. The data are representative of at least four independent experiments.

also augmented by overexpression of calcineurin and may reflect the deleterious consequences for the T cell of a supraoptimal Ca^{2+} signal. Importantly, significant reporter gene activity was detected in calcineurin tranfected cells at suboptimal concentrations of ionomycin that elicited little or no activity in control cells. Moreover, in the absence of ionomycin, transfected murine calcineurin can synergize with PMA to stimulate $\sim 30\%$ of maximal NFAT-SX and NFIL2A-SX activity. This apparent Ca^{2+}/calmodulin-independent effect of calcineurin is probably a direct consequence of overexpression of the CN-A and CN-B subunits, which together exhibit significant *in vitro* phosphatase activity in the absence of calmodulin.[38] The specificity of the effect of calcineurin was confirmed by two independent observations. First, expression of the human PP2A gene had no effect on the ionomycin dose-response curve for NFAT-SX (FIGURE 3a, open squares), and second, overexpression of calcineurin did not affect the PMA inducibility of the CsA/FK506-insensitive AP-1 reporter gene (FIGURE 3c). Thus, these results establish a previously uncharacterized role for calcineurin in T cell signal transduction events leading to IL 2 gene expression and therefore provide strong evidence supporting the simple loss of function model outlined in FIGURE 1a.

A Calcium-Independent Constitutively Active Calcineurin Mutant Can Synergize with Phorbol Ester to Activate NFAT and NFIL2A Promoter Activity

Previous studies using limited proteolysis to map functional domains in calcineurin led to the identification of a proteolyzed form of calcineurin that lacked the calmodulin binding and the C-terminal autoinhibitory domains and that exhibited Ca^{2+}-independent constitutively active phosphatase activity.[39] Using PCR, we introduced a premature stop codon into the wild-type CNAα1 cDNA at codon 397, in order to generate a calcineurin mutant (CNMUT2B) with these properties.

This mutant calcineurin was used to further probe the role of calcineurin in Ca^{2+}-dependent signaling events in T cell activation. Transfection of pBJ5-CNMUT2B into TAg Jurkat cells was able to synergize with PMA and replace the normal requirement for ionomycin in the activation of NFAT-dependent transcription (FIGURE 4a). Similar results were observed when the effects of CNMUT2B expression on NFIL2A promoter activity were measured (FIGURE 4b). Thus, a constitutively active calcineurin can synergize with PMA-derived signals to replace the normal requirement for an increase in intracellular calcium in the activation of at least two transcription factor complexes involved in IL-2 gene expression.

DISCUSSION

Collectively, the data presented here identify calcineurin as a key rate-limiting enzyme in the T cell signal transduction cascade and provide biological evidence to support the notion that the interaction of drug-isomerase complexes with calcineurin underlies the molecular basis of CsA and FK506 action.

We have shown that overexpression of murine calcineurin renders transfected cells markedly resistant to the inhibitory effects of the immunosuppressive drugs CsA and FK506. *A priori,* these findings suggest that one of the primary determinants of cellular sensitivity to these immunosuppressive drugs is likely to be the intracellular concentration of calcineurin. In this respect, T lymphocytes are known to express low levels of calcineurin,[28,40] which may, in part, explain the exquisite sensitivity of this cell lineage to CsA and FK506. Although other factors such as both the concentration and availability of immunophillins and the central, apparently nonredundant, role of calcineurin in T cell activation are also likely to be important determinants.

Furthermore, we have demonstrated that overexpression of wild-type calcineurin can enhance both NFAT- and NFIL2A-dependent transcription and that a Ca^{2+}-independent constitutively active calcineurin mutant can synergize with PMA-mediated signals to replace the normal requirement for an increase in intracellular calcium in the activation of NFAT and NFIL2A promoter activity. These data identify calcineurin as an important downstream effector of the calcium signal in T cell activation and provide direct evidence linking calcineurin to the activation of at least two transcription factor complexes that play essential roles in IL-2 gene expression[36] and possibly the expression of other lymphokine genes.[14] This establishes calcineurin as a nodal point in the transduction of signals from the early

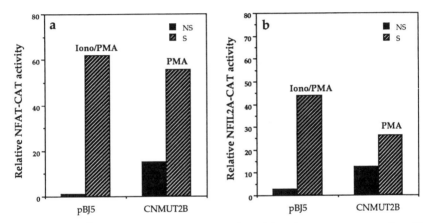

FIGURE 4. A Ca^{2+}-independent constitutively active calcineurin mutant can synergize with PMA to replace ionomycin in the activation of NFAT and NFIL2A promoter activity. TAg Jurkat cells were cotransfected with either pBJ5 or pBJ5-CNMUT2B together with NFAT-CAT (a) or NFIL2A-CAT (b). Transfected cells were either left nonstimulated (NS) or were stimulated (S) with the indicated agents and assayed for chloramphenicol acetyltransferase activity. Results are the mean of duplicate transfections and are representative of at least three independent experiments.

biochemical events that occur at the T cell membrane to gene regulatory events in the nucleus (FIGURE 5), and thereby provides a further explanation for the profound effects of CsA and FK506 on T cell activation.

How does calcineurin regulate the activity of NF-AT and NF-IL2A? NFAT is comprised of at least two components, a preexisting T-cell-specific cytosolic component and an inducible, ubiquitously expressed nuclear component.[15] This latter nuclear component is transcriptionally induced by PMA and is likely to represent members of the AP1 family of proteins.[29,41] The NFAT cytosolic component is translocated to the nucleus in response to an increase in intracellular calcium, whereupon it interacts with the nuclear component and binds to its cognate DNA binding site.[15] It is this calcium-dependent nuclear translocation event that is inhibited by CsA and FK506.[15] Thus, it is possible that calcineurin could potentially directly regulate nuclear translocation via dephosphorylation of the NF-AT cytoplasmic component. In this regard, the yeast transcription factor SW15 represents a well characterized precedent, since its cell-cycle-dependent nuclear translocation is regulated by the dephosphorylation of serine residues located within and close to its nuclear localization signal.[42] Alternatively, calcineurin may regulate NF-AT indirectly. Molecular cloning of the cytosolic component of NF-AT and identification of the relevant calcineurin substrates will be necessary to resolve these alternatives.

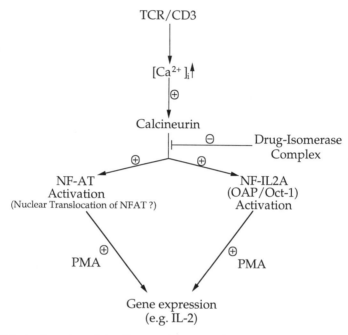

FIGURE 5. A schematic model to illustrate the proposed central role of calcineurin in T cell signal transduction. Note that we do not mean to infer from this model that calcineurin is involved in all Ca^{2+}-dependent transcriptional events in T cells, because the transcription of certain genes, although dependent upon an increase in intracellular calcium, remains insensitive to the effects of CsA and FK506.[9,12]

ACKNOWLEDGMENTS

The authors thank Dr. R. Kincaid for his generous gift of cDNAs encoding the murine CNA and CNB subunits, Dr. R. Bram for plasmids NFAT-SX and NFIL2A-SX, and Dr. J. Northrop for TAg Jurkat cells. Note that some of these results have been previously published.[30] Reprinted here in part with permission from *Nature* copyright 1992 Macmillan Magazines Limited.

REFERENCES

1. KAHAN, B. D. 1989. N. Engl. J. Med. **321:** 1725–1738.
2. THOMPSON, A. W. 1989. Immunol. Today **10:** 6–9.

3. STORB, R., H. J. DEEG, L. FISHER. *et al.* 1988. Blood **71**: 293.
4. KRONKE, M., W. LEONARD, J. DEPPER, S. ARYA, F. WONG-STAAL & R. GALLO. 1984. Proc. Natl. Acad. Sci. USA **81**: 5214–5218.
5. GRANELLI-PIPERNO, A., K. INABA & R. M. STEINMAN. 1986. J. Exp. Med. **163**: 922–937.
6. TOCCI, M. J., D. A. MATKOCICH, K. A. COLLIER, P. KWOK, F. DUMONT, S. LIN, S. KEGUDICIBUS, J. J. SIEKIERKA, J. CHIN & N. I. HUTCHINSON. 1990. J. Immunol. **143**: 718–726.
7. ALTMAN, A., K. M. COGGESHALL & T. MUSTELIN. 1990. Adv. Immunol. **48**: 227–357.
8. CRABTREE, G. R. 1989. Science **243**: 355–361.
9. MATTILA, P. S., K. S. ULLMAN, S. FIERING, M. McCUTCHEON, G. R. CRABTREE & L. A. HERZENBERG. 1990. EMBO J. **9**: 4425–4433.
10. LIN, C. S., R. C. BOLTZ, J. J. SIEKIERKA & N. H. SIGAL. 1991. Cell. Immunol. **133**: 269–284.
11. KAY, J. E., S. E. A. DOE & C. R. BENZIE. 1989. Cell. Immunol. **124**: 175–181.
12. GUNTER, K. C., S. G. IRVING, P. F. ZIPFEL, U. SIEBENLIST & K. KELLY. 1989. J. Immunol. **142**: 3286–3291.
13. EMMEL, E. A., C. L. VERWEIJ, D. B. DURAND, K. M. HIGGINS, E. LACY & G. R. CRABTREE. 1989. Science **246**: 1617–1620.
14. RANDAK, C., T. BRABLETZ, M. HERGENRÖTHER, I. SOBOTTA & E. SERFLING. 1990. EMBO J. **9**: 2529–2536.
15. FLANAGAN, W. F., B. CORTHESY, R. J. BRAM & G. R. CRABTREE. 1991. Nature **352**: 803–807.
16. BIERER, B. E., P. K. SOMERS, T. J. WANDLESS, S. J. BURAKOFF & S. L. SCHREIBER. 1990. Science **250**: 556–559.
17. DUMONT, F. J., M. R. MELINO, M. J. STARUCH, S. L. KOPRAK, P. A. FISCHER & N. H. SIGAL. 1990. J. Immunol. **144**: 1418–1424.
18. TROPSCHUG, M., I. B. BARTHELMESS & W. NEUPERT. 1989. Nature **342**: 953–955.
19. SCHREIBER, S. L. 1991. Science **251**: 283–287.
20. TAKAHASHI, N., T. HAYANO & M. SUZUKI. 1989. Nature **337**: 473–475.
21. FISCHER, G., B. WITTMANN-LIEBOLD, K. LANG, T. KIEFHABER & F. X. SCHMIDT. 1989. Nature **337**: 476–478.
22. HARDING, M. W., A. GALAT, D. E. UEHLING & S. L. SCHREIBER. 1989. Nature **341**: 758–760.
23. SIEKIERKA, J. J., S. H. Y. HUNG, M. POE, C. S. LIN & N. H. SIGAL. 1989. Nature **341**: 755–757.
24. LIU, J., J. D. FARMER, W. S. LANE, J. FRIEDMAN, I. WEISSMAN & S. L. SCHREIBER. 1991. Cell **66**: 807–815.
25. FRIEDMAN, J. & I. WEISSMAN. 1991. Cell **66**: 799–806.
26. KINCAID, R. 1993. Adv. Second Messenger Posphoprotein Res. **27**: 1–23.
27. KLEE, C. B., G. F. DRAETTA & M. J. HUBBARD. 1988. Calcineurin. *In:* Advances in Ezymology and Related Areas of Molecular Biology. A. Meister, Ed.: 149–209. John Wiley & Sons. New York, N.Y.
28. KINCAID, R. L., P. R. GIRI, S. HIGUCHI, J. TAMURA, S. C. DIXON, C. A. MARIETTA, D. A. AMORESE & B. M. MARTIN. 1990. J. Biol. Chem. **265**: 11312–11319.
29. NORTHROP, J. P., K. S. ULLMAN & G. R. CRABTREE. 1993. J. Biol. Chem. **268**: 2917–2923.
30. CLIPSTONE, N. A. & G. R. CRABTREE. 1992. Nature **357**: 695–697.
31. AUSUBEL, F. M., R. BRENT, R. E. KINGSTON, *et al.,* Eds. 1987. Current Protocols in Molecular Biology. Greene Publishing Associates. New York, N.Y.
32. SWANSON, S. K-H., T. BORN, L. D. ZYDOWSKY, H. CHO, H. Y. CHANG, C. T. WALSH & F. RUSNAK. 1992. Proc. Natl. Acad. Sci. USA **89**: 3741–3745.
33. SHENOLIKAR, S. & A. C. NAIRN. 1991. Adv. Second Messenger Phosphoprotein Res. **23**: 1–121.
34. AGOSTINIS, P., R. DERUA, S. SARNO, J. GORIS & W. MERLEVEDE. 1992. Eur. J. Biochem. **205**: 241–248.
35. UMI, H., M. IMAZU, K. MAETA, H. TSUKAMOTO, K. AZUMZ & M. TAKEDA. 1988. J. Biol. Chem. **263**: 3752–3761.
36. DURAND, D. B., J. P. SHAW, M. R. BUSH, R. E. REPLOGLE, R. BELAGEJE & G. R. CRABTREE. 1988. Mol. Cell. Biol. **8**: 1715–1724.

37. GUERINI, D. & C. B. KLEE. 1989. Proc. Natl. Acad. Sci. USA **86:** 9183–9187.
38. MERAT, D. L., Z. Y. HU, T. E. CARTER & W. Y. CHEUNG. 1985. J. Biol. Chem. **260:** 11053–11059.
39. HUBBARD, M. J. & C. B. KLEE. 1989. Biochemistry **28:** 1868–1874.
40. KINCAID, R. L., H. TAKAYAMA, M. L. BILLINGSLEY & M. V. SITKOVSKY. 1987. Nature **330:** 176–178.
41. JAIN, J., P. G. MCAFFERY, V. E. VALGE-ARCHER & A. RAO. 1992. Nature **356:** 801–804.
42. MOLL, T., G. TEBB, U. SURANA, H. ROBITSCH & K. NASMYTH. 1991. Cell **66:** 743–758.

Rapamycin Inhibits p34^{cdc2} Expression and Arrests T Lymphocyte Proliferation at the G1/S Transition

W. MICHAEL FLANAGAN[a] AND GERALD R. CRABTREE

Howard Hughes Medical Institute
Beckman Center
Stanford University Medical School
Stanford, California 94025

The macrolides FK506 and rapamycin are powerful immunosuppressants that inhibit T cell proliferation.[1] Although structurally related, FK506 and rapamycin inhibit two distinct T cell signaling pathways: T cell activation and T cell proliferation. FK506 blocks T cell activation by interfering with antigen-induced T cell receptor signaling pathways that are Ca^{2+} dependent and result in the production of lymphokines such as interleukin-2 (IL-2), an essential T cell growth factor.[2] In contrast, rapamycin inhibits T cell proliferation by blocking growth factor mediated receptor signal transduction.[3]

The intracelluar receptors for FK506 and rapamycin (called FK binding proteins, FKBP) have been identified and shown to be peptidyl-propyl *cis-trans* isomerases that catalyze the slow *cis-trans* isomerization of proline peptide bonds.[4,5] Binding of the drugs to their intracellular receptor inhibits their enzymatic activity. However, the immunosuppressive effects of the drugs results from the formation of an inhibitory complex and not the inhibition of the isomerase activity. The FK506-FKBP inhibitory complex has been demonstrated to specifically bind to and inhibit calcineurin, a Ca^{2+}-dependent serine/threonine phosphatase.[6,7] Overexpression of calcineurin relieves the immunosuppressive effects of FK506 and results in IL-2 expression.[8,9] The transcription factor NF-AT (nuclear factor of activated T cells), which is essential for expression of IL-2, is a target for FK506 action. NF-AT is formed when a calcium signal emanating from the T cell antigen receptor induces a preexisting cytoplasmic subunit to translocate to the nucleus and combine with a newly synthesized, phorbol ester inducible nuclear subunit of NF-AT. FK506 specifically blocks the translocation of the cytoplasmic component, presumably by preventing its dephosphorylation by calcineurin.[10] The nuclear component of NF-AT has been demonstrated to contain members of the *c-fos* and *c-jun* family,[11,12] while the cytoplasmic component awaits characterization.

In contrast to our understanding of the mechanism of action of FK506, we have only a partial understanding of the immunosuppressive effects of rapamycin. Initially, rapamycin was identified as a potent antifungal agent and was subsequently demonstrated to be an immunosuppressant.[13,14] The remarkable ability of rapamycin to inhibit proliferation in yeast and mammalian cells suggests that rapamycin blocks an evolutionarily conserved mechanism regulating growth.[15] While the target of the rapamycin-FKBP complex has yet to be identified, recent studies have shown that rapamycin inhibits the activation of p70 S6 kinase in IL-2-stimulated T cells and

[a]Current affiliation: Gilead Sciences, 353 Lakeside Drive, Foster City, California 94044.

31

serum-starved fibroblasts.[16-19] However, the importance of p70 S6 kinase in cell cycle progression is unknown.

In T cells, IL-2 stimulates proliferation. The binding of IL-2 to its cognate receptor initiates a phosphorylation cascade that results in the progression of cells into the DNA synthesis or S phase of the cell cycle.[20] During this highly regulated cascade of events, several cyclins and cyclin-dependent kinases are expressed and activated. Cyclins are regulatory subunits of kinases and are the key governors of cell cycle checkpoints.[21,22] Five families of cyclins have been identified to date: cyclins C, D, E, A, and B. As indicated by the name, cyclins are temporally regulated in a cell-cycle-dependent manner. Cyclins C, D, and E are expressed during the G1 phase of the cell cycle.[23] The best characterized cyclins A and B are expressed during S and G2/M phase of the cell cycle, respectively. Cyclin B forms a complex with p34[cdc2], a serine/threonine kinase, to regulate both mitotic entry and exit.[23] Cyclin A also forms a complex with p34[cdc2] during S and G2 phases of the cell cycle. Although p34[cdc2]'s main role in cell cycle progression appears to be the transition of cells through mitosis, several studies suggest that p34[cdc2] may also play an essential role in the G1 → S transition.[24-26]

In this study, we have analyzed the effects of rapamycin on the cell cycle progression of an IL-2-dependent murine T cell line (D10) and demonstrate that rapamycin blocks DNA synthesis or S phase entry of these cells. Futhermore, we report that p34[cdc2] expression is induced in IL-2-stimulated D10 cells, that rapamycin blocks the induced expression of p34[cdc2], and that this block correlates with the failure of these cells to enter S phase of the cell cycle.

MATERIAL AND METHODS

Cells

The IL-2-dependent murine helper T cell clone (D10.G4.1) was a kind gift from DNAX, Palo Alto, California. The cells were grown in RPMI 1640 containing 10% fetal calf serum (FCS), 100 U per ml penicillin, a 100 μg/ml streptomycin, 50 mM B-mercaptoethanol, and IL-2 (DNAX).

Cell Cycle Analysis

Cells were centrifuged and fixed in 70% ethanol. The fixed cells (10^7 cells/ml) were then treated with 1 mg/ml RNase A at 37°C for 30 minutes. The cellular DNA was stained with 20 μg/ml of propidium iodide for 15–30 minutes and analyzed by fluorescence-activated cell sorting.

Antibodies

Antibodies to p34[cdc2] as well as the horseradish peroxidase conjugated rabbit antimouse immunoglobulin G (IgG) were purchased from Zymed Laboratories and used at a 1:1000 dilution. The proteins were examined using chemiluminescent detection (Amersham).

RNA Analysis

Total RNA (10 μg) was isolated from D10 cells at the times indicated following stimulation with IL-2 and hybridized to ^{32}P-labeled antisense murine cdc2 riboprobe (3' Pst fragment bp 700–935) and digested as described.[27]

Immunoblot Analysis

Nuclear extracts were prepared as previously described.[10] Nuclear extracts (10 μg) were fractionated on a 10% sodium dodecyl sulfate-polyacrylamide gel electrophoresis (SDS-PAGE), transferred electrophorectically to Westran (Schleicher and Schuell), and probed with the cdc2 antibody.

RESULTS

To determine when during the cell cycle rapamycin blocked T cell proliferation, we analyzed the DNA content of cells treated with IL-2, IL-2 and FK506 (5 ng/ml), and IL-2 plus rapamycin (5 ng/ml). As shown in TABLE 1, rapamycin dramatically

TABLE 1. Rapamycin Blocks IL-2-Stimulated Progression of Cells into S Phase of the Cell Cycle[a]

	IL-2 Alone	IL-2 + FK506	IL-2 + Rapamycin
Percent G1	64	60	78
Percent S	7.4	5.9	1.7
Percent G2	12.2	11.1	5.1

[a]D10 cells were stimulated with IL-2 in the presence or absence of FK506 (5 ng/ml) or rapamycin (5 ng/ml), stained with propidium iodide, and analyzed for DNA content with a fluorescence-activated cell sorter. Values are given as percent of the total cell population.

decreased the proportion of cells entering S phase of the cell cycle. These results are consistent with previous results that demonstrated that ^{3}H-thymidine incorporation was reduced in T cells treated with rapamycin.[16,17,28] While rapamycin inhibits the percentage of cells entering S phase by approximately threefold, a population of the cells are apparently resistant to rapamycin. One interpretation is that these cells were committed to enter S phase before the addition of rapamycin and, thus, beyond the cell cycle checkpoint at which rapamycin acts.

The transition of cells from G1 into S phase of the cell cycle is tightly regulated. Growth factors, such as IL-2, induce the regulated accumulation of proteins necessary to replicate the genome. Once cells commit to S phase, growth factors can be removed and the cells will continue through mitosis. Several cyclins and cyclin-dependent kinases have been implicated in this transition including p34^{cdc2} kinase.[23] A recent study by Furukawa et al. demonstrated that the inhibition of p34^{cdc2} synthesis by antisense oligonucleotides arrested T cell proliferation at the G1 to S boundary.[24] To examine if p34^{cdc2} may play a role in IL-2-driven transition of T cells from G1 into S phase of the cell cycle, we analyzed the time course of expression of cdc2 RNA and the incorporation of ^{3}H-thymidine into DNA. As shown in FIGURE

1A, expression of cdc2 RNA is induced at 13 hours just prior to the incorporation of
^{3}H-thymidine and the onset of DNA replication. These data suggest that p34^{cdc2} is
initimately involved in the transition of cells into S phase.

To determine whether rapamycin affected p34^{cdc2} expression, D10 cells were
starved of IL-2 for 24 hours and then stimulated with IL-2 in the presence of 5 ng/ml
of rapamycin for 21 hours. Protein and RNA extracts were prepared and analyzed

A.

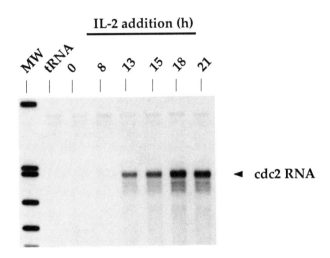

B.

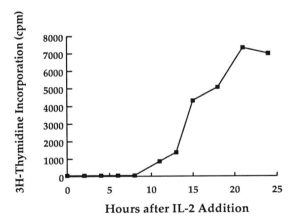

FIGURE 1. IL-2-stimulated induction of cdc2 RNA correlates with the entry into S phase of
the cell cycle. A: Time course of expression of cdc2 RNA following IL-2 stimulation of D10
T-cells. B: Time course of IL-2-induced ^{3}H-thymidine incorporation.

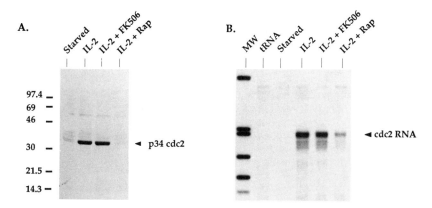

FIGURE 2. Rapamycin inhibits the IL-2-induced expression of p34[cdc2]. A: Immunoblot of p34[cdc2] from IL-2-starved and IL-2-stimulated D10 T cells in the absence or presence of FK506 (5 ng/ml) or rapamycin (5 ng/ml). B: Analysis of cdc2 RNA levels in IL-2-starved and IL-2-stimulated cells with or without addition of FK506 (5 ng/ml) or rapamycin (5 ng/ml).

for cdc2 expression. Rapamycin inhibited the appearance of p34[cdc2] (FIGURE 2A). Moreover, the accumulation of cdc2 RNA was blocked by rapamycin (FIGURE 2B), implying that rapamycin prevents the cell cycle regulated transcriptional induction of p34[cdc2]. FK506, a structural analogue of rapamycin, had no effect on p34[cdc2] expression, suggesting that the mechanism of action of rapamycin is specific. In fact, FK506 at 1000-fold molar excess to rapamycin completely reverses the effects of rapamycin on p34[cdc2] expression,[29] suggesting that rapamycin mediates its effects through FKBP, a common receptor for both FK506 and rapamycin.

DISCUSSION

The progression of mammalian cells through the cell cycle is coordinated by the action of protein kinases and their associated regulators: cyclins. A key component in this regulation is p34[cdc2], a serine/threonine kinase. The activation of the kinase results from the specific formation of the cdc2-cyclin complex, which in turn is regulated by the phosphorylation state of both components of the complex.[23] While the importance of p34[cdc2] in regulating cell proliferation is clear, its precise role during the transition of cells through G1/S is poorly understood.

The mouse cell line FT210, a p34[cdc2] temperature-sensitive mutant, arrests at the G2/M transition when shifted to the nonpermissive temperature.[30] In contrast, studies have demonstrated that the addition of cdc2-cyclin complexes from S phase cells to extracts from G1 cells resulted in the replication of DNA in the G1 extracts.[25] Furthermore, the requirement for cdc2 at the G1/S transition in yeast has been clearly demonstrated through genetic analysis.[26] These studies posit that p34[cdc2] is important in the G1 → S phase transition.

The results presented in this report are consistent with the model supporting a role for p34[cdc2] in the entry of cells into S phase of the cell cycle since p34[cdc2] was induced prior to DNA synthesis and inhibition of p34[cdc2] expression by rapamycin correlates with the T cells arresting at the G1 to S transition. In addition, our results identify expression of p34[cdc2], which is known to be intimately involved in cell cycle progression, as a target of rapamycin.

The retinoblastoma (Rb) protein, a tumor suppressor, has recently been shown to regulate p34[cdc2] expression.[31] The Rb protein is constitutively expressed during the cell cycle and is regulated by its phosphorylation state.[32] In the underphosphorylated state, the Rb protein acts as a tumor suppressor, sequesters E2F—a transcription factor that is necessary for p34[cdc2] expression—and, thus, inhibits p34[cdc2] expression. Upon hyperphosphorylation of the Rb protein, E2F is presumably able to transcribe the cdc2 gene.[33] To date, the kinase responsible for phosphorylating the Rb protein *in vivo* has not been identified, although current models suggest that cyclin E complexed with p33[cdk2] may be the physiologic kinase for Rb. Currently, we are analyzing the effect of rapamycin on the p33[cdk2]–cyclin E complex as well as the phosphorylation state of Rb.

Despite the fact that the targets of rapamycin's mechanism of action appear to be evolutionarily conserved proteins required for cell cycle progression, rapamycin's immunosuppressive effects appear to be specific: T cell proliferation is inhibited, yet fibroblasts continue to divide.[18] This paradox may be explained by the redundancy of growth factor signaling in fibroblasts (platelet-derived growth factor, PDGF; epidermal growth factor, EGF; and insulinlike growth factor, IGF), while IL-2 is not only a competence factor but also a progression factor for T cells.[20] Thus, the reliance of IL-2-dependent cells on a single signaling pathway renders these cells uniquely susceptible to rapamycin.[16]

Finally, it is clear that rapamycin will prove to be a useful tool in dissecting growth factor dependent signaling pathways. Moreover, understanding the molecular basis of the immunosuppressive properties of rapamycin will aid the development of a second generation of less toxic, more potent immunosuppressants.

SUMMARY

Rapamycin, a potent immunosuppressant and antifungal agent, inhibits an evolutionarily conserved mechanism regulating cell cycle progression. In an interluekin-2 (IL-2) dependent murine T cell, we demonstrate that rapamycin arrested T cells prior to the entry into S-phase of the cell cycle and that rapamycin inhibited the IL-2-stimulated expression of p34[cdc2], a serine/threonine kinase that is required for cells to progress through the cell cycle. The mechanism of action of rapamycin appeared specific since the structural analogue and immunosuppressant FK506 had no effect on the progression of the cells through S-phase or the expression of p34[cdc2]. These results demonstrate a rapamycin-sensitive IL-2-dependent signaling pathway in T cells and suggest that the immunosuppressive properties of rapamycin are mediated by impinging on the IL-2-induced T cell expression of p34[cdc2].

REFERENCES

1. SIGAL, N. H. & F. J. DUMONT. 1992. Annu. Rev. Immunol. **10:** 519–560.
2. SCHREIBER, S. L. & G. R. CRABTREE. 1992. Immunology Today **13:** 136.
3. DUMONT, F. J., M. J. STARUCH, S. L. KOPRAK, M. R. MELINO & N. H. SIGAL. 1990. J. Immunol. **251:** 144.
4. SIEKIERKA, J. J., S. H. Y. HUNG, M. POE, C. S. LIN & N. H. SIGAL. 1989. Nature **341:** 755.
5. HARDING, W. M., A. GALAT, D. E. UEHLING & S. L. SCHREIBER. 1989. Nature **341:** 758.
6. LIU, J., J. D. FARMER, W. S. LANE, J. FRIEDMAN, I. WEISSMAN & S. L. SCHREIBER. 1991. Cell **66:** 807–815.

7. FRIEDMAN, J. & I. WEISSMAN. 1991. Cell **66:** 799–806.
8. CLIPSTONE, N. A. & G. R. CRABTREE. 1992. Nature **357:** 695–697.
9. O'KEEFE, S. J., J. TAMURA, R. L. KINCAID, M. J. TOCCI & E. A. O'NEILL. 1992. Nature **357:** 692–694.
10. FLANAGAN, W. M., B. CORTHESY, R. J. BRAM & G. R. CRABTREE. 1991. Nature **352:** 803.
11. JAIN, J., P. G. MCCAFFREY, V. E. VALGE-ARCHER & A. RAO. 1992. Nature **356:** 801–804.
12. NORTHROP, J. P., K. S. ULLMAN & G. R. CRABTREE. 1993. J. Biol. Chem. **268:** 2917–2923.
13. SEGHAL, S. N., H. BAKER & C. VEZINA. 1975. J. Antibiot. **31:** 727–732.
14. MARTEL, R. R., J. KLICIUS & S. GALAT. 1977. Can. J. Physiol. Pharmacol. **55:** 48–51.
15. HEITMAN, J., N. R. MOVVA & M. N. HALL. 1991. Science **253:** 905.
16. KUO, C. J., J. CHUNG, D. F. FIORENTINO, W. M. FLANAGAN, J. BLENIS & G. R. CRABTREE. 1992. Nature **358:** 70.
17. CALVO, V., C. M. CREWS, T. A. VIK & B. E. BIERER. 1992. Proc. Natl. Acad. Sci. USA **89:** 7571.
18. CHUNG, J., C. J. KUO, G. R. CRABTREE & J. BLENIS. 1992. Cell **69:** 1227.
19. PRICE, D. J., J. R. GROVE, V. CALVO, J. AVRUCH & B. E. BRIERER. 1992. Science **257:** 973.
20. CANTRELL, D. A. & K. A. SMITH. 1984. Science **224:** 1312.
21. MURRAY, A. W. & M. W. KIRSCHNER. 1989. Science **246:** 614.
22. EVANS, T., E. T. ROSENTHAL, J. YOUNGBLOM, D. DISTEL & T. HUNT.1983. Cell **33:** 389.
23. CROSS, F., J. M. ROBERTS & H. WEINTRAUB. 1989. Annu. Rev. Cell Biol. **5:** 341.
24. FURUKAWA, Y., H. PIWNICA-WORMS, T. J. ERNST, Y. KANAKURA & J. D. GRIFFIN. 1990. Science **250:** 805.
25. D'URSO, G., R. L. MARRACCINO, D. R. MARSHAK & J. M. ROBERTS. 1991. Science **250:** 786.
26. FORESBURG, S. L. & P. NURSE. 1991. Annu. Rev. Cell Biol. **7:** 227–256.
27. MENDEL, D. B., L. P. HANSEN, M. K. GRAVES, P. B. CONLEY & G. R. CRABTREE. 1991. Genes Dev. **5:** 1042.
28. MORICE, W. G., G. J. BRUNN, G. WIEDERRECHT, J. J. SIEKIERKA & R. T. ABRAHAM. 1993. J. Biol. Chem. **268:** 3734–3738.
29. FLANAGAN, W. M., E. FIRPO, J. M. ROBERTS & G. R. CRABTREE. Submitted.
30. TH'NG, J. P. H., P. S. WRIGHT, J. HAMAGUCHI, M. G. LEE, C. J. NORBURY, P. NURSE & E. M. BRADBURY. 1990. Cell **63:** 313–324.
31. DALTON, S. 1992. EMBO J. **11:** 1797.
32. WEINBERG, R. A. 1991. Science **254:** 1138.
33. NEVINS, J. R. 1992. Science **258:** 424–429.

Proline Isomerases in Microorganisms and Small Eukaryotes[a]

CHARLES HEMENWAY[b] AND JOSEPH HEITMAN[b,c,d]

[b]Departments of Pathology and Pediatrics
[c]Section of Genetics, Department of Pharmacology, and the
Howard Hughes Medical Institute
Box 3546
Duke University Medical Center
Durham, North Carolina 27710

INTRODUCTION

Organ transplantation is an important therapeutic option for human end-stage kidney, liver, and heart disease, and bone marrow transplantation is widely employed to treat genetic and hematologic disorders and to rescue patients following high dose chemotherapy for cancer. Additional treatments employing cell and tissue transplants are likely to become increasingly important. Over the past decade, transplant surgery has been revolutionized by the discovery and implementation of potent immunosuppressants that can prevent rejection of foreign tissues. These compounds are small and diffuse into cells where they bind to small target receptors, the immunophilins.[1,2] These target proteins are highly conserved from bacteria to yeast to vertebrates. Studies of their role has illuminated much that is known about how these drugs act and promise to reveal novel intracellular regulatory signaling pathways.

The immunosuppressants cyclosporin A (CsA), FK506, and rapamycin prevent T-lymphocyte activation by preventing intermediate signal transduction steps required for T-cell activation.[1] CsA and FK506 block T-cell responses to antigen presentation, whereas rapamycin blocks responses to the T-cell growth factor IL-2. With drug affinity chromatography, two distinct families of binding proteins have been identified: cyclophilins bind to CsA, and FK506 binding proteins (FKBPs) bind the related macrolides FK506 and rapamycin.[3] Although these two protein families share no primary or tertiary sequence homology, both types of proteins are enzymes that catalyze an unusual reaction, *cis-trans* peptidyl-prolyl isomerization, that can be the rate-limiting step during protein folding.[4] Because drug binding inhibits this enzymatic activity, early models suggested that T-cell signal transduction pathway components required peptidyl-prolyl isomerization for function. This simple model has now been excluded by several observations. For example, analogues of CsA and the macrolides are known that potently inhibit proline isomerization *in vitro* but are not immunosuppressive *in vivo*. An alternative model, that immunophilin-drug complexes bind to and inhibit the activity of other proteins required for cell function, has now been confirmed by biochemical[5] and genetic results.[6–8] For example, the cyclophilin-CsA and FKBP-FK506 complexes directly bind and inhibit the activity of a serine-threonine specific protein phosphatase, calcineurin,[5] which participates in a critical rate-limiting step in T-cell response to antigen[9,10] by regulating the nuclear

[a]C. Hemenway is supported by the Toxicology Program and NIEHS grant no. NRSA ES07031. J. Heitman is an Assistant Investigator of the Howard Hughes Medical Institute.
[d]Author to whom correspondence should be addressed.

38

import of one subunit of the NF-AT transcription factor.[11,12] In contrast, the FKBP-rapamycin complex does not block the antigen response pathway or inhibit calcineurin. Instead, rapamycin prevents T-cell response to IL-2. Although rapamycin indirectly inhibits the activation of S6 kinase,[13,14] the role of S6 kinase, if any, is controversial and the direct target of the FKBP-rapamycin complex has not yet been identified.

Our approach has been to work with microorganisms in which we can use genetics to dissect immunosuppressant action and immunophilin functions. We have concentrated our efforts on the yeast *Saccharomyces cerevisiae* and have (1) cloned the yeast homologue of the human FKBP12 immunophilin,[15] (2) shown that mutants lacking four proline isomerases (FKBP12, and cyclophilins CPR1, CPR2, and CPR3) are viable,[16] (3) found that FK506 toxicity in yeast results from inhibition of amino acid transport, possibly by poisoning an FKBP required to fold amino acid transporters,[55] and (4) demonstrated that FKBP12 and the TOR1 and TOR2 proteins are required for rapamycin sensitivity and may regulate G1 to S phase cell cycle progression in yeast and possibly also in T-cells.[7] Further studies should shed light on cellular functions of immunophilins and the molecular mechanisms of T-cell activation.

PROLINE ISOMERASES IN PROKARYOTES

Despite their ubiquity in virtually all eukaryotes, the nature and distribution of immunophilins in prokaryotes are less clear. However, within the last several years, the cloning of prokaryotic virulence factors as well as the analysis of bacterial unidentified open reading frames has demonstrated significant homology to both FKBPs and cyclophilins. This unexpected and intriguing finding has stimulated speculation about the relationship of the known properties of eukaryotic FKBPs to the physiology and pathobiology of several important bacterial species.

The identification of proline isomerases in prokaryotes begins with *Escherichia coli,* which expresses two cyclophilins, one in the periplasm and a second in the cytoplasm.[17–19] Both exhibit proline isomerase activity and share significant homology with mammalian cyclophilins, but both are relatively insensitive to inhibition by CsA. *E. coli* cyclophilin a (the periplasmic form) contains a phenylalanine substituted for a tryptophan residue invariant in the mammalian cyclophilins. Substitution of this residue by tryptophan significantly increases sensitivity of the *E. coli* enzyme to CsA, and correspondingly, introduction of a phenylalanine at this position in human cyclophilin A renders the enzyme 75-fold less CsA sensitive.[19] That *E. coli* cyclophilins are present in both the cytoplasm and periplasm would be consistent with a role in protein folding and refolding following translocation, but this has not yet been explicitly tested.

As a part of their extensive studies on the pathogenesis of *Legionella pneumophila,*[20] Engleberg, Cianciotto, and coworkers identified a unique 24-kDa cell surface protein. Mutational studies indicated that this protein was important in the early stages of infection of human macrophages at some point after bacterial attachment to the macrophage membrane. The encoding gene was consequently designated *mip* or *m*acrophage *i*nfectivity *p*otentiator.[21] Infection of macrophages by *Legionella* is known to result in an inhibition of normal phagocytic formation, including the oxidative burst and phagosome-lysosome fusion.[20,22] Because the Mip protein is polycationic, initial hypotheses concerning the enhanced virulence associated with the protein focused on the inhibition of phagosome-lysosome fusion.[21,23] But further analysis of the *mip* gene sequence showed the predicted 120 carboxy terminal residues to be highly homologous to *Neurospora crassa* and human FKBP.[24] The possibility that the Mip protein might exhibit peptidyl-prolyl isomerase activity and that catalysis of changes in host protein folding might be important in pathogenesis was immediately noted. Studies by Fischer and associates[25] were undertaken to explore *cis/trans* prolyl isomerization of synthetic oligopeptides by the *Legionella* Mip protein. Catalytic activity was, in fact, demonstrated with a K_{cat}/K_m similar to that found for eukaryotic FKBPs, and activity was inhibited by FK506. Hence there is now good evidence that the Mip protein exhibits both sequence homology and basic enzymatic properties of the immunophilin FKBP.

In addition, characterization of a 27-kDa cell surface protein from *Chlamydia trachomatis* and hypothetical proteins encoded by cloned, unidentified open reading frames from *Neisseria meningitidis* and *Pseudomonas aeruginosa* have shown homology to both the *L. pneumophila* Mip protein and to eukaryotic FKBPs.[24,26,27] The cloned sequence of *N. meningitidis* has since been expressed and purified (as a fusion protein with maltose binding protein) and has also been shown to possess FK506 inhibitable *cis/trans* proline isomerase activity.[28]

While prokaryotic immunophilins have now been recognized, their functional significance, like those of eukaryotes, is still poorly understood. Perhaps most provocative are hypotheses concerning the *Legionella* virulence factor, the Mip protein, and the related cell surface protein of *Chlamydia*. Both organisms are intracellular pathogens whose life cycle is dependent upon evasion of cellular defense mechanisms. Although evidence is only suggestive at this point, inhibition of phagosome-lysosome fusion may be an important functional property of the Mip protein. In this regard, the modification of protein structure by catalysis of peptidyl-prolyl *cis/trans* isomerization could play a significant role.[25] Of potential significance to hypotheses attempting to explain the function of these bacterial proteins, there is now emerging evidence that in addition to cytoplasmic immunophilins, both secreted and cell surface immunophilins may be important in mediating some components of the immune response in mammals. Murine macrophages stimulated by bacterial endotoxin secrete an 18-kDa protein now designated sp18. The protein has proinflammatory/chemotactic properties both *in vitro* and *in vivo*. Interestingly, it also has N-terminal sequence homology to the cyclosporin binding protein cyclophilin. Importantly, these proinflammatory effects are inhibited by cyclosporin A but not by cyclosporin H.[29] This suggests that peptidyl/prolyl *cis-trans* isomerization is not essential for activity, as both compounds are isomerase inhibitors but only cyclosporin A has recognized immunosuppressive effects. A mammalian cell surface protein with an extracellular domain showing sequence homology to cyclophilin has also recently been identified. This 150-kDa protein is found on the surface of natural killer cells and may be important in the target recognition process.[30] As these extracellular proteins appear to be important in some of the signaling pathways of the mammalian immune response, bacterial immunophilins may be able to alter cellular signaling pathways within the host to blunt a bacteriacidal response. Even more speculative is the role of the FKBP-like proteins of *P. aeruginosa* and *N. meningitidis* as they have not yet been characterized beyond DNA sequence analysis. Nevertheless, further research in the field of prokaryotic immunophilins, especially as virulence factors, may prove to be useful in elucidating their functions in eukaryotes.

PROLINE ISOMERASES IN YEASTS

The yeast *S. cerevisiae* is known to express at least four cyclophilins: CPR1 is cytoplasmic and analogous to mammalian cyclophilin A,[31] CPR2 and CPR4 have secretory signal sequences and at least CPR2 is membrane associated, possibly within the lumen of the endoplasmic reticulum (ER),[32–34] and CPR3 is presumed to be mitochondrial, based on the presence of an N-terminal mitochondrial signal sequence and the phenotype of *cpr3* mutant strains.[16] At present, two FKBPs have been described: FKBP12 is cytosolic,[15,27,35] and FKBP13[36,37] is in the ER. At least one additional FK506-sensitive FKBP is presumed to exist in yeast, because yeast strains missing FKBP12 and FKBP13 retain partial sensitivity to FK506 growth inhibition.[15,55] Mutants lacking one or more (up to four proline isomerases) are viable, hence either enzymatic proline isomerization is not essential for viability or additional proteins substitute for the missing ones.[16] Some proline isomerase mutations do confer phenotypes: strains missing FKBP12 grow slower than isogenic wild-type strains,[15] and *cpr3* mutant strains lacking the presumptive mitochondrial cyclophilin are unable to utilize lactate as a carbon source at 37°C, which requires the mitochondrial enzyme cytochrome B2.[16] Nonetheless, these subtle phenotypes do not yet satisfactorily explain the multiplicity, abundance, ubiquity, and high degree of conservation of the proline isomerases. In this respect, the proline isomerases are reminiscent of heat shock proteins, and the recent finding that FKBP59 is the 59-kDa heat shock protein HSP59 suggests this similarity may not be coincidental.[38–40]

Appropriate yeast strains are sensitive to growth inhibition by the immunosuppressants CsA, FK506, and rapamycin. Only a few strains are sensitive to CsA (this is thought to reflect a permeability barrier) and even then only at doses beyond those used clinically (100 μg/ml).[6] CsA-resistant mutants have been described that either fail to express cyclophilin CPR1 or may express mutant forms with decreased affinity for CsA.[6] However, a detailed genetic analysis of such mutants is lacking.

A number of yeast strains are known to be FK506 sensitive.[15,41] In our strain background, diploid strains are inherently more FK506 sensitive compared to isogenic haploid strains. In addition, a number of amino acid auxotrophic mutations contribute significantly to FK506 sensitivity, and we have recently shown that FK506 impairs amino acid import in yeast cells, possibly by inhibiting an FKBP required for folding amino acid transporters.[55] The relevant FK506-sensitive FKBP for FK506 toxicity is neither FKBP12 (cytoplasmic) nor FKBP13 (ER) and remains to be identified.[55]

The target for cyclophilin-CsA and FKBP-FK506 action in T-cells is calcineurin, which is also conserved in yeast,[42–47] where it may play a role in responding to rises in intracellular calcium during pheromone response.[48] Yeast cells initially respond to pheromone by arresting in the G1 stage of the cell cycle in preparation for mating. Cells that respond but fail to find a mating partner eventually recover and reenter the cell cycle. Calcineurin is required for this recovery from mating pheromone arrest. Relatively low doses of cyclosporin A (1–10 μg/ml) also inhibit recovery from pheromone arrest, and cyclophilin CPR1 is required for this effect, suggesting that a cyclophilin-CsA complex also inhibits calcineurin in yeast.[8] FK506, in an FKBP12-dependent manner, has a similar effect, again at concentrations (0.1–1 μg/ml) significantly lower than those required to observe cell toxicity in yeast. These observations suggest that at low doses, CsA and FK506 inhibit calcineurin activity in yeast. This is unlikely to account for CsA or FK506 toxicity in yeast because calcineurin is not essential for viability. A further distinction is that CsA toxicity in yeast is thought to require cyclophilin CPR1, which is also the relevant cyclophilin for calcineurin inhibition. In contrast, an FKBP in addition to FKBP12 and FKBP13 is required for FK506 toxicity. Current models for CsA and FK506 toxicity in yeast envision that a cyclophilin-CsA complex may inhibit another protein in yeast (not calcineurin) and that FK506 interacts with an as yet unidentified FKBP and blocks growth, either by inhibiting proline isomerase activity of this FKBP or by forming a drug-protein complex that is toxic to an essential protein.

In contrast to FK506, the related macrolide rapamycin forms a complex with FKBP but does not inhibit T-cell response to antigen. Instead the FKBP-rapamycin complex interferes with T-cell response to IL-2. We therefore tested whether FK506 and rapamycin have different effects in yeast cells. Rapamycin is exceedingly toxic to yeast cells with a minimum inhibitory concentration of 50 to 100 ng/ml. Yeast strains missing FKBP12 are completely resistant to the toxic effects of rapamycin.[7,35] Because FKBP12 is required for rapamycin toxicity but not for cell viability, the toxic effects of rapamycin cannot be attributed to inhibition of FKBP12 proline isomerase activity because if this were the case, an FKBP12 disruption mutation should have the same effect as the presence of the drug. Both the protein and the drug must be present for the toxic effect, providing strong support for the toxic complex model of immunophilin immunosuppressant action. Thus rapamycin acts in a very similar way in yeast and in T-cells; the drug interacts with an abundant conserved protein in both cell types and forms a complex toxic to some other cellular component. We think that this rapamycin target is likely to be conserved between yeast and multicellular eukaryotes because rapamycin causes a specific stage-specific arrest in the cell cycle in both T-cells and in yeast at the G1 to S border.[7]

We have identified two additional proteins that participate in rapamycin action, TOR1 and TOR2.[7] Mutations in either of these genes confer rapamycin resistance. Genetic crosses between FKBP12, TOR1, and TOR2 mutants reveal a phenomenon known as nonallelic noncomplementation, which suggests the protein products interact, either physically or functionally. Based on the rapamycin-inflicted cell cycle arrest in both yeast and in T-cells, we suggest that FKBP12, TOR1, and TOR2 participate in a pathway that regulates cell cycle progression in response to growth-promoting cues, either IL-2 for T-cells and perhaps nutrients for yeast cells.

PROLINE ISOMERASES IN *DROSOPHILA*

Genetic studies in *Drosophila melanogaster* first identified the *ninaA* mutation, which impairs electrophysiological aspects of visual phototransduction, giving rise to the name *neither inactivation nor after potential*.[49] Simplistically one can consider the flies blind. *ninaA* mutant flies have reduced levels of rhodopsin, and the defect in expression is posttranslational. The *ninaA* gene encodes a cyclophilin homologue with unusual features, an *N*-terminal signal sequence and a C-terminal hydrophobic membrane domain, and tissue distribution restricted to photoreceptor cells of the eye.[50,51] In *ninaA* mutants, rhodopsin isoforms 1 and 2 fail to properly transit the secretory pathway and form aggregates and lead to a proliferation of the ER.[52] In contrast, isoforms 3 and 4 are *ninaA*-independent. The distinguishing feature is proline residues conserved between *ninaA*-dependent isoforms that are not found in *ninaA*-independent rhodopsins. Current models suggest ninaA is a proline isomerase required to fold some members of the rhodopsin family of integral membrane proteins during transit through the secretory pathway. Notably, ninaA homologues are present in vertebrates.[53]

Recently, 70 new *ninaA* alleles have been isolated from 700,000 EMS mutagenized fly lines that were screened for mutations unable to complement a *ninaA* null allele.[54] *ninaA* mutations diminish rhodopsin levels altering the structure of the ommatidia in the eye, which can be observed by shining a light on the fly eye and detecting loss of a light reflection referred to as the deep pseudopupil. Two interesting types of alleles have emerged. First, two alleles exhibit temperature-sensitive ninaA activity *in vivo,* and when the corresponding amino acid substitutions were engineered into rat cyclophilin A, the resulting protein exhibits temperature-sensitive proline isomerase activity, providing evidence that ninaA may function *in vivo* to isomerize one or more peptidyl-prolyl bonds in rhodopsins. A second subset of these *ninaA* alleles contain substitutions within the membrane spanning hydrophobic anchor of ninaA. Because several of these substitutions do not alter the overall hydrophobicity of the anchor, and would therefore not be predicted to disrupt membrane association, this hydrophobic stretch may serve some function beyond simply tethering ninaA to the membrane. One possibility is that one or more transmembrane domains of rhodopsin interact with the ninaA transmembrane domain during rhodopsin biogenesis. Further study of the *Drosophila* cyclophilin homologue ninaA should continue to further our understanding of the normal *in vivo* functions of proline isomerases.

IMPLICATIONS FOR THE ROLE OF PROLINE ISOMERASES IN PROTEIN FOLDING AND IMMUNOSUPPRESSION

We now know a great deal about the role of the immunophilins in immunosuppressant action. We know that CsA binds to cyclophilins and FK506 and rapamycin to FKBPs, that drug binding blocks proline isomerase activity but that this is not required for immunosuppression: rather immunophilin-drug complexes target additional cellular proteins. We know that calcineurin is the target for cyclophilin-CsA and FKBP-FK506 and that calcineurin plays a critical role in regulating T-cell activation by responding to increases in intracellular calcium and then possibly dephosphorylating and driving nuclear import of the T-cell-specific transcription factor NF-AT. We now know two reasons why these drugs can interact with non-T-cell-specific proteins to mediate selective effects on T-cells. First, because T-cells have relatively low levels of calcineurin compared to other tissues, lower amounts of CsA and FK506 suffice to inhibit calcineurin-dependent T-cell functions without blocking calcineurin function in other cell types. Second, the calcineurin-dependent T-cell component NF-AT is T-cell specific. In contrast, our understanding of FKBP-rapamycin action is less well defined but promises to reveal much about how cells grow in response to external signals.

In comparison, we know much less about the normal cellular functions of the proline isomerases. One is almost certain to play a fundamental basic role required of all cells involving protein folding and trafficking. In addition, proline isomerases may play more specific regulatory roles. For example, FKBPs and cyclophilins could serve to present endogenous ligands, which the immunosuppressants emulate, to regulate the functions of other proteins, such as calcineurin. Such models make the testable prediction that cyclophilin and FKBP would normally interact with and modulate the function of proteins such as calcineurin.

ACKNOWLEDGMENTS

We thank Bonnie Kissell for patient and conscientious preparation of the manuscript.

REFERENCES

1. HEITMAN, J., N. R. MOVVA & M. N. HALL. 1992. Proline isomerases at the crossroads of protein folding, signal transduction, and immunosuppression. New Biologist **4:** 448–460.

2. SCHREIBER, S. L. 1992. Immunophilin-sensitive protein phosphatase action in cell signaling pathways. Cell **70:** 365–368.
3. SCHREIBER, S. L. 1991. Chemistry and biology of the immunophilins and their immunosuppressive ligands. Science **251:** 283–287.
4. GETHING, M.-J. & J. SAMBROOK. 1992. Protein folding in the cell. Nature **355:** 33–45.
5. LIU, J., J. D. FARMER, W. S. LANE, J. FRIEDMAN, I. WEISSMAN & S. L. SCHREIBER. 1991. Calcineurin is a common target of cyclophilin-cyclosporin A and FKBP-FK506 complexes. Cell **66:** 807–815.
6. TROPSCHUG, M., I. B. BARTHELMESS & W. NEUPERT. 1989. Sensitivity to cyclosporin A is mediated by cyclophilin in *Neurospora crassa* and *Saccharomyces cerevisiae.* Nature **342:** 953–955.
7. HEITMAN, J., N. R. MOVVA & M. N. HALL. 1991. Targets for cell cycle arrest by the immunosuppressant rapamycin in yeast. Science **253:** 905–909.
8. FOOR, F., S. A. PARENT, N. MORIN, A. M. DAHL, N. RAMADAN, G. CHREBET, K. A. BOSTIAN & J. B. NIELSEN. 1992. Calcineurin mediates inhibition by FK506 and cyclosporin of recovery from α-factor arrest in yeast. Nature **360:** 682–684.
9. O'KEEFE, S. J., J. TAMURA, R. L. KINCAID, M. J. TOCCI & E. A. O'NEILL. 1992. FK-506- and CsA-sensitive activation of the interleukin-2 promoter by calcineurin. Nature **357:** 692–694.
10. CLIPSTONE, N. A. & G. R. CRABTREE. 1992. Identification of calcineurin as a key signalling enzyme in T-lymphocyte activation. Nature **357:** 695–697.
11. FLANAGAN, W. M., B. CORTHÉSY, R. J. BRAM & G. R. CRABTREE. 1991. Nuclear association of a T-cell transcription factor blocked by FK-506 and cyclosporin A, Nature **352:** 803–807.
12. MCCAFFREY, P. G., B. A. PERRINO, T. R. SODERLING & A. RAO. 1993. NF-AT$_p$, a T lymphocyte DNA-binding protein that is a target for calcineurin and immunosuppressive drugs. J. Biol. Chem. **268:** 3747–3752.
13. KUO, C. J., J. CHUNG, D. F. FIORENTINO, W. M. FLANAGAN, J. BLENIS & G. R. CRABTREE. 1992. Rapamycin selectively inhibits interleukin-2 activation of p70 S6 kinase. Nature **358:** 70–73.
14. CALVO, V., C. M. CREWS, T. A. VIK & B. E. BIERER. 1992. Interleukin 2 stimulation of p70 S6 kinase activity is inhibited by the immunosuppressant rapamycin. Proc. Natl. Acad. Sci. USA **89:** 7571–7575.
15. HEITMAN, J., N. R. MOVVA, P. C. HIESTAND & M. N. HALL. 1991. FK506-binding protein proline rotamase is a target for the immunosuppressive agent FK506 in *Saccharomyces cerevisiae.* Proc. Natl. Acad. Sci. USA **88:** 1948–1952.
16. DAVIS, E. S., A. BECKER, J. HEITMAN, M. N. HALL & M. B. BRENNAN. 1992. A yeast cyclophilin gene essential for lactate metabolism at high temperature. Proc. Natl. Acad. Sci. USA **89:** 11169–11173.
17. HAYANO, T., N. TAKAHASHI, S. KATO, N. MAKI & M. SUZUKI. 1991. Two distinct forms of peptidylprolyl-*cis-trans*-isomerase are expressed separately in periplasmic and cytoplasmic compartments of *Escherichia coli* cells. Biochemistry **30:** 3041–3048.
18. LIU, J. & C. T. WALSH. 1990. Peptidyl-prolyl *cis-trans*-isomerase from *Escherichia coli:* a periplasmic homolog of cyclophilin that is not inhibited by cyclosporin A. Proc. Natl. Acad. Sci. USA **87:** 4028–4032.
19. LIU, J., C.-M. CHEN & C. T. WALSH. 1991. Human and *Escherichia coli* cyclophilins: sensitivity to inhibition by the immunosuppressant cyclosporin A correlates with a specific tryptophan residue. Biochemistry **30:** 2306–2310.
20. CIANCIOTTO, N., B. I. EISENSTEIN, N. C. ENGLEBERG & H. SHUMAN. 1989. Genetics and molecular pathogenesis of *Legionella pneumophila,* an intracellular parasite of macrophages. Mol. Biol. Med. **6:** 409–424.
21. CIANCIOTTO, N. P., B. I. EISENSTEIN, C. H. MODY, G. B. TOEWS & N. C. ENGLEBERG. 1989. A *Legionella pneumophila* gene encoding a species-specific surface protein potentiates initiation of intracellular infection. Infect. Immun. **57:** 1255–1262.
22. HORWITZ, M. A. 1983. The legionnaires' disease bacterium (*Legionella pneumophila*) inhibits phagosome-lysosome fusion in human monocytes. J. Exp. Med. **158:** 2108–2126.
23. ENGLEBERG, N. C., C. CARTER, D. R. WEBER, N. P. CIANCIOTTO & B. I. EISENSTEIN. 1989.

DNA sequence of *mip,* a *Legionella pneumophila* gene associated with macrophage infectivity. Infect. Immun. **57:** 1263–1270.

24. BANGSBORG, J. M., N. P. CIANCIOTTO & P. HINDERSSON. 1991. Nucleotide sequence analysis of the *Legionella micdadei mip* gene, encoding a 30-kilodalton analog of the *Legionella pneumophila* mip protein. Infect. Immun. **59:** 3836–3840.

25. FISCHER, G., H. BANG, B. LUDWIG, K. MANN & J. HACKER. 1992. Mip protein of *Legionella pneumophila* exhibits peptidyl-prolyl-*cis/trans* isomerase (PPIase) activity. Mol. Microbiol. **6:** 1375–1383.

26. LUNDEMOSE, A. G., S. BIRKELUND, S. J. FEY, P. M. LARSEN & G. CHRISTIANSEN. 1991. *Chlamydia trachomatis* contains a protein similar to the *Legionella pneumophila mip* gene product. Mol. Microbiol. **5:** 109–115.

27. WIEDERRECHT, G., L. BRIZUELA, K. ELLISTON, N. H. SIGAL & J. J. SIEKIERKA. 1991. *FKB1* encodes a nonessential FK506-binding protein in *Saccharomyces cerevisiae* and contains regions suggesting homology to the cyclophilins. Proc. Natl. Acad. Sci. USA **88:** 1029–1033.

28. SAMPSON, B. A. & E. C. GOTSCHLICH. 1992. *Neisseria meningitidis* encodes an FK506-inhibitable rotamase. Proc. Natl. Acad. Sci. USA **89:** 1164–1168.

29. SHERRY, B., N. YARLETT, A. STRUPP & A. CERAMI. 1992. Identification of cyclophilin as a proinflammatory secretory product of lipopolysaccharide-activated macrophages, Proc. Natl. Acad. Sci. USA **89:** 3511–3515.

30. ANDERSON, S. K., S. GALLINGER, J. RODER, J. FREY, H. A. YOUNG & J. R. ORTALDO. 1993. A cyclophilin-related protein involved in the function of natural killer cells. Proc. Natl. Acad. Sci. USA **90:** 542–546.

31. HAENDLER, B., R. KELLER, P. C. HIESTAND, H. P. KOCHER, G. WEGMANN & N. R. MOVVA. 1989. Yeast cyclophilin: isolation and characterization of the protein, cDNA and gene. Gene **83:** 39–46.

32. FRANCO, L., A. JIMÉNEZ, J. DEMOLDER, F. MOLEMANS, W. FIERS & R. CONTRERAS. 1991. The nucleotide sequence of a third cyclophilin-homologous gene from *Saccharomyces cerevisiae.* Yeast **7:** 971–979.

33. KOSER, P. L., D. J. BERGSMA, R. CAFFERKEY, W.-K. ENG, M. M. MCLAUGHLIN, A. FERRARA, C. SILVERMAN, K. KASYAN, M. J. BOSSARD, R. K. JOHNSON, T. G. PORTER, M. A. LEVY & G. P. LIVI. 1991. The *CYP2* gene of *Saccharomyces cerevisiae* encodes a cyclosporin A–sensitive peptidyl-prolyl *cis-trans* isomerase with an N-terminal signal sequence. Gene **108:** 73–80.

34. TANIDA, I., M. YANAGIDA, N. MAKI, S. YAGI, F. NAMIYAMA, T. KOBAYASHI, T. HAYANO, N. TAKAHASHI & M. SUZUKI. 1991. Yeast cyclophilin-related gene encodes a nonessential second peptidyl-prolyl *cis-trans* isomerase associated with the secretory pathway. Transplant. Proc. **23:** 2856–2861.

35. KOLTIN, Y., L. FAUCETTE, D. J. BERGSMA, M. A. LEVY, R. CAFFERKEY, P. L. KOSER, R. K. JOHNSON & G. P. LIVI. 1991. Rapamycin sensitivity in *Saccharomyces cerevisiae* is mediated by a peptidyl-prolyl *cis-trans* isomerase related to human FK506-binding protein. Mol. Cell. Biol. **11:** 1718–1723.

36. NIELSEN, J. B., F. FOOR, J. J. SIEKIERKA, M.-J. HSU, N. RAMADAN, N. MORIN, A. SHAFIEE, A. M. DAHL, L. BRIZUELA, G. CHREBET, K. A. BOSTIAN & S. A. PARENT. 1992. Yeast FKBP-13 is a membrane-associated FK506-binding protein encoded by the nonessential gene *FKB2.* Proc. Natl. Acad. Sci. USA **89:** 7471–7475.

37. PARTALEDIS, J. A., M. A. FLEMING, M. W. HARDING & V. BERLIN. 1992. *Saccharomyces cerevisiae* contains a homolog of human FKBP-13, a membrane-associated FK506/rapamycin binding protein. Yeast **8:** 673–680.

38. YEM, A. W., A. G. TOMASSELLI, R. L. HEINRIKSON, H. ZURCHER-NEELY, V. A. RUFF, R. A. JOHNSON & M. R. DEIBEL, JR. 1992. The Hsp56 component of steroid receptor complexes binds to immobilized FK506 and shows homology to FKBP-12 and FKBP-13. J. Biol. Chem. **267:** 2868–2871.

39. LEBEAU, M.-C., N. MASSOL, J. HERRICK, L. E. FABER, J.-M. RENOIR, C. RADANYI & E.-E. BAULIEU. 1992. P59, an hsp 90-binding protein. J. Biol. Chem. **267:** 4281–4284.

40. TAI, P.-K. K., M. W. ALBERS, H. CHANG, L. E. FABER & S. L. SCHREIBER. 1992. Association of a 59-kilodalton immunophilin with the glucocorticoid receptor complex. Science **256:** 1315–1318.

41. BRIZUELA, L., G. CHREBET, K. A. BOSTIAN & S. A. PARENT. 1991. Antifungal properties of the immunosuppressant FK-506: identification of an FK-506-responsive yeast gene distinct from *FKB1*. Mol. Cell. Biol. **11:** 4616–4626.
42. CYERT, M. S. & J. THORNER. 1992. Regulatory subunit (*CNB1* gene product) of yeast Ca²⁺/calmodulin-dependent phosphoprotein phosphatases is required for adaptation to pheromone. Mol. Cell. Biol. **12:** 3460–3469.
43. CYERT, M. S., R. KUNISAWA, D. KAIM & J. THORNER. 1991. Yeast has homologs (*CNA1* and *CNA2* gene products) of mammalian calcineurin, a calmodulin-regulated phosphoprotein phosphatase. Proc. Natl. Acad. Sci. USA **88:** 7376–7380.
44. YE, R. R. & A. BRETSCHER. 1992. Identification and molecular characterization of the calmodulin-binding subunit gene (*CMP1*) of protein phosphatase 2B from *Saccharomyces cerevisiae*. Eur. J. Biochem. **204:** 713–723.
45. LIU, Y., S. ISHII, M. TOKAI, H. TSUTSUMI, O. OHKI, R. AKADA, K. TANAKA, E. TSUCHIYA, S. FUKUI & T. MIYAKAWA. 1991. The *Saccharomyces cerevisiae* genes (*CMP1* and *CMP2*) encoding calmodulin-binding proteins homologous to the catalytic subunit of mammalian protein phosphatase 2B. Mol. Gen. Genet. **227:** 52–59.
46. KUNO, T., H. TANAKA, H. MUKAI, C.-D. CHANG, K. HIRAGA, T. MIYAKAWA & C. TANAKA. 1991. cDNA cloning of a calcineurin B homolog in *Saccharomyces cerevisiae*. Biochem. Biophys. Res. Commun. **180:** 1159–1163.
47. NAKAMURA, T., H. TSUTSUMI, H. MUKAI, T. KUNO & T. MIYAKAWA. 1992. Ca²⁺/calmodulin-activated protein phosphatase (PP2B) of *Saccharomyces cerevisiae*. FEBS Lett. **309:** 103–106.
48. IIDA, H., Y. YAGAWA & Y. ANRAKU. 1990. Essential role for induced Ca²⁺ influx followed by [Ca²⁺]ᵢ rise in maintaining viability of yeast cells late in the mating pheromone response pathway. J. Biol. Chem. **265:** 13391–13399.
49. LARRIVEE, D. C., S. CONRAD, R. S. STEPHENSON & W. L. PAK. 1981. Mutation that selectively affects rhodopsin concentration in the peripheral photoreceptors of *Drosophila melanogaster*. J. Gen. Physiol. **78:** 521–545.
50. SHIEH, B.-H., M. A. STAMNES, S. SEAVELLO, G. L. HARRIS & C. S. ZUKER. 1989. The *ninaA* gene required for visual transduction in *Drosophila* encodes a homologue of cyclosporin A–binding protein. Nature **338:** 67–70.
51. SCHNEUWLY, S., R. D. SHORTRIDGE, D. C. LARRIVEE, T. ONO, M. OZAKI & W. L. PAK. 1989. *Drosophila ninaA* gene encodes an eye-specific cyclophilin (cyclosporine A binding protein). Proc. Natl. Acad. Sci. USA **86:** 5390–5394.
52. COLLEY, N. J., E. K. BAKER, M. A. STAMNES & C. S. ZUKER. 1991. The cyclophilin homolog ninaA is required in the secretory pathway. Cell **67:** 255–263.
53. STAMNES, M. A., B.-H. SHIEH, L. CHUMAN, G. L. HARRIS & C. S. ZUKER. 1991. The cyclophilin homolog ninaA is a tissue-specific integral membrane protein required for the proper synthesis of a subset of *Drosophila* rhodopsins. Cell **65:** 219–227.
54. ONDEK, B., R. W. HARDY, E. K. BAKER, M. A. STAMNES, B.-H. SHIEH & C. S. ZUKER. 1992. Genetic dissection of cyclophilin function. J. Biol. Chem. **267:** 16460–16466.
55. HEITMAN, J., A. KOLLER, J. KUNZ, R. HENRIQUEZ, A. SCHMIDT, N. R. MOVVA & M. N. HALL. 1993. The immunosuppressant FK506 inhibits amino acid import in *Saccharomyces cerevisiae*. Mol. Cell. Biol. **13:** 5010–5019.

Cyclosporins

Structure-Activity Relationships

HANS FLIRI, GOETZ BAUMANN, ALBERT ENZ,
JUERG KALLEN, MARCEL LUYTEN, VINCENT MIKOL,
RAO MOVVA, VALERIE QUESNIAUX, MAX SCHREIER,
MALCOLM WALKINSHAW, ROLAND WENGER,
GERHARD ZENKE, AND MAURO ZURINI

Sandoz Pharma AG
Preclinical Research Laboratories
CH-4002 Basel, Switzerland

Cyclosporins are a group of hydrophobic cyclic undecapeptides with a remarkable spectrum of diverse biological activities of which immunosuppression is best known (TABLE 1). The first member of the group, cyclosporin A (CS; Sandimmun[R], FIGURE 1) became available for clinical use in 1983 as a key therapeutic agent to suppress rejection of transplanted organs. Since then, the number of registered indications for this drug has steadily increased, including some pending NDA's (TABLE 2).

At the time of market introduction, very little was known about the mechanism of immunosuppressive action. CS differed from other immunosuppressive drugs in several aspects: at clinical doses, it is not cytostatic and it mainly acts on lymphocytes, affecting the myeloid and hematopoietic systems only partly or indirectly. Soon it was recognized that CS affects the activation phase of T cells required for full launch of an immune response. At the molecular level, the transcriptional activation of some early T cell activation genes is blocked[1] (TABLE 3).

Proliferative responses to growth-promoting lymphokines are only affected at much higher concentrations (reviewed by Di Padova).[2] Specific T cell transcription factors involved in activating early genes such as that of IL-2 include AP-1, AP-3, Oct-1, NFkB, and NFAT (reviewed by Schreiber).[3] It could be shown[4,5] that CS affects the function of NFAT by blocking its appearance in isolated nuclei of T cells. Inhibition of NFkB is also observed. This inhibition pattern is shared with the immunosuppressive macrolide FK506. A variety of mechanisms regulating the activity of transcription factors exists. Some transcriptional activators are regulated at the level of translocation from the cytoplasm into the nucleus. This event can be initiated by ligand binding (e.g., steroid/thyroid receptors) or by changes in the phosphorylation status, as has been shown for NFkB.[6] Others, such as NFAT, are active as heterodimers consisting of nuclear and cytoplasmic subunits, the cytoplasmic subunit requiring nuclear translocation to form the active complex.[5] For NFAT, this latter step was recently identified as the CS-sensitive event.[6]

In 1984, on the basis of high-affinity cyclosporin binding, an 18-kDa protein was isolated from bovine spleen and named cyclophilin.[7] Cyclophilin is an abundant (10–30 micromolar levels) cytosolic protein occurring in two isoforms in all tissues.[8] In view of the selective action of CS, this wide tissue distribution of cyclophilin was somehow puzzling. The discovery of cyclosporin analogues of high affinity to cyclophilin yet devoid of immunosuppressive activity (TABLE 4) added to the paradox. A search for additional members of the cyclophilin group led to the discovery of a family of highly conserved genes.[9] Four human proteins have been characterized:

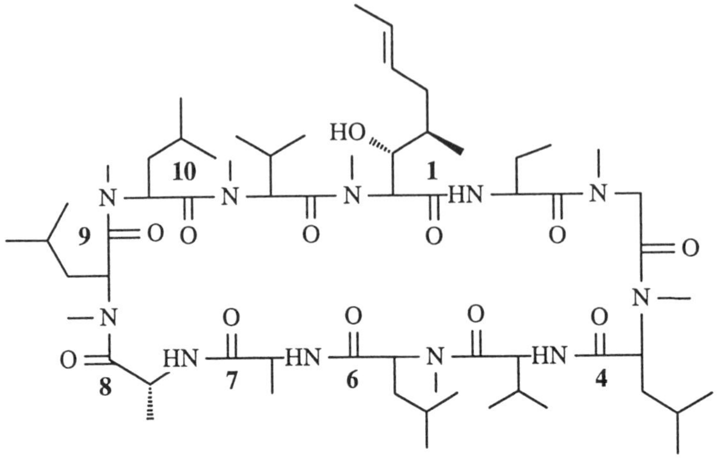

FIGURE 1. Structure of cyclosporin A (Sandimmun^R). Numbering refers to structural modifications discussed in the text.

cyclophilins A, B, C, and D.[10] In addition, cyclophilins have been found in yeast, fungi, and prokaryotic cells (reviewed in Reference 10). The wide tissue distribution, conservation, and organelle targeting of these proteins suggest important cellular functions.

In 1989, two groups investigating enzymes catalyzing protein folding isolated an enzyme from porcine kidney that was shown to be identical to cyclophilin.[11,12] In protein folding *in vitro,* two rate: determining steps are catalyzed by purified cellular enzymes: protein disulfide isomerase catalyzes thiol/disulfide interchange reactions, thereby facilitating formation of the correct set of disulfide bonds. Proteins with peptidyl prolyl *cis-trans* isomerase (PPIase) activity catalyze the otherwise slow interconversion of *cis*-X-Pro bonds to *trans*-X-Pro bonds (FIGURE 2) and can accelerate folding of proline-containing proteins *in vitro* and *in vivo.*[13]

Thus, cyclophilin has enzyme activity as peptidylprolyl isomerase (PPIase), and this PPIase activity was quickly shown to be inhibited by cyclosporin. The discovery of FKBP, the cytosolic binding protein for FK506, and the demonstration that it also possessed PPIase activity susceptible to inhibition by FK506[14–16] seemed to be compelling evidence that immunosuppression by cyclosporin (and FK506) would be the result of enzyme inhibition. However, a number of facts suggest that inhibition of PPIase activity by cyclosporin (and FK506) may not play a key role for immunosuppression, and that it is rather formation of the complex that inhibits T cell activation. This notion rests on the fact that intracellular cyclophilin concentrations are far above the IC_{50} value of cyclosporin (ca. 10–200 nM, depending on assay conditions), suggesting full inhibition of IL-2 transcription when most of cyclophilin is still unliganded and therefore active as PPIase. Secondly, some cyclosporin analogues show high cyclophilin affinity and are potent inhibitors of PPIase, yet are not immunosuppressant (TABLE 4). Finally, in certain strains of yeast cyclophilin, gene disruption results in resistance to cyclosporin.[17] Similar studies with FK506 and rapamycin, another potent immunosuppressive macrolide which binds to FKBP, showed that sensitivity of yeast to the drugs requires the presence of FKBP.[18–20]

TABLE 1. Therapeutic Indications of Cyclosporin A (Sandimmun®)

Allograft rejection	Nephrotic syndrome	Aplastic anemia[a]
Rheumatoid arthritis	Psoriasis	
Behcet's uveitis	Atopic dermatitis[a]	

[a]NDAs pending.

TABLE 2. Biological Activities of Cyclosporins

Antifungal	Immunosuppression	Tumor MDR reversal
Antiparasitic	Antiinflammatory	Antiretroviral
Insecticidal	Antiallergy	Side effects

TABLE 3. Proteins Induced upon T Cell Activation[a]

Protein	Time	Location	CS Sensitivity
c-fos	15 min	Nuclear	+
NFAT	20 min	Nuclear	+
NF$_K$B	30 min	Nuclear	+
INF-τ	30 min	Secreted	+
IL-2	45 min	Secreted	+
IL-2Rα	2 h	Membrane	+
IL-3	1–2 h	Secreted	+
IL-4	>h	Secreted	+
Others			

[a]Modified from Ryffel.[1]

TABLE 4. Cyclophilin A Affinities and Immunosuppressive IC_{50} Values of Selected Representative Cyclosporin Derivatives[a]

Cyclosporin Analogue	Cyclophilin Binding	IC_{50} In IL-2 Reporter
CsA	1	1
Me Ala^6-CS	3	46
Me Val^4-CS	0.5	>2500
Me Val^{10}-CS	120	190

[a]The values given are relative to cyclosporin A. Relative cyclophilin A affinity was measured by ELISA as described;[22] immunosuppressive activity was determined in an IL-2 reporter gene assay.[22]

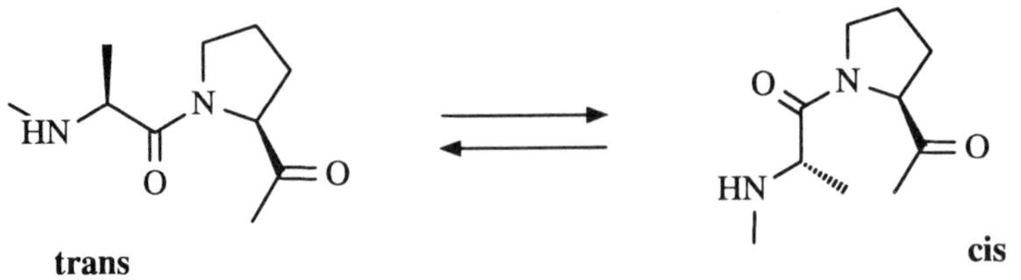

trans   **cis**

FIGURE 2. Interconversion of *cis*-ala-pro and *trans*-ala-pro isomers.

Additional support for the complexes as the toxic principle was provided by showing that FK506 and rapamycin could act as reciprocal antagonists.[21] For cyclosporins, the demonstration that cyclophilin-binding nonimmunosuppressive analogues could indeed act as competitive antagonists was possible only after the development of a highly sensitive reporter gene assay.[22] In the classical proliferation-based test systems, due to nonspecific cytostatic activity observed with all cyclosporins above micromolar concentrations, this was not possible. The inhibition of CS-induced immunosuppression by one such compound, MeVal[4]-cyclosporin, is shown in FIG-URE 3.

With the perspective that the cyclophilin-CS (or FKBP-FK506) complex may be the active species in immunosuppression, a search for proteins binding to the complexes was undertaken which culminated in the isolation of protein phosphatase 2B (calcineurin).[23] Calcineurin is a calmodulin-dependent heterodimeric protein phosphatase with specificity for serine/threonine phosphate groups. It is abundant in neural tissue but also found in lymphocytes. Calcineurin activity is the product of a multigene family.[24,25] We have investigated calcineurin phosphatase inhibition by various cyclophilin-cyclosporin complexes. Using as a substrate the peptide DLD-VPIPGRFDRRVSVAAE, phosphorylated on serine, IC_{50} values of calcineurin inhibition by the complexes of cyclosporin A with cyclophilins A, B, and C, respec-

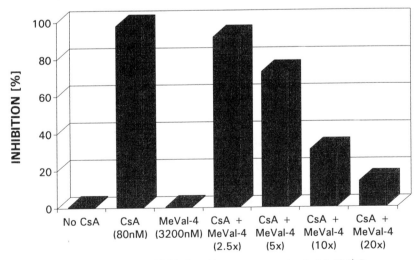

FIGURE 3. Reversal of CS-induced immunosuppression by Me Val[4]-Cs.

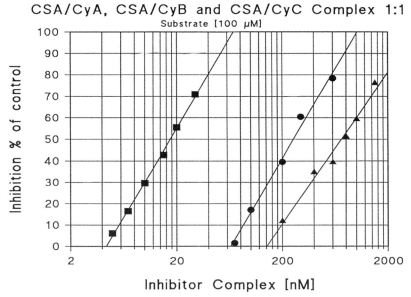

FIGURE 4. Inhibition of calcineurin by CS complexes of cyclophilins A, B, C.

tively, were obtained (FIGURE 4). The IC_{50} values obtained for the cyclophilin A and B complexes are in good agreement with parameters obtained by other groups.[26] This difference in inhibitory activity of the individual complexes could either reflect a different conformation of bound CS in the respective complex or suggest that calcineurin is interacting with both bound drug and adjacent cyclophilin surfaces.

The structure of the cyclosporin complex with cyclophilin A has been determined both by NMR[27,28] and x-ray crystallography.[29] While the crystal structure broadly confirms earlier findings provided by NMR, it also reveals new details. In the crystal, the complex forms a decamer, consisting of two pentamers in a "sandwichlike" association. Cyclosporin binds to cyclophilin with only the side chains of MeBmt[1], Abu[2], MeLeu[9], and MeVal[11] of the cyclosporin molecule making contact with cyclophilin. These residues define the binding site for cyclophilin and are identical to those predicted by the modeled structure.[30] The crystal structure also reveals the presence of a hydrogen bond between the hydroxyl group of MeBmt and the carbonyl oxygen of MeLeu[4]. The side chains of MeLeu[4], MeLeu[6], MeAla[7], MeAla[8], MeLeu[9], and MeLeu[10] make contact to two cyclophilin molecules in the decameric sandwich mediating formation of the oligomer. The fact that the majority of these amino acids are leucines is in line with the known role of leucine side chains in mediating protein-protein interactions. Some of these side chains are also likely to be primarily responsible for mediating the interaction of the cyclophilin-cyclosporin complex with calcineurin. This assumption is supported by the observed structure-activity relationship depicted in TABLE 4.

Cyclosporin, thus, is a "module" that by binding to cyclophilin confers affinity of this protein to the protein phosphatase calcineurin. The immunosuppressive species (the "drug") comprises both molecules, cyclophilin and cyclosporin. The existence of a multitude of cyclophilins and, moreover, of calcineurins likely explains the wide spectrum of biological effects displayed by this group of compounds, but at the same time makes rational attempts to improve on the immunosuppressive potency of cyclosporins or reduce side effects very difficult.

SUMMARY

Cyclosporin A (Sandimmun[R]) achieves immunosuppressive activity by complex formation with cyclophilin and subsequent binding of the binary complex to and inhibiting protein phosphatase 2B (calcineurin). Complexes of nonimmunosuppressive cyclophilin binding cyclosporin analogues do not inhibit protein phosphatase 2B, suggesting a crucial role for this enzyme in T cell activation. Binding of cyclosporin A to cyclophilins A, B, and C, respectively, results in complexes of significantly different inhibitory potency. The cyclosporin molecule thus has two functional domains, one mediating cyclophilin binding and a second one endowing affinity of the complex to calcineurin, thereby inhibiting its enzyme activity. Structure-activity studies and x-ray crystallography of cyclosporin-cyclophilin complexes indicate a crucial role of leucine side chains in positions 4 and 6 of the cyclosporin macrocycle for the calcineurin interaction.

REFERENCES

1. RYFFEL, B. 1989. Pharmacology of cyclosporine VI. Cellular activation: regulation of intracellular events by cyclosporine. Pharmacol. Rev. 41: 407–422.
2. DI PADOVA, F. A. 1989. Pharmacology of cyclosporine (Sandimmune) V. Pharmacological effects on immune function: in vitro studies. Pharmacol. Rev. 41: 373–405.
3. SCHREIBER, S. L. & G. R. CRABTREE. 1992. The mechanism of action of cyclosporin A and FK506. Immunol. Today 13(4): 136–142.
4. EMMEL, E. A., C. L. VERWEIJ, D. B. DURAND, K. M. HIGGINS, E. LACY & G. CRABTREE. 1989. Cyclosporin A specifically inhibits function of nuclear proteins involved in T cell activation. Science 246: 1617–1620.
5. FLANAGAN, W. M., B. CORTHESY, R. J. BRAM & G. CRABTREE. 1991. Nuclear association of a T-cell transcription factor blocked by FK-506 and cyclosporin A. Nature 352: 803–807.
6. SEN, R. & D. BALTIMORE. 1986. Multiple nuclear factors interact with the immunoglobulin enhancer sequences. Cell 46: 705–716.
7. HANDSCHUMACHER, R. E., M. W. HARDING, J. RICE, R. J. DRUGGE & D. SPEICHER. 1984. Cyclophilin. A specific cytosolic binding protein for cyclosporin A. Science 226: 544–547.
8. A. J. KOLETSKY, M. W. HARDING & R. E. HANDSCHUMACHER. 1986. Cyclophilin. Distribution and variant properties in normal and neoplastic tissue. J. Immunol. 137: 1054–1059.
9. HAENDLER, B., W. R. HOFER & E. HOFER. 1987. Complementary DNA for human T-cell cyclophilin. EMBO J.: 947–950.
10. WALSH, C. T., L. D. ZYDOWSKY & F. D. MCKEON. 1992. Cyclosporin A, the cyclophilin class of peptidylprolyl isomerases, and blockade of T cell signal transduction. J. Biol. Chem. 267: 13115–13118.
11. FISCHER, G., L. B. WITTMANN, K. LANGE, T. KIEFHABER & F. X. SCHMIDT. 1989. Cyclophilin and peptidyl-prolyl cis-trans isomerase are probably identical proteins. Nature 337: 476–478.
12. TAKAHASHI, N., T. HAYANO & M. SUZUKI. 1989. Peptidyl-prolyl cis-trans isomerase is the cyclosporin A binding protein cyclophilin. Nature 337: 473–475.
13. GETHING, M. J. & J. SAMBROOK. 1992. Protein folding in the cell. Nature 355: 33–45.

14. SIEKIERKA, J. J., M. J. STARUCH, S. H. HUNG & N. H. SIGAL. 1989. FK-506, a potent novel immunosuppressive agent, binds to a cytosolic protein which is distinct from the cyclosporin A–binding protein, cyclophilin. J. Immunol. **143:** 1580–1583.

15. SIEKIERKA, J. J., S. H. HUNG, M. POE, C. S. LIN & N. H. SIGAL. 1989. A cytosolic binding protein for the immunosuppressant FK-506 has peptidyl-prolyl isomerase activity but is distinct from cyclophilin. Nature **341:** 755–757.

16. HARDING, M. W., A. GALAT, D. E. UEHLING & S. L. SCHREIBER. 1989. A receptor for the immunosuppressant FK-506 is a *cis-trans* peptidyl-prolyl isomerase. Nature **341:** 758–760.

17. TROPSCHUG, M., I. B. BARTHELMESS & W. NEUPERT. 1989. Sensitivity to cyclosporin A is mediated by cyclophilin in *Neurospora crassa* and *Saccharomyces cerevisiae*. Nature **342:** 953–955.

18. KOLTIN, Y., L. FAUCETTE, D. J. BERGSMA, M. LEVY, R. CAFFERKEY, P. L. KOSER, R. K. JOHNSON & G. P. LIVI. 1991. Rapamycin sensitivity in *Saccharomyces cerevisiae* is mediated by a peptidyl-prolyl *cis-trans* isomerase related to human FK506-binding protein. Mol. Cell. Biol. **11:** 1718–1723.

19. HEITMAN, J., R. N. MOVVA, P. C. HIESTAND & M. N. HALL. 1991. FK506-binding protein proline rotamase is a target for the immunosuppressive agent FK506 in *Saccharomyces cerevisiae*. Proc. Natl. Acad. Sci. USA **88:** 1948–1952.

20. HEITMAN, J., R. N. MOVVA & M. N. HALL. 1991. Targets for cell cycle arrest by the immunosuppressant rapamycin in yeast. Science **253:** 905–909.

21. DUMONT, F. R., M. R. MELINO, M. J. STARUCH, S. L. KOPRAK, P. A. FISCHER & N. H. SIGAL. 1990. The immunosuppressive macrolides FK-506 and rapamycine act as reciprocal antagonists in murine T-cells. J. Immunol. **144:** 1418–1424.

22. BAUMANN, G., E. ANDERSEN, V. QUESNIAUX & M. K. EBERLE. 1992. Cyclosporine and its analogue SDZ IMM 125 mediate very similar effects on T-cell activation—a comparative analysis in vitro. Transplant. Proc. **24**(Suppl. 2): 43–48.

23. LIU, J., J. D. FARMER, JR., W. S. LANE, J. FRIEDMAN, I. WEISSMAN & S. L. SCHREIBER. 1991. Calcineurin is a common target of cyclophilin-cyclosporin A and FKBP-FK-506 complexes. Cell **66:** 807–815.

24. GUERINI, D. & C. B. KLEE. 1989. Cloning of human calcineurin A: evidence for two isozymes and identification of a polyproline structural domain. Proc. Natl. Acad. Sci. USA **86:** 9183–9187.

25. GUERINI, D., M. H. KRINKS, J. M. SIKELA, W. E. HAHN & C. KLEE. 1989. Isolation and sequence of a cDNA clone for human calcineurin B, the Ca^{2+}-binding subunit of the Ca^{2+}/calmodulin-stimulated protein phosphatase. DNA **8:** 675–682.

26. SWANSON, S. K.-H., T. BORN, L. D. ZYDOWSKY, H. CHO, H. CHANG, C. T. WALSH & F. RUSNAK. 1992. Cyclosporin-mediated inhibition of bovine calcineurin by cyclophilins A and B. Proc. Natl. Acad. Sci. USA **89:** 3741–3745.

27. FESIK, S. W., R. T. GAMPE, JR., T. F. HOLZMAN, D. A. EGAN, R. EDALJI, J. R. LULY, R. SIMMER, R. HELFRICH, V. KISHORF & D. H. RICH. 1990. Isotope-edited NMR of cyclosporin A bound to cyclophilin: evidence for a *trans* 9,10 amide bond. Science **250:** 1406–1409.

28. WEBER, C., G. WIDER, B. VON FREYBERG, R. TRABER, W. BRAUN, H. WIDMER & K. WUETHRICH. 1991. The NMR structure of cyclosporin A bound to cyclophilin in aqueous solution. Biochemistry **30:** 6563–6574.

29. PFLUEGL, G., J. KALLEN, T. SCHIRMER, J. N. JANSONIUS, M. G. M. ZURINI & M. D. WALKINSHAW. 1992. X-ray structure of a decameric cyclophilin-cyclosporin crystal complex. Nature **361:** 91–94.

30. SPITZFADEN, C., H.-P. WEBER, W. BRAUN, J. KALLEN, G. WIDER, H. WIDMER, M. D. WALKINSHAW & K. WUETHRICH. 1992. Cyclosporin A–cyclophilin complex formation. A model based on X-ray and NMR data. FEBS Lett. **300**(3): 291–300.

An FKBP-Rapamycin-Sensitive, Cyclin-Dependent Kinase Activity that Correlates with the FKBP-Rapamycin-Induced G1 Arrest Point in MG-63 Cells[a]

MARK W. ALBERS, ERIC J. BROWN, AKITO TANAKA,
RICHARD T. WILLIAMS,[b] FREDERICK L. HALL,[b] AND
STUART L. SCHREIBER

Department of Chemistry
Harvard University
Cambridge, Massachusetts 02138

[b]*Department of Molecular Pharmacology and Toxicology*
University of Southern California School of Medicine and Pharmacy
Los Angeles, California 90054

The natural products FK506 and rapamycin (FIGURE 1) bind the same intracellular receptors, a family of FK506 and rapamycin binding proteins (FKBPs), but cause distinct biological phenomena.[1,2] FK506 inhibits signaling emanating from T cell antigen receptors on T lymphocytes[3,4] and immunoglobulin E (IgE) Fc receptors on mast cells,[5] whereas rapamycin inhibits signaling emanating from some growth factor receptors, including interleukin-2 receptors on lymphocytes[3,4] and insulin receptors on hepatocytes[6,7] (FIGURE 2). Three lines of evidence suggest that these natural products are prodrugs that become activated upon binding to an FKBP, i.e., the binding of each ligand by FKBP results in a gain of function rather than a loss of function. First, FK506 and rapamycin reciprocally antagonize each other's action.[3,4] Second, 506BD, a nonnatural FKBP ligand (FIGURE 1), has no known biological activity but can reverse the actions of both FK506 and rapamycin.[8] Third, a strain of *Saccharomyces cerevisiae* with a null FKBP12 mutation is viable, but insensitive to both FK506 and rapamycin.[9-12] The gain-of-function model was confirmed when calcineurin, a Ca^{2+}, calmodulin protein phosphatase, was shown to bind the FKBP12-FK506 complex, but neither component alone nor the FKBP-rapamycin complex.[13] Evidence that calcineurin is an *in vivo* target of FKBP-FK506 complexes has been generated by four independent methods. The ability of analogues of FK506 to inhibit TCR-mediated signaling *in vivo* correlates with their ability to inhibit calcineurin's phosphatase activity *in vitro*.[14] Second, the phosphatase activity of calcineurin in lymphocyte extracts was shown to be inhibited by pretreatment of the cells with FK506 but not rapamycin.[15] Third, overexpression of calcineurin in Jurkat T cells

[a]Supported by the National Institutes of Health (GM-38627, awarded to SLS and a Biomedical Research Support Grant to CHLA), the National Science Foundation (DCB-9104769, awarded to FLH), and the John C. Wilson Jr. Endowment (awarded to FLH via Vernon Tolo). MWA is a Howard Hughes Medical Institute predoctoral fellow. RTW is an affiliate of the University of Queensland, Australia.

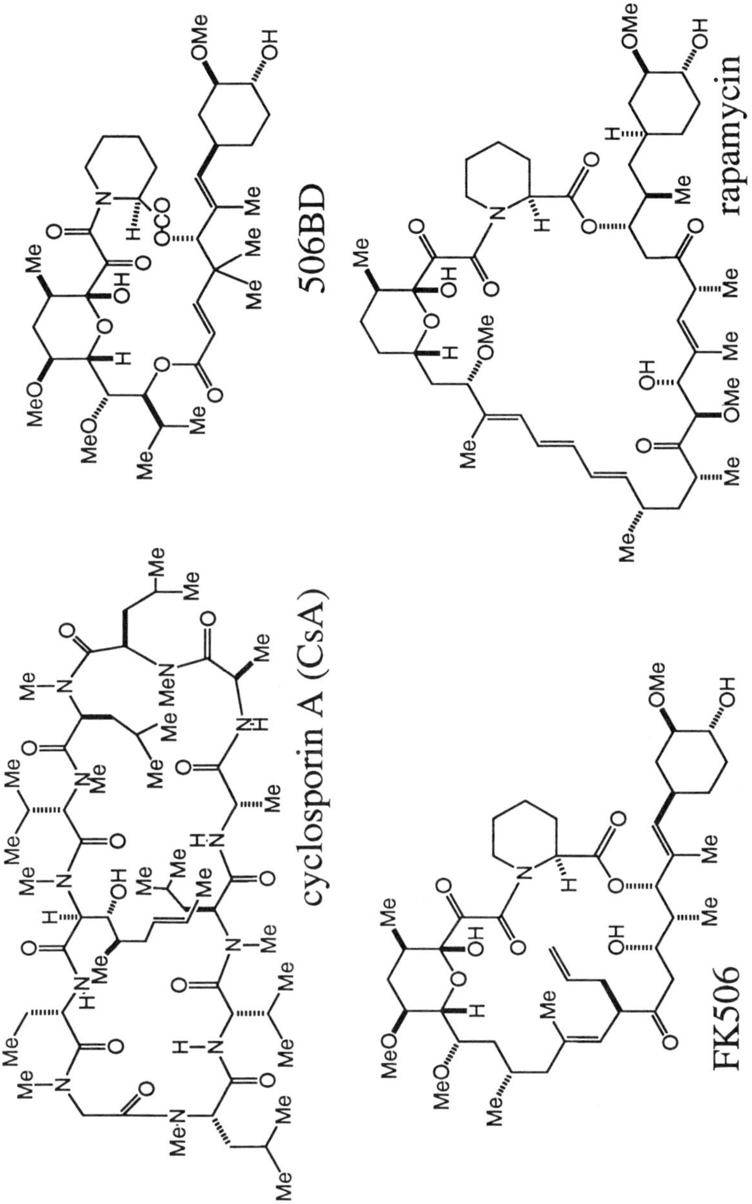

FIGURE 1. Structures of immunophilin ligands.

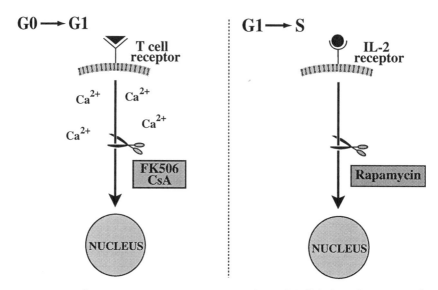

FIGURE 2. Ca^{2+}-dependent, CsA and FK506-sensitive and Ca^{2+}-independent, rapamycin-sensitive signaling pathways.

conferred decreased sensitivity to inhibition of TCR-mediated signaling by FK506.[16,17] Moreover, this study provided evidence that calcineurin lies on the signaling pathway initiated by the TCR (see Clipstone *et al.* and Wiederrecht *et al.* in this volume for more details). Fourth, an FKBP12-FK506-calcineurin complex was isolated from yeast extracts, and the formation of this complex correlated with FK506's biological activity.[12]

To date, the direct target of the FKBP-rapamycin complex remains a mystery. Nevertheless, rapamycin has been shown to prevent the phosphorylation and activation of a 70-kDa ribosomal S6 protein kinase p70[S6K] following growth factor stimulation of lymphocytes,[18,19] hepatocytes,[7] and fibroblasts;[20] this activation normally occurs within minutes following growth factor addition. Moreover, activation of p70[S6K] can be reversed within two minutes by rapamycin treatment, transforming a phosphorylated p70[S6K] to an underphosphorylated form.[20] However, all evidence gathered to date indicates that p70[S6k] is not a direct target of the FKBP12-rapamycin complex, suggesting that the phosphorylation and activation of p70[S6k] occur downstream of the direct target of the FKBP-rapamycin complex.

P70[S6k] is thought to be activated by multiple phosphorylations within an autoinhibitory region of the protein.[21] The phosphorylations presumably lower the affinity between this intramolecular inhibitor and the active site. It has been shown that the relative phosphorylation states of p70[S6k] can be estimated by differences in its electrophoretic mobility; increased phosphorylation correlates with decreased mobility on sodium dodecyl sulfate-polyacrylamide gel electrophoresis (SDS-PAGE).[22] Using this observation, Chung *et al.* have demonstrated that p70[S6k] becomes hyperphosphorylated *in vivo* following treatment of fibroblasts with the phosphatase inhibitor okadiac acid and that rapamycin prevents this phenomenon.[20] We first asked whether rapamycin inhibits a kinase activity that activates p70[S6k] or stimulates a phosphatase activity that can act on phosphorylated p70[S6k]. This experiment does not necessarily address the immediate target of FKBP-rapamycin, but likely involves the rapamycin-sensitive factor immediately upstream of p70[S6k]. Rapamycin treatment resulted in dephosphorylation of p70[S6k] in NIH3T3 fibroblasts as evidenced by its faster mobility during SDS-PAGE (FIGURE 3, lanes 2 and 3). The addition of calyculin (30 nM), a potent inhibitor of the protein phosphatases PP1 and PP2A, results in an upward mobility shift of p70[S6k] (FIGURE 3, lanes 4 and 5). This effect was prevented by pretreatment with 30 nM rapamycin (FIGURE 3, lane 6). Since calyculin places p70[S6k] in a defined, phosphorylated state, subsequent inhibition of the activating kinase by rapamycin should not affect the phosphorylation state of p70[S6k], whereas activation of a phosphatase would alter this state. When these fibroblasts were stimulated with 30 nM calyculin for 30 min and then treated with 30 nM rapamycin for 30 min, no change in the phosphorylation state of p70[S6k] was observed (FIGURE 3, lane 7). Since FKBP-rapamycin complexes do not inhibit the calyculin-sensitive phosphatases PP1 and PP2A *in vitro*,[14] this result is consistent with a model where the net effect of FKBP-rapamycin is to block an activating kinase of p70[S6k].

Since it has not been demonstrated that the activity of p70[S6k] is necessary for cell cycle progression, additional studies were carried out to characterize in more detail rapamycin's ability to cause G1 arrest. Since rapamycin is thought to block a signaling event prior to the onset of S phase, further characterization of the cell cycle arrest may provide insights into the target of rapamycin as well as signal transduction pathways required for G1 progression. A human osteosarcoma cell line MG-63 was used for these studies. These cells can be rendered quiescent by deprivation of serum growth factors for 48 hours without loss of viability,[23] and then progress together through G1 and into S phase once serum growth factors are reintroduced.

With these synchronized cells, flow cytometric analysis was performed to investigate their sensitivity to rapamycin. A histogram of the DNA content of an asynchronous population of MG-63 cells in the presence of serum is illustrated in FIGURE 4A. In this population, all the phases of the cell cycle are represented. When deprived of

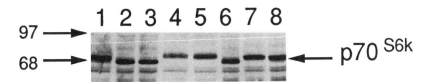

FIGURE 3. FKBP-rapamycin directly or indirectly blocks a p70[S6k] kinase. The phosphorylation state of p70[S6k] can be inferred from its relative mobility during SDS-PAGE.[22] NIH3T3 fibroblasts were grown in DMEM and 10% fetal bovine serum (FBS). These cells were rendered quiescent by culturing in DMEM and 0.5% horse serum for 48 hours. Cells were harvested by washing with Hanks Balanced Salt Solution and then with phosphate buffered saline (PBS), both preequilibrated to 4°C. The cells were lysed by incubation for 30 min at 4°C in 0.5% Triton X-100, 50 mM K-Hepes, 35 mM KCl, 1 mM Na_3VO_4, 15 mM β-glycerophosphate, 15 mM Na pyrophosphate, 4μg/ml leupeptin, 2 μg/ml aprotinin, 1 mM benzamidine, 20 nM calyculin A (LC Services), 1 mM DTT (pH 7.4). The extract was centrifuged at 14,000g for 20 min at 4°C. Protein concentration was determined by the Bradford Assay (Bio-Rad). Normalized samples were then analyzed by SDS-PAGE followed by electroblotting to Immobilon-P (Millipore), probing with a 1:5000 dilution of an anti-p70[S6k] polyclonal antibody (UBI), and visualization using the ECL immunodetection kit (Amersham). **Lane 1:** Quiescent cells. **Lane 2:** Quiescent cells treated with 30 nM rapamycin for 30 min. **Lane 3:** Quiescent cells treated with 30 nM rapamycin for 60 min. **Lane 4:** Quiescent cells treated with 30 nM calyculin A for 30 min. **Lane 5:** Quiescent cells treated with 30 nM calyculin A for 60 min. **Lane 6:** Quiescent cells treated with 30 nM rapamycin for 30 min and then with 30 nM calyculin for 30 min. **Lane 7:** Quiescent cells treated with 30 nM calyculin and then treated with 30 nM rapamycin for 30 min. **Lane 8:** Quiescent cells treated with 10% FBS for 30 min.

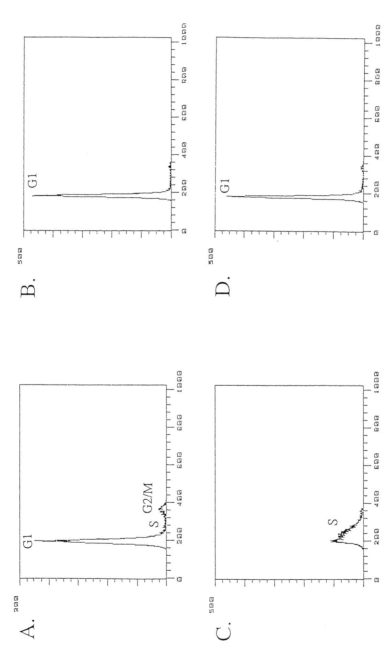

FIGURE 4. Flow cytometric analysis of MG-63 cells. **A:** Asynchronous MG-63 cells. Each histogram is number of cells versus fluorescence intensity (amount of DNA). G0/G1, S, M phase are indicated. **B:** Synchronized MG-63 cells after 48 hours of serum (growth factor) deprivation. **C:** Synchronized cells 18 hours following serum readdition. **D:** Synchronized cells 18 hours following serum readdition in presence of 50 nM rapamycin. These data indicate that rapamycin arrests MG-63 cells in G1.

serum, MG-63 cells accumulate at the G0/G1 boundary (FIGURE 4B). If serum growth factors are reintroduced for 18 hours, most of the cells have progressed through G1 and entered S phase and G2 (FIGURE 4C). Rapamycin at a concentration of 5 nM prevented synchronized cells from progressing through G1 and entering S phase following 18 hours of serum stimulation (FIGURE 4D). Furthermore, excess FK506 reversed the inhibitory effects of rapamycin treatment, indicating that rapamycin also functions in a complex with an FKBP.[24]

Flow cytometric analysis of synchronized MG-63 cells was then used to determine when cells become refractory to rapamycin treatment following serum growth factor stimulation (FIGURE 5). Addition of rapamycin at two or four hours after serum stimulation clearly inhibited S phase entry, while addition at later times had only partial effects. Rapamycin seems to block a critical event that occurs after four

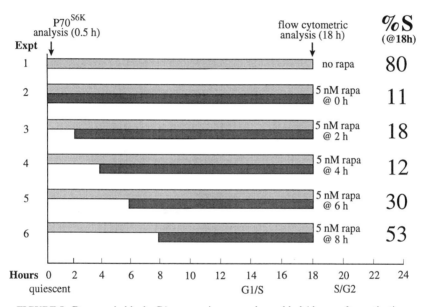

FIGURE 5. Rapamycin blocks G1 progression even when added 4 hours after activation.

hours of serum stimulation. In osteosarcoma cells, $p70^{S6k}$ remains active and phosphorylated for at least eight hours after serum stimulation.[25] Both the activation and phosphorylation of $p70^{S6k}$ were reversed by adding rapamycin at all times tested within these first eight hours of G1. In order to be consistent with the flow cytometry data summarized in FIGURE 5, if $p70^{S6k}$ activity is required for G1 progression, it must be necessary after the first four hours of serum stimulation. In other words, $p70^{S6k}$ activity in the first four hours is not sufficient to allow progression to S phase in MG-63 cells.

While the involvement of the $p70^{S6k}$ kinase activity in G1 progression remains to be determined, we initiated another series of experiments to investigate the effect of rapamycin on a protein kinase activity that has been implicated in cell cycle progression, histone H1 kinase activity of $p9^{Ckshs1}$ precipitates. $p9^{Ckshs1}$ is a protein that binds at least three cyclin-dependent kinases (cdks) (cdc2, cdk2, and cdk3) with high affinity.[26] Cdks comprise the catalytic subunits of protein kinases that are implicated by both genetic and biochemical evidence to be essential for cell cycle progression in eukaryotic cells, ranging from yeast to mammalian cells.[27,28] Cdks associate with labile regulatory subunits, termed cyclins, that activate and direct the kinase to specific substrates. The synthesis and degradation of the cyclins are precisely regulated throughout the cell cycle. During G1 phase in MG-63 cells, the sequential order of induction is that cyclin D1 precedes cyclin E which precedes cyclin A.[24,29]

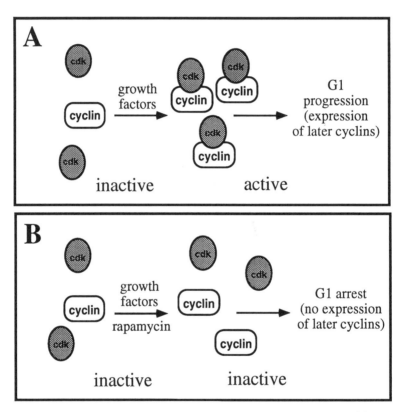

FIGURE 6. FKBP-rapamycin blocks cyclin-Cdk association and kinase activity.

In the course of these experiments, we have characterized a kinase activity that associates with p9[Ckshs1] and increases four to six hours after the addition of serum in MG-63 cells.[24] This early G1 activity was significantly inhibited by treating cells with rapamycin. Treatment with rapamycin had no effect on the expression of p34[cdc2] or p33[cdk2], but rapamycin inhibits the expression of cyclins. Cyclin D1 levels, which normally increase after four to six hours of growth factor stimulation, were slightly reduced in rapamycin-treated cells. However, the induction of cyclins E and A, which normally occurs later than eight hours after serum stimulation, was completely inhibited by rapamycin. Thus, it appears that the induction of cyclins E and A relies on signaling events that occur after the induction of cyclin D1. The correlation between cyclin D1 expression, the lack of cdk activity, and the "window" of rapamycin sensitivity is consistent with a model that cyclin D in some way participates in the critical rapamycin signaling event(s) that occurs sometime after four hours of serum stimulation.

Since cyclins are regulatory subunits of cdks, we examined the influence of rapamycin on the association of cyclin D1 with specific cdks that bind to p9^{Ckshs1}. Appreciable levels of cyclin D1 were precipitated by p9^{Ckshs1}-sepharose when it was incubated with extracts from cells that had been stimulated with serum for 6 hours. However, ~ 90% less cyclin D associated with the p9^{Ckshs1}-sepharose when similar extracts prepared from cells were pretreated with rapamycin were used.[24] Similar results were obtained using anti-cdc2 and anti-cdk2 antisera to immunoprecipitate these catalytic subunits. Thus, rapamycin prevents the association of cyclin D1, whether it is direct or indirect, with cdks that are recognized by p9^{Ckshs1} (FIGURE 6). Rapamycin may inhibit the induction of the histone H1 kinase activity in early G1 by blocking the association of cyclin D1 with this subset of cdks. To date, we have no evidence to suggest that FKBP12-rapamycin complexes interact directly with either cyclin D or the cdks recognized by p9^{Ckshs1}. The molecular mechanisms by which rapamycin prevents the association of cyclin D1 with specific cdks and the necessity of these cyclin D-associated kinase activities for G1 progression are currently under investigation.

REFERENCES

1. SCHREIBER, S. L. 1991. Science **251:** 283–287.
2. SCHREIBER, S. L. 1992. Cell **70:** 365–368.
3. BIERER, B. E., P. S. MATTILA, R. F. STANDAERT, L. A. HERZENBERG, S. J. BURAKOFF, G. CRABTREE & S. L. SCHREIBER. 1990. Proc. Natl. Acad. Sci. USA **87:** 9231–9235.
4. DUMONT, F. J., M. R. MELINO, M. J. STARUCH, S. L. KOPRAK, P. A. FISCHER & N. H. SIGAL. 1990. J. Immunol. **144:** 1418–1424.
5. HULTSCH, T., M. W. ALBERS, S. L. SCHREIBER & R. J. HOHMAN. 1991. Proc. Natl. Acad. Sci. USA **88:** 6229–6233.
6. FRANCAVILLA, A., B. I. CARR, T. E. STARZL, A. AZZARONE, G. CARRIERI & Q.-H. ZENG. 1992. Hepatology **15:** 871–877.
7. PRICE, D. J., J. R. GROVE, V. CALVO, J. AVRUCH & B. E. BIERER. 1992. Science **257:** 973–977.
8. BIERER, B. E., P. K. SOMERS, T. J. WANDLESS, S. J. BURAKOFF & S. L. SCHREIBER. 1990. Science Washington, D.C. **250:** 556–559.
9. WIEDERRECHT, G., L. BRIZUELA, K. ELLISTON, N. H. SIGAL & J. J. SIEKIERKA. 1991. Proc. Natl. Acad. Sci. USA **88:** 1029–1033.
10. KOLTIN, Y., L. FAUCETTE, D. J. BERGSMA, M. A. LEVY, R. CAFFERKEY, P. L. KOSER, R. K. JOHNSON & G. P. LIVI. 1991. Mol. Cell. Biol. **11:** 1718–1723.
11. HEITMAN, J., N. R. MOVVA & M. N. HALL. 1991. Science **253:** 905–909.
12. FOOR, F., S. A. PARENT, N. MORIN, A. M. DAHL, N. RAMADAN, G. CHREBET, K. A. BOSTIAN & J. B. NIELSON. 1992. Nature **360:** 682–684.
13. LIU, J., J. D. J. FARMER, W. S. LANE, J. FRIEDMAN, I. WEISSMAN & S. L. SCHREIBER. 1991. Cell Cambridge, Mass. **66:** 807–815.
14. LIU, J., M. W. ALBERS, T. J. WANDLESS, S. LUAN, D. A. ALBERG, P. J. BELSHAW, P. COHEN, C. MACKINTOSH, C. B. KLEE & S. L. SCHREIBER. 1992. Biochemistry **31:** 3896–3901.
15. FRUMAN, D. A., C. B. KLEE, B. E. BIERER & S. J. BURAKOFF. 1992. Proc. Natl. Acad. Sci. USA **89:** 3686–3690.
16. CLIPSTONE, N. A. & G. R. CRABTREE. 1992. Nature **357:** 695–697.
17. O'KEEFE, S. J., J. TAMURA, R. KINCAID, M. TOCCI & E. O. O'NEILL. 1992. Nature **357:** 692–694.

18. KUO, C. J., J. CHUNG, D. F. FIORENTINO, W. M. FLANAGAN, J. BLENIS & G. R. CRABTREE. 1992. Nature 358: 70–73.
19. CALVO, V., C. M. CREWS, T. A. VIK & B. BIERER. 1992. Proc. Natl. Acad. Sci. USA 89: 7571–7575.
20. CHUNG, J., C. J. KUO, G. R. CRABTREE & J. BLENIS. 1992. Cell 69: 1227–1236.
21. FERRARI, S., W. BANNWARTH, S. J. MORLEY, N. F. TOTTY & G. THOMAS. 1992. Proc. Natl. Acad. Sci. USA 89: 7282–7286.
22. KOZMA, S. C., S. FERRARI, P. BASSAND, M. SIEGMANN, N. TOTTY & G. THOMAS. 1990. Proc. Natl. Acad. Sci. USA 87: 7365–7369.
23. WILLIAMS, R. T., L. WU, D. A. CARBONARO-HALL, V. T. TOLO & F. L. HALL. 1993. J. Biol. Chem. 268: 8871–8880.
24. ALBERS, M. W., R. T. WILLIAMS, E. J. BROWN, A. TANAKA, F. L. HALL & S. L. SCHREIBER. J. Biol. Chem. (In press.)
25. ALBERS, M. W., E. J. BROWN, R. T. WILLIAMS, F. L. HALL & S. L. SCHREIBER. Unpublished results.
26. MEYERSON, M., G. H. ENDERS, C.-L. WU, L.-K. SU, C. GORKA, C. NELSON, E. HARLOW & L.-H. TSAI. 1992. EMBO J. 11: 2909–2917.
27. NORBURY, C. & P. NURSE. 1992. Annu. Rev. Biochem. 61: 441–470.
28. REED, S. I. 1992. Annu. Rev. Cell Biol. 8: 529–561.
29. HALL, F. L., R. T. WILLIAMS, L. WU, F. WU, D. CARBONARO-HALL, J. W. HARPER & D. WARBURTON. 1993. Oncogene 8: 1377–1384.

Mechanisms of Action
of Mycophenolic Acid

ANTHONY C. ALLISON, W. JOSEPH KOWALSKI,
CHRISTIAN D. MULLER, AND ELSIE M. EUGUI

Syntex Discovery Research
3401 Hillview Avenue
Palo Alto, California 94304

INTRODUCTION

The advantages and limitations of currently used immunosuppressive drugs are well known. Each drug has particular advantages as well as side effects. For example, cyclophosphamide can produce hemorrhagic cystitis;[1] cyclosporin, nephrotoxicity and hypertension;[2] and methotrexate, liver damage, pneumonitis, and bone marrow suppression.[3] In addition there are short-term and long-term effects common to many immunosuppressive drugs. In the short term, immunosuppressive drugs can increase susceptibility to virus and other infections; it is desirable that when treatment is terminated, immune function is rapidly restored, so that recovery from infections is facilitated. A long-term risk of immunosuppressive therapy is the development of lymphomas. This is well known in organ graft recipients,[4] but is observed also in patients with rheumatoid arthritis.[5] As discussed more fully below, two factors predispose to lymphoma development. One is inhibition of surveillance against outgrowth of Epstein-Barr virus transformed B-lymphocytes.[6] The second is chromosomal translocations, which can convert polyclonal B cell proliferation into frank malignancy.[7] Mutagenic effects of immunosuppressive drugs are obviously undesirable. Cyclosporin inhibits surveillance against EBV-transformed lymphocytes.[6] Cyclophosphamide[8] and azathioprine[9] have several active metabolites and mechanisms of action. Metabolites of cyclophosphamide are alkylating agents,[8] and their effects on lymphocytes are not rapidly reversible. Cyclophosphamide is mutagenic and carcinogenic.[10] Azathioprine is also mutagenic.[11] Methotrexate, which inhibits synthesis of thymididylate as well as *de novo* purine synthesis,[3] has nonselective antiproliferative effects, which are no more potent on lymphocytes than on other cell types, including hematopoietic precursors, fibroblasts, and endothelial cells.[3,12]

Hence there has been a need for a new immunosuppressive drug with reversible antiproliferative effects that are more potent on lymphocytes than on other cell types, including hematopoietic cells, and that are free of hepatotoxicity, nephrotoxicity, mutagenicity and other serious side effects. We approached the design of such a drug by identifying a metabolic pathway more susceptible to inhibition in human T- and B-lymphocytes than in other cell types. Observations on children with inherited defects of purine metabolism provided a lead.

BACKGROUND

Purine Metabolism in Lymphocytes

There are two major pathways of purine synthesis (FIGURE 1). In the *de novo* pathway, the ribose phosphate portion of purine nucleotides is derived from 5-phos-

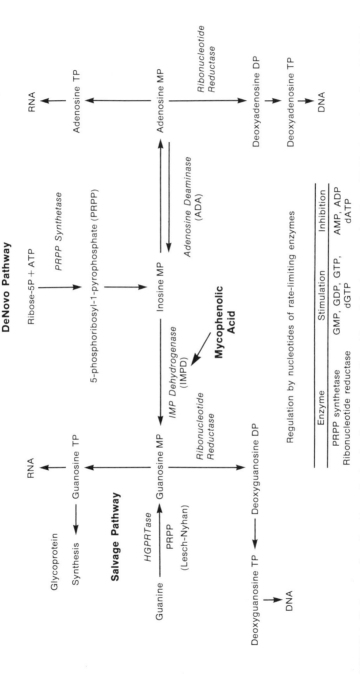

FIGURE 1. Pathways of purine biosynthesis, showing the central position of inosine monophosphate (IMP). Mycophenolic acid inhibits IMP dehydrogenase, thereby depleting GMP, GTP, and dGTP. Two rate-limiting enzymes in lymphocytes are activated by guanosine ribonucleotides and dGTP, but inhibited by AMP, ADP, and dATP, respectively.

phoribosyl-1-pyrophosphate (PRPP), which is synthesized from ATP and ribose-5-phosphate, a product of the pentose phosphate pathway. The purine ring is assembled on ribose phosphate by a series of steps, the first of which is catalyzed by glutamine-PRPP amidotransferase. PRPP is also used by the purine salvage pathways, including the major pathway catalyzed by hypoxanthine-guanine phosphoribosyltransferase (HGPRTase). Production of an adequate level of PRPP is therefore essential for synthesis of purine ribonucleotides by either pathway. Ribonucleotide diphosphates (ADP and GDP) are converted by ribonucleotide diphosphate reductase into the corresponding deoxyribonucleotides (dADP and dGDP), which are phosphorylated to produce dATP and dGTP, substrates for DNA polymerase.

Activities of key, rate-limiting enzymes, PRPP synthetase and ribonucleotide reductase, are allosterically regulated by nucleotides (FIGURE 1). In bacteria, both adenosine and guanosine nucleotides, signaling an abundance of purine nucleotides, inhibit PRPP synthetase.[13] However, we showed that this is not the case with PRPP synthetase from human lymphocytes:[14] the enzyme is inhibited by adenosine nucleotides (AMP and ADP) but activated by guanosine nucleotides (GMP, GDP, and GTP). Such regulation is a critical factor in the therapeutic strategy discussed in this paper. The overall catalytic activity of ribonucleotide reductase is decreased by binding of dATP, whereas binding of dGTP stimulates ADP reduction.[13] It follows that an excess of adenosine nucleotides, and/or depletion of guanosine nucleotides, can decrease the pool of PRPP, and that an excess of dATP and/or depletion of dGTP can inhibit ribonucleotide reductase activity, thereby decreasing the pool of substrates required for DNA polymerase activity. In other words, adequate levels of guanosine and deoxyguanosine nucleotides are required for proliferative responses of lymphocytes to antigenic and mitogenic stimulation, whereas an excess of adenosine or deoxyadenosine nucleotides would be expected to inhibit proliferation. As shown in FIGURE 1, IMP is at the branch point in purine nucleotide synthesis, since it can be converted to AMP or GMP. Two enzymes decrease levels of adenosine nucleotides relative to guanosine nucleotides: adenosine deaminase (ADA) and inosine monophosphate dehydrogenase (IMPDH). From the arguments just presented, it would be expected that both of these enzymes would be required for lymphocyte proliferation.

In 1972, Eloise Giblett and her colleagues showed that children with inherited ADA deficiency have a selective decrease in the numbers and functions of T- and B-lymphocytes in the presence of normal numbers of neutrophils, erythrocytes, and platelets and normal brain function.[15] Shortly afterwards, we showed that children lacking HGPRTase (Lesch-Nyhan syndrome) have essentially normal numbers and functions of T- and B-lymphocytes.[16] These findings led us to postulate that *de novo* purine synthesis is crucially important for proliferative responses of human T- and B-lymphocytes to mitogens, whereas the major salvage pathway catalyzed by HGPRTase is not required for lymphocyte proliferation.[16,17] Children with the Lesch-Nyhan syndrome have mental deficiency and compulsive self-mutilation, showing the importance of the salvage pathway controlled by HGPRTase for brain cells. The level of this enzyme in brain is higher than in any other tissue, whereas the activity of glutamine-PRPP amidotransferase, which catalyzes the committed step in the *de novo* pathway, is low in brain.[13] Thus cell types and tissues can be arranged according to their dependence on the *de novo* and salvage pathways of purine synthesis, with lymphocytes at one extreme, brain cells at the other, and most cell types, able to use both pathways, occupying an intermediate position.

The importance of adequate PRPP levels and of *de novo* purine synthesis in lymphocytes responding to antigenic and mitogenic stimulation is clear. We found a rapid and sustained increase in PRPP concentrations in human lymphocytes following mitogenic stimulation,[18] as well as markedly increased *de novo* purine synthesis, as shown by incorporation of ^{14}C-glycine into purine nucleotides.[19] In stimulated cells, the label is about equally distributed into pools of adenosine nucleotides on the one hand and inosine and guanosine nucleotides on the other, whereas in resting cells, synthesis of adenosine nucleotides predominates. Thus proliferation is accompanied by activation of PRPP synthetase and of IMPDH, increasing *de novo* purine synthesis and channeling it towards GMP. As discussed by Natsumeda,[20] in stimulated lymphocytes, the gene for a distinct isoform of IMPDH is activated, so the total amount of enzyme per cell is increased, in addition to allosteric regulation by nucleotides. Elevation of PRPP concentrations in human lymphocytes following PHA stimulation, and suppression of that elevation by adenosine, has also been reported by Peters *et al.*[21]

Inhibition of Inosine Monophosphate Dehydrogenase

Because of the importance of guanosine and deoxyguanosine nucleotides in activating PRPP synthetase and ribonucleotide reductase, respectively, we postulated that depletion of GMP (and consequently GTP and dGTP) by inhibiting inosine monophosphate dehydrogenase (IMPDH) would have antiproliferative effects. Furthermore, since lymphocytes rely on *de novo* purine synthesis whereas other cell types do not, antiproliferative effects produced in this way would be more potent on lymphocytes than on other cell types. Of several possible inhibitors of IMPDH, we selected for detailed study mycophenolic acid (MPA, FIGURE 2), a fermentation product of several *Penicillium* species. MPA was preferred to nucleoside analogues such as mizoribine because the latter must be phosphorylated to inhibit IMPDH, and because of the side effects of this class of compounds. The efficiency of nucleoside phosphorylation can vary in different cell types,[22] and the relevance of target cells in addition to lymphocytes (e.g., cells of the monocyte-macrophage lineage, endothelial cells, and smooth muscle cells) is described below. Nucleoside analogues frequently have undesirable effects, such as inhibiting DNA repair enzymes and producing chromosome breaks. MPA is not a nucleoside, and is a potent, noncompetitive, reversible inhibitor of eukaryotic but not prokaryotic IMP dehydrogenases.[20,23] Contrary to early reports, MPA does not inhibit GMP synthetase, the enzyme catalyzing the conversion of XMP to GMP.[20]

We soon found that MPA had the predicted cytostatic effects on lymphocytes. Dr. Peter Nelson focused synthetic effort on obtaining a derivative of MPA with improved oral bioavailability. The morpholinoethyl ester of MPA (mycophenolate mofetil, FIGURE 2) was found, unexpectedly, to have improved bioavailability in primates as compared with MPA.[24] The ester is rapidly hydrolyzed to yield MPA, both in human peripheral blood mononuclear cell cultures and *in vivo*. Mycophenolate mofetil (MM) proved suitable for pharmaceutical formulation and was selected for development. Most of our *in vivo* studies were made with MM, although comparative studies with MPA were often included. MPA is rapidly converted into the glucuronide, which is the principal metabolite. This undergoes enterohepatic recycling and is excreted in the urine.

MPA proved to have preferential effects in lymphocytes for another reason discussed by Natsumeda.[20] The type II isoform of IMPDH, which predominates in proliferating B- and T-lymphocytes, is about four times as sensitive to inhibition by MPA than is the type I isoform, expressed in most cell types.

Inhibition of Lymphocyte Proliferation

Concentrations of MPA that are readily attainable therapeutically inhibit the proliferative responses of human peripheral blood mononuclear cells to phytohemagglutinin (a T-cell mitogen), pokeweed mitogen (a T-dependent B-cell mitogen), and *Staphylococcus* protein A sepharose (a B-cell mitogen).[25] Mixed lymphocyte responses are also inhibited by MM and MPA. In all cases the IC_{50} is less than 100 nM, a concentration of drug having no antiproliferative effect on fibroblasts or endothelial cells (FIGURE 3), or on other cell types studied. Thus the drug has greater *in vitro*

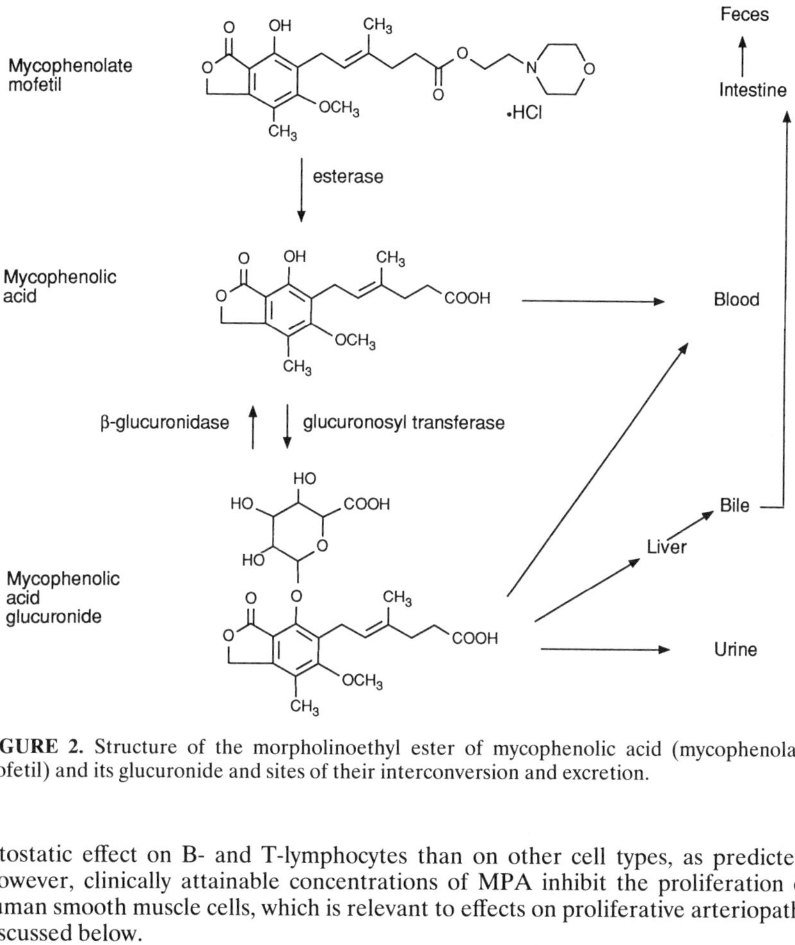

FIGURE 2. Structure of the morpholinoethyl ester of mycophenolic acid (mycophenolate mofetil) and its glucuronide and sites of their interconversion and excretion.

cytostatic effect on B- and T-lymphocytes than on other cell types, as predicted. However, clinically attainable concentrations of MPA inhibit the proliferation of human smooth muscle cells, which is relevant to effects on proliferative arteriopathy discussed below.

When added to ongoing mixed lymphocyte reactions 72 hours after initiation, MPA was still inhibitory, showing that it blocks a late event in lymphocyte responses (TABLE 1). MPA and MM also strongly inhibit proliferation of all the human T- and B-lymphocytic cell lines tested.[25] One of these lines lacks HGPRTase, which is experimentally convenient.

Intracellular Pools of GTP and dGTP

To ascertain whether the antiproliferative effects of MPA are due to depletion of GTP or of dGTP, pools of nucleotides were measured in mitogen-activated human peripheral blood mononuclear cells and human T-lymphocytic cell lines in the presence or absence of MPA, and in the presence of MPA when Guo, Gua, or dGuo were added back to the culture medium (FIGURE 4). As expected, MPA depletes

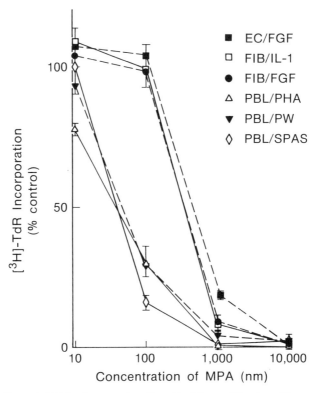

FIGURE 3. Potent inhibition by mycophenolic acid of the proliferation of human peripheral lymphocytes (PBL) responding to stimulation by a T-cell mitogen (PHA), pokeweed mitogen (PW), and a B-cell mitogen (staphylococcal protein A sepharose, SPAS).[26] Higher concentrations of MPA are required to inhibit the proliferation of human dermal fibroblasts (FIB) in response to IL-1β or human umbilical vein endothelial cells (EC) in response to basic fibroblast growth factor.

GTP and dGTP; Gua or Guo efficiently reverse depletion of GTP and less efficiently restore dGTP; dGuo efficiently reverses depletion of dGTP and less efficiently restores GTP.[26] In the MPA-treated HGPRTase-deficient T-cell line, BUC-7, dGuo restores dGTP but not GTP, as expected from metabolic pathways. Clinically attainable concentrations of MPA (1–10 μM) significantly deplete GTP in human lymphocytes and monocytes but not in neutrophils (FIGURE 5). This may be due to cellular selectivity of the inhibition of IMPDH or to a low rate of utilization of GTP in neutrophils. The consequences of this difference in cell types are discussed below.

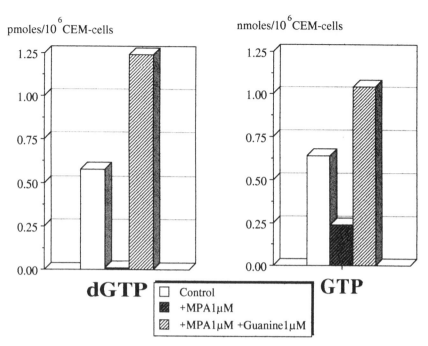

FIGURE 4. Treatment of T-lymphocytic cells (CEM) with 1 μM MPA for 6 hours depletes GTP and dGTP pools. Adding back guanine in the presence of MPA restores GTP and dGTP to levels higher than observed in the absence of MPA.[25]

The effects of these manipulations on cellular proliferation are shown in FIGURE 6. MPA or MM (1 μM) completely suppressed DNA synthesis in PHA-stimulated peripheral blood cells. Adding back 10 μM dGuo or 50 μM Guo restored DNA synthesis to control levels observed in the absence of the drug, as shown by [3]H[TdR] incorporation.[26] Neither Ado nor dAdo in any concentration tested restored DNA synthesis in MPA-treated cells or had significant effects in the absence of the drug. In HGPRTase-deficient cells treated with MPA, dGuo partially restored DNA synthesis whereas Gua or Guo did not. In cells with HGPRTase, higher concentrations of Guo than of dGuo were needed to restore DNA synthesis, in keeping with the requirement for conversion to dGTP. Thus the inhibition of DNA synthesis in

TABLE 1. Effect of Mycophenolic Acid Added at the Time of Initiation of Human MLR and 72 Hours Later

	% of Inhibition				
Time of MPA Addition	1000 nM	100 nM	10 nM	1 nM	IC_{50} nM
0 hour	98[a]	81[b]	25	4	30
72 hours	90[a]	73[b]	11	11	50
0 hour	94[a]	82[b]	−7	−27	40
72 hours	95[a]	61[b]	6	2	70

[a] $p < 0.001$.
[b] $p < 0.01$.

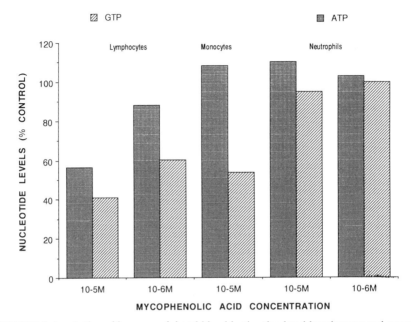

FIGURE 5. Incubation of human peripheral blood lectin-stimulated lymphocytes and monocytes with 10 μM MPA significantly depletes GTP levels whereas there is no depletion in neutrophils (N. Byars and A. C. Allison, unpublished).

MPA-treated lymphocytes is apparently due to depletion of dGTP. The findings show the metabolic selectivity of action of MPA: if the drug were acting on other enzymes or metabolic functions, or on thymidine transport, it would not have been possible to restore proliferation with Guo or dGuo. Excess dGuo inhibits DNA synthesis in the presence or absence of MPA, showing that the dGTP pool must be kept within a rather narrow optimal range.

Cytokine Production

MPA in concentrations up to 10 μM did not inhibit IL-1β formation by activated human monocytes.[25] Cyclosporin A and FK-506 inhibit early stages of lymphocyte activation, including the production of IL-2. In contrast, MM or MPA in concentrations up to 1 μM had no detectable effect on IL-2 production in mitogen-activated human peripheral blood lymphocytes.[25] These findings show that early signal transduction systems in T-lymphocytes are not inhibited by MPA, a conclusion confirmed by Dayton et al.[27]

Antibody Formation In vitro

Antibody formation by polyclonally activated human B-lymphocytes was almost completely inhibited by 100 nM MPA[25] (FIGURE 7). The capacity of MM to inhibit antibody formation in human allograft recipients is currently under investigation.

Inhibition of the Transfer of Fucose and Mannose to Glycoproteins, Including Adhesion Molecules

If depletion of GTP in lymphocytes by MPA does not impair early signal transduction in these cells, the question arises whether it has any other important metabolic consequences. The answer to that question is yes: we have defined one effect that is likely to be important *in vivo,* and there may be others. MPA-mediated depletion of GTP inhibits the transfer of fucose and mannose to glycoproteins, some

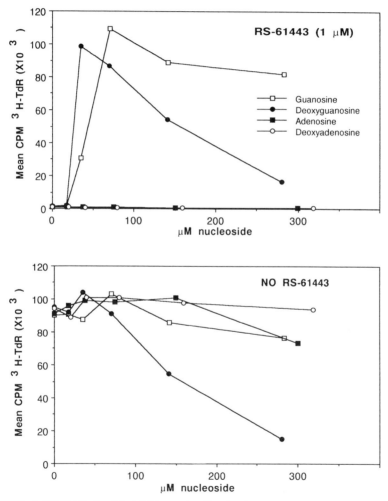

FIGURE 6. RS-61443 (1 μM) inhibits to baseline levels DNA synthesis in human PBL stimulated by PHA. Addition of deoxyguanosine, or a higher concentration of guanosine, restores DNA synthesis to levels observed in the absence of MPA. No restoration is observed following addition of adenosine or deoxyadenosine. Excess deoxyguanosine in the presence or absence of MPA decreases DNA synthesis.[26]

of which are adhesion molecules facilitating the attachment of leukocytes to endothelial cells and to target cells. By this mechanism, MPA could decrease the recruitment of lymphocytes and monocytes into sites of chronic inflammation, such as synovial tissue of patients with rheumatoid arthritis, and into sites of vascularized organ graft rejection, as well as interactions of lymphocytes with other cell types, thereby inhibiting ongoing rejection.

Recruitment of leukocytes into sites of inflammation occurs in several stages. First, a relatively weak interaction between leukocytes and endothelial cells allows leukocytes to roll along the walls of postcapillary venules and some other blood vessels rather than being swept through in the circulating blood. Second, the rolling interaction can be converted into a stronger interaction which causes the leukocytes to stick; the surfaces of leukocytes and endothelial cells are deformed sufficiently to

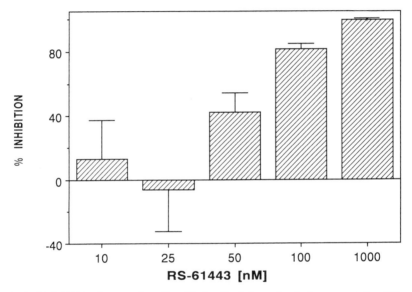

FIGURE 7. Inhibition by mycophenolic acid of antibody formation by human peripheral blood lymphocytes polyclonally activated by *Staphylococcus* protein A-sepharose.[25]

allow the leukocytes to squeeze between the endothelial cells and migrate to perivascular connective tissue. Third, the leukocytes in connective tissue respond to chemotactic stimuli by directional migration. The first two stages are mediated by adhesion molecules. Surface expression of one group of adhesion molecules, the selectins, plays a major role in the initial interaction between leukocytes and endothelial cells responsible for rolling; this interaction is a prerequisite for integrin-mediated sticking.[28,29] Selectins are so termed because of their lectinlike structures and properties. They share amino acid sequences with lectins, and their complementary ligands are fucose-containing oligosaccharides (TABLE 2).

While a great deal of attention has been given to complementary interactions of adhesion molecules in leukocytes and endothelial cells, it is clear that adhesion molecules also participate in the initiation and effector phases of immune responses. Interactions between antigen-presenting cells and lymphocytes require complemen-

TABLE 2. Adhesion Molecules on Leukocytes and Complementary Ligands on Endothelial Cells

Leukocyte	Endothelial Cell	Reference
Lacto *N*-fucapentaose III (CD15)	P-selectin (GMP-140, CD62)	37
α(2,3) sialyl, α(1,3) fucosyl lactos-aminoglycan	E-selectin (ELAM-1)	38
L-selectin (LECAM-1, MEL14)	Sialylated fucosyl oligosaccharide	29
VLA-4	VCAM-1	35

tary binding of adhesion molecules,[30] and the same is true of interactions of effector lymphocytes with target cells.[31] It follows that blocking the interactions between complementary adhesion molecules could exert immunosuppressive and antiinflammatory activity. A striking example is the administration of monoclonal antibodies against ICAM-1 and its complementary ligand LFA-1 to mice that have received cardiac allografts. Treatment with these antibodies for 6 days after transplantation induces donor-strain-specific tolerance to the alloantigens.[32]

Glycosylation of proteins and lipids occurs through nucleotide intermediates (FIGURE 8). Glucose, galactose, and their amines are transferred to dolichol phosphate and then to proteins through uridine-diphospho intermediates, whereas fucose and mannose are transferred through guanosine-diphospho intermediates.[33] We have found that in activated human peripheral blood lymphocytes, treatment with MPA significantly decreases the transfer of mannose to dolichol phosphate and to membrane glycoproteins.[34] This was shown by following labeled mannose, by measuring the expression of mannose on the surface of the cells, using a lectin specific for terminal mannose (FIGURE 9), and by measuring the terminal mannose content of different membrane glycoproteins. Immunoprecipitation studies showed that one of the lymphocyte glycoproteins affected is VLA-4, the ligand for VCAM-1 on activated endothelial cells.[35] Treatment of either T-cells or IL-1-activated endothelial cells with MPA in therapeutically attainable doses (1–10 μM) decreased

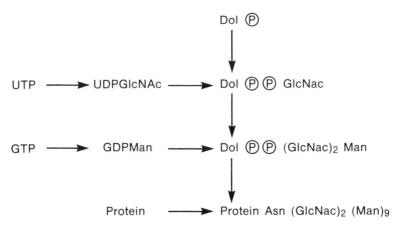

FIGURE 8. The role of sugar nucleotides and dolichol phosphate in the transfer of *N*-acetylglucosamine and mannose to asparagine residues of membrane glycoproteins. Depletion of UTP and/or GTP inhibits glycosylation.

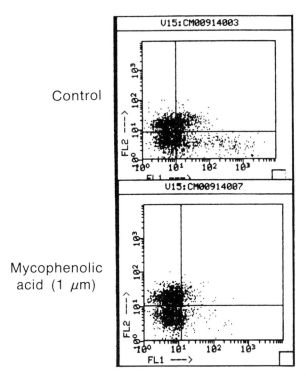

FIGURE 9. Flow cytometric measurements of the binding to human peripheral blood lymphocytes of a labeled lectin (fluorochrome 1, *Galanthus nivalis* agglutinin selective for terminal, $\alpha(1–3)$-linked mannose). The lymphocytes were stimulated for 48 hours with concanavalin A in the presence or absence of MPA added to the culture medium for the last 8 hours. MPA markedly decreases mannose available on the cells for lectin binding.[34]

lymphocyte attachment; and when both cell types were treated with MPA, the attachment was further inhibited (FIGURE 10). This effect is presumably due mainly to decreased expression of ligands for selectins on interacting cells. In addition, decreased glycosylation of VLA-4 appears to reduce its affinity for VCAM-1, even though the latter is not a selectin; perhaps the conformation of VLA-4 depends on glycosylation, as known for several glycoproteins.[36]

Inhibition of glycosylation by depletion of GTP and/or UTP is theoretically more appealing than attempting to do it by inhibitors of glycosyl transferases. There are several fucosyl and manosyl transferases with different stereospecificities, and it would be difficult to design and use inhibitors of all relevant enzymes. Such mixtures of inhibitors might well have generalized toxicity, whereas the effects of MPA are focused on lymphocytes and monocytes, the cells involved in immunologically driven inflammatory reactions. Use of recombinant adhesion molecules themselves, or of antibodies against them, is also a less attractive option since many are involved,[29] and they cannot be administered orally. For the same reasons, synthetic carbohydrate ligands are inconvenient.

Because transfer of other sugars to glycoproteins requires UDP-sugar intermediates, depletion of UTP would also be expected to decrease glycosylation. Inhibitors of pyrimidine synthesis, such as brequinar, would therefore be expected to have similar effects to those of MPA, and the two drugs should have at least additive effects on glycosylation.

Lack of Effect on Neutrophil Chemotaxis, Superoxide Production, and Microbicidal Capacity

One of the remarkable features of MM is that even chronic treatment of experimental animals and humans with immunosuppressive doses does not increase susceptibility to infections, unless the patients have also received other potent immunosuppressive treatments. We therefore ascertained whether clinically attainable concentrations of MPA affect responses of human neutrophils to chemotaxis and their capacity to produce superoxide and kill bacteria. Concentrations of MPA up to 10 μM had no demonstrable effect on any of these responses. One reason for lack of an effect in this system is the fact that 10 μM MPA does not deplete GTP in neutrophils (FIGURE 5), in contrast to lymphocytes and monocytes.

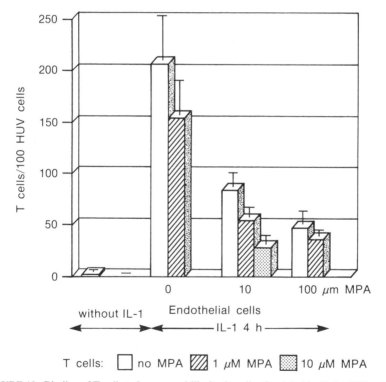

FIGURE 10. Binding of T-cells to human umbilical vein cells stimulated by IL-1α (100 ng/ml) is decreased when either the T-cells or the endothelial cells are treated with MPA. The inhibition is strongest when both cell types are treated.[34]

EFFECTS OF MYCOPHENOLIC ACID IN EXPERIMENTAL ANIMALS

Lymphocyte-Selective, Reversible Antiproliferative Effects

To ascertain whether the antiproliferative effects of MPA and MM are also lymphocyte selective *in vivo,* we injected mice subcutaneously with an antigen (ovalbumin) in adjuvant, which stimulates DNA synthesis by cells in lymph nodes of the drainage chain: while a secondary response to antigen was in progress, the mice were injected intraperitoneally with [³H]TdR. One group of mice was given MPA (100 mg/kg per day orally) while a control group received vehicle. Incorporation of [³H]TdR into DNA was measured in draining lymph nodes, spleen, and testis.[39] As shown in TABLE 3, the orally administered drug strongly inhibited DNA synthesis in the lymph nodes but had no detectable effect on DNA synthesis in the germinal cells of the testis or the basal epithelial cells of the small intestine (demonstrated by autoradiography). Effects on the spleen were intermediate, in keeping with the presence in the mouse spleen of hematopoietic cells as well as lymphocytes. Doses of MM required to prevent allograft rejection did not affect the production of neutrophils or platelets in any species. In the rat, a reversible hypoplastic anemia was observed,[40] but this has not been found in any other animal species. These observations show that the antiproliferative effects of MPA and MM are more potent on lymphocytes than on other cell types *in vivo.*

The cytostatic effects of MPA on lymphocytes are rapidly and fully reversible: peripheral blood mononuclear cells separated from the plasma of patients treated with MM respond normally to mitogenic stimulation, even when the plasma is strongly suppressive. Infections have not been a serious problem in patients treated with MM. However, if virus or other infections do occur, the drug can be withdrawn, and the immunosuppressive effects would be expected to disappear within a few days.

Inhibition of Cell-Mediated Immune Responses to Allogeneic Cells

Cytotoxic T-lymphocytes are important mediators of allograft rejection.[41] A classical model[42] was used to ascertain the effects of MPA and MM on cytotoxic T-lymphocytic responses to allogeneic cells. Tumor cells (P815, H-2^d) were injected intraperitoneally into C57B1 mice (H-2^b) to immunize them. Recipient mice were orally dosed with MPA, MM, or vehicle, and spleens were removed on day 10 or 11 for *in vitro* cytoxicity studies using ⁵¹Cr-labeled P815 target cells. This lysis is genetically restricted and largely due to cytotoxic T-cells. As shown in FIGURE 11,

TABLE 3. Effect of MPA on [³H]TdR Incorporation into DNA in Different Tissues

Tissue	Control (cpm/sample)	MPA Treated[a] (cpm/sample)	% Inhibition	p Value
Inguinal lymph node[b]	8765	528	93.9	0.000
Spleen[b]	2727	1070	60.7	0.019
Testis[c]	7435	7043	5.3	0.726

[a]50 mg/kg bid for two days.
[b]10⁷ cells.
[c]10 mg tissue.

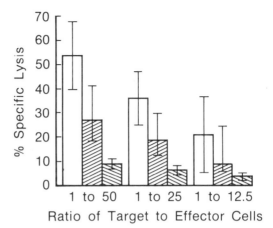

FIGURE 11. Dose-dependent inhibition of the generation of cytotoxic T-lymphocytes in mice treated with MPA.[39]

MPA inhibited in a dose-related fashion the induction of a cytotoxic T-lymphocyte response to allogeneic cells.[39]

Allogeneic tumor cells in the peritoneal cavity can be quantified and their viability assessed by capacity to grow as colonies in agar. In vehicle-treated animals, the tumor cells were found to increase rapidly for the first four days and thereafter decrease as the host immune response became effective; by the eighth day, no viable tumor cells could be recovered. In MPA-treated mice, the tumor cells continued to increase and remain viable until the animals were killed for humane reasons.[39] This is a convenient model because cytotoxic T-lymphocytes can be analyzed without complicating effects on the vasculature of allografts.

These investigations show that MM and MPA inhibit the generation of cytotoxic T-cells and the rejection of allogeneic cells. Together with our studies on inhibition of antibody formation and leukocyte homing, they provided justification for use of the drug in organ transplantation.

Inhibition of Antibody Formation

Antibody responses of rats and mice to sheep erythrocytes were analyzed by the Jerne plaque assay.[43] Administration of MM inhibited the formation of antibodies in a dose-dependent manner;[39] oral administration 30 mg/kg per day to rats virtually abolished the formation of antibodies against xenogeneic cells (FIGURE 12).

Prevention of Allograft Rejection

Collaborations were established with transplantation immunologists to ascertain whether MM can prevent the rejection of tissue and organ allografts.

Following preliminary studies in the mouse, Dr. Randall Morris and his coworkers at Stanford investigated effects of MM in Lewis rat recipients of heterotopically grafted BN hearts. Monotherapy with MM (30–40 mg/kg per day) was found to prevent rejection of the grafts; if treatment was discontinued after 50 days, all of the hearts in the animals receiving the higher dose survived in good functional condition indefinitely.[40] When such animals were challenged in the absence of further immuno-suppression with donor-strain atrial tissue beneath the renal capsule, it continued to beat indefinitely, whereas atrial tissue from a third-party strain (ACI) was promptly rejected.[44] Thus, short-term treatment with MM could induce a state of donor-specific tolerance. In these animals, mixed lymphocyte responses of recipient to donor-strain lymphocytes were significantly lower than in untreated recipients, whereas responses to third-party cells were normal.

The second finding was that when MM and cyclosporin A were used together, their effects were at least additive without any demonstrable increase in toxicity.[40] Since the drugs act by different mechanisms, this was not surprising. The third finding was that if the first dose of MM was delayed until the fifth day following transplantation, by which time there is a marked mononuclear cell infiltrate into the graft and edema, the heart could still be preserved in good functional condition indefinitely.[40] When azathioprine or cyclosporine was given under comparable conditions, it could not prevent rejection. This finding suggested that MM might be efficacious for the treatment of rejection crises.

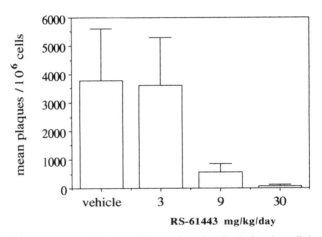

FIGURE 12. Dose-dependent inhibition of the number of antibody-forming cells in the spleens of rats immunized with sheep red blood cells and treated with MPA.[39]

As discussed at this meeting, Hao and her colleagues found that MM prolongs survival of pancreatic islet allografts in rodents. Some immunosuppressive drugs preventing allograft rejection in rodents have failed to do so in large animal models and man. Activity in dogs has proven to be a useful predictor of efficacy in humans. We were therefore pleased when studies in the laboratory of Dr. Hans Sollinger, University of Wisconsin, showed that MM was effective in the dog renal allograft model.[45] Monotherapy with MM (40 mg/kg per day) markedly prolonged graft survival, but combined therapy (MM 20 mg/kg per day, cyclosporin A 5 mg/kg per day and methylprednisolone 0.1 mg/kg per day) was more efficacious than either modality alone. There was no nephrotoxicity, hepatotoxicity, or bone marrow suppression. The only serious toxicity in the dog was in the small intestine, and may be attributable to the large volume of concentrated bile secreted by the dog; efficient enterohepatic recycling of MPA glucuronide exposes the intestine to high a concentration of the drug. Such intestinal toxicity is not observed in any other species of animal. Later studies showed that MM can reverse acute renal allograft rejection in dogs.[46] While treatment with steroid bolus therapy could only temporarily halt rejection in some dogs, MM reversed rejection and prevented subsequent rejection episodes.

These studies in experimental animals showed the efficacy of MM in preventing and treating allograft rejection without limiting toxicity or increased susceptibility to infections. They provided the experimental basis on which studies in human organ transplant recipients were undertaken.

EFFECTS OF MYCOPHENOLATE MOFETIL IN HUMANS

The pharmacokinetic profile showed that twice daily oral administration of MM provided immunosuppressive doses of MPA throughout the day and night in several experimental animals. Extensive toxicology studies showed that the drug is not mutagenic, does not produce chromosome aberrations, and does not have limiting toxicity even when given for long periods to nonhuman primates in higher doses than are required for human therapy.

An open-label study was undertaken in patients with severe rheumatoid arthritis not responsive to cyclooxygenase inhibitors, methotrexate, and long-acting antirheumatic drugs. Dose escalation studies showed that oral MM in doses up to 1.5 g twice daily was well tolerated, with no nephrotoxicity, hepatotoxicity, myelosuppression, or other limiting side effects. The principal side effect is gastrointestinal intolerance, not associated with erosion. Continued treatment with 1 g to 1.5 g MM twice daily induced remissions in two-thirds of rheumatoid arthritis patients,[47] which was maintained for more than one year;[8] infections were not limiting. Some clinical benefit was observed within two months of treatment, but the condition of most patients improved with further treatment between the third and fourth month, suggesting that immunosuppressive effects were being reinforced by long-acting antirheumatic activity, as predicted. A multicenter, placebo-controlled, double-blind trial of two doses of MM in patients with rheumatoid arthritis is in progress.

Several studies of MM in human recipients of organ transplants are in progress.[48] The preliminary findings are encouraging: in a triple regime with cyclosporine and low-dose steroids in renal allograft recipients, MM seems to be superior to azathioprine in preventing early rejection episodes (17% as compared with 60%). MM can reverse ongoing rejection in the majority of renal, cardiac, and hepatic allograft recipients even when high-dose steroids and OKT3 have been ineffective.[49]

Proliferative Arteriopathy Associated with Chronic Rejection

Now that acute rejection can be reasonably well controlled, chronic rejection is emerging as the major limitation of long-term allograft survival.[50,51] Chronic rejection is associated with a proliferative and obliterative arteriopathy, attributed to proliferation of smooth muscle cells and fibroblasts, first observed in small and medium-sized arteries and later throughout the arterial tree of transplanted hearts, kidneys, and livers.[52] The lesions in graft recipients are usually generalized, and the intimal thickening is concentric; whereas in the general population, atherosclerotic lesions tend to be focal and asymmetric and foam cells are more prominent. The pathogenesis of proliferative arteriopathy in grafts is complex: some authorities believe that it is predominantly mediated by T-lymphocytes,[53] others that antibodies against donor antigens play a pathogenetic role;[51] probably both humoral and cellular mechanisms are involved. Several growth factors could stimulate proliferation of smooth muscle cells in the neointima. For example, activated macrophages release IL-1β, IL-6, and platelet-derived growth factor. Activated endothelial cells release basic fibroblast growth factor, IL-6, and endothelins. It is therefore a better therapeutic strategy to inhibit the end result (proliferation of arterial smooth muscle cells) than to attempt to inhibit the production or effects of individual cytokines.

A major objective of transplantation immunologists is to define a therapy that prevents chronic as well as acute rejection. MPA inhibits T-lymphocytic responses, is a better inhibitor of antibody formation than cyclosporin, and, acting over a long period, reduces IL-1 production by macrophages. Perhaps more important, clinically

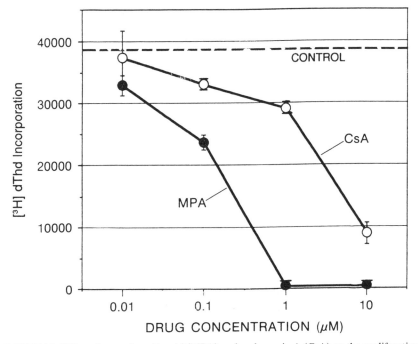

FIGURE 13. Effect of mycophenolic acid (MPA) and cyclosporin A (CsA) on the proliferation of human arterial smooth muscle cells in culture (J. Kowalski and A. C. Allison, unpublished).

attainable concentrations of MPA (1 to 10 μM) inhibit the proliferation of human arterial smooth muscle cells in culture (FIGURE 13). The dose-response curve is similar to that for fibroblasts and endothelial cells (FIGURE 5). Clinically attainable concentrations of cyclosporin and of brequinar do not inhibit smooth muscle cell proliferation. Similar results have been obtained by others;[54] the only other immuno-suppressive drug in development with this activity is rapamycin.[54]

The possibility that MM might be superior to currently used therapies for the prevention of chronic rejection was explored, using rat heterotropic heart allo-grafts.[44] In this model, moderate doses of cyclosporin A do not prevent arteriopathy, and low or moderate doses of FK506 prevent mononuclear cell infiltration of the myocardium but not graft coronary disease. Only a highly toxic dose of azathioprine was able to prevent arteriopathy in grafts examined one month after transplantation. Even in long-term recipients of MM, the incidence and severity of proliferative arteriopathy were low compared to that in recipients of other drugs.[44]

A rat aortic allograft model was also studied.[55] Three months after aortic allografting, the intima showed marked proliferation, which was not seen when syngeneic aortas were grafted. MM significantly decreased proliferation, whereas cyclosporine and brequinar did not. Accelerated proliferative vasculopathy has also been observed in primate cardiac xenografts (cynomolgus hearts into baboon recipients) maintained with cyclosporine, azathioprine, and methylprednisolone.[55] As discussed at this meeting, when MM was used instead of azathioprine in triple therapy, survival of cardiac xenografts was improved and the coronary arteries remained in good condition.

Thus, MM is so far unique among immunosuppressive drugs in clinical use for allograft recipients, in preventing arterial smooth muscle cell proliferation. Furthermore, the drug more effectively prevents proliferative arteriopathy in rat and primate allografts. What is found in rats and nonhuman primates may also be applicable to humans. If so, MM maintenance therapy may, by inhibiting proliferative arteriopathy, allow retention of allografts in good condition for long periods. This would be a useful contribution for several reasons, one being the shortage of organs available for transplantation.

Effects on B-Lymphocytes Transformed by Epstein-Barr Virus

It is well documented that in organ graft recipients, there is an increased incidence of non-Hodgkin's lymphomas.[4] In patients with rheumatoid arthritis receiving some immunosuppressive therapies, an excess of lymphomas is also observed.[5] The majority of malignancies in organ graft recipients are polyclonal B-cell lymphomas, and Epstein-Barr virus (EBV) driven proliferation of B-lymphocytes is widely accepted as playing a pathogenetic role.[57] EBV infects B-lymphocytes and induces them to proliferate; responding T-lymphocytes are able to lyse EBV-transformed B-lymphocytes in a genetically restricted fashion and to produce TNF and interferon-γ, which has antiviral activity.[6] Infectious mononucleosis is the overt form of this lymphoproliferation and resolution. Cyclosporine does not oppose proliferation of EBV-transformed B-lymphocytes but inhibits T-cell-mediated surveillance, thereby allowing polyclonal B-cell hyperproliferation.[6]

Transplant recipients receiving high-dose cyclosporin A have shown a spectrum of disorders ranging from benign polyclonal hyperplasias to frankly malignant B-lymphomas.[57] Some of the lymphomas have regressed following reduction of immunosuppressive therapy.[4,57] Reduced doses of cyclosporine in recent years have decreased lymphoma risk, not abolished it. With regard to the distinction between benign polyclonal B-cell hyperproliferation and frank lymphoma development, evidence has accumulated that chromosomal translocation, including *myc*/Ig translocation, favors the latter.[7,58] Thus simultaneous use of cyclosporine (which allows B-cell hyperproliferation) and of a drug that increases the frequency of chromosomal abnormalities could increase the probability of lymphoma development. Azathioprine is mutagenic,[9] and mizoribine (bredinin) induces chromosome breakage.[59] In contrast, MPA does not increase the incidence of point mutations or chromosome breaks in any of the situations studied.

We have investigated the effects of MPA, in clinically attainable concentrations (1 to 10 μM), on interactions of EBV and human B-lymphocytes.[60] Early events, including expression of EB nuclear antigen-2 and latent membrane protein-1, were unaffected. However, even 1 μM MPA inhibited the proliferation of newly infected or established EBV-transformed B-cell lines or of Burkitt lymphoma lymphoblasts in culture. Following withdrawal of MPA five days postinfection, long-term lymphoblastoid cells grew out, indicating that MPA was cytostatic, and did not block cell growth transformation. Further, MPA did not inhibit lytic EBV infection or late EBV gene expression. Thus in organ graft recipients, MPA would be expected to inhibit the proliferation of EBV-transformed B-lymphocytes, thereby decreasing the probability of late lymphoma development. In patients with lymphomas that have spread to the central nervous system, MPA would probably not provide any protection because of failure to pass the blood-brain carrier.

DIFFERENCES BETWEEN MM AND OTHER DRUGS INHIBITING PURINE SYNTHESIS

The most obvious comparisons are with azathioprine and with mizoribine, which has been used as an immunosuppressive in Japan. Both drugs inhibit purine synthesis, but the mechanisms involved are different. Azathioprine and 6-mercaptopurine (6-MP) are converted to the IMP analogue 6-thioinosinic acid, which inhibits several enzymes of purine synthesis: IMPDH, PRPP-amidotransferase, and adenylosuccinate synthetase.[61] In lymphocytes, 6-MP inhibits proliferation by depletion of adenosine rather than guanosine nucleotides; addition of adenosine restores lymphocyte proliferation.[27] An azathioprine metabolite is incorporated into DNA in the form of thioguanosine.[9] It is not surprising that azathioprine is mutagenic.[11] Inhibition by azathioprine is not reversed by either guanosine or adenosine, so that azathioprine metabolites are not selective inhibitors of IMPDH.[27] In head-to-head comparisons, MM is obviously more efficacious than azathioprine even when the latter is used in maximal tolerated doses, e.g., in treatment of ongoing rejection of cardiac allografts in rats,[40] and in the prevention of allograft rejection in humans.[48]

Mizoribine (bredinin) is an imidazole nucleoside, which when phosphorylated is a selective inhibitor or IMPDH.[62] Suppression of lymphocyte proliferation by mizoribine is reversed by guanosine except when concentrations of the drug are high, which suggests that there is reasonable selectivity for IMPDH.[27] However, the efficiency of phosphorylation of nucleosides can vary in different cell types,[22] and the importance of inhibition of IMPDH in monocytes, endothelial cells, and smooth muscle cells is obvious. Moreover, phosphorylated nucleosides can inhibit DNA repair mechanisms, which may explain why many chromosome breaks are observed in mizoribine-treated cells.[59] MPA does not require phosphorylation for activity, nor does it produce chromosome breaks. Thus, MPA has effects on the desired cell types and may have a better safety profile for long-term use than mizoribine.

FUTURE APPLICATIONS OF MYCOPHENOLATE MOFETIL

The observations in experimental animal and in human recipients of MM are converging to provide a guide to probable early clinical applications of the drug.

Cyclosporine Sparing

The nephrotoxicity and other side effects of cyclosporin A are well known. While these may be reduced to some extent by using the new cyclosporins, it is unlikely that they will be eliminated altogether. Any combination therapy that allows doses of cyclosporine to be lowered while preventing allograft rejection should decrease side effects. In several experimental animal models, including cardiac allografts in the rat[40,44] and kidney allografts in the dog,[45] combined therapy with MM allows doses of cyclosporine to be reduced while preventing allograft rejection. In humans, MM combined with cyclosporine and low-dose prednisone decreases the incidence of rejection to 17% in comparison with 60% in the absence of MM.[48] While it has not yet been formally shown that MM has cyclosporine-sparing effects, that is a likely prediction from the data now available.

Treatment of Ongoing Rejection

One of the remarkable properties of MM is its capacity to reverse ongoing rejection. This was demonstrated in several experimental animal models, including cardiac allografts in the rat[40] and renal allografts in the dog.[46] MM has now been used for the treatment of refractory rejection in more than 150 patients, including recipients of kidneys, heart, and liver allografts in a multicenter study. The overall rate of reversion is around 70%. Phase III trials for this indication are ongoing.

Maintenance Therapy of Organ Graft Recipients

A long-term application of MM would be for maintenance therapy of allografts, possibly as monotherapy or in combination with a low-dose glucocorticoid. MM has several advantages over cyclosporine for maintenance therapy of organ graft recipients. In experimental animals, allograft rejection can be prevented using MM alone. This has been demonstrated in several experimental animal models, e.g., pancreatic islet allografts in the mouse and cardiac allografts in rats.[40,44] Liver allografts in three humans have been retained in good functional condition using MM with low-dose prednisone but no cyclosporine; in a fourth patient, a low maintenance dose of cyclosporine was also given.[63]

The long-term benefits of maintenance therapy using MM without cyclosporine, or with a low dose of cyclosporine, are obvious. First is the reduced nephrotoxicity, hypertension, and other side effects of cyclosporine. Second is the decreased risk of proliferative arteriopathy associated with chronic rejection, where MM appears to have unique advantages. Third is the low risk of lymphoma development. Although the findings in experimental animals are strongly suggestive, careful examination of patients treated with MM over several years will be required to establish that extrapolation to humans is valid.

ACKNOWLEDGMENTS

Dr. Peter Nelson's chemical syntheses and the collaboration of our immunology staff (A. Mirkovich and S. Almquist) made the basic research program possible. Outside collaboration with Drs. H. Sollinger, K. Lafferty, and R. Morris showed the efficacy of the drug in transplantation models. Syntex experts in toxicology, formulation, clinical studies, and regulatory affairs were all essential for the later stages of the program. In particular, Dr. Robert Kauffman's supervision of the trials in human organ graft recipients and Dr. Ronald Goldblum's supervision of trials in rheumatoid arthritis patients are carrying the program to a successful conclusion. We are indebted to Dr. Caroline Alfieri for permission to quote observations on effects of MPA on interactions of EBV with B-lymphocytes.

REFERENCES

1. LEVINE, L. A. & D. F. JARRARD. 1993. Treatment of cyclophosphamide-induced hemorrhagic cystitis with intravesical carboprost tromethamine. J. Urol. **149:** 719–723.
2. BENNETT, W. M. & J. P. PULLIAM. 1983. Cyclosporine nephrotoxicity. Ann. Intern Med. **99:** 851–854.
3. JOLIVET, J., K. H. COWAN, G. A. CURT, N. J. CLENDENINN & B. A. CHABNER. 1983. The pharmacology and clinical use of methotrexate. N. Engl. J. Med. **309:** 1094–1104.
4. PENN, I. 1988. Tumors of the immunocompromised patient. Annu. Rev. Med. **39:** 63–73.
5. BAKER, G. L., L. E. KAHL & B. C. ZEE. 1987. Malignancy following treatment of rheumatoid arthritis with cyclophosphamide: a long-term case-control follow-up study. Am. Med. **83:** 1–9.
6. RICKINSON, A. B., M. ROWE, I. J. HART, Q. Y. YAO, L. E. HENDERSON, H. ROBIN & M. A. EPSTEIN. 1984. T-cell-mediated regression of "spontaneous" and Epstein-Barr virus-induced B-cell transformation *in vitro:* studies with cyclosporin A. Cell. Immunol. **87:** 646–658.
7. KLEIN, G. & E. KLEIN. 1989. How one thing has led to another. Annu. Rev. Immunol. **7:** 1–34.
8. CLARKE, L. & D. J. WAXMAN. 1989. Oxidative metabolism of cyclophosphamide: identification of the hepatic monooxygenase catalysts of drug activation. Cancer Res. **49:** 2344–2450.
9. ELION, G. B. 1989. The purine path to chemotherapy. Science **244:** 41–47.
10. DE NEVE, W., F. VALERIOTE, M. EDELSTEIN, C. EVERETT & M. BISCHOFF. 1989. *In vitro* DNA cross-linking by cyclophosphamide: comparison of human chronic lymphocytic leukemia cells with mouse L1210 leukemia and normal bone marrow cells. Cancer Res. **49:** 3452–3456.
11. HERLIA, P., L. MURELLI, M. SCOTTI, M. PAOLINI & G. CANTELLI-FONTI. 1988. Organ specific activation of azathioprine in mice: role of liver metabolism in mutation induction. Carcinogenesis **9:** 1011–1023.
12. HIRATA, S., T. MATSUHARA, R. SAURA, H. TATEISHI & K. HIROHATA. 1989. Inhibition of *in vitro* vascular endothelial cell proliferation and *in vivo* vascularization by low-dose methotrexate. Arthritis Rheum. **32:** 1065–1073.
13. STRYER, L. 1988. Biosynthesis of nucleotides. *In* Biochemistry. 3rd edit.: 602– 626. W. H. Freeman. New York, N.Y.
14. GARCIA, R. C., P. LEONI & A. C. ALLISON. 1977. Control of phosphoribosyl pyrophosphate synthesis in human lymphocytes. Biochem. Biophys. Res. Commun. **77:** 1067–1073.
15. GIBLETT, E. R., J. E. ANDERSON, F. COHEN & H. J. MEUWISSEN. 1972. Adenosine deaminase deficiency of two patients with severely impaired cellular immunity. Lancet **2:** 1067–1069.
16. ALLISON, A. C., T. HOVI, R. W. E. WATTS & A. D. B. WEBSTER. 1975. Immunological observations on patients with the Lesch-Nyhan syndrome, and on the role of *de novo* purine synthesis in lymphocyte transformation. Lancet **2:** 1179–1183.
17. ALLISON, A. C., T. HOVI, W. E. WATTS & A. D. B. WEBSTER. 1977. The role of *de novo* purine synthesis in lymphocyte transformation. Ciba Found. Symp. Purine Pyrimidine Metab. **48:** 207–223.
18. HOVI, T., A. C. ALLISON & J. ALLSOP. 1975. Rapid increase of phosphoribosyl pyrophosphate concentration after mitogenic stimulation of lymphocytes. FEBS Lett. **55:** 291–293.
19. HOVI, T., A. C. ALLISON, O. RAIVIO & A. VAHERI. 1977. Purine metabolism and control of cell proliferation. Ciba Found. Symp. Purine Pyrimidine Metab. **48:** 225–248.
20. NATSUMEDA, Y. & S. F. CARR. Human type I and II IMPDH as drug targets. Ann. N.Y. Acad. Sci. (This volume.)
21. PETERS, G. J., A. OOSTERHOF & J. H. VERKAMP. 1982. Effects of adenosine and

deoxyadenosine on PHA-stimulation of lymphocytes of man, horse and pig. Int. J. Biochem. **14:** 377–385.

22. RICHMAN, D. D., R. S. KORNBLUTH & D. A. CARSON. 1987. Failure of dideoxynucleosides to inhibit IIIV replication in cultured human macrophages. J. Exp. Med. **166:** 1144–1149.

23. FRANKLIN, T. J. & J. M. COOK. 1969. The inhibition of nucleic acid synthesis by mycophenolic acid. Biochem. J. **113:** 515–524.

24. LEE, W. A., L. GU, R. MIKSZTAL, N. CHU, K. LEUNG & P. H. NELSON. 1990. Bioavailability improvement of mycophenolic acid through amino ester derivitization. Pharm. Res. **7:** 161–166.

25. EUGUI, E. M., S. ALMQUIST, C. D. MULLER & A. C. ALLISON. 1991. Lymphocyte-selective cytostatic and immunosuppressive effects of mycophenolic acid *in vitro:* role of deoxyguanosine nucleotide depletion. Scand. Immunol. **33:** 161–173.

26. ALLISON, A. C., S. J. ALMQUIST, C. D. MULLER & E. M. EUGUI. 1991. *In vitro* immunosuppressive effects of mycophenolic acid and an ester prodrug. RS-16443. Transplant. Proc. **23**(Suppl. 2): 10–14.

27. DAYTON, J. S., L. A. TURKA, C. B. THOMPSON & B. S. MITCHELL. 1992. Comparison of the effects of mizoribine with those of azathioprine, 6-mercaptopurine, and mycophenolic acid on T-lymphocyte proliferation and purine ribonucleotide metabolism. Mol. Pharmacol. **41:** 671–676.

28. LAWRENCE, M. B. & J. A. SPRINGER. 1991. Leukocytes roll on a selectin at physiologic flow rates: distinction from and prerequisite for adhesion through integrins. Cell **65:** 859–865.

29. LASKY, L. A. 1992. Selectins: interpreters of cell-specific carbohydrate information during inflammation. Science **258:** 964–969.

30. ALTMANN, D. M., N. HOGG, J. TROWSDALE & D. WILKINSON. 1989. Cotransfection of ICAM-1 and HLA-DR reconstitutes human antigen-presenting function in mouse L cells. Nature Lond. **338:** 512–514.

31. GREGORY, C. D., R. J. MURRAY, C. F. EDWARDS & A. B. RICKINSON. 1988. Downregulation of cell adhesion molecules LFA-3 and ICAM-1 in Epstein-Barr virus–positive Burkitt's lymphoma underlies tumor cell escape from virus-specific T cell surveillance. J. Exp. Med. **167:** 1811–1824.

32. ISOBE, M., H. YAGITA, K. OKUMURA & A. IHARA. 1992. Specific acceptance of cardiac allograft after treatment with antibodies to ICAM-1 and LFA-1. Science **255:** 1125–1127.

33. KORNFELD, R. & S. KORNFELD. 1980. Structure of glycoproteins and their oligosaccharide units. *In* Biochemistry of Glycoproteins and Proteoglycans W. J. Lennarz, Ed.: 1– 137. Plenum. New York, N.Y.

34. ALLISON, A. C., W. J. KOWALSKI, C. J. MULLER, R. V. WATERS & E. M. EUGUI. 1993. Mycophenolic acid and brequinar inhibitors of purine and pyrimidine synthesis, block the glycosylation of adhesion molecular. Transplant. Proc. **47:** 67–70.

35. ELICES, M., L. OSBORN, Y. TAKADA, C. CRAUSE, S. LUHOWSKY, M. HEMLER & R. R. LOBB. 1990. VCAM-1 on activated endothelium interacts with the leukocyte integrin VLA-4 at a site distinct from the fibronectin binding site. Cell **60:** 577–584.

36. RADEMACHER, T. W., R. B. PAREKH & R. A. DWEK. 1988. Glycobiology. Annu. Rev. Biochem. **57:** 785–838.

37. LARSEN, E., T. PALABRICA, S. SAJER, G. E. GILLBERT, D. D. WAGNER, B. C. FURIE & B. FURIE. 1990. PADGEM-dependent adhesion of platelets to monocytes and neutrophils is mediated by lineage-specific carbohydrate, LNFIII (CD15). Cell **63:** 465–475.

38. TIEMEYER, M., S. J. SWLEDLER, M. ISHIHARA, M. MORELAND, H. SCHWEINGRUBER, P. HIRTZER & B. K. BRADLEY. 1991. Carbohydrate ligands for endothelial leukocyte adhesion molecule 1. Proc. Natl. Acad. Sci. USA **88:** 1138–1142.

39. EUGUI, E. M., A. MIRKOVICH & A. C. ALLISON. 1991. Lymphocyte-selective antiproliferative and immunosuppressive effects of mycophenolic acid in mice. Scand. Immunol. **33:** 175–183.

40. MORRIS, R. E., E. G. HOYT, M. P. MURPHY, E. M. EUGUI & A. C. ALLISON. 1990. Mycophenolic acid morpholinoethylester (RS-61443) is a new immunosuppressant that

prevents and halts heart allograft rejection by selective inhibition of T- and B-cell purine synthesis. Transplant. Proc. **22**: 1659–1662.

41. ROSENBERG, A. S. & A. SINGER. 1992. Cellular basis of skin graft rejection: an *in vivo* model of immune-mediated tissue destruction. Annu. Rev. Immunol. **10**: 333–358.

42. BRUNNER, K. T., J. MAUEL, J. C. CERROTINI & B. CHAPUIS. 1968. Quantitative assay of the lytic interaction of murine lymphoma cells on ^{51}Cr-labelled allogeneic target cells *in vivo*: inhibition by isoantibody and drugs. J. Immunol. **14**: 181–196.

43. JERNE, N. K. & A. A. NORDIN. 1963. Plaque formation in agar by single antibody-producing cells. Science **140**: 405–407.

44. MORRIS, R. E., J. WANG, J. R. BLUM, T. FLAVIN, M. P. MURPHY, S. J. ALMQUIST, N. CHU, Y. L. TAM, M. KALOOSTIAN, A. C. ALLISON & E. M. EUGUI. 1991. Immunosuppressive effects of the morpholinoethyl ester of mycophenolic acid (RS-61443) in rat and nonhuman primate recipients of heart allografts. Transplant. Proc. **23**(Suppl. 2): 19–25.

45. PLATZ, K. P., H. W. SOLLINGER, D. A. HULLETT, D. E. ECKHOFF, E. M. EUGUI & A. C. ALLISON. 1990. RS-61443, a new, potent immunosuppressive agent. Transplantation **51**: 27–31.

46. PLATZ, K. P., D. E. ECKHOFF, W. O. BECHSTEIN, Y. SUZUKI & H. W. SOLLINGER. 1991. RS-61443 for reversal of acute rejection in canine renal allografts. Surgery **110**: 736–741.

47. SCHIFF, M. H., R. GOLDBLUM & M. M. C. REES. 1990. 2-Morpholino-ethyl mycophenolic acid (ME-MPA) in the treatment of refractory rheumatoid arthritis (RA). Arthritis Rheum. **33**: s-155.

48. SOLLINGER, H. W., M. H. DEIERHOI, F. O. BELZER, A. DIETHELM & R. S. KAUFFMAN. 1992. RS-61443—a phase I clinical trial and pilot rescue study. Transplantation **53**: 428–432.

49. SOLLINGER, H. W., F. O. BELZER, M. H. DEIERHOI, *et al.* 1993. RS-61443 (mycophenolate mofetil). A multicenter study for refractory kidney transplant rejection. Am. Surg. **216**: 513–516.

50. FOSTER, M. C., P. W. WENHAM, P. A. ROWE, R. P. BERDEN, A. G. MORGAN, R. E. COTTON & R. W. BLAMEY. 1989. The later results of renal transplantation and the importance of chronic rejection as a cause of graft loss. Ann. R. Coll. Surg. Engl. **71**: 44–47.

51. PALMER, D. C., C. C. TSAI, S. T. ROODMAN, J. E. CODD, L. W. MILLER, J. E. SAFARIAN & G. A. WILLIAMS. 1985. Heart graft atherosclerosis. Transplantation **39**: 385–392.

52. FOEGH, M. L. 1990. Chronic rejection-graft arteriosclerosis. Transplant. Proc. **22**: 119–122.

53. BILLINGHAM, M. E. 1989. Graft coronary disease: the lesions and the patients. Transplant. Proc. **21**: 3665–3666.

54. GREGORY, C. R., R. E. PRATT, P. HUIE, R. SHORTHOUSE, V. J. DZAU, M. E. BILLINGHAM & R. E. MORRIS. 1993. Effects of treatment with cyclosporine, FK506, rapamycin, mycophenolic acid, or deoxyspergaulin on vascular muscle proliferation *in vitro* and *in vivo*. Transplant. Proc. **25**: 770–771.

55. STEELE, D. M., D. A. HULLETT, W. O. BECHSTEIN, W. J. KOWALSKI, L. S. SMITH, F. KENNEDY, A. C. ALLISON & H. W. SOLLINGER. 1993. Effects of immunosuppressive therapy in the rat aortic allograft model. Transplant. Proc. **25**: 754–755.

56. MCMANUS, R. P., D. P. O'HAIR, J. B. HUNTER & R. KAMAROWSKI. 1992. Spectrum of vascular changes in primate cardiac xenografts. Transplant. Proc. **24**: 619–623.

57. HANTO, D. W., K. J. GAJL-PECZALSKIA, G. FRIZZERA, *et al.* 1983. Epstein-Barr virus (EBV)-induced polyclonal B-cell lymphoproliferative diseases occurring after renal transplantation. Clinical, pathological and virologic findings and implications for therapy. Am. Surg. **193**: 356–369.

58. KORSMEYER, S. S. 1992. Chromosomal translocations in lymphoid malignancies reveal novel protooncogenes. Annu. Rev. Immunol. **10**: 785–808.

59. SAKAGUCHI, K., M. TSUJINO & M. YOSHIZAWA. 1975. Action of bredinin on mammalian cells. Cancer Res. **35**: 1643–1648.

60. ALFIERI, C., A. C. ALLISON & E. KIEFFE. Effect of mycophenolic acid on Epstein-Barr virus infection of human B-lymphocytes. Antimicrob. Agents Chemother. (Submitted.)

61. WOLBERG, G. 1988. Antipurines and purine metabolism. Handbook Exp. Pharm. **85**: 517–533.

62. KOYAMA, H. & M. TSUJI. 1983. Genetic and biochemical studies on the activation and cytotoxic mechanism of bredinin, a potent inhibitor of purine biosynthesis in mammalian cells. Biochem. Pharmacol. **32:** 35–47.
63. FREISE, C. E., M. HEBERT, R. W. OSORIO, B. NIKOLAI, J. R. LAKE, R. S. KAUFFMAN & J. P. ROBERTS. 1993. Maintenance immunosuppression with prednisolone and RS-61443 alone following liver transplantation. Transplant. Proc. **25:** 1758–1759.

Human Type I and II IMP Dehydrogenases as Drug Targets

YUTAKA NATSUMEDA[a] AND STEPHEN F. CARR

Institute of Biochemistry and Cell Biology
Syntex Discovery Research
3401 Hillview Avenue
Palo Alto, California 94303

INTRODUCTION

IMP dehydrogenase (IMPDH; EC 1.1.1.205) catalyzes the conversion of IMP to XMP at the IMP metabolic branch point in the *de novo* purine nucleotide synthetic pathway. The activity of IMPDH and channeling of IMP into *de novo* guanylate synthesis in cells have been shown to be enhanced in a manner that is closely linked with cell proliferation.[1,2] IMPDH has proven to be a target for anticancer, antiviral, antiparasitic, and immunosuppressive chemotherapy.[3-6] The mechanism of action of IMPDH inhibitors has been attributed to the decrease in intracellular concentrations of guanine nucleotides, especially GTP and dGTP in the target cells.[3,4,7-9] Human IMPDH was regarded as a single molecular species until the recent discovery of two isoforms derived from different genes.[10] The discoveries of IMPDH isoforms and of their differential regulation during neoplastic transformation, lymphocyte activation, and cancer cell differentiation have attracted attention as a possible novel basis for isozyme-selective chemotherapy.[10-13] This review compares the properties of human type I and type II IMPDHs from the standpoint of drug targeting.

STRIKING DIFFERENCES IN THE EXPRESSION OF IMPDH ISOFORMS

Northern blot analyses using specific cDNA probes for type I and type II IMPDHs demonstrated that type I mRNA was the dominant species in human normal leukocytes and lymphocytes, whereas type II predominated over type I in human ovarian tumor cells, leukemic cell lines K562 and HL-60, and leukemic cells from patients with different types of leukemia.[10-13] The increase in type II mRNA expression positively correlated with an increase in IMPDH activity in these leukemic cells.[12] Moreover, a close linkage of the up regulation of type II IMPDH with cell proliferation was demonstrated in several different experimental systems. The low level of type II mRNA in normal lymphocytes was up regulated markedly by phytohemagglutinin stimulation or by Epstein-Barr viral transformation.[13] Conversely, the enhanced levels of type II IMPDH mRNA, protein, and total IMPDH activity in leukemic cells and melanoma cells were down regulated during differentiation induced by retinoic acid, 12-*O*-tetradecanoylphorbol-13-acetate or dimethyl sulfoxide.[12-17] By contrast, type I IMPDH mRNA was constitutively expressed in the various states of cell proliferation and differentiation.[12,13] Enhanced expression of type II IMPDH was also demonstrated in solid tumors and cancer cell lines at mRNA and protein levels.[11,18]

[a]Present affiliation: Schering-Plough K.K., 2-3-7 Hiranomachi, Chuo-ku, Osaka 541, Japan.

88

Differentiation of neoplastic cells is associated with the down regulation of type II IMPDH resulting in decreases in *de novo* GTP biosynthesis and intracellular concentrations of GTP. In fact, the activity of IMPDH decreased during differentiation induced by retinoic acid, even though retinoic acid did not directly inhibit IMPDH activity.[14] Moreover, inhibitors of IMPDH that directly blocked *de novo* GTP biosynthesis strongly induced differentiation of various kinds of neoplastic cells.[7,8,13,14,16,17] The decrease in concentrations of GTP in the cells was demonstrated to be critical in differentiation induced by an IMPDH inhibitor such as mycophenolic acid, tiazofurin, or selenazofurin: exogenous guanine or guanosine, a precursor for salvage synthesis of GMP, restored the GTP pools and blocked the differentiation.[7,8,14] However, the mechanisms involved in differentiation induced by retinoic acid or dimethyl sulfoxide seemed to be different from that resulting from IMPDH inhibition: exogenous guanosine failed to block differentiation.[8,14] When the cells were treated with an IMPDH inhibitor, type II IMPDH expression changed in a biphasic fashion. Since type II IMPDH expression is inversely regulated by intracellular guanine nucleotide concentrations,[19] the inhibition of IMPDH, which was

TABLE 1. Expression of Human Type I and Type II IMPDHs during Cell Proliferation and Differentiation[a]

	IMPDH Isoforms	
Cell Types and Conditions	Type I	Type II
Normal lymphocytes		
Phytohemagglutinin stimulation	No change	Up
Epstein-Barr viral transformation	No change	Up
Cancer cells		
Induction of differentiation	No change	Down
Depletion of intracellular GTP		
(Early response)	No change	Up
(Late response, differentiation)	No change	Down
Expansion of intracellular GTP	No change	Down

[a]In mature normal lymphocytes, type I IMPDH is the dominant species. However, in actively proliferating cancer cells, type II predominates over type I. Up and Down indicate up regulation and down regulation, respectively.

followed by depletion of guanine nucleotides, initially up regulated type II IMPDH.[13,16,17] Subsequently, the type II isoform was down regulated during differentiation with retardation of cell proliferation.[13,16,17] However, the steady-state level of type I IMPDH mRNA remained constant.[13] The expression levels of type I and type II IMPDHs during cell proliferation and differentiation are summarized in TABLE 1.

STRUCTURAL DIFFERENCES AND SIMILARITIES BETWEEN IMPDH ISOFORMS

Human type I and type II IMPDH cDNAs encode the same size proteins of 514 amino acids with 84% sequence identity.[10] Human type II IMPDH has a similar primary structure to mouse and chinese hamster IMPDHs in which only 6 and 7 amino acids are replaced, respectively.[10,20,21] The difference between the human type I and type II IMPDH sequences is much more extensive: 84 out of 514 amino acids are substituted.[10] Out of the 84 amino acid changes, 52 are conservative substitutions and 32 diverge with respect to their chemical properties.[10]

The consensus nucleotide-binding motif of β-α-β has been predicted in *Escherichia coli* IMPDH on the basis of steric and physicochemical properties of amino acids from pattern searches of protein-sequence databases.[22] The domains are located from Asp-319 to Lys-349 in human IMPDHs, and the sequences are well conserved in IMPDHs from seven different species reported (FIGURE 1).[10,20,21,23,24] The nucleotide-binding domain includes a cysteine which is the only sulfhydryl group conserved in the seven different sequences (FIGURE 1). It is interesting to note that the IMP binding site has been suggested to include a thiol group, which reacts with 6-chloro-IMP to form a thioether bond with C-6 of the purine ring, and thereby inactivates IMPDH, as shown for the bacterial and mammalian enzymes.[25,26]

Human I	DGLRV**GMGCGSIC**I**C**ITQE**V**MAC**GRPQ**G**TA**VYK
Human II	DALRV**GMGSGSIC**I**C**ITQE**V**LAC**GRPQ**A**TA**VYK
Mouse	DALRV**GMGSGSIC**I**C**ITQE**V**LAC**GRPQ**A**TA**VYK
Hamster	DALRV**GMGCGSIC**I**C**ITQE**V**LAC**GRPQ**A**TA**VYK
L. donovani	DGIRI**GMGSGSIC**I**C**ITQE**V**LAC**GRPQ**A**TA**VYK
B. subtilis	DVVKV**GIGPGSIC**T**C**TRV**V**AGV**GV**P**QITA**IYD
E. coli	SAVKV**GIGPGSIC**T**C**TRI**V**TGV**GV**P**QITA**VAD

FIGURE 1. Consensus nucleotide-binding motif of β-α-β in seven different IMPDHs. The segment was first predicted in *E. coli* IMPDH by Bork and Grunwald.[22] Amino acid residues shown in bold are conserved in IMPDHs from seven different species. The underlined Cys is the only cysteine residue conserved in the sequences of seven different IMPDHs.

KINETIC PROPERTIES OF HUMAN TYPE I AND II IMPDHs

In our preliminary attempts to purify human type I and type II IMPDHs from native sources, we encountered difficulties in separating the two isoforms. Therefore, to compare kinetic properties, the respective human IMPDHs were expressed as recombinant nonfusion proteins in *E. coli*.[32] To avoid contamination by the endogenous *E. coli* IMPDH, the enzymes were expressed in an IMPDH-deficient strain, H712, and purified to homogeneity, as judged by sodium dodecyl sulfate-polyacrylamide gel electrophoresis (SDS-PAGE). The final enzyme preparations were also homogeneous under nondenaturing conditions and constituted a tetrameric structure, as judged by glycerol gradient centrifugation. We also found that the lacZ'-IMPDH fusion proteins expressed and purified under the same conditions included a monomeric form and many different sizes of aggregated forms in addition to a tetramer. The tetrameric quaternary structure of the nonfusion human IMPDHs expressed in *E. coli* is identical to that of IMPDH purified from rat hepatoma 3924A.[27]

In the studies using the recombinant nonfusion enzymes, human type I and type II IMPDHs both exhibited an ordered Bi-Bi mechanism in which IMP binds to the free enzyme first, followed by NAD. After the formation of products, NADH is released followed by XMP, as proposed previously in studies with IMPDHs purified from various different sources.[27–30] Both IMPDH isoforms showed similar affinities for the substrates. K_m values for type I and type II IMPDHs were 18 and 9 μM, respectively, for IMP, and 46 and 32 μM, respectively, for NAD. Sensitivities to inhibition by the products, NADH and XMP, were also similar for the two isoforms. The K_i values of type I and II IMPDHs were 102 and 90 μM, respectively, for NADH, and 80 and 94 μM, respectively, for XMP. The IMPDH isoforms also had similar turnover numbers at 37°C of approximately 1 mol transformed/second per mol of enzyme subunit. The pH profiles of the isoforms were slightly shifted relative to one another with pH optima of 7.7 and 7.9 for type I and type II, respectively.

DIFFERENT SENSITIVITIES OF HUMAN IMPDH ISOFORMS TO MYCOPHENOLIC ACID

The striking differences in type I and type II IMPDH gene expression suggest that the two isoforms may play different biological roles in *de novo* guanine nucleotide synthesis and have different regulatory mechanisms. Also, the proliferation-linked expression of the type II isoform suggests that development of type-II-specific drugs may provide improved selectivity against target cells in anticancer and immunosuppressive chemotherapy.

The inhibitiory effects by mycophenolic acid, an immunosuppressive agent, were also compared with the recombinant nonfusion human IMPDHs. Mycophenolic acid inhibited noncompetitively with respect to each substrate, IMP and NAD, suggesting that mycophenolic acid binds to the enzyme after a ternary complex is formed of enzyme, IMP, and NAD. This inhibitory mechanism was the same for both isoforms. However, type II IMPDH (K_i = 9.5 nM) was 3.9-fold more sensitive to mycophenolic acid than the type I isoform (K_i = 37 nM). The selective inhibition of type II IMPDH may explain in part the relatively mild side effects of mycophenolate mofetil, a prodrug of mycophenolic acid, observed in phase I clinical trials.[31]

REFERENCES

1. NATSUMEDA, Y., T. IKEGAMI, K. MURAYAMA & G. WEBER. 1988. *De novo* guanylate synthesis in the commitment to replication in hepatoma 3924A cells. Cancer Res. **48:** 507–511.
2. JACKSON, R. C., G. WEBER & H. P. MORRIS. 1975. IMP dehydrogenase, an enzyme linked with proliferation and malignancy. Nature **256:** 331–333.
3. TRICOT, G. J., H. N. JAYARAM, E. LAPIS, Y. NATSUMEDA, C. R. NICHOLS, P. KNEEBONE, N. HEEREMA, G. WEBER & R. HOFFMAN. 1989. Biochemically directed therapy of leukemia with tiazofurin, a selective blocker of inosine 5'-phosphate dehydrogenase activity. Cancer Res. **49:** 3696–3701.
4. STREETER, D. G., J. T. WITKOWSKI, G. P. KHARE, R. W. SIDWELL, R. J. BAUER, R. K. ROBINS & L. N. SIMON. 1973. Mechanism of action of 1-β-D-ribofuranosyl-1,2,4-triazole-3-carboxamide (Virazole), a new broad spectrum antiviral agent. Proc. Natl. Acad. Sci. USA **70:** 1174–1178.
5. WANG, C. C., R. VERHAM, H.-W. CHEN, A. RICE & A. L. WANG. 1984. Differential effects of inhibitors of purine metabolism on two trichomonad species. Biochem. Pharmacol. **33:** 1323–1329.
6. NELSON, P. H., E. EUGUI, C. C. WANG & A. C. ALLISON. 1990. Synthesis and immunosuppressive activity of some side-chain variants of mycophenolic acid. J. Med. Chem. **33:** 833–835.
7. OLAH, E., Y. NATSUMEDA, T. IKEGAMI, Z. KOTE, M. HORANYI, J. SZELENYI, E. PAULIK, T. KREMMER, S. R. HOLLAN, J. SUGAR & G. WEBER. 1988. Induction of erythroid differentiation and modulation of gene expression by tiazofurin in K-562 leukemia cells. Proc. Natl. Acad. Sci. USA **85:** 6533–6537.

8. SOKOLOSKI, J. A., O. C. BLAIR & A. C. SARTORELLI. 1986. Alterations in glycoprotein synthesis and guanosine triphosphate levels associated with the differentiation of HL-60 leukemia cells produced by inhibitors of inosine 5'-phosphate dehydrogenase. Cancer Res. **46:** 2314–2319.

9. LUI, M. S., M. A. FADERAN, J. J. LIEPNIEKS, Y. NATSUMEDA, E. OLAH, H. N. JAYARAM & G. WEBER. 1984. Modulation of IMP dehydrogenase activity and guanylate metabolism by tiazofurin (2-β-D-ribofuranosylthiazole-4-carboxamide). J. Biol. Chem. **259:** 5078–5082.

10. NATSUMEDA, Y., S. OHNO, H. KAWASAKI, Y. KONNO, G. WEBER & K. SUZUKI. 1990. Two distinct cDNAs for human IMP dehydrogenase. J. Biol. Chem. **265:** 5292–5295.

11. KONNO, Y., Y. NATSUMEDA, M. NAGAI, Y. YAMAJI, S. OHNO, K. SUZUKI & G. WEBER. 1991. Expression of human IMP dehydrogenase types I and II in *Escherichia coli* and distribution in human normal lymphocytes and leukemic cell lines. J. Biol. Chem. **266:** 506–509.

12. NAGAI, M., Y. NATSUMEDA, Y. KONNO, R. HOFFMAN, S. IRINO & G. WEBER. 1991. Selective up-regulation of type II inosine 5'-monophosphate dehydrogenase messenger RNA expression in human leukemias. Cancer Res. **51:** 3886–3890.

13. NAGAI, M., Y. NATSUMEDA & G. WEBER. 1992. Proliferation-linked regulation of type II IMP dehydrogenase gene in human normal lymphocytes and HL-60 leukemic cells. Cancer Res. **52:** 258–261.

14. YAMAJI, Y., Y. NATSUMEDA, Y. YAMADA, S. IRINO & G. WEBER. 1990. Synergistic action of tiazofurin and retinoic acid on differentiation and colony formation of HL-60 leukemia cells. Life Sci. **46:** 435–442.

15. COLLART, F. C. & E. HUBERMAN. 1990. Expression of IMP dehydrogenase in differentiating HL-60 cells. Blood **75:** 570–576.

16. KIGUCHI, K., F. R. COLLART, C. HENNING-CHUBB & E. HUBERMAN. 1990. Induction of cell differentiation in melanoma cells by inhibitors of IMP dehydrogenase: altered patterns of IMP dehydrogenase expression and activity. Cell Growth Differ. **1:** 259–270.

17. KIGUCHI, K., F. R. COLLART, C. HENNING-CHUBB & E. HUBERMAN. 1990. Cell differentiation and altered IMP dehydrogenase expression induced in human T-lymphoblastoid leukemia cells by mycophenolic acid and tiazofurin. Exp. Cell Res. **187:** 47–53.

18. COLLART, F. R., C. B. CHUBB, B. L. MIRKIN & E. HUBERMAN. 1992. Increased inosine-5'-phosphate dehydrogenase gene expression in solid tumor tissues and tumor cell lines. Cancer Res. **52:** 5826–5828.

19. GLESNE, D. A., F. R. COLLART & E. HUBERMAN. 1991. Regulation of IMP dehydrogenase gene production by its end products, guanine nucleotides. Mol. Cell. Biol. **11:** 5417–5425.

20. COLLART, F. R. & E. HUBERMAN. 1988. Cloning and sequence analysis of the human and chinese hamster inosine-5'-monophosphate dehydrogenase cDNAs. J. Biol. Chem. **263:** 15769–15772.

21. TIEDEMAN, A. T. & J. M. SMITH. 1991. Isolation and sequence of a cDNA encoding mouse IMP dehydrogenase. Gene **97:** 289–293.

22. BORK, P. & C. GRUNWALD. 1990. Recognition of different nucleotide-binding sites in primary structures using a property-pattern approach. Eur. J. Biochem. **191:** 347–358.

23. WILSON, K., F. R. COLLART, E. HUBERMAN, J. R. STRINGER & B. ULLMAN. 1991. Amplification and molecular cloning of the IMP dehydrogenase gene of *Leishmania donovani.* J. Biol. Chem. **266:** 1665–1671.

24. KANZAKI, N. & K. MIYAGAWA. 1990. Nucleotide sequence of the *Bacillus subtilis* IMP dehydrogenase gene. Nucleic Acids Res. **18:** 6710.

25. BROX, L. W. & A. HAMPTON. 1968. Inosine 5'-phosphate dehydrogenase. Kinetic mechanism and evidence for selective reaction of the 6-chloro analog of inosine 5'-phosphate with a cysteine residue at the inosine 5'-phosphate site. Biochemistry **7:** 2589–2596.

26. ANDERSON, J. H. & A. C. SARTORELLI. 1969. Inhibition of inosinic acid dehydrogenase by 6-chloropurine nucleotide. Biochem. Pharmacol. **18:** 2737–2745.

27. YAMADA, Y., Y. NATSUMEDA & G. WEBER. 1988. Action of the active metabolites of tiazofurin and ribavirin on purified IMP dehydrogenase. Biochemistry **27:** 2193–2196.

28. ANDERSON, J. H. & A. C. SARTORELLI. 1968. Inosinic acid dehydrogenase of sarcoma 180 cells. J. Biol. Chem. **243:** 4762–4768.

29. HOLMES, E. W., D. M. PEHLKE & W. N. KELLEY. 1974. Human IMP dehydrogenase,
     kinetics and regulatory properties. Biochim. Biophys. Acta **364**: 209–217.
30. HUPE, D. J., B. A. AZZOLINA & N. D. BEHRENS. 1986. IMP dehydrogenase from the
     intracellular parasitic protozoan *Eimeria tenella* and its inhibition by mycophenolic acid.
     J. Biol. Chem. **261**: 8363–8369.
31. DEIERHOI, M. H., H. W. SOLLINGER, A. G. DIETHELM, F. O. BELZER & R. S. KAUFFMAN.
     1993. One-year follow-up results of a phase I trial of mycophenolate mofetil (RS61443)
     in cadaveric renal transplantation. Transplant. Proc. **25**: 693–694.
32. CARR, S. F., E. PAPP, J. WU & Y. NATSUMEDA. Characterization of human type I and type
     II IMP dehydrogenases. J. Biol. Chem. **268**. (In press.)

Immunosuppression by Discodermolide

ROSS E. LONGLEY,[a] SARATH P. GUNASEKERA,[a]
DENISE FAHERTY,[b] JOHN MCLANE,[b]
AND FRANCIS DUMONT[c]

[a]Division of Biomedical Marine Research
Harbor Branch Oceanographic Institution
5600 U.S. No. 1, North
Fort Pierce, Florida 34946

[b]Department of Immunopharmacology
Hoffmann-LaRoche Inc.
340 Kingsland Street
Nutley, New Jersey 07110-1199

[c]Immunology Research
Merck Institute for Therapeutic Research
Merck Sharp & Dohme Research Laboratories
Rahway, New Jersey 07065-0900

INTRODUCTION

The discovery of novel immunomodulatory agents from natural product sources has been largely confined to the systematic screening of extracts obtained from terrestrial plants and microorganisms.[1-2] A few exceptions, notably didemnin B[3] and the bryostatins,[4] comprise the sum total experience of the discovery of immunosuppressive and immunostimulatory compounds derived from marine organisms. Recently, we described the *in vitro*[5] and *in vivo*[6] immunosuppressive activities of a novel compound, discodermolide, which was derived from a marine sponge, *Discodermia dissoluta,* and isolated following a bioassay guided approach.[7] The compound possessed potent *in vitro* immunosuppressive activity in both murine and human lymphocyte stimulation assays and demonstrated remarkable immunosuppression in an experimental model of graft vs. host disease (GVHR). In our efforts to begin to determine the exact mechanism of action by which discodermolide suppresses immune responsiveness, we discovered that the compound exerted antiproliferative activity toward a number of cell lines of different tissue types and origin. In the present article, we will summarize the work to date regarding discodermolide's immunosuppressive activity and we will describe the compound's ability to block proliferation in lymphoid and nonlymphoid cells and correlate the effect with changes we have observed in cell cycling patterns observed in T hybridoma cells treated with the compound.

INITIAL STUDIES DEMONSTRATING SUPPRESSION OF *IN VITRO* MURINE IMMUNE RESPONSES BY DISCODERMOLIDE

Discodermolide is a polyhydroxylated lactone which was isolated from the marine sponge *Discodermia dissoluta* using a bioassay-guided approach[7] (FIGURE 1). The pure compound suppressed the two-way murine mixed lymphocyte response

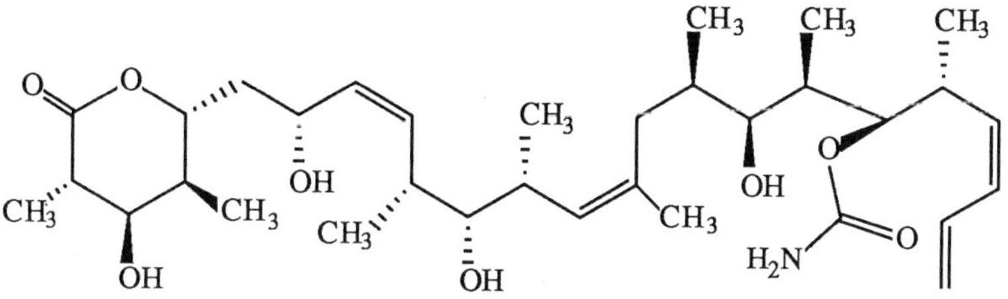

FIGURE 1. Molecular structure of discodermolide.

(MLR), concanavalin (Con A) stimulation of splenocytes, and the induction of proliferation of purified murine T cells by the combination of phorbol ester (PMA) and the calcium ionophore ionomycin at subnanomolar concentrations (TABLE 1). Discodermolide was not toxic to unstimulated lymphocytes at concentrations greater than 1.26 μM. Discodermolide had little to no effect on IL-2 production and no effect on IL-2 mRNA expression of PMA-ionomycin-stimulated T lymphocytes. In collaboration with Francis Dumont at Merck, we found that discodermolide was capable of inhibiting the proliferation of T cells induced by three distinct modes of activation (FIGURE 2). This effect of discodermolide is in contrast to what his laboratory originally reported for cyclosporin A (CsA) or FK506; both of which compounds suppress responses induced by Con A or PMA + ionomycin, but not that induced by IL-2 + PMA.[8]

As indicated above, while discodermolide had only a slight effect on IL-2 production of PMA-ionomycin-stimulated cells, the effects of the compound on the expression of the IL-2 receptor were more dramatic. Using the rat monoclonal antibody 7D4 (specific for the 55-kDa IL-2 receptor) and a fluorescently conjugated goat antirat immunoglobulin M (IgM), cells were stained for IL-2 receptor and examined using fluorescence microscopy. A high percentage of discodermolide-treated cells expressed "dim" fluorescence which quenched rapidly compared to non-drug-treated, positive controls and the negative (unstimulated) controls (TABLE 2). These cells also appeared to have already undergone "blast transformation," indicating activation had already taken place. The remaining 24% of these cells expressed a bright, partial to full ring fluorescence and were "blast"-like in appearance, similar to positive, activated controls. Subsequently, we examined similar 7D4 stained cultures that had been incubated with discodermolide, using flow cytometric analyses. The histogram in FIGURE 3 confirms our earlier microscopic observations in that both the total number and fluorescence intensity of discodermolide-treated cells expressing the 7D4 antibody were reduced compared to stimulated, non-drug-treated control cultures. These results suggest that discodermolide-treated cells have

TABLE 1. Effect of Discodermolide on *In Vitro* Murine Lymphocyte Responses

Assay	EC_{50}
MLR	0.240 μM
Concanvalin A (Con A)	0.190 μM
PMA-ionomycin	0.009 μM
Toxicity (to unstimulated lymphocytes)	> 1.26 μM
IL-2 production	Little to no effect
IL-2 mRNA expression	No effect

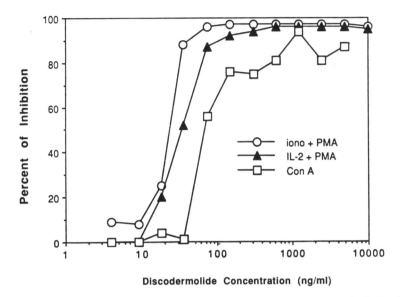

Discodermolide Concentration (ng/ml)

FIGURE 2. Effect of discodermolide on proliferative responses of murine splenic T cells. Mouse splenic T cells were purified by nylon wool column separation. Cell suspensions in RPMI 1640 medium supplemented with 10% fetal calf serum were placed as 0.2 ml/well aliquots in flat-bottom 96-well microculture plates. For Con A stimulation (5.0 μg/ml), cells were cultured at 1×10^6 cells/ml. For ionomycin (250 ng/ml) plus PMA (10 ng/ml) or IL-2 (100 U/ml) plus ionomycin, 5×10^5 cells/ml were cultured. Discodermolide was dissolved at 10 mg/ml in absolute ethanol and stored as 100-μl aliquots at −70°C until use. Plates were incubated for 3 days and 2 μCi of tritiated thymidine was added during the last 4 h of incubation. Cultures were harvested, and the incorporated radioactivity determined by liquid scintillation counting.

TABLE 2. Effect of Discodermolide on IL-2 Production and IL-2 Receptor Expression of Murine T Lymphocytes[a]

Culture[b]	Discodermolide	IL-2 (U/ml)[c]	IL-2 Receptor[d]	
T + PMA + ionomycin	−	68.9	+[e]	(94%)[f]
T + PMA + ionomycin	+	44.0	+,+/−	(24%), (76%)
T + PMA + CsA + ionomycin	−	4.0	+	(>99%)
T cells alone	−	<1.0	−	(<1%)

[a] Purified T lymphocytes were obtained by plastic adherence and nylon wool depletion.

[b] T lymphocytes (2.5×10^6) were incubated with PMA (12.4 ng/ml) and ionomycin (3.13 μg/ml), with or without discodermolide (0.08 μM) or CsA (0.08 μM) at 37°C for 24 h.

[c] Supernatants were analyzed for IL-2 production using the IL-2-independent cell line, CTLL-2. Results are expressed as units of IL-2 per milliliter (U/ml).

[d] Purified T-cells were stained for the IL-2 receptor using rat monoclonal antibody, 7D4 and fluorescein-conjugated goat anti-rat IgM.

[e] Bright ring fluorescence designated as "+;" Dull, rapidly quenching fluorescence designated as "+/−."

[f] Percentage of 7D4 positive cells.

a reduced density of the low-affinity, p55-associated IL-2 receptor and that an associated mechanism of action of discodermolide might include the modulation of such a receptor. This possibility is being further explored in our laboratory.

ADDITIONAL STUDIES ON THE IMMUNOSUPPRESSION OF *IN VITRO* MURINE IMMUNE RESPONSES BY DISCODERMOLIDE

In collaboration with Bill Benjamin, Denise Faherty, and John McLane at Hoffmann-LaRoche, discodermolide was evaluated in several murine immune re-

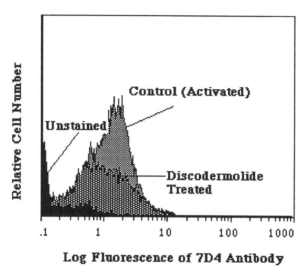

Log Fluorescence of 7D4 Antibody

FIGURE 3. Effect of discodermolide on IL-2 receptor expression of PMA-ionomycin stimulated murine T cells. Mouse splenic T cells were purified by nylon wool column separation. Cell suspensions in RPMI 1640 medium supplemented with 10% fetal calf serum and antibiotics were placed as 2 ml/well aliquots in flat-bottom 24-macrowell tissue culture plates in the presence of PMA (12.4 ng/ml) and ionomycin (0.313 mM), with or without discodermolide (0.080 μM) at 37°C for 48 h. Cells were collected and washed three times with tissue culture medium. The resulting cell pellet was adjusted to 1×10^6 cells/ml in phosphate-buffered saline with 0.01% sodium azide plus 1% fetal calf serum (PBS/FCS-azide) and stained with 5.0 μg of fluorescein conjugated anti-7D4 monoclonal antibody (Pharmingen) for 60 min at 4°C. Cells were washed three times with PBS/FCS-azide and resuspended in one ml of the solution. Cells were analyzed for green fluorescence using a Coulter EPICS ELITE flow cytometer with 488 nM excitation from a 10 mW argon laser. Dead cells were identified with propidium iodide and were gated out during the analyses. A total of 10,000 cells were analyzed for each group (control activated, discodermolide treated, and unstained activated).

sponse models, including stimulus-induced proliferative and cytokine secretion response assays. In addition, they examined antigen-specific and innate responses of freshly isolated splenocytes. The results of their study are presented in TABLE 3. Discodermolide suppressed the cytolytic responses of C57BL/6 splenocytes that had been cocultured with irradiated BALB/c splenocytes for 6 days and allowed to react with P-815 cells added on day 6, with an IC_{50} of 37 nM which was identical to that

TABLE 3. Effect of Discodermolide and Cyclosporin A on Murine *In Vitro* Immune Responsiveness

Immune Response		IC_{50} $(nM)^a$	Toxicity $(nM)^a$
Cytolytic T cell generation		37	100
	CsA	37	
Lymphokine activated killer cell induction		56	100
	CsA	No effect	
Auto-Th$_1$ Cell IL-2 secretion		200	1000
	CsA	< 1	
Il-1-Induced Th$_2$ cell proliferation		10–100	100^b
	CsA	1 μM	
Allo-induced Th$_2$ cell proliferation		20	> 30,000
	CsA	70	

^{a} Best response.
^{b} Toxic to cells at 100 nM, no effect at 10 nM.

induced by CsA. Toxicity of the discodermolide was approximately 100 nM. In a similar fashion, discodermolide suppressed (IC_{50} = 56 nM) the activity of lymphokine activate killer cells (LAK) of C57BL/6 mice generated by culture of splenocytes with 500 units/ml of recombinant human IL-2 for three days and assayed for the ability to lyse chromium-labeled YAC cells. Toxicity was approximately 100 nM. By contrast and as expected, CsA did not suppress LAK cell generation and associated activity. C8A3 is an autoreactive T cell hybrid which secretes IL-2 in response to syngeneic non–T cells, such as the F6 B cell line, comprising an auto–T helper$_1$ subset activation system. In the presence of 200 nM of discodermolide, these cells failed to secrete IL-2 into the supernatant after a 24-h incubation. CsA effectively suppressed their response at concentrations less than 1 nM. Two additional cell lines were tested for sensitivity to discodermolide. One clone, D10.N4.M, proliferates in response to exogenous IL-1 and comprises an IL-1-induced Th$_2$ subset model system. Increasing concentrations of discodermolide were added to cultures of these cells, and the proliferative response in the presence and absence of increasing concentrations of IL-1 (up to 10 pM) was measured for the last 6 h of a 72-h assay. Discodermolide inhibited the proliferation of these cells in a range of 10–100 nM. The 100-nM concentration of discodermolide, however, proved to be toxic. CsA was inhibitory at 1 μM but not at 0.3 μM. The other subclone, D10.G4.1, also proliferates in response to IL-1 and, in addition, responds to allogeneic stimulator cells and comprises the allo-induced Th$_2$ subset model system. For this allogeneic induction of proliferation, D10.G4.1 cells were cocultured with irradiated splenocytes from C57BL/6 mice in the presence of discodermolide or CsA. Proliferation was measured by thymidine incorporation during the last 6 h of a 24-h culture period. Again, discodermolide inhibited the proliferation of D10.G4.1 cells, with an IC_{50} of 20 nM. No reduction in viability of the cells was noted, even with concentrations as high as 30 μM. CsA inhibited the response as well, with an IC_{50} of 70 nM. These results, taken together, indicated that discodermolide was an effective, nontoxic immunosuppressive agent that inhibited immune responsiveness at the nanomolar level in a number of murine lymphocyte activation models.

STUDIES ON THE IMMUNOSUPPRESSION OF *IN VITRO*
HUMAN IMMUNE RESPONSES BY DISCODERMOLIDE

Additional collaborative studies with the Hoffmann-La Roche group focused on the effects of discodermolide on human immune cell responsiveness. Specifically, they examined the effects of discodermolide on mitogen responsiveness of human peripheral blood lymphocytes (PBL) and the cytokine-dependent proliferation of a T cell line. The results of this study are presented in TABLE 4. Cultures of PBL with either Con A or phytohemmagglutinin as stimulating agents were established on day 0 in the presence or absence of various concentrations of discodermolide or CsA. During the last 4 h of a 72-h culture period, tritiated thymidine was added to the cultures as a measure of cellular proliferation. In a second experiment, discodermolide or CsA was added on day 3 following Con A or PHA initiation of the culture and the plates processed the next day (72 h) as above. Discodermolide or CsA, when added on day 0, suppressed the responses of both Con A- and PHA-stimulated PBL, with IC_{50}s of 12 nM and 57 nM for PHA- and Con A–induced proliferation, respectively. Discodermolide was not toxic at concentrations up to 10,000 nM. In experiments where discodermolide or CsA was added on day 3 following initiation of the cultures, discodermolide still inhibited the responses. However, higher concentrations were needed to achieve equivalent, 50% inhibition for PHA (IC_{50} = 53 nM) but not for Con A–induced responsiveness (IC_{50} = 36 nM). CsA was no longer inhibitory when added on day 3. These results indicated that discodermolide was effective in inhibiting cell proliferation even after activation of PBL had taken place.

Two subclones of a human T cell line, Kit 225, originally derived from a patient with T cell chronic lymphocytic leukemia, one IL-2 dependent and the other IL-2 independent, were used to further investigate discodermolide's immunosuppressive activity. Kit 225 cells were incubated with various concentrations of discodermolide or CsA for 24 h. Tritiated thymidine was then added, and the cultures incubated for an additional 5 h. For the IL-2-dependent clone, 10 units/ml of human recombinant IL-2 was added when the cultures were established. The results in TABLE 4 show that the proliferation of both clones was inhibited by discodermolide (IC_{50} = 21 nM and 14 nM for IL-2-dependent and IL-2-independent Kit 225 cells, respectively). CsA did not inhibit the proliferation of either of the subclones.

TABLE 4. Effect of Discodermolide and Cyclosporin A on Human *In Vitro* Immune Responsiveness

Immune Response	IC_{50} (nM)[a]	Toxicity (nM)[a]
PHA-induced T cell proliferation	12[b]	> 10,000
Con A–induced T cell proliferation	57[b]	> 10,000
PHA-induced T cell proliferation (day 3)	53[c]	ND[d]
Con A–induced T cell proliferation (day 3)	36[c]	ND
Kit 225 IL-2-dependent T cell proliferation	21[c]	ND
Kit 225 IL-2-independent T cell proliferation	14[c]	ND

[a] Best response.
[b] Inhibition by cyclosporin A.
[c] No inhibition by cyclosporin A.
[d] Not determined.

EFFECT OF DISCODERMOLIDE ON THE CONSTITUTIVE
PROLIFERATION OF LYMPHOID AND NONLYMPHOID
CELL LINES OF MURINE OR HUMAN ORIGIN

Because of the apparent nonselectivity regarding discodermolide's ability to block lymphoid cell proliferation induced by a number of different immune stimuli, the effects of discodermolide on the inhibition of constitutive proliferation of a number of lymphoid and nonlymphoid cell lines of mouse or human origin were investigated. The results are presented in TABLE 5. For the murine lymphoid lines, the 70Z/3, a pre–B cell line, and the EL-4 thymoma, a pre–T lymphoma, were incubated in the presence of varying concentrations of discodermolide or CsA. After 24 h, tritiated thymidine was added and the cultures incubated for an additional 16 h. Discodermolide inhibited the proliferation of both cell lines, with IC_{50}s of 3 nM and 30 nM for 70Z/3 and EL-4 cells, respectively. CsA also inhibited the proliferation of

TABLE 5. Effect of Discodermolide on Constitutive Proliferation of Murine and Human Cell Lines

Immune Response	IC_{50} (nM)[a]	Toxicity (nM)[a]
Murine:lymphoid[b]		
70Z/3 pre-B proliferation	3	10
EL-4 thymoma proliferation	30	100
Murine:nonlymphoid[b]		
Swiss 3T3 proliferation	37	ND[c]
BMSC 8.3 proliferation	50	ND
BMSC 8.6 proliferation	84	ND
BMSC 25.4 proliferation	59	ND
F7 fibroblast proliferation	60	ND
Human:nonlymphoid[b]		
Normal fibroblast proliferation	15	> 3000

[a] Best response.
[b] Cyclosporin A activity: 100 nM for 70Z/3, 500 nM for EL-4, no inhibition for 3T3 and BMSC lines up to 1 μg/ml, not tested in F7, no inhibition for human fibroblasts up to 3 μM.
[c] Not determined.

these cell lines, but at concentrations that were 16 to 30 times higher compared to discodermolide. For the nonlymphoid murine cell lines, Swiss 3T3 fibroblasts, three bone marrow stromal cell lines (BMSC) derived from C57BL/6 mice, and a fibroblast line (F7) derived from neonatal "steel" mice were used. Cultures were established for each of the cell lines for an initial 12-h incubation period. Varying concentrations of discodermolide were then added, and the cells incubated for an additional 50 hr, the last 12 h in the presence of tritiated thymidine. CsA was assayed in a similar fashion using all cell lines except for F7. The results show that the IC_{50} values were very similar for all cell lines tested (ranges from 37–84 nM). CsA did not inhibit the proliferation of any of the cell lines tested at concentrations up to 1 μM. In addition, normal human foreskin fibroblasts were similarly exposed to various concentrations of discodermolide and their proliferation measured. The results show that these human cells were very sensitive to the antiproliferative effects of discodermolide with an $IC_{50} = 15$ nM. Interestingly, discodermolide did not affect viable cell recovery (toxicity) at concentrations of the compound up to 3.0 μM. A similar result of discodermolide's apparent preferential noncytotoxic property towards human cells was also observed in the PHA- or Con A–stimulated PBLs (TABLE 4). These results indicate that discodermolide's immunosuppressive mechanism of action is linked to its ability to inhibit cellular proliferation. However, this antiproliferative activity is not specific to any cell type (lymphoid vs. nonlymphoid). Discodermolide, on the other hand, appears to be especially nontoxic in human cells in the 3–10 mM range, in contrast to its potent inhibition of cellular proliferation in the nM range.

EFFECT OF DISCODERMOLIDE ON CELL CYCLE PROGRESSION AND COMPARISON WITH DOXORUBICIN

Since the apparent mechanism of action of discodermolide included inhibition of cellular proliferation in a wide range of cell types, cell cycle studies were initiated in order to try to pinpoint a specific phase within the cell cycle in which discodermolide was exerting this effect. In addition, the known antiproliferative agent doxorubicin (formerly Adriamycin) was used as a comparison standard. We used murine DO11.10 T hybridoma cells as cell cycle targets for discodermolide. Cell cycle analyses were performed as follows: DO11.10 cells were incubated in the presence or absence of varying concentrations of discodermolide or doxorubicin for 3, 5, or 24 h. Cells were harvested and stained either with propidium iodide (PI) alone (50 μg/ml) which stains DNA of only dead cells or with PI together with 0.1% Nonidet P-40 detergent plus 0.7 mg/ml of RNAse according to the method of Vindelov.[9] This procedure permeabilizes live cells and allows entry of PI to stain DNA (propidium iodide also stains double-stranded RNA, so RNAse is included in the preparation to exclude this possibility). Stained preparations were analyzed on a Coulter EPICS ELITE with 488 nM excitation with the dead cells excluded by back gating of PI preparations without detergent on forward and side scatter histograms. Fluorescence measurements and resulting DNA histograms were collected from 10,000 PI-stained cells at an emission wavelength of 690 nM. Raw histogram data were further analyzed using a cell cycle analysis program (Multicycle, Phoenix Flow Systems). The results of these experiments are shown in FIGURE 4. Control cultures of DO11.10 cells show a characteristic pattern of cell cycling. Approximately 68% of the control cells comprise the G_1 phase of the cell cycle while approximately 31% of the cells comprise the S phase. Only approximately 1% of these cells are demonstrable in the G_2/M phase in asynchronous cultures at any one time mainly due to high proliferative rate of DO11.10 cells (FIGURE 4A). Cells incubated in the presence of 1.0 μg/ml (1.68 μM) of discodermolide for only 3 h already begin to show shifts in percentages of cell in each phase of the cycle. The percentages of cells in G_1 decreased (from 68% to 52%), while the percentages of cells in S and G_2/M increased (from 31% to 40% and 1% to 8% for S and G_2/M phases, respectively) (FIGURE 4B). By 5 h, the percentage of cells in G_1 had decreased further to 40%. However, S phase cells began also to show a decrease in percentage (35%) but with a concomitant increase in the percentage of G_2/M cells (24%) (FIGURE 4C). At 24 h post–culture initiation with discodermolide, the percentage of cells in G_1 phase had fallen further to 25% and those in S to 16%. However, the percentage of cells in G_2/M had risen even further to 58% (FIGURE 4D). These results show that discodermolide prevented the normal cycling of cells through various phases of the cell cycle. FIGURE 5 shows a comparison of discodermolide's DNA histogram pattern with that obtained with DO11.10 cells cultured with 0.5 μg/ml of doxorubicin for 24 h. Although the patterns are not exactly identical, it is clear from these histograms that both discodermolide (FIGURE

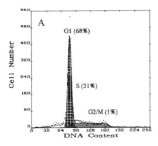

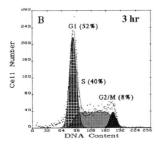

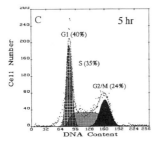

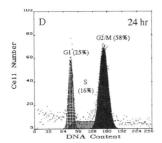

FIGURE 4. Effect of discodermolide on cell cycle progression. DO11.10 T hybridoma cells (1×10^6 cells/ml) were cultured in RMPI 1640 medium supplemented with 10% fetal calf serum and antibiotics as 1.0 ml aliquots in 24-well macroculture plates in the presence or absence of 1.0 μg/ml (1.68 μM) discodermolide for 3, 5, and 24 h. At the end of each incubation period, cells were removed from culture wells and washed three times in tissue culture medium. The final pellet was resuspended in 1.0 ml of PBS/FCS-azide buffer containing 50 μg/ml of propidium iodide (PI). A volume of 0.5 ml of this suspension was removed and added to 0.5 ml of Vindelov's modified PI solution containing 70 mg/ml RNase, 0.1% Nonidet P-40, 6 mg/ml of NaCl, and 5 mg/ml PI. Both tubes were incubated on ice for 15 min prior to flow cytometric analyses. Excitation was at 488 nM using a 10 mW argon laser and emission monitored at 690 nM. Dead cells (identified by the PI only preparation) were identified and gated out using forward scatter vs. side scatter parameters. DNA histogram data were collected on 10,000 cells. Raw histogram data were analyzed for DNA cell cycle using commercial software (Multicycle, Phoenix Flow Systems). Numbers in parentheses indicate percentage of cells in each phase of the cycle.

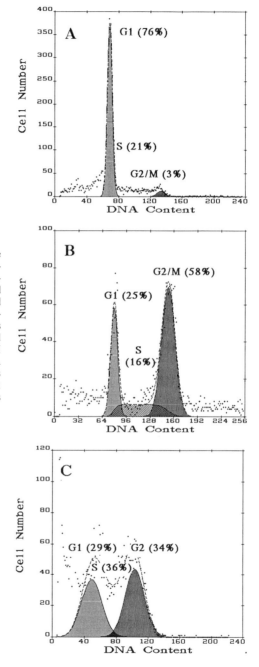

FIGURE 5. Comparison of cell cycle kinetics of discodermolide- or doxorubicin-treated cells. DO11.10 hybridomas (1×106 cells/ml) were incubated as 1 ml cultures with either 1.0 µg/ml of discodermolide or 0.5 µg/ml of doxorubicin in 24-well macroculture plates at 37°C for 24 h. Cells were collected from each culture and stained with PI solutions, and flow cytometric DNA cell cycle analyses were performed as described in FIGURE 4. Numbers in parentheses indicate percentage of cells in each phase of the cycle.

5B) and doxorubicin (FIGURE 5C) blocked the progression of cells from G_2/M back to G_1 as indicated by a depletion of cells in G_1 and S phases and a "piling up" of cells in G_2/M. It appears, then, that discodermolide blocks cells in the G_2/M phase of the cell cycle, a mechanism that is consistent with that observed and reported by ourselves and others[10-14] for doxorubicin.

REVERSIBILITY OF DISCODERMOLIDE'S BLOCKING OF CELL CYCLE PROGRESSION

We were further interested to determine if the discodermolide block was reversible. DO11.10 cells were cultured for 24 h in the presence or absence of 1.0 $\mu g/ml$ (1.68 μM) of discodermolide. Control and discodermolide-treated cultures were then harvested, washed three times with tissue culture media, and cultures reestablished in the absence of discodermolide. At time intervals of 24 h and 48 h postreculture, cells were harvested, stained with PI, and cell cycle analysis performed as described above. FIGURE 6B shows that cells cultured 24 h after removal of discodermolide begin to show cycling patterns by increasing numbers of G_1 (36%) and S (21%) phase cells and corresponding decreasing numbers of G_2/M (43%). Cells cultured for 48 h post removal of discodermolide had almost completely recovered "normal" cycling patterns, with control percentages of G_1 cells (61% for discodermolide treated vs. 60% for control) and the percentages of S and G_2/M returning to control values (FIGURE 6C). These results indicate that the G_2/M block mediated by discodermolide appears to be indeed reversible.

DISCUSSION

Important criteria to be considered in the discovery of immunomodulators from natural sources, in our case, the marine environment, should include requirements that the compound of interest be nontoxic *in vitro* with potency in the nanomolar range, demonstration of comparable activity in human cells, a unique mechanism of action, and a degree of *in vivo* immunosuppression without appreciable toxicity in an appropriate model. Discodermolide fulfills all but one of the above criteria. Discodermolide exhibits potent suppression of mitogen-stimulated and allogeneic-induced proliferation of lymphoid cells and associated cell lines derived from both mice and humans. Concentrations of discodermolide required to achieve such levels of suppression mirror closely those observed with CsA *in vitro* (nanomolar amounts) and are not cytotoxic for lymphocytes per se. An interesting aspect of these studies is the apparent lack of cytotoxicity of the compound for human lymphocytes and associated cell lines compared to that observed for the murine system. The exact nature of this apparent selective "noncytotoxicity" for human cells is being explored further in our laboratory. Our initial *in vivo* studies[5] also revealed discodermolide's potent *in vivo* activity in the suppression of the graft vs. host reaction, using the Simonsen splenomegaly assay, indicating the bioavailability of the compound *in vivo*.

Our initial studies demonstrating the modulation of the expression of the p55-associated IL-2 receptor by discodermolide[4] and subsequent confirmation of these studies using flow cytometric analyses suggested a possible specific mechanism of action by which discodermolide was mediating its immunosuppressive effects. This prompted a more thorough biological evaluation of the compound in additional cell lines of different tissue types and origins. The studies reported herein point to an additional important criterion not considered above, i.e., the immunosuppressive

FIGURE 6. Effect of washout experiments on the reversibility of discodermolide's blocking of the cell cycle. Cultures of DO11.10 cells (1 × 106 cells/ml) were established in 24-well macroculture plates in the presence or absence of 1.0 μg/ml (1.68 μM) discodermolide, and the plates incubated for 24 h. At the end of this period, cells were collected from all wells and washed three times in tissue culture medium. The cell concentration was adjusted to 1 × 106 cells/ml in fresh tissue culture medium without discodermolide, and the cells reincubated at 37°C for 24 h. Cells were collected from some cultures, stained with PI solutions, and subjected to DNA cell cycle analysis (so designated at 24 h postcultures). The remainder of the cells were allowed to incubate for an additional 24 h at 37°C and were then subsequently collected, stained with PI solutions, and subjected to DNA flow cytometric cell analysis as indicated in FIGURE 4. Numbers in parentheses indicate percentage of cells in each phase of the cycle.

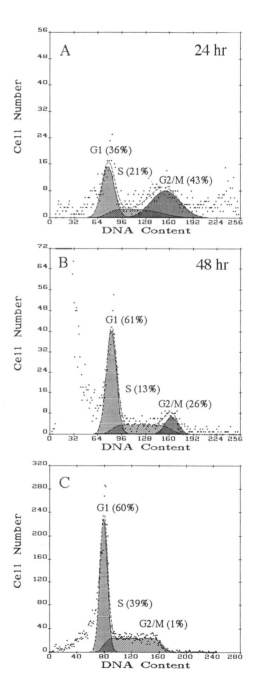

compound of interest should exhibit a mechanism specific to immune cells. Our results show that the immunosuppressive activity mediated by discodermolide was due to its antiproliferative activity which could be additionally demonstrated on nonlymphoid cells as well. While this apparent nonselective property of discodermolide would make it a less desirable compound to be considered as an immunosuppressive agent, its relative nontoxic effects compared to its potent antiproliferative effects prompted us to further examine the exact nature of this curious mechanism.

DNA analyses using flow cytometry are an accurate and convenient way to determine the effects of agents on cycling populations of cells. Our studies reported here show that discodermolide treatment of cells induced a block in the proliferation of DO11.10 T-hybridoma cells at the G_2/M interface as evidenced by cells progressing through G_1 and S phases with a G_2/M cell "pile-up" and no return to G_1. DNA synthesis appeared not to be blocked immediately, as cells continued to progress from G_1 (containing a 2n complement of DNA) through S (containing 2n + X DNA) to G_2/M (containing 4n DNA). Forward scatter vs. side scatter histogram data (data not shown) indicated that these G_2/M phase cells contained twice the amount of DNA and were larger compared to their G_1 counterparts. Thus, it appears that the discodermolide block prevents cells from cycling back to G_1. The discodermolide block demonstrated in our studies proved to be reversible in that cells recovered normal cycling patterns following removal of the compound. The exact point at which discodermolide exerts this block during mitosis (prophase, anaphase, telephase, metaphase), however, has not been determined and is the subject of current investigation in our laboratory.

Doxorubicin and anthracyclines are know to stabilize protein-DNA intermediates during relaxation of supercoiled DNA, and topoisomerase II activity (DNA gyrase) has been shown to be necessary for unlinking double-stranded sister chromosomes prior to their segregation and cell division.[15] The possibility exists that an interuption of topoisomerase II activity by discodermolide could be the biochemical lesion responsible for the G_2/M block observed in discodermolide-treated cells that possess a 4n complement of DNA. This would explain, in part, the inability of discodermolide-treated cells to "cycle back" to G_1. We are currently investigating the possible effects of discodermolide on topoisomerase II activity.

SUMMARY

In summary, discodermolide, a novel, marine-derived compound, is a potent *in vitro* and *in vivo* immunosuppressive agent. Discodermolide blocks cellular proliferation in lymphoid and nonlymphoid cells. This blocking action is not due to cytotoxicity. Blockage of cell proliferation by discodermolide appears to occur at the G_2/M interface of the cell cycle, similar to that observed with other types of antiproliferative drugs (i.e., doxorubicin). The cell cycle block appears to be reversible, as cells recover normal cycling patterns within 48 h after removal of the compound. Additional work with this compound is targeted towards determining the exact nature of discodermolide's mitotic block and is currently under way.

ACKNOWLEDGMENTS

The authors wish to thank Dr. Robert W. Wallace for his thoughtful discussion and critical review of the manuscript and Ms. Amy Brinson for her excellent technical expertise. This is Harbor Branch Oceanographic Inst. publication no. 971.

REFERENCES

1. BALANDRIN, M. F., J. A. KLOCKE, E. S. WURTELE & W. H. BOLLINGER. 1985. Natural plant chemicals: sources of industrial and medicinal materials. Science **228:** 1154–1160.
2. KINO, T., H. HATANAKA, M. HASHIMOTO, M. NISHIYAMA, T. GOTO, M. OKUHARA, M. KOHSAKA, H. AOKI & H. IMANAKA. 1987. FK-506, a novel immunosuppressant isolated from a Streptomyces. J. Antibiotics **40:** 1249–1255.
3. MONTGOMERY, D. W. & C. F. ZUKOSKI. 1985. Didemnin B: a new immunosuppressive cyclic peptide with potent activity in vitro and in vivo. Transplantation **40:** 49–56.
4. TRENN, G., G. R. PETTIT, H. TAKAYAMA, J. HU-LI & M. V. SITKOVSKY. 1988. Immunomodulating properties of a novel series of protein kinase C activators. The bryostatins. J. Immunol. **140**(2): 433–439.
5. LONGLEY, R. E., D. CADDIGAN, D. HARMODY, M. GUNASEKERA & S. P. GUNASEKERA 1991. Discodermolide: a new marine-derived immunosuppressive compound. I. In vitro studies. Transplantation **52:** 650–656.
6. LONGLEY, R. E., D. CADDIGAN, D. HARMODY, M. GUNASEKERA & S. P. GUNASEKERA. 1991. Discodermolide: a new marine-derived immunosuppressive compound. II. In vivo studies. Transplantation **52:** 656–661.
7. GUNASEKERA, S. P., M. GUNASEKERA, R. E. LONGLEY & G. K. SCHULTE. 1990. Discodermolide, a new bioactive polyhydroxylated lactone from the marine sponge, *Discodermia dissoluta.* J. Org. Chem. **55:** 4912–4915.
8. DUMONT, F. J., M. J. STARUCH, S. L. KOPRAK, M. R. MELINO & N. H. SIGAL. 1990. Distinct mechanisms of suppression of murine T cell activation by the related macrolides FK-506 and rapamycin. J. Immunol. **144:** 251–258.
9. VINDELOV, L. L. 1977. Microfluorimetric analysis of nuclear DNA in cells from tumors and cell suspensions. Virchow's. Arch. B. Cell. Pathol. **24:** 227–242.
10. SUZUKI, M. 1992. Flow cytometric analysis of effects of chemohormonal agents on the cell cycle distribution of MCF-7 cells. Nippon Geka Gakkai Zasshi **93**(1): 71–80.
11. NAKATA, B., Y. S. CHUNG, H. YOKOMATSU, T. SAWADA, T. KUBO, Y. KONDO, K. SATAKE & M. SOWA. 1992. Flow cytometric bromodeoxyuridine/DNA analysis of hyperthermia and/or adriamycin for human pancreatic adenocarcinoma cell line Capan-2. Jpn. J. Cancer Res. **83**(5): 477–482.
12. SUPINO, R., M. MARIANI, A. COLOMBO, E. PROSPERI, A. C. CROCE & G. BOTTIROLI. 1992. Comparative studies on the effects of doxorubicin and differentiation inducing agents on B16 melanoma cells. Eur. J. Cancer **28A**(4–5): 778–783.
13. NGUYEN, H. N., B. U. SEVIN, H. AVERETTE, J. PERRAS, M. UNTCH, R. RAMOS, D. DONATO & M. PENALVER. 1992. Comparative evaluation of pirarubicin and adriamycin in gynecologic cancer cell lines. Gynecol. Oncol. **45**(2): 164–173.
14. LEONCE, S., A. PIERRE, M. ANSTETT, V. PEREZ, A. GENTON, J. P. BIZZARI & G. ATASSI. 1992. Effects of a new triazinoaminopiperidine derivative on adriamycin accumulation and retention in cells displaying P-glycoprotein-mediated multidrug resistance. Biochem. Pharmacol. **44**(9): 1707–1715.
15. LOCK, R. B. & W. E. ROSS. 1987. DNA topoisomerases in cancer therapy. Anti-Cancer Drug Design **2:** 151–164.

Brequinar Sodium, Mycophenolic Acid, and Cyclosporin A Inhibit Different Stages of IL-4- or IL-13-Induced Human IgG4 and IgE Production *In Vitro*

CHIA-CHUN J. CHANG, GREGORIO AVERSA,
JUHA PUNNONEN, HANS YSSEL, AND JAN E. DE VRIES

DNAX Research Institute of Molecular and Cellular Biology
Human Immunology Department
901 California Avenue
Palo Alto, California 94304-1104

INTRODUCTION

Allergen-specific IgE antibodies are important mediators of allergic reactions. Induction of IgE synthesis by human B cells requires IL-4 and contact mediated costimulatory signals delivered by activated CD4[+] T-helper cells.[1] One of these T-helper signals is provided by interactions between the CD40 ligand (CD40L), transiently expressed on CD4[+] T-helper cells following activation, and CD40, which is constitutively expressed on B cells.[2-5] Recently, we cloned and expressed a novel cytokine IL-13 which, like IL-4, induces naive surface immunoglobulin D[+] (sIgD[+]) B cells to switch to IgG4 and IgE producing cells.[5-7]

Brequinar sodium (BQ) is a noncompetitive inhibitor of dihydroorotate dehydrogenase, an enzyme required for *de novo* pyrimidine synthesis. Mycophenolic acid (MPA) inhibits inosine monophosphate (IMP) dehydrogenase, which results in the depletion of GTP and the inhibition of DNA synthesis. Because of their capacity to inhibit DNA synthesis, both BQ and MPA have been shown to have immunosuppressive effects *in vitro* and *in vivo*.[8-10] However, their effects on productive T-B cell interactions, resulting in cytokine-driven immunoglobulin (Ig) isotype switching and Ig production, have not been documented.

In the present study, the effects of BQ and MPA on IL-4- and IL-13-induced IgG4 and IgE synthesis are investigated and their effects are compared to those of cyclosporin A (CsA). It is shown that BQ inhibits IgG4 and IgE synthesis in a dose-dependent fashion, whereas MPA and CsA, depending on the concentrations used, had either inhibitory or enhancing effects. In addition, the effects of these compounds on IL-4-induced B cell proliferation and T cell activation and proliferation, CD40L expression, and cytokine production by T cells were investigated.

MATERIALS AND METHODS

Reagents

Purified human rIL-4 was provided by Schering-Plough Research (Bloomfield, N.J.), purified human rIL-13 was prepared by Dr. S. Menon (DNAX), PE-conjugated mAb against CD3, CD4, CD8, CD14, CD16, CD56 were obtained from Becton Dickinson (San Jose, Calif). The purified anti-CD40 mAb89 (IgG1) was kindly provided by Dr. J. Banchereau (Schering-Plough, Dardilly, France). The CD40-Ig fusion protein was obtained by fusion of the cDNA segments encoding the extracellular domain of CD40 to cDNA fragments encoding human IgG1 and kindly provided by Dr. J.-P. Galizzi (Schering-Plough, Dardilly, France). CsA was purchased from Sandoz Pharmaceuticals (Basel, Switzerland). Purified phytohemagglutinin (PHA) was purchased from Wellcome Diagnostics (Dartford, United Kingdom), concanavalin A (Con A) was obtained from Pharmacia (Uppsala, Sweden). MPA and BQ were kindly provided by Dr. Anthony C. Allison (Palo Alto, Calif.). MPA and BQ were dissolved in dimethyl sulfoxide (DMSO) (Sigma Chemical Co., St. Louis, Mo.) and PBS (JRH Biosciences, Lenexa, Kans.), respectively, and further diluted in PBS to the concentrations indicated.

Cells

Peripheral blood mononuclear cells (PBMC) were isolated from heparinized blood from healthy donors by centrifugation over Histopaque-1077 (Sigma). Splenocytes were isolated from patients undergoing splenectomy due to trauma. Highly purified B cells were obtained by negative sorting of splenocytes as described.[5,7] An aliquot of the sorted cells was reanalyzed by FACS after staining with CD20-FITC (anti-Leu-16) or isotype control mAb. The sorted cells were always > 98% CD20[+].

Culture Conditions for Ig Production

Five $\times$ 10^4 highly purified B cells/well or 1 $\times$ 10^5 PBL/well were cultured in round bottomed 96-well plates (Linbro, McLean, Va.) in a final volume of 0.2 ml of Yssel's medium supplemented with 10% FCS and 10 $\mu g/ml$ ultrapure transferrin (Pierce Chemical Co., Rockford, Ill.). Anti-CD40 mAb (20 $\mu g/ml$), rIL-4 (400 U/ml), or rIL-13 (400 U/ml), CsA, MPA, and BQ were added at the onset of the cell cultures as indicated. Cultures were performed in triplicates and incubated 14 days at 37°C in 5% CO_2. At the end of the incubation period, the supernatants from each of three wells were harvested and pooled, or assayed individually for Ig isotype determination by ELISA as previously described.[5,7] The sensitivities of the ELISA were determined with calibrated standards from Behring (Marburg, Germany), and found to be 0.2 ng/ml for IgE and IgG4, and 0.5–1 ng/ml for total IgG, IgM, and IgA.

Cell Proliferation Assays

PBMC or highly purified B cells were cultured for 5 days in U-bottom 96-well Linbro plates at a density of 1 $\times$ 10^5 or 5 $\times$ 10^4 cells/well respectively in Yssel's medium supplemented with 10% FCS (Hyclone, Logan, Utah), in a final volume of 0.2 ml. To each well, rIL-4 (400 U/ml) or rIL-13 (400 U/ml), anti-CD40 (20 $\mu g/ml$), and the compounds were added as indicated. One μCi of tritiated thymidine ([^{3}H]TdR) was added to each well during the last 16 hours of culture and [^{3}H]TdR incorporation was measured as described.[5] For T cell proliferation assay, PBMC (10^5 cells/well) were activated by PHA (1 $\mu g/ml$) in Yssel's medium supplemented with 10% FCS, and the immunosuppressive compounds were added as indicated. After incubating for 4 days, the proliferation assay was performed as described above. The results are expressed as cpm of [³H]TdR incorporation and represent the mean of triplicate cultures.

Cytokine Production

Cytokine-containing supernatants were prepared from two CD4⁺ T cell clones as described.[11] T cell clone B21 belongs to the Th0 subset,[12] whereas the T cell clone NP12 is a CD4⁺ T cell clone of the Th2 subset, specific for the major house dust mite allergen *Der p*I.[11] Briefly, for cytokine production, 10^6 resting cloned T cells were cultured in 24 well plates (Linbro) in a volume of 1 ml of Yssel's medium supplemented with 1% human AB⁺ serum for 24 h in the presence of Con A (10 μg/ml). After this activation period, supernatants were harvested and cytokine production was determined by cytokine-specific ELISAs using mAbs specific for IL-2, IL-4, IL-5, IFN-γ, and GM-CSF as described.[11] The sensitivity of these assays varied between 50 and 100 pg/ml.

Detection of CD40 Ligand

For measuring CD40L expression, the CD4⁺ T cell clone B21 was activated for 6 h by the calcium ionophore A23187 (500 ng/ml) in combination with the phorbol ester TPA (1 ng/ml) (both purchased from Calbiochem, La Jolla, Calif.). The activated T cell clone was then incubated with a biotinylated CD40-Ig fusion protein for 30 min at 4°C, and subsequently stained with phycoerythrin-labeled streptavidin (Becton-Dickinson, San Jose, Calif.). The cells were analyzed by an FACScan® (Becton-Dickinson).

RESULTS

MPA, BQ, and CsA Modulate IgE Synthesis

MPA, BQ, and CsA added at various concentrations to cultures of PBMC modulated IL-4-induced IgE synthesis differently. CsA had dual effects. CsA was suppressive at a concentration of 10^{-6} M, whereas it consistently enhanced IgE synthesis at 10^{-7} M and 10^{-8} M (FIGURE 1). The strongest enhancing effects were generally observed at concentrations of 10^{-7} M. MPA showed similar dual effects. It completely suppressed IL-4-induced IgE synthesis at concentrations of 10^{-4}–10^{-6} M, whereas it generally had enhancing effects at concentrations of 10^{-7} and 10^{-8} M. Interestingly, BQ suppressed IgE production at all concentrations (10^{-4}–10^{-8} M) tested, although generally only partial inhibition was observed at 10^{-8} M. These results indicate that MPA and BQ are potent in inhibiting IgE synthesis equally as CsA and that BQ, in contrast to CsA or MPA, had no enhancing effects on IgE production at the range of concentrations tested.

The compounds had comparable effects on IL-13-induced IgE synthesis by PBMC (FIGURE 2). CsA again was only inhibitory at 10^{-6} M, whereas it enhanced IL-13-induced IgE synthesis at 10^{-7} and 10^{-8} M. MPA blocked IgE synthesis at a concentration of 10^{-4}–10^{-7} M, but potentiated IL-13-induced IgE synthesis at 10^{-8} M. The strongest suppressive effects were again observed with BQ, which inhibited IL-13-induced IgE synthesis at all concentrations (10^{-4}–10^{-8} M) tested.

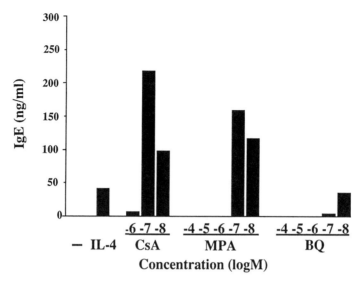

FIGURE 1. Effects of different concentrations of CsA, MPA, and BQ on IL-4-induced IgE synthesis by PBMC. For IgE determination, the supernatants of the triplicate cultures were pooled.

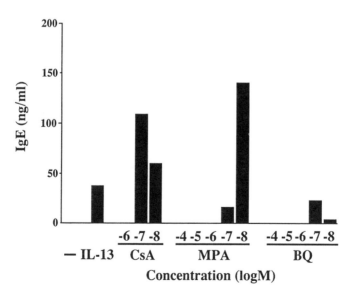

FIGURE 2. Effects of different concentrations of CsA, MPA, and BQ on IL-13-induced IgE synthesis by PBMC.

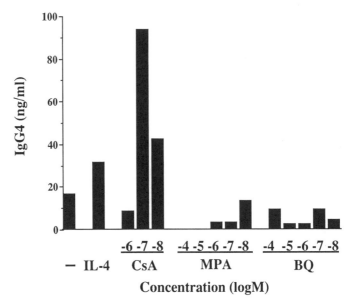

FIGURE 3. Effects of different concentrations of CsA, MPA, and BQ on IL-4-induced IgG4 synthesis by PBMC.

MPA, BQ, and CsA Modulate IgG4 Synthesis

IL-4 and IL-13 induce human B cells also to switch to IgG4 producing cells.[13] In FIGURES 3 and 4, it is shown that MPA, BQ, and CsA also modulate IL-4- and IL-13-induced IgG4 synthesis by PBMC. With the exception of MPA, the effects were generally comparable to those described for IgE. CsA was clearly inhibitory at 10^{-6} M, and again had enhancing effects at 10^{-8} M, whereas BQ and MPA blocked IgG4 production at all concentrations tested. Generally, partial inhibitory effects of MPA and BQ were observed at 10^{-8} M. These results indicate that the modulating effects of MPA on induction of IgG4 synthesis differ from those on induction of IgE synthesis. In the latter situation, MPA generally had enhancing effects at lower concentrations.

Effects of MPA, BQ, and CsA on Anti-CD40-Induced IgE Synthesis

Anti-CD40 mAbs either in their soluble form, or presented by L cells transfected with FcγII receptors (CD32), have been shown to induce IgE synthesis.[14,15] To determine whether the modulating effects of MPA, BQ, and CsA on IgE synthesis were due to direct effects on B cells, or whether they were indirectly mediated by other cells present in the PBMC cultures, the compounds were tested in a culture system in which highly purified B cells were stimulated by anti-CD40 mAbs, i.e., in the absence of T cells and monocytes. In FIGURE 5, it is shown that CsA and BQ inhibit IgE synthesis in this culture system in a dose-dependent fashion. In contrast to CsA, MPA had dual effects in this culture system. Complete blocking of IgE synthesis was observed at 10^{-5} and 10^{-6} M, whereas MPA at concentrations of 10^{-7}

M generally had slight enhancing effects. Comparable results were obtained with IL-13-induced IgE synthesis by B cells costimulated by anti-CD40 mAbs (not shown).

Collectively, these results indicate that these immunosuppressive compounds inhibit IL-4- and IL-13-induced IgE synthesis by directly acting on the B cells.

Effects of MPA, BQ, and CsA on the Proliferation of PBMC

Under the present culture conditions, IL-4 and IL-13 induced considerable levels of spontaneous proliferation of PBMC, which was inhibited by MPA, BQ, and CsA in a dose-dependent fashion (FIGURES 6 and 7). CsA strongly blocked IL-4- and IL-13-induced cell proliferation at a concentration of 10^{-6} M, the same concentration at which it blocked IgE synthesis. At CsA concentrations of 10^{-7} and 10^{-8} M, a partial inhibition of the proliferative responses was observed. In contrast, these CsA concentrations enhanced IgE synthesis, indicating that there is no correlation between cell proliferation and induction of IgE synthesis. On the other hand, BQ did not significantly inhibit cell proliferation at concentrations of 10^{-6}–10^{-8} M, although these concentrations were strongly inhibitory for IL-4- and IL-13-induced IgG4 and IgE synthesis. These results indicate that the inhibitory effects of BQ on IgE production were not directly related to the inhibition of B cell proliferation. Even at concentrations of 10^{-4} and 10^{-5} M, BQ had only partial inhibitory effects on cell proliferation. MPA strongly blocked cell proliferation at 10^{-4}–10^{-6} M, but had no, or modest, effects at 10^{-7} and 10^{-8} M, suggesting that the inhibitory effects of MPA on IgE production correlated with inhibition of cell proliferation. Since both T and B cells were induced to proliferate under these culture conditions, the results indicate that these compounds can inhibit the proliferation of both cell types.

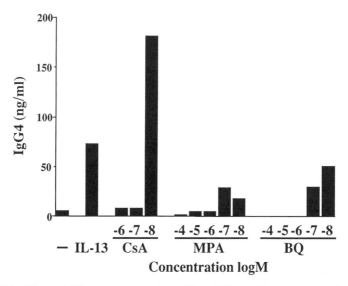

FIGURE 4. Effects of different concentrations of CsA, MPA, and BQ on IL-13-induced IgG4 synthesis by PBMC.

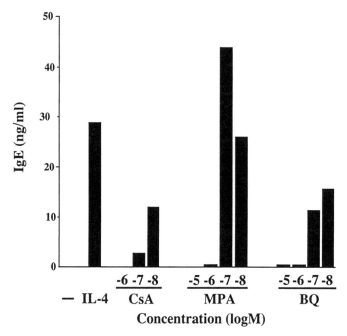

FIGURE 5. Effects of CsA, MPA, and BQ on IL-4-induced IgE synthesis in cultures of highly purified B cells costimulated by anti-CD40 mAbs.

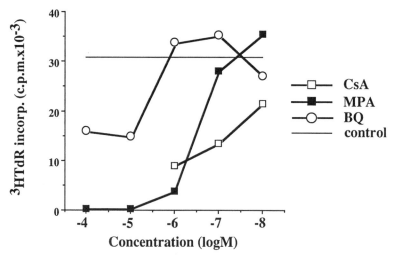

FIGURE 6. Effects of CsA, MPA, and BQ on IL-4-induced proliferation of PBMC. Results are expressed as mean cpm of triplicate cultures. Standard deviations were always <5%.

Effects of MPA, BQ, and CsA on B and T Cell Proliferation

To determine the role of MPA, BQ, and CsA on the proliferative responses of B and T cells in more detail, the effects of these compounds were tested on purified B cells stimulated by anti-CD40 mAbs and IL-4, or on PBMC stimulated by PHA. In FIGURE 8 it is shown that MPA at 10^{-5}–10^{-6} M, had strong inhibitory effects on B cell proliferation, whereas it was ineffective at concentrations of 10^{-7} and 10^{-8} M. These results are consistent with the inhibitory effects of MPA on Ig production and further support the notion that these are probably due to direct inhibitory effects on B cell proliferation. The inhibitory activities of CsA, and particularly of BQ on B cell proliferation induced by anti-CD40 and IL-4 were less pronounced. Moderate, inhibitory effects were only observed at the highest concentrations of 10^{-5} M of BQ and 10^{-6}–10^{-7} M CsA. BQ was not inhibitory at 10^{-6} M, confirming that its inhibition of IgG4 and IgE synthesis did not correlate with reduced B cell proliferation.

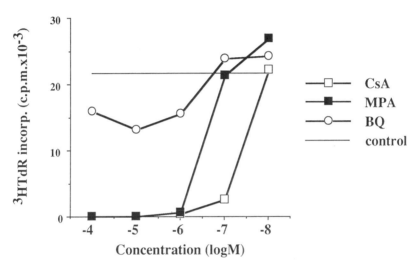

FIGURE 7. Effects of CsA, MPA, and BQ on IL-13-induced proliferation of PBMC.

Both MPA and CsA strongly blocked the proliferative responses of PHA activated T cells (FIGURE 9). More than 90% inhibition was observed at concentrations of 10^{-6} M. Similarly, as observed for its effects on B cell proliferation, BQ had only a partial inhibitory effect on T cell proliferation at 10^{-4}–10^{-5} M, and failed to block T cell proliferation at lower concentrations.

Effects of MPA, BQ, and CsA on CD40L Expression

Recently, it had been shown that interactions between CD40L, transiently expressed on CD4+ T-helper cells following activation, and CD40 constitutively expressed on B cells, are involved in IL-4- and IL-13-induced IgG4 and IgE production.[2,5,7] To determine whether the inhibitory effects of MPA, BQ, and CsA on Ig isotype production were associated with down regulatory effects on CD40L

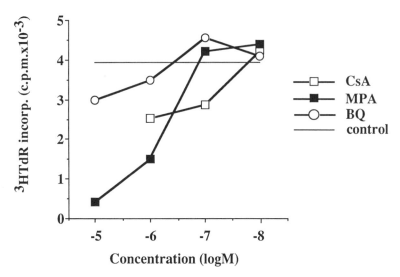

FIGURE 8. Effects of CsA, MPA, and BQ on the proliferation of highly purified B cells cultured in the presence of IL-4 and anti-CD40 mAbs.

expression, the effects of these compounds on CD40L induction on the Th0 like, CD4[+] T cell clone B21 activated by TPA and ionomycin were investigated. As shown in FIGURE 10, only CsA had a dose-dependent inhibitory effect on CD40L induction. Complete inhibition of CD40L expression was observed at the highest CsA concentration of 10^{-6} M, indicating that the down regulatory effects of CsA on CD40L expression seem to be directly associated with its inhibitory effects of productive T-B

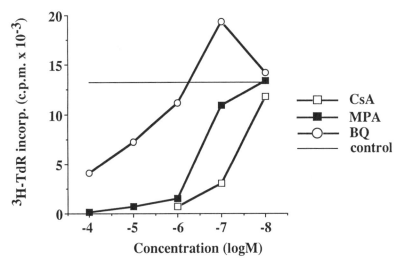

FIGURE 9. Effects of CsA, MPA, and BQ on the proliferation of PHA-activated PBMC.

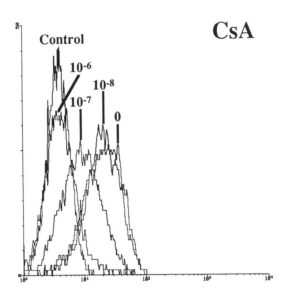

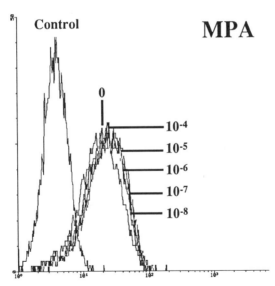

FIGURE 10. Effects of CsA and MPA on CD40L expression on the CD4[+] T cell clone B21 following activation by calcium ionophore and TPA for 6 hours. CD40L expression was measured by FACS analysis.

cell interactions, leading to IgG4 and IgE synthesis. However, it has to be noted that CsA, at a concentration of 10^{-7} M, partially blocked CD40L expression, but enhanced IL-4- or IL-13-induced IgE synthesis. In contrast, MPA and BQ were completely ineffective in these 6-hour assays, even at the highest concentrations tested. CsA had similar inhibitory effects on CD40L expression on the Th2-like CD4+ T cell clone NP12, whereas MPA and BQ again were ineffective (not shown). These results indicate that no differences were observed in modulation of CD40L expression between Th0 and Th2 T cell clones.

Effects of MPA, BQ, and CsA on Cytokine Production

Although IL-4 and IL-13 are the only cytokines capable of inducing IgG4 and IgE synthesis, many other cytokines have been found to modulate this process. IFN-γ,

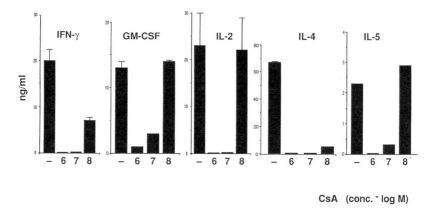

CsA   (conc. - log M)

FIGURE 11. Effects of various concentrations of CsA on cytokine production by the CD4+ T cell clone B21. B21 (10^6 cells/ml) was activated for 24 hours by Con A (10 μg/ml), whereafter cytokine production was measured in the supernatants. Results are expressed mean ± standard deviation of triplicate cultures.

IFN-α, TGF-β, and IL-10 inhibit IL-4-induced IgE synthesis, whereas IL-5, IL-6, and TNF-α have enhancing effects.[1] It is well established that CsA inhibits cytokine production by activated T cells. In FIGURE 11 it is shown that CsA effectively inhibits IFN-γ, GM-CSF, IL-2, IL-4, and IL-5 production by the human CD4+ T-helper clone B21, belonging to the Th0 subset, activated by ConA for 24 hours. Similarly, IL-4 and IL-5 production by the Th2 T-cell clone NP12 was completely blocked by CsA (not shown). In contrast, MPA and BQ tested over a concentration range of 10^{-5}–10^{-8} M, failed to significantly modulate cytokine production by both T cell clones (results not shown). These results confirm that MPA and BQ do not interfere with the early activation and signaling pathways resulting in cytokine production.

DISCUSSION

In the present study, we demonstrate that the immunosuppressive drugs MPA, BQ, and CsA inhibit both IL-4- and IL-13-induced IgG4 and IgE production *in vitro*.

BQ efficiently inhibited IgG4/IgE production, and generally even at concentrations of 10^{-8} M, strong inhibitory effects were observed. CsA and MPA were less potent, and had dual effects when added to cultures of PBMC. Although both compounds blocked IgG4/IgE synthesis at concentrations of 10^{-4} M for CsA, and 10^{-4}–10^{-6} M for MPA, enhancing effects were observed at lower concentrations. Interestingly, comparable dual effects of CsA have been described in mouse models, in which low doses of CsA enhanced Ag-specific IgE production *in vitro,* whereas higher doses were suppressive.[16]

CsA can also potentiate IgE production *in vivo.* CsA administered at concentrations of 5–150 mg/kg was found to selectively enhance antigen-specific IgE antibody production in mice *in vivo.*[17] On the other hand, most studies thus far indicate that CsA predominantly has immunosuppressive effects on Ig production both *in vitro* and *in vivo.*[18] In a previous report, it has been shown that CsA at 1 μg/ml inhibits both spontaneous and IL-4-induced IgE synthesis by tonsillar MNC, which is consistent with the present data. However, CsA was not tested at lower concentrations in that study.[19]

The enhancing effects of CsA on induction of Ag-specific IgE synthesis were found to correlate with a reduced production of IFN-γ,[18] which has been shown to strongly counteract IL-4-induced IgE synthesis both *in vivo* and *in vitro.*[1,20] Inhibition of IFN-γ production by CsA may also contribute to the enhanced IgG4/IgE production observed at a concentration of 10^{-7} M, since at this concentration, CsA blocked T cell proliferation and IFN-γ production by these cells, but had only partial inhibitory effects on B cell proliferation, induced by anti-CD40 mAbs and IL-4. The enhanced IgG4/IgE synthesis observed at a CsA concentration of 10^{-7} M also suggests that reduced levels of CD40L expression are still sufficient for productive T-B cell interactions, resulting in Ig production, since these CsA levels induced reductions in CD40L expression on activated T cell clones. However, it cannot be excluded that additional T and B cell surface molecules contribute to B cell differentiation.[21] CsA at 10^{-6} M strongly inhibited IgG4/IgE synthesis by PBMC, which was associated with complete inhibition of CD40L expression, T cell activation, cytokine production, and T and B cell proliferation induced by anti-CD40 mAbs and IL-4.

In contrast to CsA and MPA, BQ strongly inhibited IL-4- or IL-13-induced IgG4/IgE production by PBMC, or purified B cells costimulated by anti-CD40 mAbs, at concentrations of 10^{-6}–10^{-7} M, which did not (or only modestly) inhibit T or B cell proliferation. These results suggest that there is no absolute correlation between inhibition of B cell differentiation and Ig production and T or B cell proliferation by BQ and that B cell differentiation might occur in the absence of extensive B cell proliferation. BQ did not affect the induction of CD40L expression or cytokine production by activated T cell clones at any of the concentrations tested, indicating that BQ does not affect early events leading to T cell activation and cytokine production. The mechanisms of its inhibitory effects on Ig production remain to be determined. One possibility is that exhaustion of the pyrimidine nucleotide pools may become a limiting factor only in long-term assays, such as the present Ig-production assays, which require incubation periods of minimally 12 days in order to obtain optimal Ig production levels, whereas IgG4/IgE production is first observed after 7–9 days of culture.[20,22] This may also explain why BQ (at the highest concentrations of 10^{-4}–10^{-5} M) has only partial inhibitory effects in the T or B cell proliferation assays, which required incubations of 3 and 5 days respectively. The same hypothesis may explain the ineffectiveness of BQ in suppressing CD40L induction and cytokine production, which required 6 hours and 24 hours respectively, and which occur in the absence of proliferation. However, the inhibition of T and B cell proliferation at high doses of BQ is compatible with the lymphopenia observed in patients receiving BQ at the maximal tolerated dose, indicating that BQ also blocks T and B cell development and expansion in *vivo*.[23]

MPA is a potent inhibitor of T and B cell proliferation.[8,9] MPA was particularly effective and more powerful than CsA in inhibiting anti-CD40-induced B cell proliferation. Overall, its direct inhibitory effects on B cell proliferation correlated with its inhibitory effects on IL-4- or IL-13-induced IgG4/IgE production. However, since MPA, like BQ, does not interfere with T cell activation and IFN-γ production, its enhancing effects on IgE production by PBMC observed at low concentrations are presently difficult to explain. One assumption could be that MPA inhibits IFN-γ synthesis, or the production of another suppressor factor by T cells, at later stages of the culture.

Collectively, our data indicate that relatively high concentrations of BQ, CsA, and MPA inhibit IL-4- or IL-13-dependent IgG4 and IgE production at different stages of the induction process. In addition, it is shown that both CsA and MPA, at lower concentrations, can enhance IL-4- or IL-13-induced IgE synthesis. Whether CsA and MPA at a certain dose range also can enhance human antigen specific IgE responses *in vivo,* thereby enhancing allergic reactions, remains to be established.

SUMMARY

We investigated the effect of cyclosporin A (CsA), mycophenolic acid (MPA), and brequinar sodium (BQ) on human IgG4 and IgE synthesis induced by IL-4 or IL-13. BQ inhibited IL-4 and IL-13-induced IgG4 and IgE synthesis in cultures of peripheral blood mononuclear cells (PBMC) or highly purified B cells costimulated by anti-CD40 mAbs in a dose-dependent fashion. CsA and MPA had either suppressive or enhancing effects depending on the concentrations tested. Interestingly, BQ inhibited IgG4 and IgE synthesis at concentrations of 10^{-6}–10^{-8} M, which did not affect T or B cell proliferation, indicating that the inhibitory effects of BQ on Ig production were not directly related to inhibition of T or B cell proliferation. In contrast, the inhibitory effects of MPA on Ig production were directly associated with inhibitory effects on T and B cell proliferation. CsA blocked T and B cell proliferation at the same concentration (10^{-7} M) which enhanced IgG4 and IgE synthesis, indicating that reduction in T or B cell proliferation correlated with enhanced IgE production. CsA also inhibited CD40 ligand expression and IL-2, IL-4, IL-5, IFN-γ, and GM-CSF production by activated CD4+ T cell clones, whereas MPA and BQ were ineffective, indicating that these compounds do not inhibit early events in T cell activation. Collectively, our data indicate that BQ, MPA, and CsA block different stages of the IgG4 and IgE production process. In addition, we observed that CsA and MPA, in contrast to BQ, at lower concentrations can also have potentiating effects on the production of these Ig isotypes.

REFERENCES

1. DE VRIES, J. E., J-F. GAUCHAT, G. G. AVERSA, J. PUNNONEN, H. GASCAN & H. YSSEL. 1991. Regulation of IgE synthesis by cytokines. Curr. Opin. Immunol. **3:** 851–858.
2. ARMITAGE, R. J., W. C. FANSLOW, L. STROCKBINE, T. A. SATO, K. N. CLIFFORD, B. M. MACDUFF, D. M. ANDERSON, S. D. GIMPEL, S. T. DAVIS, C. R. MALISZEWSKI, E. A. CLARK, C. A. SMITH, K. H. GRABSTEIN, D. COSMAN & M. K. SPRIGGS. 1992. Molecular and biological characterization of a murine ligand for CD40. Nature **357:** 80–82.

3. SPRIGGS, M. K., R. J. ARMITAGE, L. STROCKBINE, K. N. CLIFFORD, B. M. MACDUFF, T. A. SATO, C. R. MALISZEWSKI & W. C. FANSLOW. 1992. Recombinant human CD40 ligand stimulates B cell proliferation and immunoglobulin secretion. J. Exp. Med. **176:** 1543–1550.

4. HOLLENBAUGH, D., L. S. GROSMAIRE, C. D. KULLAS, N. J. CHALUPNY, S. BRAESCH-ANDERSEN, R. J. NOELLE, I. STAMENKOVIC, J. A. LEDBETTER & A. ARUFFO. 1992. The human T cell antigen gp39, a member of the TNF gene family, is a ligand for the CD40 receptor: expression of a soluble form of gp39 with B cell costimulatory activity. EMBO J. **11:** 4313–4321.

5. COCKS, B., R. DE WAAL MALEFYT, J.-P. GALIZZI, J. E. DE VRIES & G. AVERSA. 1993. IL-13 induces proliferation and differentiation of human B cells activated by the CD40 ligand. Int. Immunol. **5:** 657–663.

6. MCKENZIE, A. N. J., J. A. CULPEPPER, R. DE WAAL MALEFYT, F. BRIERE, J. PUNNONEN, G. AVERSA, A. SATO, W. DANG, B. G. COCKS, S. MENON, J. E. DE VRIES, J. BANCHEREAU & G. ZURAWSKI. 1993. Interleukin-13, a novel T cell-derived cytokine that regulates monocyte and B cell function. Proc. Natl. Acad. Sci. USA **90:** 3735–3739.

7. PUNNONEN, J., G. AVERSA, B. G. COCKS, A. N. J. MCKENZIE, S. MENON, G. ZURAWSKI, R. DE WAAL MALEFYT & J. E. DE VRIES. 1993. Interleukin-13 induces interleukin-4-independent IgG4 and IgE synthesis and CD23 expression by human B cells. Proc. Natl. Acad. Sci. USA **90:** 3730–3734.

8. EUGUI, E. M., S. J. ALMQUIST, C. D. MULLER & A. C. ALLISON. 1991. Lymphocyte-selective cytostatic and immunosuppressive effects of mycophenolic acid *in vitro:* role of deoxyguanosine nucleotide depletion. Scand. J. Immunol. **33:** 161–173.

9. EUGUI, E. M., A. MIRKOVICH & A. C. ALLISON. 1991. Lymphocyte-selective antiprolifera-tive and immunosuppressive effects of mycophenolic acid in mice. Scand. J. Immunol. **33:** 175–183.

10. CRAMER, D. V., F. A. CHAPMAN, B. D. JAFFEE, E. A. JONES, M. KNOOP, G. HREHA-EIRAS & L. MAKOWKA. 1992. The effect of a new immunosuppressive drug, brequinar sodium, on heart, liver and kidney allograft rejection in the rat. Transplantation **53:** 303–308.

11. YSSEL, H., K. E. JOHNSON, P. V. SCHNEIDER, J. WIDEMAN, A. TERR, R. KASTELEIN & J. E. DE VRIES. 1992. T cell activation-inducing epitopes of the house dust mite allergen *Der p* I. J. Immunol. **148:** 738–745.

12. M. G. RONCAROLO, H. YSSEL, J.-L. TOURAINE, R. BACCHETTA, L. GEBUHRER, J. E. DE VRIES & H. SPITS. 1988. Antigen recognition by MHC-incompatible cells of a human mismatched chimera. J. Exp. Med. **168:** 2139–2152.

13. GASCAN, H., J.-F. GAUCHAT, M.-G. RONCAROLO, H. YSSEL, H. SPITS & J. E. DE VRIES. 1991. Human B cell clones can be induced to proliferate and switch to IgE and IgG4 synthesis by IL-4 and a signal provided by activated CD4+ T cell clones. J. Exp. Med. **173:** 747–750.

14. GASCAN, H., J.-F. GAUCHAT, G. AVERSA, P. VAN VLASSELAER & J. E. DE VRIES. 1991. Anti-CD40 monoclonal antibodies or CD4+ T cell clones and IL-4 induced IgG4 and IgE switching in purified B cells via different signaling pathways. J. Immunol. **147:** 8–13.

15. ROUSSET, F., E. GARCIA & J. BANCHEREAU. 1991. Cytokine-induced proliferation and immunologlobulin production of human B lymphocytes triggered through their CD40 antigen. J. Exp. Med. **173:** 705–710.

16. CHEN, S.-S., Q. LI, E. PEARLMAN & W.-H. CHEN. 1992. Dual mechanisms of potentiation of murine antigen-specific IgE production by cyclosporin A *in vitro.* J. Immunol. **149:** 762–767.

17. CHEN, S.-S., G. STANESCU, A. R. MAGALSKI & Y. QIAN. 1989. Cyclosporin A is an adjuvant in murine IgE antibody responses. J. Immunol. **142:** 4225–4232.

18. SIEKIERKA, J. J. & N. H. SIGAL. 1992. FK-506 and cyclosporin A: immunosuppressive mechanism of action and beyond. Curr. Opin. Immunol. **4:** 548–552.

19. RENZ, H., B. D. MAZER & E. W. GELFAND. 1990. Differential inhibition of T and B cell function in IL-4-dependent IgE production by cyclosporin A and methylprednisolone. J. Immunol. **145:** 3641–3646.

20. PENE, J., F. ROUSSET, F. BRIERE, I. CHRETIEN, J. Y. BONNEFOY, H. SPITS, T. YOKOTA, N. ARAI, K. ARAI, J. BANCHEREAU & J. E. DE VRIES. 1988. IgE production by normal

human lymphocytes is induced by interleukin 4 and suppressed by interferons gamma and alpha and prostaglandin E2. Proc. Natl. Acad. Sci. USA **85:** 6880–6884.

21. AVERSA, G., J. PUNNONEN & J. E. DE VRIES. 1993. The 26 kd transmembrane form of TNF-α on activated CD4+ T-cell clones provides a costimulatory signal for human B cell activation. J. Exp. Med. **177:** 1575–1585.

22. GAUCHAT, J.-F., D. A. LEBMAN, R. L. COFFMAN, H. GASCAN & J. E. DE VRIES. 1990. Structure and expression of germline ε transcripts in human B cells induced by IL-4 to switch to IgE production. J. Exp. Med. **172:** 463–473.

23. PETERS, G. J., G. SCHWARTSMANN, J. C. NADAL, E. J. KAURENSSE, C. J. VAN GROENINGEN, W. J. VAN DER VIJGH & H. M. PINEDO. 1990. *In vivo* inhibition of the pyrimidine *de novo* enzyme dihydroorotic acid dehydrogenase by brequinar sodium in mice and patients. Cancer Res. **50:** 644–649.

Deoxyspergualin

Mechanism of Action Studies of a Novel Immunosuppressive Drug

MARK A. TEPPER

Bristol Myers Squibb Pharmaceutical Research Institute
3005 First Avenue
Seattle, Washington 98121

INTRODUCTION

15-Deoxyspergualin (DSG, 1-amino-19-guanidine-11-hydroxy-4,9,12-triaza-nonadecane-10,13-dione) (FIGURE 1) is a synthetic analogue of the antitumor antibiotic spergualin produced by *Bacillus laterosporus* and discovered in the early 1980s at the Institute of Microbial Chemistry in Japan.[1] Spergualin was originally discovered while screening for natural products that inhibited the foci formation of Rous sarcoma virus (RSV) transformed chick embryo fibroblasts. After an extensive synthetic effort of over 400 spergualin analogues; DSG was selected for further development because of its greater potency and broader dose range compared to spergualin.

Initial preclinical studies with DSG focused on its antitumor properties. DSG was found to be active in animal tumor models including L1210, B16, P388, and P815.[2] Based on activity in these models, phase I clinical trials of DSG were initiated by the National Cancer Institute (NCI). DSG was well tolerated in these studies at doses up to 2000 mg/m[2].

In addition to its antitumor activity, DSG was shown in animal models to exhibit strong immunosuppressive activity.[3-8] *In vivo* immunosuppressive activities reported for DSG included suppression of autoimmune disease, prolongation of survival of transplant allografts, induction of transplant tolerance, reversal of allograft rejection, inhibition of antibody responses, and suppression of delayed-type hypersensitivity (DTH). As monotherapy, in most of these models (except antibody and DTH), DSG's activity is comparable to other agents given alone. However, DSG in combination therapy has exhibited exceptional activity for prevention of transplant rejection, and in some models has induced long-term tolerance.[9-11] In humans, DSG has proven effective for prevention and treatment of solid organ rejection.[12] Reischensperner *et al.* have combined DSG therapy with cyclosporine A and observed exceptionally long survival (> 150 days) in a kidney allograft model in baboons.[9]

Recently, Pittman *et al.* have reported that the combination of DSG and polyclonal rabbit anti–thymocyte globulin (R-ATG) can induce long-term survival of pig pancreatic islets transplanted into rats.[13] This exceptional activity of DSG in combination with ATG to suppress the rejection of transplanted pancreatic islets cells has been observed in the human setting as well.

Gores *et al.* reported recently that the transplant of combined cadaveric islets and kidneys[14] into diabetic patients treated with induction therapy of DSG followed by quadruple immunosuppressive therapy resulted in the maintenance of an insulin-independent state for greater than six months. Treatment with DSG in this study was for only 10 days. These results suggest that DSG may exhibit unique activity at

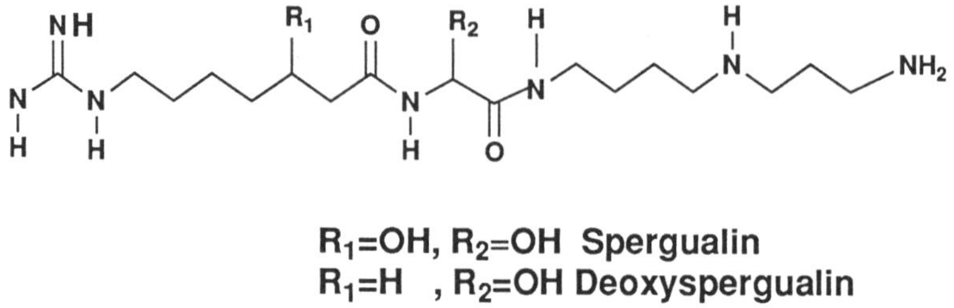

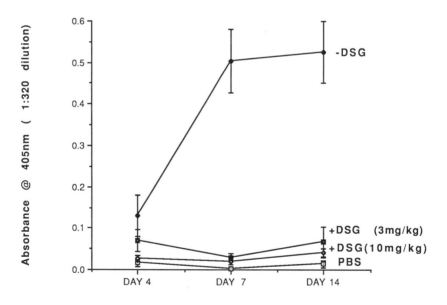

R_1=OH, R_2=OH Spergualin
R_1=H , R_2=OH Deoxyspergualin

FIGURE 1. Chemical structure of 15-deoxyspergualin and spergualin.

protecting islets from inflammatory as well as immune-mediated distruction. Similar studies suggest that neither CsA nor FK506 elicits islet protection.[11]

Finally, one model where DSG is particularly effective when administered alone is the suppression of the antibody response to foreign protein antigens.[15,16] As seen in FIGURE 2 DSG is a potent inhibitor of the primary antibody response to the immunogenic protein keyhole limpet hemocyanin (KLH) in mice, inhibiting the IgG antibody titer by greater than 90%. We have also shown that DSG inhibits the antibody response to an immunotoxin in mice even upon repeated immunotoxin injection for 7 days. In humans, an NCI sponsored clinical trial recently reported that

FIGURE 2. Inhibition of antibody response by deoxyspergualin. Mice were immunized with keyhole limpet hemocyanin (KLH) protein (500 μg) and treated for three days with DSG (intraperitonial administration) at 3 and 10 mg/kg. Mice were bled on day 4, 7, and 14 and anti-KLH antibody levels determined as described.[18] PBS-treated animals did not receive any KLH.

DSG suppressed the human antimouse antibody response (HAMA) to a murine monoclonal antibody.[17]

While DSG clearly exhibits promising immunosuppressive properties in animal models, the precise mechanism of action of DSG is poorly understood. A variety of cellular immunological effects have been reported. These include diminished release of superoxide and lysosomal enzymes by monocytes,[13] modulation of IL-1 production,[18–20] suppression of antibody formation,[15,21] inhibition of alloreactive secondary CTL induction,[22] down regulation of MHC class II or class I antigens,[19,20] and decreased expression of IL-2R.[23,24] Recently, DSG has been shown to specifically bind to Hsc70, a constitutively expressed member of the heat shock protein 70 (Hsp70) family[25] which has a role in the binding and intracellular transport of antigenic peptides.[26–28] This manuscript gives an overview of DSG's actions on T lymphocytes, B lymphocytes, and monocytes and addresses our current understanding of DSG's mechanism of action relative to other immunosuppressive agents under development.

MECHANISM OF ACTION STUDIES

DSG Effects on T Cells

The activity of DSG has been investigated at the cellular level in numerous *in vitro* models of immune function.[29–32] Unfortunately, *in vitro* studies have been hampered by the fact that DSG is metabolized to toxic aldehydes by polyamine oxidases (PAO) found in fetal calf serum.[33] Lack of attention to this fact has led to several reports of a direct effect of DSG on T cell proliferation *in vitro*.[29–31] In our lab, in the absence of PAOs, DSG has no effect on mitogen-induced T cell proliferation.[30] DSG does, however, exhibit immunosuppressive activity *in vitro* in alloantigen-driven human mixed lymphocyte responses (MLR) in the absence of PAOs. Inhibition of the MLR by DSG, however, reaches a maximum at 70%, with DSG showing the same activity when added either at the beginning of the culture or 24 hours later. CsA, on the other hand, inhibits proliferation > 95%, but only when added at the initiation of the culture. Activity of CsA to inhibit lymphocyte proliferation drops off rapidly after initiation of the immune response. Since IL-2 production is inhibited by CsA, it follows that DSG does not act via this mechanism. Studies of the effects of DSG on cytokine expression in the MLR have revealed no changes in levels of either IL-2 or interferon-gamma. Furthermore, DSG does not bind to cyclophilin or FK506-binding protein and has no activity at inhibiting their rotamase activity (personal communication, S. Schrieber, C. T. Walsh), clearly suggesting a different molecular target for DSG's actions.

In order to determine whether DSG acts via the CD4+ T cell subset or the CD8+ population, studies were performed to examine IL-2 receptor expression on CD4+ and CD8+ T cells from peripheral lymphocytes in DSG-treated mixed lymphocyte cultures. The results of this study revealed a reduction of IL-2 receptor expression in both CD4+ and CD8+ cells suggesting that DSG is not specific for inhibition of either subpopulation. Additional studies on T lymphocyte effects suggest that DSG is a potent inhibitor of cytotoxic T cell generation when added to an *in vitro* culture of CTL induction.[30,32] However, DSG does not interfere with effector function of already established CTLs. These results taken together suggest that DSG does not act on a single population of T cells.

Finally, DSG has been reported to suppress the delayed type hypersensitivity (DTH) response to sheep red blood cells (SRBC) *in vivo*.[34] In this study, mice were immunized with SRBC and treated for 3 days with 10 mg/kg of DSG. Upon footpad rechallenge with SRBC, DSG-treated mice exhibited complete suppression of the DTH response. DSG added at the time of SRBC rechallenge had no effect on the effector phase of the DTH response. Thus DSG appears to act by interfering with the development of effector cells rather than on the expression of effector function.

Recently studies have been initiated to address the activity of DSG on lymphocyte development. These studies showed that DSG exhibits inhibitory activity by exerting a cytostatic effect on hematopoiesis. This result suggests that the effects of DSG on inhibiting the cell-mediated immune responses may be due to a cytostatic effect of DSG on effector cell development. The practical outcome of these studies is that the cytostatic properties of DSG may be useful as a myeloprotective agent.[35] Mice treated with cytotoxic anticancer agents and DSG show a higher number of bone marrow colony forming units after chemotherapy.

DSG Effects on B Cells

One of the most notable activities of DSG is its potent ability to suppress the humoral immune response. Mice given DSG for 3 days at a dose between 1 and 10 mg/kg show a dose-dependent inhibition of plaque-forming antibody-producing cells to SRBC immunization. Mice immunized with keyhole limpet hemocyanin (KLH) protein and treated for three days with DSG at 3 and 10 mg/kg also exhibit almost complete suppression of the antibody response[15] (FIGURE 2). Likewise, mice treated with multiple doses (10 mg × 7 d) of an immunotoxin (anti-Tac-LysPE40) and treated with DSG at a dose of 5 mg/kg for 21 days exhibit complete suppression of antibodies to both the *Pseudomonas* exotoxin and the anti-Tac antibody.[16] While DSG inhibits the antibody response to the above-mentioned T-cell-dependent antigens, DSG also inhibits dose dependently the antibody response to the T-independent antigens DNP-LPS and DNP-ficoll.[34] Additionally, DSG inhibits the response of athymic mice to these same T-independent antigens. Taken together these results suggest that humoral suppression by DSG is not dependent on direct effects of DSG on T cells but may be due to suppression of B cell or antigen presenting cell functions.

Because of the potent activity of DSG at inhibiting the humoral response *in vivo* (> 90% suppression),[15] we have examined the direct effects of DSG on B cell function. In this study, antibody-producing and -secreting B cell myelomas and hybridomas were examined for the effects of DSG on constitutive antibody production. DSG did not inhibit the antibody secretion from any of these isotype-specific myelomas and hybridomas.[36] With many stages of B cell differentiation at which DSG could potentially interfere, our studies next focused on earlier stages of B cell differentiation.

We examined the activity of DSG on a murine pre–B cell line, 70Z/3.12.[45] This cell line, when induced by lipopolysaccharide (LPS) or interferon-gamma, up regulates the synthesis of immunoglobulin kappa light chain and as a consequence expresses IgM on its surface.[37] Mu heavy chain expression in this cell line is constitutively turned on. 70Z/3 cells were incubated with DSG at 5 mg/ml for 24, 48, or 72 hours in RPMI1640 +10% fetal calf serum + 1 mM aminoguanidine a (polyamine oxidase inhibitor) followed by LPS at 1 mg/ml for 24 h. These cells were then incubated at 4°C with FITC-labeled antibodies to kappa or IgM and analyzed by fluorescent activated cell sorting. The results of this study showed that DSG blocked both the LPS and IFN-gamma induced expression of kappa in 70Z/3.12 cells that were preincubated with DSG. This effect was specific for kappa expression, as neither MHC class I nor CD45 levels were affected by DSG pretreatment. Additionally, when 70Z/3.12 cells were pretreated with CsA, there was no effect on kappa expression.

Since kappa expression in 70Z cells is transcriptionally regulated, we next looked at the effect of DSG on kappa and mu mRNA expression. When cells were pretreated with DSG for 72 hours there was a > 10-fold inhibition of kappa mRNA expression in both LPS and IFN-gamma induced cells. In contrast the level of mu heavy chain and B-actin mRNA was unchanged. Therefore, we concluded that DSG affects the activation of differentiation specific genes, such as kappa, in this pre–B cell line. This prompted us to look next at the activation of the transcription factors responsible for activating kappa light chain expression.

In 70Z/3.12 cells, kappa expression is under the regulation of the transcription factors NF-KB, Oct-1, and Oct-2.[38] NF-KB and Oct-2 activation was examined by gel retardation assays. When cells were pretreated with DSG for 72 hours, there was essentially complete inhibition of LPS-induced NF-KB and OCT-2 activation. This inhibition of NF-KB and OCT-2 activation was exhibited as a reduction in the amount of these transcription factors in the nucleus and the cytoplasm. Thus, DSG appears to have effects on these pre–B cells at the stage of pre–B cell (sIgM$^-$) to immature B cell (sIgM$^+$) differentiation. Interference with differentiation of pre–B cell into surface IgM expressing immature B cells could explain, at least in part, the inhibitory effect of DSG on antibody production. Further studies will be needed to determine if other stages of B cell differentiation are affected.

DSG Effects on Monocytes

Although precise elucidation of DSG's properties have been confounded by *in vitro* degradation in the presence of fetal calf serum, reports suggest that DSG inhibits macrophage functions, such as generation of superoxide radicals and hydrolytic enzymes; expression of MHC class II antigens; and secretion of IL-1β. However, many of these studies have not been duplicated in the absence of PAOs.

Recently, we have observed that DSG inhibits the T cell proliferative response to conventional antigens (i.e., those requiring processing), but not to superantigens. To determine whether DSG exerted its inhibitory effect at the level of the antigen-presenting monocyte or at the level of the antigen-responding T cell, we isolated purified subpopulations of T cells and monocytes. Each subpopulation was preincubated separately with DSG for 48 h. Monocytes were subsequently pulsed for 16 h with antigen (tetanus toxoid, TT, or toxic shock syndrome toxin, TSST-1). T cell proliferation to antigen was examined after 6 d in culture. Preincubation of T cells with DSG for 48 h had only a minimal effect on the capacity of the T cells to proliferate in response to autologous monocytes pulsed with TT or TSST-1. In the same experiment, monocytes were preincubated for 48 h with DSG, then pulsed with TT or TSST-1, washed (3×), irradiated, and examined for their capacity to induce proliferation of autologous T cells. Preincubation with DSG strongly inhibited the capacity of monocytes to present TT antigen to T cells, but had no effect on TSST-1 superantigen induced T cell activation. The expression of MHC class II antigen on DSG pretreated monocytes was not affected. Furthermore, DSG did not interfere with costimulatory signals such as secretion of IL-1 and IL-6 or interaction between the accessory cell surface molecule B7 and the T cell antigen CD28. Studies with peptide-specific T cell clones showed similar results with DSG not inhibiting T cell proliferation in response to peptide challenge, whereas proliferation of T cells to native antigen, requiring antigen processing, was inhibited. Thus we have shown that

DSG inhibits the capacity of purified monocytes to present to T cells conventional antigens but not superantigens, suggesting a direct effect of DSG on the ability of APCs to present antigen.

BIOCHEMICAL MECHANISM OF ACTION OF DSG

Although the precise biochemical mechanism of action of DSG has not been determined, recent studies aimed at identifying the intracellular target of DSG have revealed some exciting results. These studies showed, using the biochemical approach of immobilizing methoxyDSG to an affinity column, that DSG specifically binds to Hsc70, a constitutively expressed member of the heat shock protein 70 (Hsp70) family.[25] To quantitate binding constants (K_d) of DSG to Hsp70 and Hsp90, we utilized the technique of capillary zone electrophoresis.[39] The binding constants of DSG for mammalian Hsp70 and Hsp90 were observed to be 4 μM and 5 μM respectively. These concentrations fall within the pharmacologic range of DSG levels in man[40] and suggest that the K_d of Hsps for DSG is sufficient for *in vivo* binding. Interestingly, binding affinities of active and inactive DSG analogues to Hsp70 and Hsp90 were found to correlate well with immunosuppressive activity.

How is it that DSG binding to Hsp70 and Hsp90 proteins can result in immune suppression? One possible explanation is that Hsp70 plays a role in the binding and intracellular transport of antigenic peptides within the antigen presenting cell.[26-28] Supporting this theory are several reports suggesting that Hsps contain a peptide binding groove very similar to MHC molecules.[41] Our data, discussed earlier in this report, show that DSG inhibits the capacity of monocytes to present antigen to T cells; thus it is plausible that DSG interferes with antigen processing and presentation by interfering with the loading of peptides onto MHC molecules. In that respect, DSG could represent a true peptide mimetic.

Alternatively, another possible explanation of how DSG's immunosuppressive activity may be related to binding to Hsps is through the association of Hsp70 and Hsp90 in a complex with the glucocoricoid receptor, Hsp59, and possibly cyclophilin.[42-44] This observation links the immunosuppressive activities of cyclosporine A, FK506, steroids, and DSG through a potentially common biochemical pathway. This pathway involves the formation of a complex between these proteins with the ultimate activation of the glucocorticoid receptor occurring via interactions with Hsps 59, 70, and 90 and their ligands. At our current level of understanding, however, we cannot say how DSG might interfere with this pathway. It is intriguing to think that these unrelated immunosuppressive agents bind to different proteins found in a common complex and act via some related mechanism. Perhaps, Hsps represent a new class of immunophilins which bind DSG and exert their own immunosuppressive activity.

Over the last decade, the discovery of new immunosuppressive agents has increased dramatically. DSG represents a novel immunosuppressive agent with unique activities and a novel mechanism of action. FIGURE 3 is a schematic showing our current understanding of the cellular mechanism of action of DSG and many of the other known immunosuppressive agents. These immunosuppressive agents have mechanisms of action that fall into four classes: early activation gene inhibitors, purine and pyrimidine biosynthesis inhibitors, costimulation inhibitors, and antigen-processing inhibitors.

Cyclosporine A, FK506, and rapamycin fall into the first class, having effects on the early activation of T cells. CsA and FK506 act at the molecular level by binding to immunophilins and inhibiting their *cis-trans* prolyl isomerase (PPIase) activity. It is not clear whether suppression of PPIase activity is responsible for the activity of these agents. Another mechanism by which these agents may exert their immunosuppressive properties is via binding the protein phosphatase calcineurin. At the cellular level both cyclosporine and FK506 are believed to act by inhibiting T cell proliferation via blocking IL-2 production. Rapamycin, on the other hand, is also an inhibitor

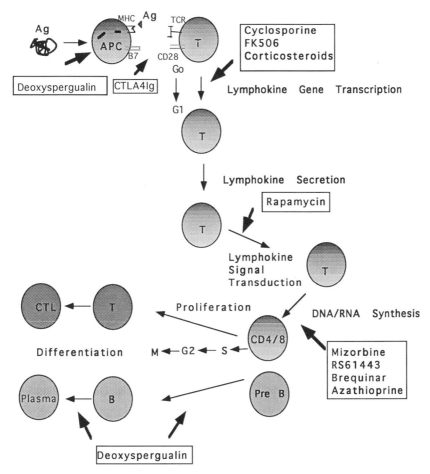

FIGURE 3. Schematic of the mechanism of action of Deoxyspergualin and other immunosuppressive drugs.

of T cell proliferation, but is believed to interfere with IL-2 signaling mechanisms instead of inhibiting IL-2 production. Steroids, although exhibiting multiple actions, appear to work in part by inhibiting T cell activation as well.

The second class of immunosuppressive agents, depicted in FIGURE 3, work at the molecular level by inhibiting purine and pyrimidine biosynthesis. These agents include Mizorbidine, micophenolic acid (RS61443), Brequinar, and azathioprine. Inhibition of purine and pyrimidine biosynthesis results in a block in DNA synthesis of rapidly dividing T and B cells. These agents act at the cellular level by interfering with the proliferation and development of T and B cells. Many of these agents have exhibited excellent *in vivo* immunosuppressive activity.

A new class of immunosuppressive agent shown in FIGURE 3 interferes with the costimulatory signal necessary for activation of the T cell. These agents include a fusion protein of the CD28 homologue, CTLA-4, and human Ig called CTLA4-Ig. Its mechanism of action is believed to result from interference with the required CTLA4/B7 costimulatory interaction between the T cell and the APC needed for optimal T cell proliferation. Studies have shown that *in vivo,* this agent can induce antigen-specific nonresponsiveness.[45]

Finally, at our current level of understanding, it appears that DSG exerts its immunosuppressive effects by interfering with the differentiation of effector cells, including cytotoxic T cells and antibody-producing B cells. Additionally, DSG may interfere with antigen processing. The molecular mechanism of action of DSG may be due to its interaction with the Hsps. Certainly, more studies are needed before we fully understand DSG's mechanism of action.

REFERENCES

1. TAKEUCHI, T., H. IINUMA, S. KUNIMOTO, T. MASUDA, M. ISHIZUKA, M. TAKEUCHI, M. HAMADA, H. NAGANAWA, S. KONDO & H. UMEZAWA. 1981. A new antitumor antibiotic, spergualin: isolation and antitumor activity. J. Antibiot. **34:** 1619.

2. K. NISHIKAWA, C. SHIBASAKI, K. TAKAHASHI, T. NAKAMURA, T. TAKEUCHI & H. UMEZAWA. 1986. Antitumor activity of spergualin: a novel antitumor antibiotic. J. Antibiot. **39:** 1461–1466.

3. SCHORLEMMER, H. U., G. DICKNEITE & F. R. SEILER. 1990. Treatment of acute rejection episodes and induction of tolerance in rat skin allotransplantation by 15-deoxyspergualin. Transplant. Proc. **22:** 1626.

4. REICHENSPURNER, H., A. HILDEBRANDT, P. A. HUMAN, D. H. BOEHM, A. G. ROSE, J. A. ODELL, B. REICHART & H. U. SCHORLEMMER. 1990. 15-Deoxyspergualin for induction of graft nonreactivity after cardiac and renal allotransplantation in primates. Transplantation **50:** 181.

5. NEMOTO, K. 1991. Deoxyspergualin in lethal murine graft vs. host disease. Transplantation **51:** 712.

6. SCHORLEMMER, H. U. & F. R. SEILER. 1990. Therapy of human multiple sclerosis MS disease modifying activity of 15-deoxyspergualin on acute and chronic relapsing experimental allergic encephalomyelitis EAE. Immunobiology **181:** 236–237.

7. SCHORLEMMER, H. U., R. R. BARTLETT, R. SCHLEYERBACH, G. DICKNEITE, F. R. SEILER & A. G. BEHRINGWERKE. 1989. Immunosuppressive therapy of experimental autoimmune diseases like rheumatoid arthritis and systemic lupus erythematosus by 15-deoxyspergualin. Int. J. Immunother. **5:** 9–20.

8. SCHORLEMMER, H. U., R. R. BARTLETT & F. R. SEILER. 1990. Curative effect of 15-deoxyspergualin on the development of SLE-like autoimmune disease in MRL-LPR mice. Immunobiology **181:** 222.

9. REICHENSPURNER, H., A. HILDEBRANDT, P. A. HUMAN, D. H. BOEHM, A. G. ROSE, H. U. SCHORLEMMER & B. REICHART. 1990. 15-Deoxyspergualin after cardiac and renal allotransplantation in primates. Transplant. Proc. **22:** 1618–1619.

10. UENO, M., Y. NAKAJIMA, M. SEGAWA, M. HISANAGA, H. YABUUCHI, A. YOSHIMURA & H. NAKANO. 1992. Immunosuppressive effect in combination therapy of cyclosporine-A, FK-506, and 15-deoxyspergualin on pancreatic-islet xenotransplantation. Transplant. Proc. **24:** 638–640.

11. JINDAL, R. M., M. A. TEPPER, K. SOLTYS, F. YOST, E. BEER & S. I. CHO. Effect of

deoxyspergualin on the endocrine function of the rat pancreas. Transplantation. (In press.)

12. AMEMIYA, H., S. SUZUKI, T. OTAK, K. TAKAHASHI, T. SONODA, et al. 1991. Multicenter clinical trial of anti-rejection post therapy with deoxyspergualin kidney transplantations. Int. J. Clin. Pharm. Res. 11: 175.

13. PITTMAN, K., J. THOMAS & F. THOMAS. 1992. Reduction of primary nonfunction in discordant pancreas islet xenografts. Transplant. Proc. 24: 649–650.

14. GORES, P., J. S. NAJARIAN, E. STEPHANIAN, LLOVERAS, S. L. KELLEY & D. E. R. SUTHERLAND. 1993. Insulin independence in type 1 diabetes after transplantation of unpurified islets from single donor with 15-deoxyspergualin. Lancet 341: 19–20.

15. TEPPER, M. A., B. PETTY, I. BURSUKER, R. PASTERNAK, J. CLEAVELAND, B. SCHACTER & G. L. SPITALNY. 1991. Inhibition of antibody production by the immunosuppressive agent, 15-deoxyspergualin. Transplant. Proc. 23: 1, 328–331.

16. PAI, L., M. A. TEPPER, D. J. FITZGERALD, B. SCHACTER, G. L. SPITALNY & I. PASTAN. 1990. Inhibition of antibody response to Pseudomonas exotoxin (PE) and an immunotoxin containing Pseudomonas exotoxin by 15-deoxyspergualin in mice. Cancer Res. 50: 7750–7753.

17. DHINGRA, K., H. FRITSCHE, J. L. MURRAY, A. F. LOBUGLIO, M. B. KHAZELI, S. L. KELLEY, M. A. TEPPER, D. GREENE, D. BOOSER, A. BUZDAR, M. RUBER, L. GUTIERREZ & G. HORTOBAGYI. Suppression of human anti-mouse antibody response to murine monoclonal antibody L6 by deoxyspergualin: a phase I study. Proceedings of the 5th International Workshop on Breast Cancer Research and Immunology. (In press.)

18. NEMOTO, K., F. ABE, T. NAKAMURA, M. ISHIZUKA, T. TAKEUCHI & H. UMEZAWA. 1987. Blastogenic responses and the release of interleukins 1 and 2 by spleen cells obtained from rat skin allograft recipients administered with 15-deoxyspergualin. J. Antibiot. 40: 1062.

19. WAAGA, A. M., K. ULRICHS, M. KRZYSMANSKI, J. TREUMER, M. L. HANSMANN, R. ROMMEL & W. MULLER-RUCHHOLTZ. 1990. The immunosuppressive agent 15-deoxyspergualin induces tolerance and modulates MHC-antigen expression and interleukin-1 production in the early phase of rat allograft responses. Transplant. Proc. 22: 1613.

20. TAKASU, S., K. SAKAGAMI, F. MORISAKI, T. KAWAMURA, M. HAISA, T. OIWA, M. INAGAKI, H. HASUOKA, Y. KUROZOMI & K. ORITA. 1991. Immunosuppressive mechanism of 15-deoxyspergualin on sinusoidal lining cells in swine liver transplantation: suppression of MHC class II antigens and interleukin-1 production. J. Surg. Res. 51: 165.

21. LEVENTHAL, J. R., H. C. FLORES, S. A. GRUBER, J. FIGUEROA, J. L. PLATT, J. C. MANIVEL, F. H. BACH, A. J. MATAS & R. M. BOLMAN. 1992. Evidence that 15-deoxyspergualin inhibits natural antibody production but fails to prevent hyperacute rejection in a discordant xenograft model. Transplantation 54: 26.

22. NISHIMURA, K. & T. TOKUNAGA. 1989. Mechanism of action of 15-deoxyspergualin. I. Suppressive effect on the induction of alloreactive secondary cytotoxic T lymphocytes in vivo and in vitro. Immunology 68: 66.

23. KERR, P. G. & R. C. ATKINS. 1989. The effects of deoxyspergualin on lymphocytes and monocytes in vivo and in vitro. Transplantation 48: 1048.

24. JIANG, H., S. TAKAHARA, Y. TAKANO, M. MACHIDA, A. IWASAKI, Y. KOKADO, H. KAMEOKA, A. MOUTABARRIK, M. ISHIBASHI & T. SONODA. 1990. In vitro immunosuppressive effect of deoxymethylspergualin. Transplant. Proc. 22: 1633.

25. NADLER, S. G., M. A. TEPPER, B. SCHACTER & C. E. MAZZUCCO. 1992. Interaction of the immunosuppressant deoxyspergualin with a member of the Hsp70 family of heat shock proteins. Science 258: 484.

26. VANBUSKIRK, A., B. L. CRUMP, E. MARGOLIAH & S. K. PIERCE. 1989. A peptide binding protein having a role in antigen presentation is a member of the Hsp70 heat shock family. J. Exp. Med. 170: 1799.

27. HIGHTOWER, L. E. 1991. Heat shock, stress proteins, chaperones, and proteotoxicity. Cell 66: 191.

28. GETHING, M. J. & J. SAMBROOK. 1992. Protein folding in the cell. Nature 355: 33.

29. KERR, P. G. & R. C. ATKINS. 1989. The effects of deoxyspergualin on lymphocytes and monocytes in vivo and in vitro. Transplantation 48: 1048–1052.

30. TEPPER, M. A., S. G. NADLER, C. MAZZUCCO, C. SINGH & S. L. KELLEY. 1993. Mechanism of action of 15-deoxyspergualin, a novel immunosuppressive drug. Ann. N.Y. Acad. Sci. 685: 136–147.

31. FALK, W., K. ULRICHS & W. MULLER-RUCHHOLTZ. 1987. 15-Deoxyspergualin (a new guanidine-like drug) blocks T lymphocyte proliferation. Transplant. Proc. 19: 4239–4240.

32. FUJII, H., T. TAKADO, N. KYUICHI, A. FUMINORI, A. FUJII, J. E. TALMADGE, T. TAKEUCHI. 1992. Deoxyspergualin, a novel immunosuppressant, markedly inhibits human mixed lymphocyte reaction and cytotoxic T-lymphocyte activity in vitro. Int. J. Immunopharmacol. 14: 731–737.

33. KUNIMOTO, S., C. NOSAKA, C. Z. XU & T. TAKEUSHI. 1989. Serum effect on cellular uptake of spermidine, spergualin, 15-deoxyspergualin, and their metabolites by L5178Y cells. J. Antibiot. 42: 116.

34. MAKINO, M., M. FUJIWARA, H. WATANABE, T. AOYAGI & H. UMEZAWA. 1987. Immunosuppressive activities of deoxyspergualin. II. The effect on the antibody responses. Immunopharmacology 14: 115–122.

35. NEMOTO, K., Y. SUGAWARA, M. OGINO, T. MAE, F. ABE & T. TAKEUCHI. 1992. Myeloprotective activity of deoxyspergualin: influence on splenic colony-forming cell injury and antitumor activity of mitomycin C in mice. Jpn J. Cancer Res. 83: 789–793.

36. STERBENZ, K. G. & M. A. TEPPER. Effects of 15-deoxyspergualin on the expression of surface immunoglobulin in 70Z/3.12 murine pre-B cell line. Ann. N.Y. Acad. Sci. 685: 205–206.

37. MAINS, P. E. & C. H. SIBLEY. 1983. LPS-nonresponsive variants of the mouse B cell lymphoma, 70Z/3: isolation and characterization. Som. Cell Genet. 9: 699–720.

38. SEN, R. & D. BALTIMORE. 1986. Inducibility of kappa immunoglobulin enhancer–binding protein NF-KB by a posttranslational mechanism. Cell 47: 921–928.

39. NADEAU, K., S. N. NADLER, M. SAULNIER, M. A. TEPPER & C. WALSH. Quantitation of the interaction of the immunosuppressant deoxyspergualin and analogs with Hsp70 and Hsp90. J. Biol. Chem. (In press.)

40. MUINDI, J. F., S. J. LEE, L. BALTZER, A. JAKUBOWSKI, H. I. SCHER, L. A. SPRANCMANIS, C. M. RILEY, D. VANDER VELDE & C. W. YOUNG. 1991. Clinical pharmacology of deoxyspergualin in patients with advanced cancer. Cancer Res. 51: 3096–3101.

41. RIPPMANN, F., W. R. TAYLOR, J. B. ROTHBARD & N. M. GREEN. 1991. A hypothetical model for the peptide binding domain of hsp70 based on the peptide binding domain of HLA. EMBO J. 10: 1053–1059.

42. YEM, A. W., A. G. TOMASSELLI, R. L. HEINRIKSON, H. Z. NELLY, V. A. RUFF, R. A. JOHNSON & M. R. DEIBEL. 1992. The Hsp56 component of the steroid receptor complexes binds to immobilized FK506 and shows homology to FKBP-12 and FKBP-13. J. Biol. Chem. 267: 2868–2871.

43. TAI, P. K., M. W. ALBERS, H. CHANG, L. E. FABER & S. L. SCHREIBER. 1992. Association of a 59-kilodalton immunophilin with the glucocorticoid receptor complex. Science 256: 1315–1318.

44. SCHREIBER, S. L. 1991. Chemistry and biology of the immunophilins and their immunosuppressive ligands. Science 251: 283.

45. LINSLEY, P. S., P. M. WALLACE, J. JOHNSON, M. G. GIBSON, J. GREENE, J. LEDBETTER, C. SINGH & M. A. TEPPER. 1992. Immunosuppression in vivo by a soluble form of the CTLA-4 T cell activation molecule. Science 257: 792.

The IL-1β Converting Enzyme as a Therapeutic Target

DOUGLAS K. MILLER,[a] JIMMY R. CALAYCAY,[b]
KEVIN T. CHAPMAN,[c] ANDREW D. HOWARD,[a]
MATTHEW J. KOSTURA,[d] SUSAN M. MOLINEAUX,[e]
AND NANCY A. THORNBERRY[f]

[a] Department of Biochemical and Molecular Pathology
[b] Department of Analytical Biochemistry
[c] Department of Medicinal Chemical Research
[d] Department of Cellular and Molecular Pharmacology
[e] Department of Molecular Immunology
[f] Department of Biochemistry
Merck Research Laboratories
Post Office Box 2000
Rahway, New Jersey 07065-0900

INTRODUCTION

Interleukin-1β (IL-1β) and interleukin-1α (IL-1α) are proinflammatory cytokines that promote leukocyte infiltration, prostaglandin synthesis, joint swelling, and tissue destruction.[1–8] IL-1α and IL-1β are members of a family of cytokines that also includes the IL-1 receptor antagonist protein (IL-1RA; see FIGURE 1), all of which are synthesized most prominently by monocytic cells. In contrast to the agonist activity of IL-1α and IL-1β,[9] IL-1RA is a strict antagonist on IL-1 receptors. It is synthesized on membrane-bound polysomes and exported via the classical endoplasmic reticulam (ER)/Golgi route where it becomes glycosylated. IL-1α and IL-1β, on the other hand, both lack leader sequences and are found in cytoplasm.[10–14] IL-1β is released from cells following stimulation, and it is the major agonist form of IL-1 found in biological fluids during diseased states.[15,16] In contrast, IL-1α remains largely intracellular in spite of its synthesis at significant levels.[13,17] IL-1RA is also released from stimulated cells, but its appearance in blood is delayed relative to that of IL-1β. Because IL-1RA is produced at about 100-fold higher concentrations than IL-1β, it may serve to decrease IL-1β activity.[18]

The importance of IL-1 as a target for antiinflammatory therapy is shown by the efficacy of IL-1RA, soluble IL-1R, and antiIL-1 receptor monoclonal antibodies in several animal models of human disease.[19–23] For example, PMN infiltration, swelling, and tissue necrosis were reduced in a rabbit model of inflammatory bowel disease by IL-1RA. Mortality was drastically reduced in murine graft vs host disease with the use of IL-1RA. Truncated soluble IL-1 receptors showed efficacy in reducing the swelling in cat adjuvant arthritis and blocking allograft rejection in mice.[24] Monoclonals against the IL-1 receptor have also been shown to block PMN extravasation and acute phase protein synthesis in mice.[25]

The importance of IL-1β as the primary form of IL-1 responsible *in vivo* has been confirmed recently by the discovery of pox virus proteins that are specific for IL-1β. A pox virus protein, similar in structure to soluble type II IL-1 receptors, bound only IL-1β and not IL-1α. Production of this protein by the virus reduced the cell-

	IL-1α	IL-1β	IL-1RA
Major Cell Source	Macrophage	Macrophage	Macrophage
Biosynthesis	31 KDa Cytoplasm	31 KDa Cytoplasm	18-22 KDa Golgi-CHO
Proteolytic Processing for Activation	−	+ (17.5 KDa) Asp^{116}-Ala^{117}	−
Receptor Active Form	31 KDa Agonist	17.5 KDa Agonist	22 KDa Antagonist
Secreted *in vitro*	−	+	+
Presence in Disease States (CSF, Synovial Fluid)	+	+++	++++

FIGURE 1. Characteristics of the IL-1 family of molecules binding to IL-1 receptors.

mediated immune response induced by the infection, suggesting that the host response was primarily IL-1β mediated.[26,27]

ROLE OF ICE IN IL-1 ACTIVATION

While both IL-1β and IL-1α are synthesized as 31-kDa forms, only IL-1α is active on IL-1 receptors without further processing; IL-1β must first be processed from its inactive 31-kDa cytoplasmic precursor form (pIL-1β) to an active 17.5-kDa mature form (mIL-1β).[9,17,28] A unique cytoplasmic enzyme thus far found only in monocytic cells has been identified, termed IL-1β converting enzyme (ICE).[29–34] ICE cleaves the Asp^{116}-Ala^{117} bond of pIL-1β to generate the mIL-1β (see FIGURE 2). It also cleaves pIL-1β at a secondary cleavage site Asp^{27}-Gly^{28} to form small amounts of a 28-kDa fragment which can be further processed to the 17.5-kDa form. In contrast, ICE does not appear to cleave other proteins containing Asp-X linkages.[30] ICE is essential for the generation of mIL-1β: cells lacking ICE activity even when transfected with pIL-1β do not form active mIL-1β.[35,36] Another protein, crmA, synthesized by pox viruses provides additional support for the intracellular role of ICE in mIL-1β formation: this serpin inhibits the processing of pIL-1β by ICE.[37] No enzyme has been found to specifically process IL-1α, although calpain has been shown to cleave IL-1α.[38] Because IL-1α remains largely cell associated and is not normally secreted, its appearance on the outside of cells may be associated with cell death.[13,39] The presence of a processed extracellular active 17-KDa form of IL-1α may result from cleavage by other proteases ("bystander proteases") at, for example, the Phe^{118}-Leu^{119} bond[1,40] (see also Reference 41).

No mIL-1β is found inside cells, and little pIL-1β is found outside cells in the absence of cell damage. Pulse-chase analysis indicates that there is a precursor-product relationship between intracellular pIL-1β and secreted mIL-1β.[13,42] Thus, the cleavage of pIL-1β must be closely associated with the secretion of mIL-1β. The unusual mechanism of synthesis, posttranslational modification, and cellular export of IL-1β presents a number of potential sites for therapeutic interdiction. Because of the substrate specificity of ICE, development of an inhibitor for ICE represents a unique opportunity to develop a small molecule inhibitor of mIL-1β formation.

CHARACTERIZATION OF ICE ENZYMATIC ACTIVITY

To determine the minimum recognition sequence of ICE, a 14-amino-acid peptide spanning the Asp-Ala cleavage site of pIL-1β, NEAYVHDAPVRSLN, as well as series of amino-terminal or carboxy-terminal truncations were prepared. These peptides were used as substrates for ICE, and their relative activity (V_{max}/K_m) was compared[34] (FIGURE 3, top). The results indicated that residues beyond P1' were not required, and at P1' only a methylamine substituent was necessary. At least four residues to the left of the cleavage site were necessary for activity; no cleavage activity was observed when the Tyr was removed.

Using a pentapeptide to further characterize the relative activity of individual amino acids in the sequence, it was determined that Ac-Tyr-Val-Ala-Asp-Gly was recognized best by ICE (FIGURE 3, bottom). Asp is absolutely required at the P1 position; glutamate at this position is cleaved only slightly. Small aliphatic residues (Gly and Ala) are preferred in P1'. Substitutions in P2 are well tolerated, Val is preferred in P3, and hydrophobic residues are preferred in P4. To facilitate rapid, sensitive measurement of ICE, a fluorometric assay utilizing Ac-Tyr-Val-Ala-Asp-amino-4-methylcoumarin (AcYVAD-AMC) as a substrate was subsequently employed.[34]

ICE was found to be a thiol protease based upon its inhibition by a number of thiol selective reagents such as *N*-ethyl maleimide and iodoacetic acid (TABLE 1). It was not inhibited by inhibitors of serine or aspartyl proteases such as PMSF, leupeptin, or pepstatin. While ICE activity was not inhibited by EDTA, addition of *o*-phenanthroline resulted in inhibition after a prolonged incubation, suggesting that ICE might be a metalloprotease. This inhibition was reversed by high (10 mM) but not low (0.1 mM) DTT. The addition of copper increased the rate of inhibition, and

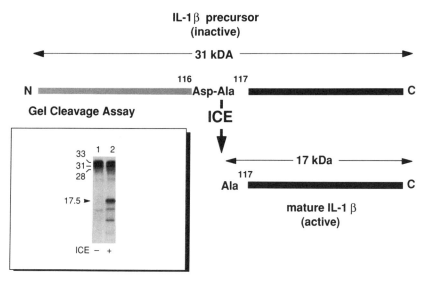

FIGURE 2. Cleavage of the IL-1β precursor by ICE to generate mIL-1β. Inset, autoradiograph of an SDS-PAGE gel of 31-kDa ³⁵S-Met *in vitro* translated pIL-1β cleaved by ICE to 17.5-kDa mIL-1β.[30]

the simultaneous addition of EDTA prevented any inhibition. These results suggested that the o-phenanthroline inhibition of ICE occurred by a metal-catalyzed oxidation of a labile thiol.[34]

Definitive evidence that ICE was a cysteine protease came from potent inhibition by a peptide diazomethylketone (L-707,509) and a peptide aldehyde[34] (L-709,049; FIGURE 4). Addition of 250 nM of a peptide diazomethylketone resulted in time-dependent and complete inhibition of ICE activity, but this was prevented by saturating levels of the AcYVAD-AMC substrate ($70 \times K_m$; $K_m = 14$ μM). Addition of a high concentration of the substrate after inhibition had occurred did not relieve the inhibition, indicating that the inhibition was irreversible. The peptide aldehyde

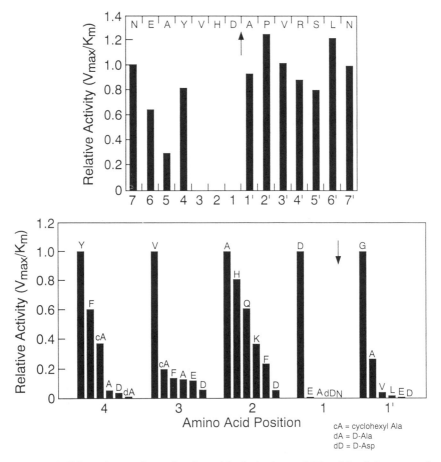

FIGURE 3. Effect of truncation and amino acid substitution on ICE activity. Substrates and products were separated by RP-HPLC and quantitated. Top, ICE activity (V_{max}/K_m) of either N- or C-terminally truncated peptides of the 14-mer pIL-1β spanning peptide NEAYVH-DAPVRSLN; activity was expressed relative to that of the 14-mer defined as 1.0. Bottom, ICE activity of a pentapeptide with the indicated amino acid substitutions; activity was expressed relative to Ac-YVADG defined as 1.0.

TABLE 1. Inhibition of YVAD-AMC Cleavage by Inhibitors of Various Classes of Proteases[a]

Class	Reagent	Inhibition
Serine	PMSF (1 mM)	0 ± 2
	DFP (1 mM)	6 ± 8
	leupeptin (1 mM)	1 ± 2
Aspartyl	Pepstatin (0.1 mM)	0 ± 2
Thiol	NEM (1 mM)	99 ± 1
	Iodoacetate (1 mM)	99 ± 5
	E-64 (1 mM)	0 ± 1
Metallo	EDTA (10 mM)	13 ± 10
	OPA[b] (1 mM) $t_{1/2}$ = 60 min)	98 ± 3
	OPA (1 mM) + 10 μM Cu^{2+} ($t_{1/2}$ = 1 min)	99 ± 3
	OPA + EDTA	10 ± 10
	OPA + 10 mM DTT	10 ± 10
	OPA + 0.1 mM DTT	98 ± 3

[a]Assays were done at the indicated concentration of inhibitors and expressed as a percentage of uninhibited activity. Inhibitors included phenylmethylsulfonylfluoride (PMSF), diisopropyl-fluorophosphate (DFP), *N*-ethyl maleimide (NEM, and 1,10 (*ortho*)-phenanthroline (OPA).
[b]O-Phenanthroline inhibits ICE via metal catalyzed oxidation.

L-709,049 was also a competitive inhibitor of ICE activity, but saturating levels of substrate added after inhibition had occurred could reverse the inhibition. A competitive substrate peptide hydroxylamine (L-700,018) could also inhibit ICE cleavage, as shown here using *in vitro* translated ^{35}S-Met-labeled pIL-1β (FIGURE 5). ICE was not inhibited by a specific elastase inhibitor (L-680,833).[51]

PURIFICATION AND STRUCTURE OF ACTIVE ICE

Active ICE was purified to homogeneity by conventional ion exchange and reverse phase high-performance liquid chromatography (RP-HPLC) techniques[43] as well as with an inhibitor affinity column.[34] Because the P2 position in ICE substrates was relatively insensitive to substitution (FIGURE 3), a reversible peptide aldehyde inhibitor was prepared with Lys in place of Ala in P2. The Ac-YVAD-CHO was coupled via a spacer arm to Sepharose 4B (FIGURE 6) to generate a specific affinity matrix. Crude dialyzed THP.1 cytosol or a partially purified DEAE pool of that cytosol was allowed to bind to the column and extensively washed. ICE was specifically eluted with 100 μM L-709,049, and found to contain by sodium dodecyl sulfate-polyacrylamide gel electrophoresis (SDS-PAGE) two tightly associated proteins at 20 and 10 KDa (termed p20 and p10 respectively) in a 1:1 ratio (FIGURE 6). To recover active ICE, the L-709,049 bound ICE was first incubated with oxidized glutathione (to form a stable, inactive enzyme-glutathione conjugate) and hydroxyl-amine (to destroy the aldehyde inhibitor). Secondly, after desalting, DTT was added to remove the glutathione and generate the active enzyme.

Because the ICE active site thiol is more than 10-fold more reactive than ordinary thiols, the Cys could be readily labeled with ^{14}C-iodoacetate. Since the alkylation was competitive with substrate, saturating levels of substrate could prevent the labeling. As shown in FIGURE 7A, ICE inhibition could be almost totally achieved with 100

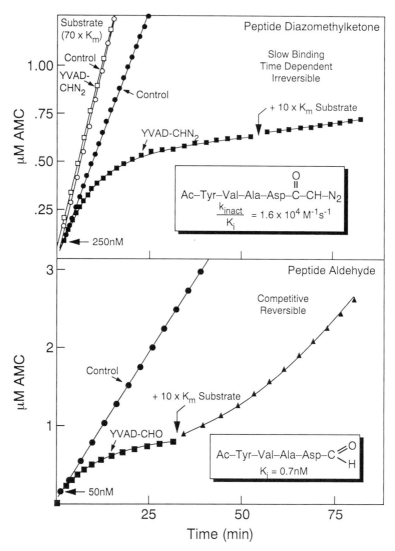

FIGURE 4. Inhibition of ICE by the thiol protease inhibitors Ac-YVAD-diazomethyketone (L-707,509, top) and aldehyde (L-709,049, bottom) using AcYVAD-AMC at its K_m (14 μM). (Taken from Thornberry *et al.*[34] with permission.)

μM iodoacetic acid at 40 min. Under these conditions in the absence of substrate, the p20 protein was selectively labeled (FIGURE 7B). With saturating amounts of substrate where no enzyme inhibition was observed, no p20 labeling occurred. Isolation of the p20 followed by tryptic cleavage and C_8 RP-HPLC separation of the resultant peptides led to the identification of a single labeled peptide (FIGURE 7C) which had the sequence Val-Ile-Ile-Ile-Gln-Ala-(^{14}C)Cys.

After obtaining sequence of tryptic and Asp.N peptides of the p20 and p10 proteins, degenerate oligonucleotides were used to PCR ICE cDNA fragments. These were used to screen a THP.1 monocytic cell cDNA library for full-length cDNA clones. All clones cross-hybridized with probes to both p20 and p10, indicating that both ICE proteins were encoded on a single mRNA. The resultant open reading frame encoded a 45-kDa protein (p45; FIGURE 8) which contained a 13-kDa polypeptide N-terminal to the p20 and a 2-kDa peptide separating the p20 from the p10 which were not found on the isolated active enzyme (FIGURE 9). No sequence homology to other Cys proteases or other proteins in the protein databank was observed.[34] The human cDNA was used to clone out the mouse[44,45] and rat[46] forms of the enzyme (FIGURE 8). All three proteins contained the active site Cys with considerable stretches of amino acid identity particularly in the p10 region where there was 81% amino acid identify between the mouse and human proteins. Identity was less in the p20 region (62%) and still less in the pro domain (53%).[44] An alternatively cleaved, 1.6-kDa higher molecular weight form of the p20, termed p22, was in some cases purified along with the p20 protein (FIGURE 9).[43] All four cleavage sites generating the p20, p22, and p10 proteins followed Asp residues, perhaps indicating autoprocessing of the p45.[34]

The p45 form of ICE is the major form of ICE found in monocytic cells as determined by immunoblots with antibodies generated to affinity purified human ICE. Extracts of p45 have, however, no detectable pIL-1β cleavage activity. Only after dialysis or short incubations at 30°C, when p45 is cleaved to the p20/p10 form of the enzyme, is significant pIL-1β cleavage activity seen.[47] Both p20 and p10 are necessary for ICE activity; ion exchange column fractions of cytoplasmic extracts containing p20 in the absence of p10 contain no ICE activity.[43]

Expression in COS-7 cells of the p45 ICE protein resulted in generation of pIL-1β cleavage activity that could be inhibited by the peptide aldehyde inhibitor L-709,049 (FIGURE 10). An [116]Asp to Ala mutant of pIL-1β was not a substrate for

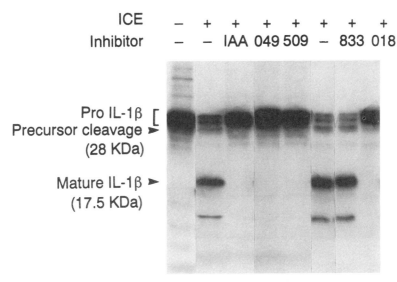

FIGURE 5. Inhibition of ICE cleavage of ^{35}S-Met-labeled pIL-1β by various inhibitors. **IAA,** iodoacetic acid, 5 mM; **049,** L-709,049, AcYVAD-CHO, 0.5 μM; **509,** L-707,509, AcYVAD-CN$_2$, 10 μM; **833,** L-680,833[51], 5 μM; **018,** L-700,018, AcYVAD-NHOH, 0.5 mM.

the recombinant ICE.[34] Expression of human p45 in *Escherichea coli* or *baculovirus* systems, followed by purification on the peptide aldehyde affinity column resulted in the purification of both p20 and p10 in 1:1 ratios.[48] Presumably the N-terminal domain of the p45 is necessary for proper folding of the p20 and p10 proteins;

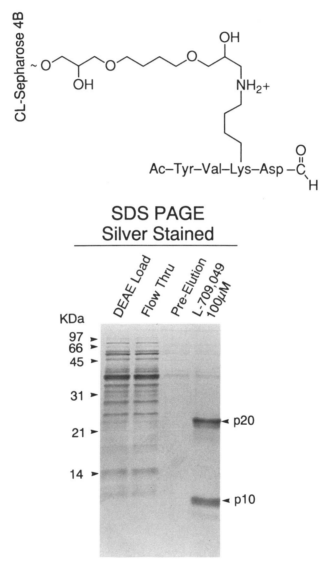

FIGURE 6. Affinity purification of ICE. **Top:** A peptide aldehyde affinity matrix was prepared by coupling AcYVKD-CHO to Sepharose 4B as shown.[34] **Bottom:** Silver-stained SDS-PAGE of fractions from an affinity column purification beginning with a partially purified DEAE fraction of ICE.[43] The load, the flowthrough fraction, a column fraction after extensive washing, and the proteins eluted by 100 μM L-709,049 are shown.

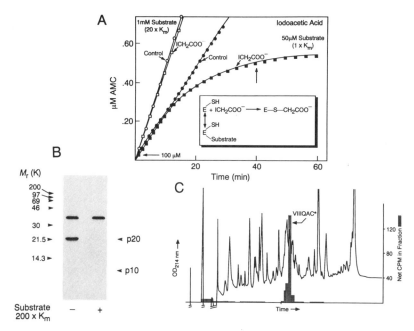

FIGURE 7. Inhibition of ICE by ^{14}C-iodoacetic acid and its labeling of the active site Cys. **A:** Kinetic analysis of iodoacetic acid inhibition of ICE using 100 μM iodoacetic acid and its competition by saturating substrate. **B:** Under conditions of 99% inhibition of ICE (40 min), the p20 protein found in a partially purified sulfopropyl-HPLC fraction of active[43] THP.1 ICE was labeled and identified following SDS-PAGE and autoradiography.[34] **C:** C_8-RP-HPLC chromatography of the tryptic peptides of the p20 labeled with ^{14}C-iodoacetic acid (the p20 was purified by C_4-RP-HPLC prior to trypsin cleavage). Only one peptide was labeled, and sequencing of this peptide revealed that the active site Cys was found in a sequence VIIIQAC.[43]

coexpression of isolated p20 and p10 together in *E. coli* did not produce any active enzyme.[48] The activity of the recombinant enzyme was comparable to that of the native THP.1 enzyme: the ICE inhibitor affinity column yielded similar amounts of isolated enzyme for the same amount of activity units applied. Occasionally a processed form of p10, termed p7, presumably also formed by autocatalysis, could be copurified on the affinity column.[48] This form could also be generated in small amounts in highly purified fractions of THP.1 ICE where it contained substantially less activity.[43]

EFFECT OF INHIBITION OF ICE ON IL-1β SECRETION FROM MONOCYTES

To determine the effect of ICE inhibitors on mIL-1β production in human monocytes, ^{35}S-Met labeled heparinized blood was stimulated with heat-killed *Staphylococcus aureus* which has been shown to promote both rapid synthesize of pIL-1β as well as rapid release extracellularly of mIL-1β.[49] When this stimulation was performed on cells preincubated with the peptide aldehyde inhibitor L-709,049, mIL-1β release was inhibited in a dose-responsive fashion with an IC_{50} of about 2 μM (FIGURE 11). In contrast, the addition of a control peptide aldehyde with a D-Ala residue in the P3 position (K_i = 1.5 μM vs. K_i = 0.8 nM for L-709,049) resulted in little observable inhibition of mIL-1β release.[34] The specificity of this inhibition for IL-1β release was shown by the lack of inhibition of TNFα, IL-6, or IL-8 release by the same cells (FIGURE 12).

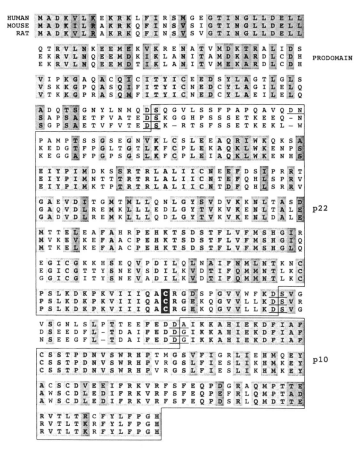

FIGURE 8. The amino acid sequence of human, mouse, and rat ICE. ICE was cloned as described,[34,44,46] and the aligned open reading frame is shown. Shaded areas indicate amino acids of identity or close similarity. The boxed in regions correspond to the sequence contained within the p22 and p10 proteins. The active site Cys is shown in black. Sites of cleavage to form the individual p22, p20, and p10 proteins are underlined.

DISCUSSION

We have succeeded in purifying, characterizing, and expressing ICE, a unique Cys protease from monocytic cells that cleaves pIL-1β at the Asp^{116}-Ala^{117} bond. That ICE is a cysteine protease is shown by its sensitivity to known nonspecific thiol

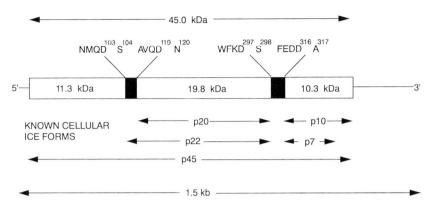

FIGURE 9. Structural organization of the human ICE precursor protein (p45) and the sites of cleavage found in ICE forms identified in THP.1 cells and recombinant expression systems, including p22, p20, p10, and p7, a truncated form of p10.

alkylating agents such as NEM and iodoacetic acid, and its insensitivity to Ser, Asp, or metalloprotease inhibitors. More definitively, such specific agents as tetrapeptide aldehydes or diazomethylketones inhibit ICE, while, in contrast, a truncated carbo-benzyloxy aspartyl diazomethylketone is 10,000-fold less potent as an ICE inhibitor.[34] Furthermore, the replacement of the active site Cys with Ala totally eliminates any ICE activity.[50] The minimum recognition sequence for ICE is a relatively small

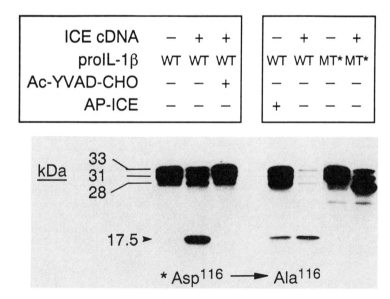

FIGURE 10. Functional expression of active recombinant ICE expressed in COS-7 cells. Extracts of cells transfected with human p45 ICE were incubated with ^{35}S-Met-labeled wild-type pIL-1β (WT) or a Ala[116] mutant of IL-1β (MT) in the presence or absence of affinity purified ICE (taken from Reference 34 with permission). The resultant samples were separated by SDS-PAGE and visualized by autoradiography.

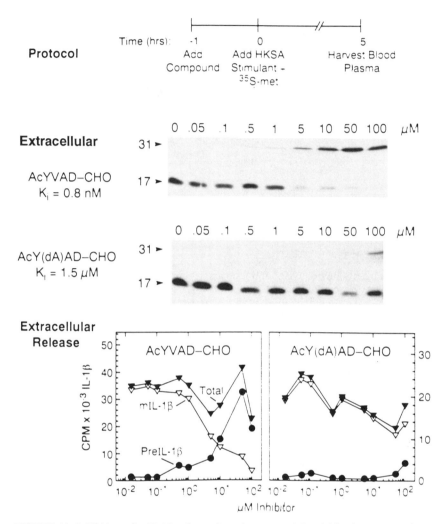

FIGURE 11. Inhibition of mIL-1β release from human peripheral blood monocytes by a peptide aldehyde inhibitor (Ac-YVAD-CHO) or a relatively inactive D-Ala control peptide (AcYdAAD-CHO). ^{35}S-Met-labeled heparinized blood was preincubated with indicated concentrations of the inhibitor for 1 h, followed by a 5-h incubation with heat-killed *Staphylococcus aureus*. The plasma was removed and immunoprecipitated with antiIL-1β antiserum, and the immunoprecipitates were separated by SDS-PAGE and subjected to autoradiography. Radioimaging of the individual bands is shown at the bottom (Taken from Reference 34 with permission).

tetrapeptide characterized most prominently by the absolute necessity for an Asp in P1 and secondarily by the need for a relatively large hydrophobic group in P4. ICE bears no homology to other known Cys or Ser proteases; the original observation of active site sequence similarity to Ser proteases[34] was not borne out when the mouse and rat sequences were obtained[44-46] in that the Ser289 was replaced by a Lys.

ICE itself appears to require processing before it can become active. While it is synthesized as a 45-kDa protein and is the predominant cellular form seen in monocytic cells, it has no detectable pIL-1β cleavage activity until removal of a precursor domain of about 13 kDa and a 2-kDa intervening piece between the p20 and p10 proteins. Exactly how and where this processing occurs is not known, but all of the cleavage sites are preceded by Asp residues. Because purified ICE can cleave the p45 precursor, it is possible that this processing is autocatalytic.[34]

Whereas active ICE is a complex of freely dissociable inactive monomers,[34] there is no evidence that the p20 and p10 polypeptides themselves are freely dissociable from one another. Simultaneous expression of both p10 and p20 in *E. coli* does not generate active ICE.[48] Furthermore, purification by ion exchange columns of active ICE from THP.1 cytoplasmic extracts has shown no evidence for p10 separate from p20.[43] What is seen is that p10 is susceptible to proteolysis, and that p20 is found associated not only with intact p10, but also with a lower molecular weight C-terminally cleaved form of p10 (p7) forming an ICE complex with reduced activity. p20 can also be found with all of the p10 removed, in which case no ICE activity is seen.[43] Thus, the p10 part of ICE is clearly needed for ICE activity. Not surprisingly, it is the most conserved portion of ICE (FIGURE 8).

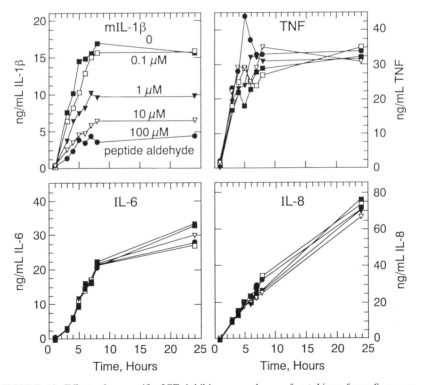

FIGURE 12. Effect of a specific ICE inhibitor on release of cytokines from *S. aureus*–stimulated human peripheral blood monocytes. Various concentrations of the peptide aldehyde inhibitor (AcYVAD-CHO) were preincubated with cells as described in FIGURE 13, and the supernatants were analyzed by ELISA for IL-1β, TNFα, IL-6, or IL-8 release.

We have shown that specific inhibitors of ICE can be synthesized; the peptide aldehyde inhibitor affinity column will purify active ICE from THP.1 cytosol in a single step. Furthermore, this inhibitor can inhibit release of mIL-1β from activated monocytes without preventing the release of TNFα, IL-6, or IL-8. Even though inhibition of ICE inhibits cellular pIL-1β processing, pIL-1β secretion from the monocytic cell is unaffected (see FIGURE 13); that is, secretion occurs independently of processing. A critical issue, then, in the development of a therapeutic ICE inhibitor is whether or not pIL-1β might be processed by "bystander proteases" at sites of inflammation to yield an active product with activity similar to mIL-1β. Secondly, there is the question of whether other cytokines such as TNFα or IL-1α released from damaged cells might be sufficient to maintain the inflammatory response.

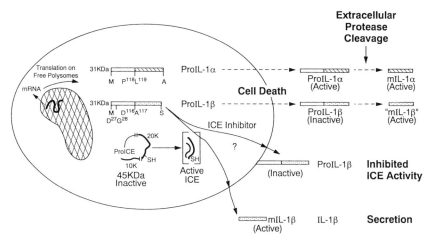

FIGURE 13. Schema of IL-1 processing and secretion. IL-1α and IL-1β are synthesized as 31-kDa cytoplasmic precursor proteins. The precursors are ordinarily not released from cells except following cell damage or death, at which time they could be potentially cleaved by other proteases. The 31-kDa IL-1β is normally processed to the 17.5-kDa mIL-1β by an active form of ICE that is itself activated from a 45-kDa precursor. Cleavage of pIL-1β occurs independently of mIL-1β secretion, since inhibition of ICE cleavage results in extracellular accumulation of pIL-1β.

ACKNOWLEDGMENTS

We thank Drs. John Schmidt and Michael Tocci for their support and critical comments concerning these studies.

REFERENCES

1. SCHMIDT, J. A. & M. J. TOCCI. 1990. *In* The Handbook of Experimental Pharmacology I. Peptide Growth Factors and Their Receptors. M. Sporn & A. Roberts, Eds: **95:** 473–521. Springer Verlag. Berlin, Germany.
2. DINARELLO, C. A. 1988. FASEB J. **2:** 108–115.

3. PETTIPHER, E. R., G. A. HIGGS, & B. HENDERSON. 1986. Proc. Natl. Acad. Sci. USA **83:** 8749–8753.
4. STIMPSON, S. A., F. G. DALLDORF, I. G. OTTERNESS & J. H. SCHWAB. 1988. J. Immunol. **140:** 2964–2969.
5. HOM, J. T., A. M. BENDELE & D. G. CARLSON. 1988. J. Immunol. **141:** 834–841.
6. EASTGATE, J. A., N. C. WOOD, F. S. DI GIOVINE, J. A. SYMONS, F. M. GRINLINTON & G. W. DUFF. 1988. Lancet **ii:** 706–709.
7. WADA, H., S. TAMAKI, M. TANIGAWA, M. TAKAGI, Y. MORI, A. DEGUCHI, N. KATAYAMA, T. YAMAMOTO, K. DEGUCHI & S. SHIRAKAWA. 1991. Thromb. Haemostasis **65:** 364–368.
8. STARNES, J. 1991. Semin. Hematol. **28:** 34–41.
9. MOSLEY, B., D. L. URDAL, K. S. PRICKETT, A. LARSEN, D. COSMAN, P. J. CONLON, S. GILLIS & S. K. DOWER. 1987. J. Biol. Chem. **262:** 2941–2944.
10. GIRI, J. G., P. T. LOMEDICO & S. B. MIZEL. 1985. J. Immunol. **140:** 343–349.
11. AURON, P. E., S. J. WARNER, A. C. WEBB, J. G. CANNON, H. A. BERNHEIM, K. J. MCADAM, L. J. ROSENWASSER, G. LOPRESTE, S. F. MUCCI & C. A. DINARELLO. 1987. J. Immunol. **138:** 1447–1456.
12. SINGER, I. I., S. SCOTT, G. L. HALL, G. LIMJUCO, J. CHIN & J. A. SCHMIDT. 1988. J. Exp. Med. **167:** 389–407.
13. HAZUDA, D. J., J. C. LEE & P. R. YOUNG. 1988. J. Biol. Chem. **263:** 8473–8479.
14. HAZUDA, D., R. L. WEBB, P. SIMON & P. YOUNG. 1989. J. Biol. Chem. **264:** 1689–1693.
15. GRASSI, J., C. J. ROBERGE, Y. FROBERT, P. PRADELLES & P. E. POUBELLE. 1991. Immunol. Rev. **119:** 125–145.
16. AOTSUKA, S., K. KAKAMURA, T. NAKANO, M. KAWAKAMI, M. GOTO, M. OKAWA-TAKATSUJI, M. KINOSHITA & R. YOKOHARI. 1991. Ann. Rheumat. Dis. **50:** 27–31.
17. LONNEMANN, G., S. ENDRES, J. W. M. VAN DER MEER, J. G. CANNON, K. M. KOCH & C. A. DINARELLO. 1989. Eur. J. Immunol. **19:** 1531–1536.
18. GRANOWITZ, E. V., A. A. SANTOS, D. D. POUTSIAKA, J. G. CANNON, D. W. WILMORE, S. M. WOLFF & C. A. DINARELLO. 1991. Lancet **338:** 1423–1424.
19. AREND, W. P. 1990. Prog. Growth Factor Res. **2:** 193–205.
20. DINARELLO, C. S. & R. C. THOMPSON. 1991. Immunol. Today **12:** 404–410.
21. DINARELLO, C. A. 1992. Semin. Immunol. **4:** 133–145.
22. OHLSSON, K., P. BJORK, M. BERGENFELDT, R. HAGEMAN & R. C. THOMPSON. 1990. Nature **348:** 550–552.
23. SMITH, R. J., J. E. CHIN, L. M. SAM & J. M. JUSTEN. 1991. Arthritis Rheumatism **34:** 78–83.
24. FANSLOW, W. 1990. Science **248:** 739–742.
25. MCINTYRE, K. W., G. J. STEPAN, K. D. KOLINSKY, W. R. BENJAMIN, J. M. PLOCINSKI, K. L. KAFFKA, C. A. CAMPEN, R. A. CHIZZONITE & P. L. KILIAN. 1991. J. Exp. Med. **173:** 931–939.
26. SPRIGGS, M. K., D. E. HRUBY, C. R. MALISZEWSKI, D. J. PICKUP, J. E. SIMS, R. M. L. BULLER, & J. VANSLYKE. 1992. Cell **71:** 145–152.
27. ALCAMI, A. & G. L. SMITH. 1992. Cell **71:** 153–167.
28. LIMJUCO, G., S. GALUSKA, J. CHIN, P. CAMERON, J. BOGER & J. A. SCHMIDT. 1986. Proc. Natl. Acad. Sci. USA **83:** 3972–3976.
29. KOSTURA, M. J., M. J. TOCCI, G. LIMJUCO, J. CHIN, P. CAMERON, A. G. HILLMAN, N. A. CHARTRAIN & J. A. SCHMIDT. 1989. Proc. Natl. Acad. Sci. USA **86:** 5227–5231.
30. HOWARD, A. D., M. J. KOSTURA, N. THORNBERRY, G. J. F. DING, G. LIMJUCO, J. WEIDNER, J. P. SALLEY, K. A. HOGQUIST, D. D. CHAPLIN, R. A. MUMFORD, J. A. SCHMIDT & M. J. TOCCI. 1991. J. Immunol. **147:** 2964–2969.
31. BLACK, R. A., S. R. KRONHEIM, M. CANTRELL, M. C. DEELEY, C. J. MARCH, K. S. PRICKETT, J. WIGNALL, P. J. CONLON, D. COSMAN, T. P. HOPP, *et al.* 1988. J. Biol. Chem. **263:** 9437–9442.
32. BLACK, R. A., S. R. KRONHEIM & P. R. SLEATH. 1989. Febs. Lett. **247:** 386–390.
33. SLEATH, P. R., R. C. HENDRICKSON, S. R. KRONHEIM, C. J. MARCH & R. A. BLACK. 1990. J. Biol. Chem. **265:** 14526–14528.
34. THORNBERRY, N. A., H. G. BULL, J. R. CALAYCAY, K. T. CHAPMAN, A. D. HOWARD, M. J. KOSTURA, D. K. MILLER, S. M. MOLINEAUX, J. R. WEIDNER, J. AUNINS, K. O. ELLISTON, J. M. AYALA, R. J. CASANO, J. CHIN, G. J.-F. DING, L. A. EGGER, E. P. GAFFNEY, G.

LIMJUCO, O. C. PALYHA, S. M. RAJU, A. M. ROLANDO, J. P. SALLEY, T. T. YAMIN, T. D. LEE, J. E. SHIVELY, M. MACCOSS, R. A. MUMFORD, J. A. SCHMIDT & M. J. TOCCI. 1992. Nature **356:** 768–774.

35.   YOUNG, P. R., D. J. HAZUDA & P. L. SIMON. 1988. J. Cell Biol. **107:** 447–456.
36.   FUHLBRIGGE, R. C., S. M. FINE, E. R. UNANUE & D. D. CHAPLIN. 1988. Proc. Natl. Acad. Sci. USA **85:** 5649–5653.
37.   RAY, C. A., R. A. BLACK, S. R. KRONHEIM, T. A. GREENSTREET, P. R. SLEATH, G. S. SALVESEN & D. J. PICKUP. 1992. Cell **69:** 597–604.
38.   KOBAYASHI, Y., K. YAMAMOTO, T. SAIDO, H. KAWASAKI, J. J. OPPENHEIM & K. MATSU-SHIMA. 1990. Proc. Natl. Acad. Sci. USA **87:** 5548.
39.   HOGQUIST, K. A., E. R. UNANUE & D. D. CHAPLIN. 1991. Proc. Natl. Acad. Sci. USA **88:** 8485–8489.
40.   CAMERON, P. M., G. A. LIMJUCO, J. CHIN, L. SILBERSTEIN & J. A. SCHMIDT. 1986. J. Exp. Med. **164:** 237–250.
41.   DINARELLO, C. A. 1991. Blood **77:** 1627–1652.
42.   DIGIOVINE, F. S., J. A. SYMONS & G. W. DUFF. 1991. Immunol. Lett. **29:** 211–218.
43.   MILLER, D. K., J. M. AYALA, L. A. EGGER, S. M. RAJU, T.-T. YAMIN, G. J.-F. DING, E. P. GAFFNEY, A. D. HOWARD, O. C. PALYHA, A. M. ROLANDO, J. P. SALLEY, N. A. THORNBERRY, J. R. WEIDNER, J. H. WILLIAMS, K. T. CHAPMAN, J. JACKSON, M. J. KOSTURA, G. LIMJUCO, S. M. MOLINEAUX, R. A. MUMFORE & J. R. CALAYCAY. 1993. J. Biol. Chem. **268:** 18062–18069.
44.   MOLINEAUX, S. M., F. J. CASANO, A. M. ROLANDO, E. P. PETERSON, G. LIMJUCO, J. CHIN, P. R. GRIFFIN, J. R. CALAYCAY, G. J.-F. DING, T.-T. YAMIN, O. C. PALYHA, S. LUELL, D. FLETCHER, D. K. MILLER, A. D. HOWARD, N. A. THORNBERRY & M. J. KOSTURA. 1993. Proc. Natl. Acad. Sci. USA **90:** 1809–1813.
45.   NETT, M., D. CERRETTI, R. BLACK & D. CHAPLIN. 1992. FASEB J. **6:** A2056.
46.   SHIVERS, B. D., D. A. GIEGEL & K. M. KEANE. 1993. J. Cell. Biochem. **17B:** 119.
47.   MILLER, D. K., J. M. AYALA, E. BAYNE, K. CHAPMAN, J. CHIN, S. DONATELLI, L. A. EGGER, A. HOWARD, M. KOSTURA, S. M. MOLINEAUX, A. M. ROLANDO & T. T. YAMIN. 1993. FASEB. J. **7:** A267.
48.   HOWARD, A. D., O. C. PALYHA, G. J.-F. DING, E. P. PETERSON, J. C. CALAYCAY, P. R. GRIFFIN, R. A. MUMFORD, A. B. LENNY, D. K. ROBINSON, S. WANG, M. SILBERKLANG, C. LEE, W. SUN, J. M. AYALA, L. A. EGGER, D. K. MILLER, S. M. RAJU, T. T. YAMIN, J. JACKSON, K. T. CHAPMAN, J. A. SCHMIDT, M. J. TOCCI & N. A. THORNBERRY. 1993. J. Cell. Biochem. **17B:** 146.
49.   SCHINDLER, R., B. D. CLARK & A. A. DINARELLO. 1990. J. Biol. Chem. **265:** 10232–10237.
50.   HOWARD, A. D., G. J.-F. DING, A. M. ROLANDO, O. C. PALYHA, E. P. PETERSON, F. J. CASANO, E. K. BAYNE, S. DONATELLI, J. M. AYALA, L. A. EGGER, D. K. MILLER, S. M. RAJU, T. T. YAMIN, J. JACKSON, K. T. CHAPMAN, N. A. THORNBERRY, J. A. SCHMIDT, M. J. TOCCI & S. M. MOLINEAUX. 1993. J. Cell. Biochem. **17B:** 113.
51.   KNIGHT, W. B., B. G. GREEN, P. GALE, R. CHABIN, A. MAYCOCK, W. M. WESTLER, H. WESTON, C. DORN, P. FINKE, W. HAGMANN, J. HALE, J. LIESCH, M. NAVIA, S. SHAH, D. UNDERWOOD & J. B. DOHERTY. Biochemistry **31:** 8160–8170.

Bicyclic Imidazoles as a Novel Class of Cytokine Biosynthesis Inhibitors

J. C. LEE,[a] A. M. BADGER,[a] D. E. GRISWOLD,[b]
D. DUNNINGTON,[a] A. TRUNEH,[a] B. VOTTA,[a]
J. R. WHITE,[a] P. R. YOUNG,[c] AND P. E. BENDER[d]

[a]Department of Cellular Biochemistry
[b]Department of Respiratory and Inflammation Pharmacology
[c]Department of Molecular Genetics
[d]Department of Medicinal Chemistry
SmithKline Beecham Pharmaceuticals
709 Swedeland Road
Post Office Box 1539
King of Prussia, Pennsylvania 19406

INTRODUCTION

Cytokines in Health and Disease

The network of immune and inflammatory responses is comprised of a variety of cell types and mediators acting as intercellular signaling molecules. These molecules (collectively termed lymphokines and cytokines) regulate the growth, differentiation, and function of a variety of target cells (for review, see Arai et al.).[1] A large number of these molecules have been identified and fully characterized. The availability of these proteins through recombinant DNA technology allows the elucidation of many important pathways operating in immune and inflammatory responses. The interleukins and colony stimulating factors represent the two major families of cytokines, each comprised of a multitude of molecules with unique or overlapping biological properties. Understanding the structure and function of these molecules has provided new and important insight into the fundamental biology of immunity and inflammation. The study of cytokines involved in hematopoietic cell-cell interaction and the resulting inflammatory sequelae has led to the identification of new strategies for the development of more effective medicines for the treatment of a variety of autoimmune and inflammatory diseases.

Interleukin-1 (IL-1) and tumor necrosis factor (TNF) are two of the most studied proinflammatory cytokines.[2,3] These cytokines and others (e.g., IL-6 and IL-8) have been suggested to play important roles in mediating many chronic inflammatory diseases, such as rheumatoid arthritis,[4] inflammatory bowel disease, and psoriasis.

Strategies for Therapeutic Modulation of Cytokine Expression

Studies of the biosynthesis of and cellular responses to these cytokines suggest at least three strategies to suppress cytokine expression and/or action and to effect pharmacological intervention in various disease states.[5] These strategies encompass receptor antagonism, blockade of target cell signaling pathways, and biosynthesis inhibition. While receptor antagonists, such as IL-1 receptor antagonist (IL-1RA),[6] soluble IL-1 receptor,[7] chimeric TNF-receptor-Ig-molecule,[8] and neutralizing monoclonal antibodies to the various cytokines, may prove to be feasible therapeutic entities, they all suffer from the disadvantage of being proteinaceous macromolecules and must therefore be administered parenterally, a potential disadvantage in treating chronic inflammatory conditions. Nonetheless, these molecules provided crucial tools to test the hypothesis that these cytokines are involved in various disease states and that antagonism of these molecule will be beneficial. To date, no orally active low molecular weight cytokine receptor antagonist has been identified. Strategies aimed at identifying specific second-messenger targets for cytokines have been elusive. An increasing number of recent reports have appeared in the literature suggesting that discovering low molecular weight inhibitors of cytokine production is not only conceivable but achievable as well.

The earliest compounds that showed cytokine synthesis inhibition activity were the glucocorticoids.[9] Recently, an increasing number of low molecular weight organic molecules have been implicated in the regulation of cytokine biosynthesis at the transcriptional, translational, or posttranslational (processing) level. TABLE 1

TABLE 1. Examples of Cytokine Synthesis Inhibitors

Pharmacological Class	Compound	Reference
Antiarthritic	Auranofin	Chang et al.[71]
	Tenidap	Otterness et al.[72]
Glucocorticoid	Dexamethasone	Lee et al.[9]
	Mometasone furoate	Barton et al.[73]
Antioxidant	Probucol	Ku et al.[74]
	Miscellaneous	DeForge et al.[75]
Lipoxygenase inhibitors	BW755C	Dinarello et al.[13]
Phosphodiesterase inhibitor	Pentoxifylline	Chao et al.[76]
	Rolipram	Semmler et al.[30]
Cyclic nucleotides		Endres et al.[29]
Natural product	Tetrandrine	Ferrante et al.[77]
	Chlarithromycin	Takeshita et al.[78]
Cytokine	IL-10	Malefyt et al.[79]

lists a representative group of chemically and functionally diverse compounds that have been shown to inhibit cytokine production. While these compounds are known to inhibit cytokine production, there has been a paucity of information on their molecular targets and the correlation, if any, between *in vitro* and *in vivo* effects. An additional complexity has been the lack of appropriate animal models to define the pharmacological profile of such agents.

In addition to providing a new perspective in the management of inflammatory diseases, this group of structurally diverse compounds[5,10] provides crucial probes to gain further insight into the molecular events in cytokine biosynthesis. Glucocorticoids inhibit cytokine production largely at the transcriptional level.[9] Some antiarthritic drugs, such as auranofin[12] and penicillamine,[11] have been reported to inhibit cytokine production by as yet unknown mechanisms. Lipoxygenase inhibitors, at high concentrations, have also been shown to modulate IL-1 production in human monocytes.[13]

These earlier findings prompted us to examine the effect of a member of the bicyclic imidazole class of compounds, SK&F 86002 (dihydroimidazo thiazolines), on IL-1 production.[14] This compound was found to have a potent inhibitory effect on LPS stimulated human monocyte IL-1 production (IC_{50} = 1.3 ± 1 μM). The compound, when tested at its IC_{50}, had no appreciable general effects on DNA, RNA, or protein synthesis. Furthermore, its inhibitory effect on IL-1 production was independent of the stimuli used and was also observed in other cell types (e.g., synovial cells) (unpublished observations). Optimal inhibition was observed when the cells were pretreated or treated with the compound early in the induction phase (<2 hours) of IL-1 expression. Both IL-1 isoforms were inhibited to a similar extent, as was TNF production.[15,16] Unlike the novel inhibitors of pro-IL-1 processing,[17] SK&F 86002 had no direct IL-1 convertase inhibitory activity (unpublished observations).

This communication will provide an updated overview of the pharmacology of SK&F 86002 and its metabolites SK&F 104343 (sulfone); SK&F 86096 (sulfide); and SK&F 105809, the prodrug of SK&F 105561 (sulfide) as novel cytokine biosynthesis inhibitors. The emphasis will be placed on IL-1 and TNF production *in vitro* and *in vivo*.

CHEMISTRY CONSIDERATIONS

Our initial approach to the design of novel, imidazole-containing antiinflammatory agents was to combine the structurally related pharmacophores of the antiinflammatory agent Flumizole[18] or Tiflamizole[19] with the immunomodulatory agent Levamisole,[20] leading to the class of fused bicyclic 2,3-dihydroimidazo[2,1-b]thiazoles (see FIGURE 1 for structures). The proposed structural additivity of these pharmacophores would be expected to result in agents possessing both antiinflammatory and immunomodulatory activity. Maximization of SAR with respect to the inhibition of adjuvant-induced arthritis and stimulation of low-grade oxazolone-induced contact sensitivity resulted in SK&F 81114, which demonstrated the desired hybrid pharmacological profile.[21]

Replacement of one of the substituted phenyl rings of SK&F 81114 with a 4-pyridyl ring afforded SK&F 86002 after only limited SAR maximization, and achieved a significant improvement in compound absorption and *in vivo* pharmacology.[22,23] Many of the 2,3-dihydroimidazo[2,1-b]thiazole analogues inhibited eicosanoid metabolism in 5-lipoxygenase and cyclooxygenase enzyme assays; however, few analogues demonstrated potent IL-1 synthesis inhibition in human monocytes and no eicosanoid-inhibitory or cytokine suppressive correlation was found.[16] Among the inhibitors of IL-1 synthesis, SK&F 86002 exhibited greater potency than either its sulfoxide (SK&F 86096) or sulfone (SK&F 104343) products of oxidative metabolism,[24,25] while an isomer of SK&F 86002, SK&F 86055, formed as a by-product in the original synthetic route, was of much reduced potency (TABLE 2).

A second series of bicyclic imidazoles, the 6,7-dihydro-[5H]-pyrrolo[1,2-a]imidazoles, was investigated, replacing the cyclic sulfur atom of the imidazothiazole with a methylene (CH_2) group. SK&F 105561 and its sulfoxide, SK&F 105809, have been the most extensively studied compounds in this series.[26-28] The inactive prodrug, SK&F 105809, is reductively metabolized to the active IL-1 inhibitor SK&F 105561 *in vivo* which is also active *in vitro* (TABLE 2). Via oxidative metabolism, the sulfoxide is subsequently converted to the sulfone *in vivo*, SK&F 105942, which is inactive *in vitro*.

IN VITRO PHARMACOLOGY

Effect on Eicosanoid Biosynthesis

The imidazothiazolines (SK&F 86002 and metabolites, SK&F 86096 and SK&F 104343) and the imidazopyrroles (SK&F 105809 and metabolites, SK&F 105561 and SK&F 105942) have a spectrum of effects on eicosanoid metabolism. SK&F 86002

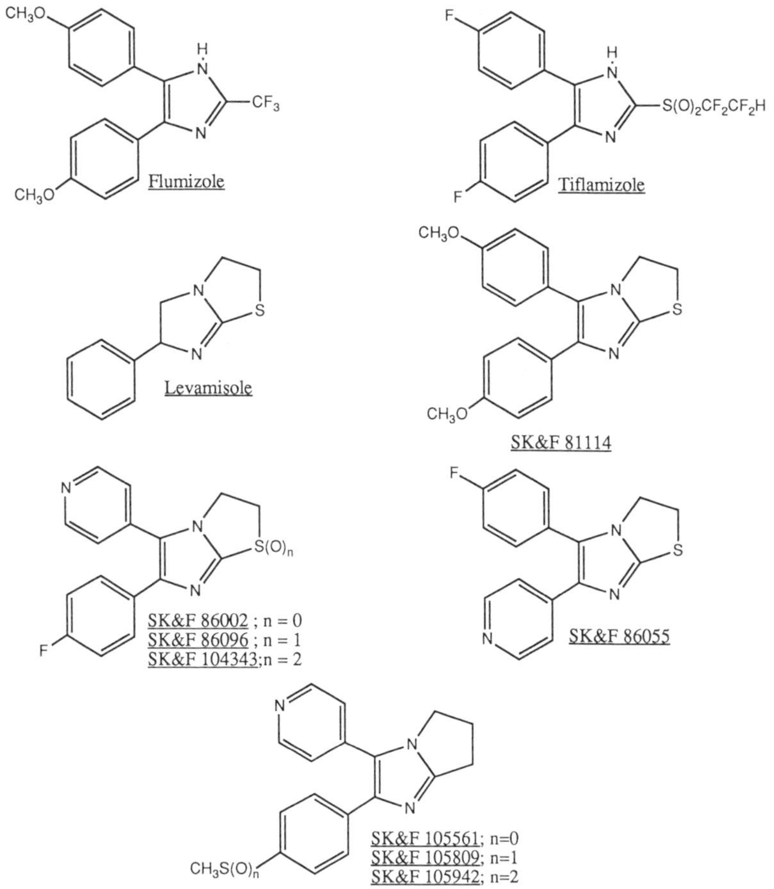

FIGURE 1. Chemical structures of bicyclic imidazoles discussed in this communication.

was found to be an inhibitor of 5-lipoxygenase, a key enzyme in the formation of leukotrienes. In addition, these molecules inhibit cyclooxygenase activity. This latter activity was expected, since it had been seen with earlier, chemically related molecules (e.g., flumizole). As seen in TABLE 3, SK&F 86002, the sulfide parent, has a relatively potent ability to inhibit isolated 5-LO enzyme prepared as a high-speed

TABLE 2. Effect of Bicyclic Imidazoles on IL-1 and TNF Production in Human Monocytes[a]

Compound	IL-1 β (IC_{50} μM)	TNF α (IC_{50} μM)
SK&F 86002 (parent)	0.5	0.4
SK&F 86096 (sulfoxide)	3.6	3.5
SK&F 104343 (sulfone)	> 5	5
SK&F 105809 (prodrug)	Inactive	Inactive
SK&F 105561 (sulfide)	2.7	3
SK&F 105942 (sulfone)	Inactive	Inactive

[a]Freshly isolated human monocytes were treated with various agents 1 hour prior to stimulation with LPS (50 ng/ml) and 16-hour culture supernatants were assessed for cytokine content by cytokine-specific enzyme-linked immunoassays. IC_{50}s were determined from a dose-response curve using regression analysis. Inactive = greater than 10 μM.

supernatant of RBL-1 cells (IC_{50} 10 μM). In contrast, the sulfoxide (SK&F 86096) and sulfone (SK&F 104343) metabolites have reduced 5-LO inhibitory activity (IC_{50}s of 50 and 22 μM, respectively). In the case of SK&F 105809, the profile of activity is complicated by the fact that the parent sulfoxide is a prodrug for the active sulfide metabolite (SK&F 105561, IC_{50} = 3 μM). The sulfone, SK&F 105942, does not have significant activity. The mechanism of 5-LO inhibition is unknown; however, judging from the kinetic profile, there is no inhibition of the lag phase that has been associated with redox-based inhibitors (unpublished observations). The inhibition seen with SK&F 105561 is reversible and may have a competitive component, since the IC_{50} varies inversely with the arachidonic acid concentration used.[27]

The activity seen with isolated 5-LO was also seen in whole cells. Using human monocytes stimulated with calcium ionophore (A23187), SK&F 86002 has an IC_{50} of 12 μM in inhibiting leukotriene production, while the sulfoxide and sulfone inhibit with IC_{50}s of 22 and 14 μM, respectively. In the case of SK&F 105809, no activity was observed; however, the active metabolite, SK&F 105561, inhibited quite well (IC_{50} = 2 μM). As in the case of the isolated enzyme, the sulfone metabolite (SK&F 105942) was inactive. Thus both classes of bicyclic imidazoles inhibited leukotriene biosynthesis, with the most potent compound being the active metabolite of SK&F 105809.[26,27]

The inhibition of cyclooxygenase activity has also been evaluated. The initial studies on SK&F 86002 using sheep seminal vesicle enzyme indicated little inhibition of prostaglandin H (PGH) synthase activity (IC_{50} = 120 μM). Subsequent work with

TABLE 3. Effect of Bicyclic Imidazoles on 5-Lipoxygenase Activity and LTB$_4$ Production[a]

Compound	RBL-1 5-LO (IC_{50} μM)	Human Monocyte LTB$_4$ (IC_{50} μM)
SK&F 86002 (parent)	10	12
SK&F 86096 (sulfoxide)	50	22
SK&F 104343 (sulfone)	22	14
SK&F 105809 (prodrug)	Inactive	Inactive
SK&F 105561 (sulfide)	3	2
SK&F 105942 (sulfone)	Inactive	Inactive

[a]RBL-1 high-speed supernatant 5-LO activity was determined by oxygen electrode. Monocyte LTB$_4$ production was stimulated by calcium ionophore (A23187).

SK&F 105561 indicated that the cyclooxygenase inhibitory activity was dependent upon the presence of peroxidase activity and improved from 100 μM to 3 μM with the addition of glutathione peroxidase.[26,27] This result complicates any interpretation but suggests that these compounds are not potent, classical inhibitors of PGH synthase 1. Inhibition of prostanoid production by A23187-stimulated human monocytes revealed considerably more activity. SK&F 86002 inhibited PGE_2 production with an IC_{50} of 1 μM, while the sulfoxide and sulfone were less effective (IC_{50}s of 8 and 14 μM, respectively). Similarly, SK&F 105561 inhibited PGE_2 production with an IC_{50} of 0.1 μM, and the parent and sulfone metabolite were inactive[23] (TABLE 4). Because of the peroxidase dependency, it is not known whether the observed inhibition of prostanoid production is consistent with the inhibition of PGH synthase 1 or due to other mechanisms.

Effect on Cytokine Production Is cAMP Independent

The expression of proinflammatory cytokines may be differentially regulated. It has been well documented that elevation of cAMP levels in human monocytes through direct (activation of adenylate cyclase) or indirect [inhibition of cyclic

TABLE 4. Effect of Bicyclic Imidazoles on Cyclooxygenase Activity and PGE_2 Production[a]

Compound	PGH Synthase (IC_{50} μM)	Human Monocyte (IC_{50} μM)
SK&F 86002 (parent)	120	1
SK&F 86096 (sulfoxide)	—	8
SK&F 104343 (sulfone)	—	14
SK&F 105809 (prodrug)	Inactive	Inactive
SK&F 105561 (sulfide)	100 (3^b)	0.1
SK&F 105942 (sulfone)	Inactive	Inactive

[a]Ram seminal vesicle PGH synthase was utilized, and enzyme activity was determined using an oxygen electrode. Human monocytes were stimulated with calcium ionophore (A23187).
[b]The IC_{50} was determined in the presence of glutathione peroxidase.

nucleotide phosphodiesterase (PDE)] mechanisms suppresses LPS-induced TNF but not IL-1 production under identical experimental conditions.[29,30] We sought to investigate whether SK&F 86002 and related analogues also inhibit LPS-induced IL-1 and TNF production via a cAMP-dependent mechanism. These compounds were found to be generally weak phosphodiesterase inhibitors (<30% inhibition at 10 μM against various PDE isoenzymes) (unpublished observations), and did not affect cAMP levels in human monocytes alone or in the presence of LPS. In contrast, prostaglandin E_2, which elevated cellular cAMP levels by activating adenylate cyclase, inhibited TNF but not IL-1 production, primarily at the transcriptional level.[31,32] Taken together, these results indicate that the bicyclic imidazoles inhibit both IL-1 and TNF in a cAMP-independent manner.

Specificity of Cytokine Inhibition

Among the multitude of cytokines produced by human monocytes stimulated with LPS, IL-1 and TNF production were inhibited to the same extent by the bicyclic imidazoles.[16] The similar IC_{50} values of the compounds for IL-1 and TNF inhibition were surprising because the two cytokines were unrelated in terms of their respective biosynthetic pathways. Inhibition of IL-6 and IL-8 was also observed and was most pronounced when the monocytes were stimulated with lower concentrations of LPS (unpublished observations). Otherwise, a higher drug concentration is required to achieve similar levels of inhibition as for IL-1 and TNF. Interestingly, granulocyte colony stimulating factor, IL-1RA, and alpha interferon production were not inhibited.[15] In addition, up regulation of CD14 expression by vitamin D3 treatment of human monocytes was also unaffected (unpublished results).

Inhibition of TNF Production **In Vitro**

SK&F 86002 inhibited TNF production from LPS-stimulated, oil-elicited C57/BL6 murine peritoneal macrophages with an IC_{50} that averaged 5 to 8 µM (FIGURE 2 top). In these experiments, the compounds were added 60 min prior to LPS and remained for the entire culture period of 4 h, at which time the supernatants were collected for evaluation of TNF levels by ELISA. Suppression of TNF levels was also observed when the mouse macrophage cell line RAW 264.7 was stimulated with LPS. As with the murine peritoneal macrophage population, the IC_{50} was 5 µM.[33] SK&F 86002 inhibition of TNF production from mouse peritoneal macrophages was about 50% at nontoxic concentrations. In human monocyte cultures, SK&F 86002 was a more effective inhibitor of TNF production (IC_{50} = 0.5 µM) than in RAW cells. (FIGURE 2 bottom).

The prodrug SK&F 105809 and its active sulfide metabolite, SK&F 105561, were also evaluated for their TNF inhibitory effects on human monocytes stimulated with LPS. As expected, SK&F 105809 was devoid of activity, whereas SK&F 105561 demonstrated potent inhibition with an IC_{50} of about 0.5 µM (FIGURE 3).[34] In summary, these bicyclic imidazoles inhibit TNF production from both murine and human monocyte cultures. Their activity on human monocytes, however, is 5 to 10-fold better than that on mouse cells.

Inhibition of IL-8 Production in Human Endothelial Cells

Interleukin-8 (NAP-1/IL-8) is a proinflammatory cytokine with neutrophil chemotactic activity.[35,36] This molecule is also chemotactic for a subset of T-cells[37] and promotes PMN degranulation, Mac-1 up regulation, and CR1 expression. IL-8 is produced by several cell types including mononuclear cells, fibroblasts, keratinocytes, and endothelial cells. It has been proposed that the production of IL-8 by endothelial cells may act as an activation signal for neutrophils.[38] IL-8 production in human umbilical-vein-derived endothelial cells (HUVEC) can initially be observed at two hours after stimulation with LPS or selected cytokines and continues for up to 24–48 hours. SK&F 86002 and SK&F 105561 inhibited the IL-1 or TNF-induced production of IL-8 in endothelial cells in a dose-dependent manner (TABLE 5). As expected, the inactive prodrug of SK&F 105561, SK&F 105809, was without effect. In addition, the glucocorticoid, dexamethasone, and phosphodiesterase IV inhibitor rolipram failed to significantly inhibit release at concentrations up to 10 µM with or without preincubation. This suggests that the PDE IV isozyme may not be an important regulator of IL-8 production in HUVEC. Furthermore, northern blot analysis for IL-8 production in HUVEC indicated that SK&F 86002 did not affect the induced steady-state IL-8 mRNA levels, suggesting that the pyridinyl imidazole compounds may act at a posttranscriptional level (see below).

Mechanism of Action of Bicyclic Imidazoles on IL-1β and TNFα Biosynthesis

These bicyclic imidazoles may inhibit cytokine biosynthesis at one or more of the following levels: transcription, mRNA stability, splicing, export to the cytosol, translation, protein processing, protein stability, or secretion. We have examined the effect of SK&F 86002 in primary human monocytes and in the human monocytic cell

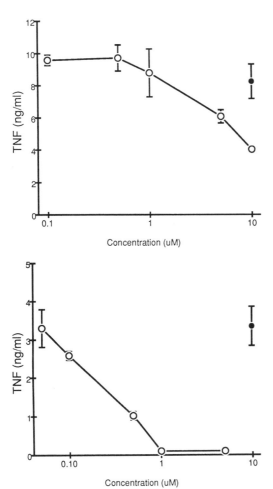

FIGURE 2. **Top:** Effect of SK&F 86002 on TNF production in LPS stimulated oil-elicited C57/BL6 murine peritoneal macrophages. **Bottom:** Effect of SK&F 86002 on TNF production in LPS stimulated human monocytes. LPS control (filled circles); SK&F 86002 treated (open circles). Cells were pretreated with the compound 1 hour prior to LPS. TNF in the 18 hour culture supernatant was determined by ELISA. Data shown are mean and standard deviation.

line THP-1. In each case, LPS at 0.5–1 μg/ml was used as a stimulus for cytokine induction. Northern blots of RNA extracted from monocytes showed no effect of SK&F 86002 (at 5 μM) on IL-1β mRNA, but a 2-fold reduction in TNFα message levels. In the same cells, IL-1β protein was inhibited by more than 2-fold, while TNFα was diminished by more than 10-fold, as measured by western blot.[39] No effect of SK&F 86002 was seen on transcript size or on the levels of intracellular versus

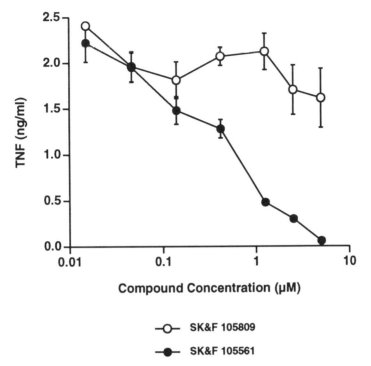

Compound Concentration (μM)

—O— SK&F 105809

—●— SK&F 105561

FIGURE 3. Effect of SK&F 105809 (prodrug) and SK&F 105561 (active metabolite) on TNF production in human monocytes. SK&F 105809 (filled circles); SK&F 105561 (open circles). Monocytes were pretreated with the compounds 1 hour prior to LPS (10 ng/ml). TNF in the 18 hour culture supernatant was determined by ELISA. Data shown are mean and standard deviation. (Reprinted from Reference 34 with permission from the publisher.)

secreted protein for either cytokine. Furthermore, SK&F 86002 did not alter the half-life of IL-1β as determined by ^{35}S-methionine pulse-chase experiments, but did affect the translation rate.[39]

In THP-1 cells, 1–5 μM SK&F 86002 had no effect on TNFα mRNA levels but decreased TNFα protein production by almost 2-fold (unpublished observations).

TABLE 5. Effect of Bicyclic Imidazoles on IL-8 Production in Human Umbilical Cord Vein Derived Endothelial Cells (HUVEC) Induced by IL-1[a]

Drug Conc.	Percent Inhibition of IL-8 Release				
	SK&F 86002	SK&F 105561	SK&F 105809	Dexamethasone	Rolipram
10 μM	65	63	10	20	10
1 μM	38	34	2	15	8
0.1 μM	15	8	0	2	8

[a]HUVEC cells were stimulated with rH-IL-1 (1 ng/ml) in the absence or presence of various compounds for 6 hours. Culture supernatants were harvested, and IL-8 content assessed by ELISA.

No effect of the compound was seen on the rates of induction or decay of TNFα mRNA. The results suggest that SK&F 86002 inhibits IL-1β and TNFα synthesis at the translational level. To confirm this hypothesis, we compared the kinetics of action of SK&F 86002 with those of a fast-acting inhibitor of transcription, actinomycin D, and of translation, anisomycin. In these experiments, parallel cultures of THP-1 cells were simultaneously activated with LPS and individual cultures were treated with compounds at various times after stimulation. All cultures were harvested at 2.5 hours post-LPS, and secreted TNFα levels were measured by an enzyme-linked immunosorbent assay. The results showed that SK&F 86002 kinetics coincided with those of anisomycin rather than actinomycin D, suggesting that SK&F 86002 inhibits a step close to the time of onset of TNFα mRNA translation.

Previous studies have shown that LPS stimulates synthesis of TNFα at both the transcriptional[40] and translational levels.[41] Translational regulation appears to involve sequences in the TNFα 5' and 3' untranslated regions, and in particular, an AU-rich motif that has also been linked to control of mRNA stability.[42] This sequence motif is also present in IL-1β. Although it is not apparent from existing models of eukaryotic translation[43] how sequences at the 3' end of the message could control the translation process, the phenomenon clearly deserves further study. The availability of compounds such as SK&F 86002 should facilitate elucidation of the molecular mechanisms that govern translational efficiency of cytokine mRNAs.

Effect on an In Vitro Model of Bone Resorption

The role of cytokines in bone remodeling has been recently reviewed.[44] Specifically, both interleukin-1 (IL-1) and tumor necrosis factor (TNF) have been demonstrated to stimulate bone resorption both *in vitro*[45,46] and *in vivo*.[47,48] These cytokines appear to stimulate both osteoclastic resorption, most likely via an accessory cell,[49] and the proliferation of osteoclast precursors.[50] Recently, Pacifici and colleagues have demonstrated a relationship between cytokine production and postmenopausal osteoporosis. Peripheral blood monocytes from high turnover osteoporotics produced more IL-1 than did monocytes from low turnover patients.[51] Furthermore, monocytes from osteoporotic patients treated with estrogen, a therapy which has been shown to reduce bone loss, produced significantly less IL-1 than did untreated patients.[52,53] These observations suggest that pharmacological modulation of cytokine production may prove efficacious in the treatment of diseases involving excessive bone remodeling.

In this regard, we asked whether SK&F 86002 would inhibit bone resorption. Using an *in vitro* fetal rat long bone organ culture system, which was first described by Raisz,[54] to quantitate bone resorption, SK&F 86002 dose-dependently (IC$_{50}$ approx. 1 μM) inhibited parathyroid hormone (PTH) stimulated bone resorption. This inhibition was reversible and independent of the stimulus employed in a manner analogous to the inhibition of IL-1 production in human monocyte cultures as described previously. The precise mechanism by which SK&F 86002 inhibits bone resorption remains to be definitively demonstrated. However, comparative pharmacological evidence strongly suggests that the inhibition of bone resorption is related to the cytokine inhibitory activity of SK&F 86002. Only compounds of this class that inhibited cytokine production (e.g., SK&F 105561) were shown to inhibit bone resorption. Additional evidence derives from the observation that selective cyclooxygenase (e.g., indomethacin, naproxen), lipoxygenase (e.g., phenidone), and dual

CO/LO inhibitors (e.g., SK&F 81114, SK&F 86055) were all inactive in this organ culture system (Votta *et al.,* manuscript in preparation).

Effect on Parameters of Immune Responses In Vitro

Although the effect of the pyridinyl imidazole compounds on production of IL-1 and TNF by cells of the myeloid lineage is now well established, very little has been described regarding their effects on antigen-specific responses of T lymphocytes. The question remained whether these compounds also have immunosuppressive activity, apart from their antiinflammatory effects. In order to address this question, we evaluated the effect of a series of these compounds on *in vitro* parameters of immune function, including mixed lymphocyte response (MLR), antigen-specific IL-2 production by T cells, and T cell proliferation.

To evaluate the effect of compounds on IL-2 production, a murine T cell hybridoma, which responds to allo stimulation by producing IL-2, was used. Briefly, a murine T cell hybridoma cell line expressing T cell receptors specific for H-2D^d was transfected with human CD4 (huCD4) and expresses functional HuCD4.[55] These T

TABLE 6. Effects on Immune Functions *In Vitro*[a]

Compound	IL-2 Production	MLR	Response to Soluble Antigen
FK506	+ + +	+ + +	+ + +
CsA	+ +	+ +	+ + +
Rapamycin	–	+ + +	+ + +
Dexamethasone	ND	+ +	ND
SK&F 86002	–	–	–
SK&F 104351	–	–	–
SK&F 105561	–	–	–

[a] –, No inhibition; + +, moderate inhibition; + + +, potent inhibition; ND, not determined

cell transfectants (I.1.B3) secrete IL-2 when cocultured with DAP3 cells, a murine fibroblast line transfected with H-2D^d and HLA-DR or HLA-DP. IL-2 production is dependent on the engagement of the TCR and huCD4 by their counterreceptors on the antigen presenting DAP3 cells, H-2D^d and MHC class II molecules.

As a positive control, IL-2 production by the murine T cell hybridoma was inhibited by nanomolar to subnanomolar concentrations of the immunosuppressive agents cyclosporin A (CsA) and FK506, but not rapamycin. In contrast, the pyridinyl imidazole compounds SK&F 86002, SK&F 105561, SK&F 104351 had very little effect on IL-2 production, even at concentrations of 10 μM and above.

The compounds were also evaluated for their effects on the response of T cells from human peripheral blood (TABLE 6). These compounds were tested for inhibition of T cell proliferation in a three-way mixed leukocyte response (MLR) using peripheral blood mononuclear cells obtained from Blood Bank buffy coats. CsA and FK506, rapamycin, and dexamethasone are potent blockers of this response, with complete inhibition being achieved with low nanomolar to subnanomolar concentrations. None of the bicyclic imidazole compounds exhibited a significant effect on MLR responses. They also fail to inhibit IL-2 production in activated T cells. Similar observations were also made in human peripheral blood T cell responses to soluble antigen. Although CsA, FK506, and rapamycin were potent blockers of T cell proliferation in response to the recall antigen tetanus toxoid, none of the bicyclic imidazole compounds had any effect.

All the above observations (TABLE 6) demonstrate that, unlike CsA, FK506, and rapamycin or the steroid dexamethasone, the bicyclic imidazoles do not have direct immunosuppressive activity mediated via inhibition of T cell functions. They block neither IL-2 production from T cells, nor the downstream responses including T cell proliferation. Since these compounds have no effect on preformed or basally expressed IL-1 or TNF, which presumably may play a role in immunoregulation, these results strongly support the notion that these compounds are not immunosuppressive and yet exert potent antiinflammatory effects. These observations are also consistent with the selectivity for IL-1 and TNF production in inflammatory settings that is distinct from the lymphokine network in T cells.

TABLE 7. Inhibition of Eicosanoid Metabolism by SK&F 86002 and SK&F 105809 in the Whole Animal[a]

Compound	LTB$_4$ Production (ED$_{50}$ mg/kg, po)	PGE$_2$ Production (ED$_{50}$ mg/kg, po)
SK&F 86002	~50	~50
SK&F 105809	41	15

[a]Eicosanoids were extracted from arachidonic acid inflamed ears, fractionated by high performance liquid chromatography, and the appropriate fractions assayed by radioimmunoassay.

These *in vitro* observations are also corroborated by *in vivo* studies with SK&F 86002, SK&F 104351, and the orally active prodrug analogue of SK&F 105561, SK&F 105809. No immunosuppressive activity was observed with any of these drugs *in vivo* under conditions where they can be shown to have antiinflammatory effects (unpublished results).

IN VIVO PHARMACOLOGY

Inhibition of Eicosanoid Metabolism

The effect of these compounds on eicosanoid metabolism was examined in the intact animal in two ways. First, their ability to inhibit LTB$_4$ or LTC$_4$ production in *ex vivo* stimulated blood was determined. SK&F 86002 and SK&F 105809 did not significantly inhibit calcium-ionophore-stimulated leukotriene production but did inhibit PGE$_2$ and HHT production (data not shown). Second, the effect on arachidonic acid–induced LTB$_4$ and PGE$_2$ production in inflamed mouse ear tissue was examined. SK&F 86002 inhibited LTB$_4$ production and PGE$_2$ production (ED$_{50}$s ~ 50 mg/kg, po).[23] In the case of SK&F 105809, the ED$_{50}$s for inhibition of LTB$_4$ and PGE$_2$ production were 41 and 15 mg/kg, po, respectively (TABLE 7). The lack of effect of these compounds with ionophore stimulation may be due to platelet arachidonate "cross-feeding" since use of zymosan as a stimulant revealed inhibition of LTB$_4$ production with SK&F 105809 (ED$_{50}$ 60 mg/kg, po).[27] These results suggest that the bicyclic imidazoles were able to inhibit leukotriene biosynthesis *in vivo*, albeit with modest potency. The inhibition of prostanoid synthesis was also apparent.

TABLE 8. Inhibition of Arachidonic Acid–Induced Inflammation by SK&F 86002 and SK&F 105809[a]

Compound	Inhibition of Edema (ED_{50} mg/kg, po)	Inhibition of MPO (ED_{50} mg/kg, po)
SK&F 86002	27	54
SK&F 105809	44	44

[a]Arachidonic acid (2 mg) was applied to the ears of Balb/c mice. The edematous response at one hour was measured using a thickness gauge, and the myeloperoxidase activity was extracted from the ear tissue and read spectrophotometrically.

Antiinflammatory Activity

Given a profile of activity of the bicyclic imidazoles that includes inhibition of cytokine production and eicosanoid metabolism, it was a clear expectation that these compounds would possess substantial antiinflammatory activity. This was examined in several models. We chose model systems that were relatively insensitive to cyclooxygenase inhibitors because we wanted to ascertain the unique activities of these molecules, i.e., the inhibition of inflammatory cytokine and leukotriene production. These compounds were the first nonantioxidant inhibitors to block arachidonic acid–induced inflammation following oral administration in the mouse. The ED_{50} for SK&F 86002 was 27 mg/kg, po for inhibition of the edematous response and 54 mg/kg, po for inhibition of neutrophil influx as measured by myeloperoxidase determination.[56] SK&F 105809 inhibited edema and the myeloperoxidase response with an ED_{50} of 44 mg/kg, po.[26] While it is likely that this response largely reflects inhibition of leukotriene synthesis, recent data implicating TNF as a mediator of neutrophil infiltration[57] raise the possibility of inhibition of cytokine release and/or synthesis as a contributing mechanism (TABLE 8).

Inhibition of inflammatory cell infiltration has been a hallmark of this class of compounds and was also demonstrable using carrageenan- and/or monosodium urate crystal–induced peritonitis in the mouse. SK&F 86002 had an ED_{50} of 44 mg/kg and 70 mg/kg, po in these models, respectively.[56] In comparison, SK&F 105809 had an ED_{50} of 72 and 64 mg/kg, po, respectively[26] (TABLE 9).

Analgesic Activity

An additional property of this class of compounds is analgesia. The analgesic activity is most easily demonstrated in mouse abdominal constriction assays using either acetic acid or phenylbenzoquinone (PBQ). Potent activity was observed for SK&F 105809 (ED_{50} 19 mg/kg, po) which was approximately equivalent to the

TABLE 9. Inhibition of Neutrophil Influx by SK&F 86002 and SK&F 105809[a]

Compound	Monosodium Urate (ED_{50} mg/kg, po)	Carrageenan (ED_{50} mg/kg, po)
SK&F 86002	70	44
SK&F 105809	64	72

[a]Monosodium urate crystals or carrageenan was injected intraperitoneally and washouts taken 2 h later. Neutrophils were counted by Coulter Counter and differential staining.

TABLE 10. Analgesic Effects of SK&F 105809[a]

Compound	PBQ Assay (ED_{50} mg/kg, po)	Randall-Selitto Assay (ED_{50} mg/kg, po)
SK&F 105809	19	86

[a]Phenylbenzoquinone was injected intraperitoneally, and the abdominal constrictions in CD1 mice counted for one hour. Randall-Selitto was done using brewer's yeast inflamed rat paw, and pain threshold was determined using a dolometer.

activity seen with ibuprofen. SK&F 105809 also has significant activity in the Randall-Selitto analgesia model but with a considerably higher ED_{50} (86 mg/kg, po), particularly in comparison to the cyclooxygenase inhibitor ibuprofen (37 mg/kg, po) (TABLE 10). Given the modest cyclooxygenase inhibitory activity of SK&F 105809, it is difficult to attribute this analgesia exclusively to that mechanism.[58] In light of the hyperalgesia induced by IL-1 and LTB_4, it is possible that inhibition of cytokine and leukotriene production/release contributed to the activity observed.

Antiarthritic Activity

SK&F 86002 (50 mg/kg per day/po) was found to markedly inhibit the disease severity (62%, $p < 0.05$) and acute phase reactant response (55%, $p < 0.05$) in collagen-induced arthritis in DBA/1LacJ mice.[59] This model is relatively insensitive to the action of cyclooxygenase inhibitors. That SK&F 86002 is rapidly converted to the sulfone which is the active principle in inhibiting inflammatory cytokine production *in vivo* may explain the antiarthritic effects. Similar results have been observed with SK&F 105809 (60 mg/kg, tid) where an 89% reduction in disease severity and a 67% inhibition of acute phase reactant response were observed[28] (TABLE 11).

Inhibition of TNF Production and Protection from Lethality In Vivo

In a manner similar to that used in addressing the question of *in vivo* inhibition of eicosanoid metabolism, data were generated to demonstrate *in vivo* inhibition of inflammatory cytokine production. Lipopolysaccharide (LPS) was utilized as a stimulus in the mouse. Following the intraperitoneal injection of LPS, a peritoneal washout was obtained and levels of tumor necrosis factor were analyzed by ELISA. The improved activity of SK&F 104343, the sulfone metabolite of SK&F 86002, is

TABLE 11. Effect of SK&F 86002 and SK&F 105809 in Collagen-Induced Arthritis in DBA/1LacJ Mice[a]

Compound	Disease Severity (% Inhibition)	Serum Amyloid P (% Inhibition)
SK&F 86002 50 mg/kg per day, po	62 ($p < 0.05$)	55 ($p < 0.05$)
SK&F 105809 60 mg/kg, tid, po	89 ($p < 0.001$)	67 ($p < 0.001$)

[a]Mice were treated with SK&F 86002 for one week following the rechallenge with collagen. With SK&F 105809, mice were administered compound for 14 days after the onset of significant disease.

notable, since upon chronic dosing, the sulfone is the predominant species *in vivo* (TABLE 12). This result suggests that cytokine inhibition may be an important feature of SK&F 86002 in the treatment of chronic inflammatory models (such as collagen-induced arthritis).

We also used a murine model of endotoxin shock in which animals are injected with LPS in combination with D-galactosamine (D-gal).[60] In this model, high levels of serum TNF (3–5 ng/ml) are observed 1 h following the injection of LPS.[34] Oral administration of SK&F 86002[61] or SK&F 105809[34] 30 or 60 min prior to the injection of LPS results in a dose-dependent suppression of serum TNF levels, the IC_{50} for both of the compounds being 10 mg/kg. A representative experiment using SK&F 105809 is shown in FIGURE 4 top. Concentrations of 10, 30, and 100 mg/kg inhibit serum TNF levels; whereas 3 mg/kg is inactive. Mice treated with these compounds also survive the lethal effect of LPS administration in this model, and the protective effect correlates with the inhibition of serum TNF levels. These results are shown in FIGURE 4 bottom where 100% protection from lethality is provided at the 100 mg/kg dose and 90% survival at 30 mg/kg. Animals treated with 10 and 3 mg/kg had survival rates of 20 and 10%, respectively.

TABLE 12. Effect of Bicyclic Imidazoles on TNF Production *In Vivo*[a]

Compound	Inhibition of TNF (ED_{50} mg/kg, po)
SK&F 86002 (parent)	32
SK&F 104343 (sulfone)	17
SK&F 105809 (prodrug)	48

[a]TNF production was stimulated in Balb/c mice by the intraperitoneal injection of LPS. Peritoneal washouts were obtained 2 h later, and the contents assayed for TNF by ELISA assay.

CONCLUSIONS AND PERSPECTIVES

The bicyclic imidazoles as noted herein represent a novel class of antiinflammatory compounds with potent inhibitory effects on cytokine production. These compounds display a wide range of antiinflammatory, analgesic, and antiarthritic activities. However, not all the activities can be totally attributed to the inhibition of eicosanoid production. These compounds are dissimilar to classical NSAIDs, both in terms of potency as well as direct effect on cyclooxygenase or lipoxygenase enzymes. There exists an apparent discrepancy in the IC_{50}s determined using broken cell enzyme assay and the intact monocyte assay measuring eicosanoid products.

No significant effects on immune functions have been observed. Particularly in the case for IL-1, it has been postulated that this cytokine, among its many biological activities, is essential as a hematopoietic and immunoregulatory molecule. The lack of obvious immunosuppressive effects despite the potent inhibition of IL-1 and TNF is encouraging for future clinical development of these compounds.

The bicyclic imidazole compounds described herein, other than the glucocorticoids, are exceptional in their ability to inhibit IL-1 and TNF production in various *in vivo* models, most notably in the murine model of endotoxic shock. This dramatic effect correlates with survival and protection from endotoxic shock related mortality. Equally exciting and perhaps holding even greater promise is the observation that these compounds also inhibit bone resorption in a rat fetal long bone organ culture system. The precise mechanism by which the bicyclic imidazoles inhibit PTH-induced bone resorption is not known. Since a large body of information suggests that a number of cytokines, especially IL-1, are proresorptive, it is reasonable to postulate that one plausible mechanism is the inhibition of cytokine production. Bone loss in osteoporotic or osteoarthritic patients is known to be independent of an inflammatory response. The potential for a clinical utility for these compounds to treat noninflammatory connective tissue diseases involving the pharmacological modulation of cytokine expression is an intriguing one. Also of import is the

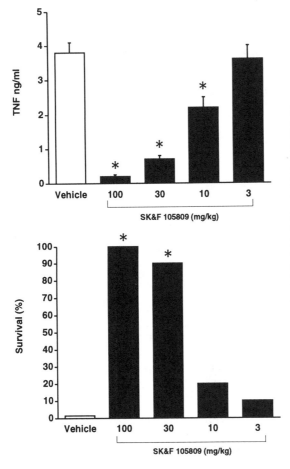

FIGURE 4. Top: Suppression of serum TNF levels in LPS-induced endotoxemic mice by oral administration of SK&F 105809. Vehicle or SK&F 105809 was administered po 0.5 hour before challenge. TNF was determined in serum collected 1 hour after challenge. $*p < 0.05$ by HSD test. **Bottom:** Protective effect of SK&F 105809 in LPS/D-galactosamine-induced endotoxic shock mortality. Vehicle or SK&F 105809 was administered po 0.5 hour before challenge. Survival assessed at 48 h following iv challenge. $*p < 0.05$ by Fisher's exact test. (Reprinted from Reference 34 with permission from the publisher.)

antiarthritic activity seen in the mouse collagen-induced arthritis model. This activity is not explained by eicosanoid inhibition, and the bicyclic imidazole compounds discussed here are among the most effective aside from the bona fide immunosuppressives. These results suggest their potential utility in both osteoarthritis and rheumatoid arthritis and may allow the treatment of the underlying disease process rather than merely the symptoms.

The first-generation bicyclic imidazole compounds described herein have inhibitory effects on several, but not all, cytokines examined. The susceptible cytokines share little in common structurally and perhaps functionally. However, they are strikingly similar in the biochemical control of their expression.[62,63] Biosynthesis of these cytokines is tightly regulated both at the transcriptional and the translational levels. Their mRNAs contain a common motif in the 3′ UTR region.[64,65] Taken together, there appear to be sufficient similarities between the biosynthetic regulation pathways of many cytokines that may allow a plausible explanation of how the bicyclic imidazoles may act.

A number of novel concepts regarding the molecular events leading to cytokine production in inflammatory situations have emerged recently, including a possible role of protein phosphorylation and dephosphorylation.[66,67] This is supported by the stimulatory effects of phosphatase inhibitors okadaic acid and calyculin A on IL-1 and TNF expression. How these biochemical events stimulated cytokine expression is not well understood and deserves further studies.

These first-generation compounds suffer from a number of apparent shortcomings. These compounds are not selective in inhibiting cytokine production, since they are also inhibitors of arachidonic acid metabolism. While they have reasonable potency (low μM range), a significant increase in the potency is required to allow a more detailed study of their mechanisms of action and establish a meaningful structure-activity relationship to identify the pharmacophore.

Since most of the available animal models of inflammation are sensitive to inhibitors of eicosanoid production, it is not readily apparent what pharmacological profile would be expected of compounds that selectively inhibit proinflammatory cytokine production. Indeed, short of a novel *in vivo* model that is unresponsive to classical NSAIDs, it would be difficult to demonstrate convincingly the pharmacological effect of the IL-1/TNF inhibitory component. Since IL-1, and to a lesser extent TNF, is hyperalgesic and both cytokines are potent inducer of chemokines and adhesion molecules, it is tempting to speculate that these inhibitors would also have analgesic and antiedematous activity irrespective of eicosanoid inhibitory activity. It is thus crucial to obtain second-generation compounds with increased potency (nanomolar range) and selectivity (for cytokine inhibition). It is equally important to devise a suitable animal model(s) to demonstrate unequivocally the utility of such compounds. Transgenic or gene knock-out animals such as the TNF transgenic mouse model,[68] in which spontaneous arthritic disease was observed, may serve as useful models for hypothesis testing. Furthermore, with more selective and potent compounds, it should be possible to design suitable radiolabeled chemical probes to identify molecular target(s) responsible for cytokine inhibition. Such an approach has been used in the study of immunosuppressive macrolides[69] and the 5-lipoxygenase translocation inhibitor.[70] The elucidation of the ligand-target structure, perhaps at the atomic level through x-ray crystallography or nuclear magnetic resonance analyses, may greatly enhance our ability to embark on the rational design of clinically useful candidates. In addition, the availability of these cytokine biosynthesis inhibitors will provide useful tools to further understand regulation of cytokine expression at the molecular level.

ACKNOWLEDGMENTS

We thank Drs. J. Adams, F. Drake, and K. Esser for reviewing this manuscript; Dr. B. Metcalf for his encouragement and support; excellent technical support of the following individuals: J. Laydon, M. Reddy, W. Prichett, A. Hand, P. McDonnell, L. Hillegass, L. Martin, J. Breton, E. Webb, and D. Olivera, and Drs. S. Kassis and U. Prabhakar for helpful discussions.

REFERENCES

1. ARAI, K., F. LEE, A. MIYAJIMA, S. MIYATAKE, N. ARAI & T. YOKOTA. 1990. Cytokines: coordinators of inflammatory responses. Annu. Rev. Biochem. **59:** 783–836.

2. DINARELLO, C. A. 1991. Interleukin-1 and interleukin-1 antagonism. Blood **77**(8): 1627–1652.

3. AREND, W. P. & J.-M. DAYER. 1990. Cytokines and cytokine inhibitors or antagonists in rheumatoid arthritis. Arthritis Rheumatism **33**(3): 305–315.

4. DAYER, J.-M. & S. DEMCZUK. 1984. Cytokines and other mediators in rheumatoid arthritis. Springer Semin. Immunopathol. **7:** 387–413.

5. BENDER, P. E. & J. C. LEE. 1989. Pharmacological modulation of interleukin-1. Ann. Rep. Med. Chem. **25:** 185–193.

6. AREND, W. P., F. G. JOSLIN, R. C. THOMPSON & C. H. HANNUM. 1989. An interleukin 1 inhibitor from human monocytes: production and characterization of biological properties. J. Immunol. **143:** 1851–1858.

7. FANSLOW, W. C., J. E. SIMS, H. SASSENFELD, P. J. MORRISSEY, S. GILLIS, S. K. DOWER & M. B. WIDMER. 1990. Regulation of alloreactivity *in vivo* by a soluble form of the interleukin-1 receptor. Science **248:** 739–742.

8. PEPPEL, K., D. CRAWFORD & B. BEUTLER. 1991. A tumor necrosis factor (TNF) receptor–IgG heavy chain chimeric protein as a bivalent antagonist of TNF activity. J. Exp. Med. **174:** 1483–1489.

9. LEE, S. W., A. P. TSOU, H. CHAN, J. THOMAS, K. PETRIE, E. M. EUGUI & A. C. ALLISON. 1988. Glucocorticoids selectively inhibit the transcription of interleukin-1 gene and decrease the stability of IL-1 β mRNA. Proc. Natl. Acad. Sci. USA **85:** 1204–1208.

10. COOPER, K. & H. MASAMUNE. 1992. Cytokine modulation as a medicinal chemistry target. Ann. Rep. Med. Chem. **27:** 209–218.

11. RORDORF-ADAM, C., J. LAZDINS, K. WOODS-COOK, E. ALTERI, R. HENN, T. GEIGER, U. FEIGE, H. TOWBIN & F. ERARD. 1989. An assay for the detection of interleukin-1 synthesis inhibitors: effects of anti-rheumatic drugs. Drugs Exp. Clin. Res. **15**(8): 355–362.

12. DANIS, V. A., A. J. KULESZ, D. S. NELSON & P. M. BROOKS. 1990. The effect of gold sodium thiomalate and auranofin on lipopolysaccharide-induced interleukin-1 production by blood monocytes *in vitro:* variation in healthy subjects and patients with arthritis. Clin. Exp. Immunol. **79:** 335–340.

13. DINARELLO, C. A., I. BISHAI, L. ROSENWASSER & F. COCEANI. 1984. The influence of lipoxygenase inhibitors on the *in vitro* production of human leukocyte pyrogen and lymphocyte activity factor (IL-1). Int. J. Immunopharm. **6:** 43–50.

14. LEE, J. C., D. E. GRISWOLD, B. VOTTA & N. HANNA. 1988. Inhibition of monocyte IL-1 production by the anti-inflammatory compound, SK&F 86002. Int. J. Immunopharm. **10:** 835–843.

15. LEE, J. C., L. REBAR & J. T. LAYDON. 1989. Effect of SK&F 86002 on cytokine production by human monocytes. Agents Actions **27**(3–4): 277–279.

16. LEE, J. C., B. VOTTA, B. J. DALTON, D. E. GRISWOLD, P. E. BENDER & N. HANNA. 1990. Inhibition of human monocyte IL-1 production by SK&F 86002. Int. J. Immunotherapy **6**(I): 1–12.

17. THORNBERRY, N. A., H. G. BULL, J. R. CALAYCAY, K. T. CHAPMAN, A. D. HOWARD, M. J. KOSTURA, D. K. MILLER, S. M. MOLINEAUX, J. R. WEIDNER, J. AUNINS, K. O. ELLISTON, J. M. AYALA, F. J. CASANO, J. CHIN, G. J.-F. DING, L. A. EGGER, E. P. GAFFNEY, G. LIMJUCO, O. C. PALYHA, S. M. RAJU, A. M. ROLANDO, J. P. SALLEY, T. YAMIN, T. D. LEE, J. E. SHIVELY, M. MACCROSS, R. A. MUMFORD, J. A. SCHMIDT & M. J. TOCCI. 1992. A novel heterodimeric cysteine protease is required for interleukin-1 β processing in monocytes. Nature **356:** 768–774.

18. LOMBARDINO, J. G. & E. H. WISEMAN. 1974. Preparation and antiinflammatory activity of some nonacidic trisubstituted imidazoles. J. Med. Chem. **17:** 1182–1188.

19. CHERKOFSKY, S. C. & T. R. SHARPE. 1980. Anti-inflammatory 4,5-diaryl-2-(substituted-thio)imidazoles and their corresponding sulfoxides and sulfones. U.S. Patent 4,190,666.

20. RAEYMAEKERS, S. H. M., F. T. N. ALLEWIJN, J. VANDERBERK, P. J. A. DEMOEN, T. T. T.

VAN OFFENWERT & P. A. J. JANSEN. 1966. Novel broad-spectrum anthelmintics. Tetramisole and related derivatives of 6-arylimidazo[2,1-b]thiazole. J. Med. Chem. **9:** 545–551.

21. BENDER, P. E., D. T. HILL, P. H. OFFEN, K. RAZGAITIS, P. LAVANCHY, O. D. STRINGER, B. M. SUTTON, D. E. GRISWOLD, M. J. DIMARTINO, D. T. WALZ, I. LANTOS & C. B. LADD. 1985. 5,6-Diaryl-2,3-dihydroimidazo[2,1b]thiazoles. Isomeric 4-pyridyl and 4-substituted phenyl derivatives. J. Med. Chem. **28:** 1169–1177.

22. LANTOS, I., P. E. BENDER, K. S. RAZGAITIS, B. M. SUTTON, M. J. DIMARTINO, D. E. GRISWOLD & D. T. WALZ. 1984. Antiinflammatory activity of 5,6-diaryl-2,3-dihydroimidazo-[2,1-b]thiazoles. Isomeric 4-pyridyl and 4-substituted phenyl derivatives. J. Med. Chem. **27:** 72–75.

23. GRISWOLD, D. E., P. J. MARSHALL, E. F. WEBB, R. GODFREY, M. J. DIMARTINO, H. M. SARAU, J. NEWTON, JR., J. G. GLEASON, G. POSTE & N. HANNA. 1987. SK&F 86002: a structurally novel anti-inflammatory agent that inhibits lipoxygenase- and cyclooxygenase-mediated metabolism of arachidonic acid. Biochem. Pharm. **36:** 3463–3470.

24. BENDER, P. E., D. E. GRISWOLD, N. HANNA & J. C. LEE. 1988. Inhibition of interleukin-1 production by monocytes and/or macrophages. U.S. Patent 4,794,114.

25. NEWTON, J. F., L. P. YODIS, D. KEOHANE, K. ECKARDT, R. DEWEY, J. DENT & B. MICO. 1989. Pharmacokinetics and metabolism of SK&F 86002 in male and female sprague-dawley rats. Drug Metab. Disp. **17**(2): 174–179.

26. GRISWOLD, D. E., P. J. MARSHALL, J. C. LEE, E. F. WEBB, L. M. HILLEGASS, J. WARTELL, J. NEWTON, JR. & N. HANNA. 1991. Pharmacology of the pyrroloimidazole, SK&F 105809-II. Antiinflammatory activity and inhibition of mediator production *in vivo*. Biochem. Pharm. **42**(4): 825–831.

27. MARSHALL, P. J., D. E. GRISWOLD, J. BRETON, E. F. WEBB, L. M. HILLEGASS, H. M. SARAU, J. NEWTON, JR., J. C. LEE, P. E. BENDER & N. HANNA. 1991. Pharmacology of the pyrroloimidazole, SK&F 105809-I. Inhibition of inflammatory cytokine production and of 5-lipoxygenase- and cyclooxygenase-mediated metabolism of arachidonic acid. Biochem. Pharm. **42**(4): 813–824.

28. HANNA, N., P. J. MARSHALL, J. NEWTON, JR., L. SCHWARTZ, R. KIRSH, M. J. DIMARTINO, J. ADAMS, P. BENDER & D. E. GRISWOLD. 1990. Pharmacological profile of SK&F 105809, a dual inhibitor of arachidonic acid metabolism. Drugs Exp. Clin. Res. **16:** 137–147.

29. ENDRES, S., H. J. FULLER, B. SINHA, D. STOLL, C. A. DINARELLO, R. GERZER & P. C. WEBER. 1991. Cyclic nucleotides differentially regulate the synthesis of tumor necrosis factor α and interleukin-1 β by human mononuclear cells. Immunology **172:** 56–60.

30. SEMMLER, J., H. WACHTEL & S. ENDRES. The specific type IV phosphodiesterase inhibitor rolipram suppress tumor necrosis factor production by human mononuclear cells. Int. J. Immunopharm. (In press)

31. KASSIS, S., J. C. LEE & N. HANNA. 1989. Effects of cAMP levels on IL-1 production in human monocytes. Agents Actions **27**(3–4): 274–276.

32. KASSIS, S., U. PRABHAKAR & J. C. LEE. Inhibition of interleukin-1 (IL-1) and tumor necrosis factor (TNF) production by the pyridinyl imidazole compounds is independent of cAMP elevating mechanisms. Agents Actions. (In press.)

33. OLIVERA, D. L., J. T. LAYDON, L. HILLEGASS, A. M. BADGER & J. C. LEE. Effects of pyridinyl imidazole compounds on murine TNF-α production. Agents Action. (In press.)

34. OLIVERA, D. L., K. M. ESSER, J. C. LEE, R. G. GREIG & A. M. BADGER. 1992. Beneficial effects of SK&F 105809, a novel cytokine-suppressive agent, in murine models of endotoxin shock. Circ. Shock **37:** 301–306.

35. YOSHIMURA, T. & N. YUHKI. 1991. Neutrophil attractant/activation protein-1 and monocyte chemoattractant protein-1 in rabbit. cDNA cloning and their expression in spleen cells. J. Immunol. **146**(10): 3483–3488.

36. STRIETER, R. M., S. L. KUNKEL, H. J. SHOWELL, D. G. REMICK, S. H. PHANS, P. H. WARD & R. M. MARKS. 1989. Endothelial cell gene expression of neutrophil chemotactic factor by TNFα, LPS and IL-1β. Science **243:** 1467–1469.

37. COLDITZ, F. G. & D. L. WATSON. 1992. The effect of cytokines and chemotactic agonists on the migration of T lymphocytes into skin. Immunology **76**: 272–278.

38. ROT, A. 1992. Endothelial cell binding of NAP-1/IL-8: role in neutrophil emigration. Immunol. Today **13**: 291–294.

39. YOUNG, P., P. McDONNELL, D. DUNNINGTON, A. HAND, J. LAYDON & J. LEE. Bicyclic imidazoles inhibit IL-1 and TNF production at the protein level. Agents Actions. (In press.)

40. SHAKHOV, A. N., M. A. COLLART, P. VASSALI, S. A. NEDOSPASOV & C. V. JONGENEEL. 1990. Kappa B–type enhancers are involved in lipopolysaccharide-mediated transcriptional activation of the tumor necrosis factor alpha gene in primary macrophages. J. Exp. Med. **171**(1): 35–47.

41. BEUTLER, B., J. HAN, V. KRUYS & B. P. GIROIR. 1992. Coordinate regulation of TNF biosynthesis at the levels of transcription and translation. *In* Tumor Necrosis Factors: the Molecules and Their Emerging Role in Medicine. B. Beutler, Ed.: 561–574. Raven Press. New York, N.Y.

42. SHAW, G. & R. KAMEN. 1986. A conserved AU-rich sequence from the 3′ untranslated region of gm-CSF mRNA mediates selective mRNA degradation. Cell **46**(5): 659–667.

43. KOZAK, M. 1989. The scanning model for translation: an update. J. Cell. Biol. **108**(2): 229–241.

44. MacDONALD, B. R. & M. GOWEN. 1992. Cytokines and bone. Br. J. Rheumatol. **31**: 149–155.

45. GOWEN, M. & G. R. MUNDY. 1986. Action of recombinant interleukin-1, interleukin-2 and interferon gamma on bone resorption *in vitro*. J. Immunol. **136**: 2478–2482.

46. BERTOLINI, D. R., G. E. NEDWIN, T. S. BRINGMAN, D. D. SMITH & G. R. MUNDY. 1986. Stimulation of bone resorption and inhibition of bone formation *in vitro* by human necrosis factors. Nature **319**: 515–518.

47. SABATINI, M., B. BOYCE, T. AUFDERMORTE, L. BONEWALD & G. R. MUNDY. 1988. Infusion of interleukin-1 α and β causes hypercalcemia in normal mice. Proc. Natl. Acad. Sci. USA **83**: 5235–5239.

48. TASHIJIAN, A. H., E. F. VOEKEL, M. LAZZARO, D. GOAD, T. BOSMA & L. LEVINE. 1987. Tumor necrosis factor α (cachectin) stimulates bone resorption in mouse calvaria via a prostaglandin-mediated mechanism. Endocrinology **120**: 2029–2036.

49. THOMPSON, B. M., G. R. MUNDY & T. J. CHAMBERS. 1987. Tumor necrosis factors α and β induce osteoblastic cells to stimulate bone resorption. J. Immunol. **138**: 775–779.

50. PFEILSCHIFTER, J., C. CHENU, A. BIRD, G. R. MUNDY & G. D. ROODMAN. 1989. Interleukin-1 and tumor necrosis factor stimulate the formation of human osteoclast-like cells. J. Bone Miner. Res. **4**: 113–118.

51. PACIFICI, M., L. RIFAS, S. TEITLEBAUM, E. SLATOPOLSKY, R. McKRACKEN, M. BERGFELD, W. LEE, L. V. AVIOLI & W. A. PECK. 1987. Spontaneous release of interleukin-1 from human blood monocytes reflects bone formation in idiopathic osteoporosis. Proc. Natl. Acad. Sci. USA **84**: 4616–4620.

52. PACIFICI, M. L., R. RIFAS, R. McKRACKEN, I. VERED, C. McMURTRY, L. V. AVIOLI & W. A. PECK. 1989. Ovarian steroid treatment blocks a postmenopausal increase in blood monocyte interleukin-1 release. Proc. Natl. Acad. Sci. USA **86**: 2398–2401.

53. PACIFICI, M., C. BROWN, E. PUSHCHEK, E. FRIEDRICH, E. SLATOPOLSKY, D. MAGGIO, R. McKRACKEN & L. V. AVIOLI. 1991. Effect of surgical menopause and estrogen replacement on cytokine release from human blood mononuclear cells. Proc. Natl. Acad. Sci. USA **88**: 5134–5138.

54. RAISZ, L. G. 1965. Bone resorption in tissue culture. Factors influencing the response to parathyroid hormone. J. Clin. Invest. **44**: 103–116.

55. LAMARRE, D. 1989. Class II MHC molecules and the HIV gp120 envelope protein interact with functionally distinct regions of the CD4 molecule. EMBO J. **8**(11): 3271–3277.

56. GRISWOLD, D. E., S. HOFFSTEIN, P. J. MARSHALL, E. F. WEBB, P. E. BENDER & N. HANNA. 1989. Inhibition of inflammatory cell infiltration by bicyclic imidazoles, SK&F 86002 and SK&F 104493. Inflammation **13**: 727–739.

57. ZHANG, Y., B. F. RAMOS & B. A. JAKSCHIK. 1992. Neutrophil recruitment by tumor necrosis factor from mast cells in immune complex peritonitis. Science **258**: 1957–1959.

58. GRISWOLD, D. E., P. MARSHALL, L. MARTIN, E. F. WEBB & B. ZABKO-POTAPOVICH. 1991. Analgetic activity of SK&F 105809, a dual inhibitor of arachidonic acid metabolism. Agents Actions Suppl. **32**: 113–117.
59. GRISWOLD, D. F., L. M. HILLEGASS, P. C. MEUNIER, M. J. DIMARTINO & N. HANNA. 1988. Effect of inhibitors of eicosanoid metabolism in murine collagen-induced arthritis. Arthritis Rheumatism **31**: 1406–1412.
60. GALANOS, C., M. A. FREUDENBERG & W. REUTTER. 1979. Galactosamine-induced sensitization to the lethal effects of endotoxin. Proc. Natl. Acad. Sci. USA **76**: 5939–5943.
61. BADGER, A. M., D. L. OLIVERA, J. E. TALMADGE & N. HANNA. 1989. Protective effect of SK&F 86002, a novel dual inhibitor of arachidonic acid metabolism, in murine models of endotoxic shock: inhibition of tumor necrosis factor as a possible mechanism of action. Circ. Shock **27**: 51–61.
62. HAN, J., T. BROWN & B. BEUTLER. 1990. Endotoxin-responsive sequences control cachectin/ tumor necrosis factor biosynthesis at the translational level. J. Exp. Med. **171**: 465–475.
63. KRUYS, V., O. MARINX, G. SHAW, J. DESCHAMPS & G. HUEZ. 1989. Translational blockade imposed by cytokine-derived UA-rich sequences. Science **245**: 852–855.
64. CAPUT, D., B. BEUTLER, K. HARTOG, R. THAYER, S. BROWN-SHIMER & A. CERAMI. 1986. Identification of a common nucleotide sequence in the 3′-untranslated region of mRNA molecules specifying inflammatory mediators. Proc. Natl. Acad. Sci. USA **83**: 1670–1674.
65. KRUYS, V., B. BEUTLER & G. HUEZ. 1990. Translational control mediated by UA-rich sequences. Enzyme **44**: 193–202.
66. SUNG, S. & J. A. WALTERS. 1993. Stimulation of interleukin-1 α and interleukin 1 β production in human monocytes by protein phosphatase 1 and 2A inhibitors. J. Biol. Chem. **268**(8): 5802–5809.
67. SUNG, J. S., J. A. WALTERS & S. M. FU. 1992. Stimulation of tumor necrosis factor α production in human monocytes by inhibitors of protein phosphatase 1 and 2A. J. Exp. Med. **176**: 897–901.
68. KEFFER, J., L. PROBERT, H. CAZLARIS, S. GEORGOPOULOS, E, KASLARIS, D. KIOUSSIS & G. KOLLIAS. 1991. Transgenic mice expressing human tumor necrosis factor: a predictive genetic model of arthritis. EMBO J **10**: 4025–4031.
69. HARDING, M. W., A. GALAT, D. E. UEHLING & S. L. SCHREIBER. 1989. A receptor for the immunosuppressant FK506 is a *cis-trans* peptidyl-prolyl isomerase. Nature **341**: 758–760.
70. MILLER, D. K., J. W. GILLARD, P. J. VICKERS, S. SADOWSKI, C. LEVEILLE, J. A. MANCINI, P. CHARLESON, R. A. F. DIXON, W. FORD-HUTCHINSON, R. FORTIN, J. Y. GAUTHIER, J. RODKEY, R. ROSEN, C. ROUZER, I. S. SIGAL, C. D. STRADER & J. F. EVANS. 1990. Identification and isolation of a membrane protein necessary for leukotriene production. Nature **343**: 278–281.
71. CHANG, D.-M., P. BAPTISTE & P. H. SCHUR. 1990. The effect of antirheumatic drugs on interleukin 1 (IL-1) activity and IL-1 and IL-1 inhibitor production by human monocytes. J. Rheumatol. **17**: 1148–1157.
72. OTTERNESS, I. G., M. L. BLIVEN, J. T. DOWNS, E. J. NATOLI & D. C. HANSON. 1991. Inhibition of interleukin 1 synthesis by Tenidap; a new drug for arthritis. Cytokine **3**(4): 277–283.
73. BARTON, B. E., J. P. JAKWAY, S. R. SMITH & M. I. SIEGEL. 1991. Cytokine inhibition by a novel steroid, mometasone furoate. Immunopharmacol. Immunotoxicol. **13**(3): 251–261.
74. KU, G., N. S. DOHERTY, J. A. WOLOS & R. L. JACKSON. 1988. Inhibition by Probucol of interleukin-1 secretion and its implication in artherosclerosis. Am. J. Cardiol. **62**: 77B–81B.
75. DEFORGE, L. E., J. C. FANTONE, J. S. KENNEY & D. G. REMICK. 1992. Oxygen radical scavengers selectively inhibit interleukin 8 in human whole blood. J. Clin. Invest. **90**(11): 2123–2129.
76. CHAO, C. C., S. HU, K. CLOSE, C. S. CHOI, T. W. MOLITOR, W. J. NOVICK & P. K. PETERSON. 1992. Cytokine release from microglia; differential inhibition by pentoxifylline and dexamethasone. J. Infect. Dis. **166**: 847–853.

77. FERRANTE, A., W. K. SEOW, B. ROWAN-KELLY & Y. H. THONG. 1990. Tetrandrine, a plant alkaloid, inhibits the production of tumor necrosis factor α (cachectin) by human monocytes. Clin. Exp. Immunol. **80:** 232–235.
78. TAKESHITA, K., I. YAMAGISHI, M. HARADA, S. OTOMO, T. NAKAGAWA & Y. MIZUSHIMA. 1989. Immunological and anti-inflammatory effects of chlarithromycin: inhibition of interleukin 1 production of murine peritoneal macrophages. Drugs Exp. Clin. Res. **15**(11/12): 4025–4031.
79. MALEFYT, R. D. W., J. ABRAMS, B. BENNETT, C. G. FIGDOR & J. E. DE VRIES. 1991. Interleukin 10 (IL-10) inhibits cytokine synthesis by human monocytes: an autoregulatory role of IL-10 produced by monocytes. J. Exp. Med. **174:** 1209–1220.

Coordinate Inhibition by Some Antioxidants of TNFα, IL-1β, and IL-6 Production by Human Peripheral Blood Mononuclear Cells

ELSIE M. EUGUI, BARBARA DELUSTRO,
SUSSAN ROUHAFZA, ROBERT WILHELM,
AND ANTHONY C. ALLISON[a]

Syntex Discovery Research
3401 Hillview Avenue
Palo Alto, California 94304

INTRODUCTION

Currently used antiinflammatory drugs include glucocorticoids and cyclooxygenase inhibitors. They have limiting side effects such as the widespread metabolic effects on bone and other target tissues of glucocorticoids and the gastrointestinal erosion produced by nonsteroidal antiinflammatory drugs. There is need for antiinflammatory drugs with novel modes of action. Our strategy has been to identify small molecules that can inhibit the expression of genes for proinflammatory cytokines and concurrently augment expression of the interleukin-1 receptor antagonist. Cytokines with proinflammatory and catabolic effects include TNFα and IL-1β. These cytokines contribute to the pathogenesis of inflammation, as well as cartilage and bone destruction, by several mechanisms.[1-3] TNFα and IL-1β induce the expression on endothelial cells of adhesion molecules required for recruitment of leukocytes into inflammatory sites.[4] The cytokines induce the production of PGE_2 by synovial fibroblast-type cells[5] and of PGI_2 by endothelial cells;[6] these prostaglandins are vasodilators and comediators of pain and increased vascular permeability. The same cytokines induce the production by chondrocytes of neutral metalloproteinases that can degrade cartilage matrix,[7] and they induce resorption of bone;[8] these processes contribute to joint erosion in patients with rheumatoid arthritis (RA). The role of IL-6 in the pathogenesis of RA is less well defined: however, the cytokine is a cofactor for T-lymphocyte differentiation[9] and in the production of immunoglobulins by B-lymphocytes in RA synovial tissue.[10] Activated T-lymphocytes[11] and immune complexes[12] are thought to contribute to pathogenesis of RA. Moreover IL-6 can act synergistically with IL-1 in augmenting bone erosion.[13]

A cytokine cascade, involving sequentially TNFα, IL-1β, IL-6, and IL-8, has been described in the synovium of patients with RA. In cultures of RA synovial tissue and derived cells, neutralization of TNFα with antibody decreases production of IL-1β,[14] and neutralization of IL-1 with antibody or the IL-1 receptor antagonist decreases production of IL-6 and IL-8.[15] Nevertheless, several effects of TNFα occur independently of IL-1,[1] and several effects of IL-1 occur independently of IL-6 and IL-8.[2,3] Administration of antibodies neutralizing TNFα[16] or of the interleukin-1 receptor

[a] Present address: 2513 Hastings Drive, Belmont, California 94002.

antagonist (IL-ra)[2,17] is reported to improve the clinical condition of patients with RA, confirming the importance of TNFα and IL-1 in pathogenesis. However, the antibody and receptor antagonist are expensive and difficult to administer on a continuous basis. Antibodies against TNFα[18] and IL-1ra[19] produce only marginal protective effects in a nonhuman primate model of endotoxic shock, suggesting that inhibiting the action of individual cytokines is insufficient for good therapy. For these reasons, our research has been directed towards the identification of a small molecule that can inhibit, in a coordinate fashion, the production by monocyte-macrophage lineage cells of TNFα, IL-1β, and IL-6. By "small molecule" we mean a synthetic organic compound of relative molecular mass 400 or less that is not a natural product such as a peptide, lipid, or sugar.

The potential therapeutic utility of a drug inhibiting cytokine production in a coordinate manner is clear: the question arises whether such a strategy is feasible. We chose to investigate antioxidants because of evidence that compounds of this general class can inhibit the activation of transcription factors NFκB[20,21] and AP-1,[22,23] which are required for induced expression of cytokine genes.[1,24,25] Furthermore, it had been reported that the antioxidants butylated hydroxyanisole,[26] N-acetyl cysteine,[27] and probucol[28,29] suppress the production of TNFα and IL-1β by mouse peritoneal and splenic macrophages and human promonocytic cell lines. Quinolones, quinoline-derived antibiotics, have also been shown to decrease IL-1 production by human peripheral blood monocytes (PBM) in a dose-related manner.[30] The moderately lipophilic antioxidant 2-octadecyl ascorbic acid reduces mortality in a mouse model of endotoxemia,[31] and the 21-aminosteroid tirilazad mesylate, which has antioxidant activity,[32] mitigates clinical manifestations of endotoxemia in neonatal calves.[33]

These are examples of small antioxidant molecules inhibiting the production of individual cytokines and attenuating septic shock. We have investigated the problem more systematically, comparing effects of different types of antioxidants on the production of TNFα, IL-1β, and IL-6 in cultured human monocytes activated by LPS and in other ways. Comparative studies in another cell type were also made. Some antioxidants, but not others, were found to be potent inhibitors of the production of all three cytokines in monocytes but not in fibroblasts. The *in vitro* observations were then confirmed by *in vivo* experiments in mice. The molecular basis of antioxidant-mediated inhibition was analyzed, showing that antioxidants can inhibit the activation of transcription factors NFκB and AP-1 and the transcription of cytokine genes, as reported separately in this meeting.[34]

MATERIALS AND METHODS

All the procedures and reagents have been described.[35] In brief, human peripheral blood mononuclear cells (PBM) were separated by Ficoll-paque gradient and enriched in monocytes by adherence to plastic or by rosetting out T-lymphocytes with aminoethylthiouronium bromide–treated sheep erythrocytes. PBM were cultured either in polypropylene tubes ($5 \times 10^5/1$ ml per tube) or in 12-well plates (1 ml/well) in RPMI-1640 supplemented with 5% human AB serum. Cultures were stimulated with lipopolysaccharide (LPS, 20 μg/ml), with or without drugs, and incubated overnight at 37°C in 5% CO_2. The supernatants were harvested, and the cell pellets were resuspended in RPMI medium, and freeze-thawed five times to prepare lysates. All samples were stored frozen ($-20°C$) until ready for cytokine determination. ELISA assays for human IL-1β, TNFα, and IL-6 have also been described.[35,36]

To test the effect of drugs on cytokine production *in vivo*, two assays were used as described previously.[35] In brief, mouse peritoneal macrophages were elicited by intraperitoneal (ip) injection of thioglycolate medium (40.5 g/l, 1 ml) and after 3 days the animals were challenged with 10–15 μg LPS/mouse. Drugs were administered before and after LPS challenge (−18 h, −30 min, and +2 h). Four hours after LPS injection, the animals were sacrificed and peritoneal exudate cells were collected. Replicate samples (2×10^6 cells) were either cultured overnight and supernatants collected for IL-1β determination, or they were freeze-thawed immediately after harvesting to prepare cell lysates. All samples were stored at −20°C until ready to measure IL-1β by ELISA.[35]

In the other assay, circulating levels of TNFα and IL-1β were measured in plasma collected at intervals following a lethal dose of LPS. Mice were treated with test compounds 30 min before LPS injection (200 μg/mouse, ip), and blood samples were

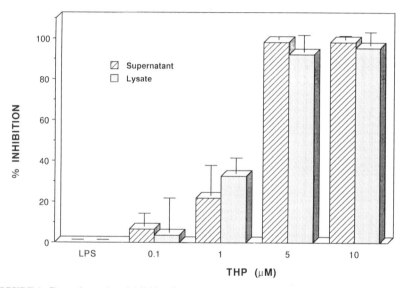

FIGURE 1. Dose-dependent inhibition by tetrahydropapaveroline (THP) of the production of IL-1β in human peripheral blood mononuclear cells activated by LPS. Means and standard errors of intracellular (lysate) and extracellular cytokines are shown.[35]

collected 1½ h after LPS administration for TNFα assay.[35] Mice were given a second dose of drug 2 h after LPS injection, and blood samples were collected 2 h later for IL-1β assay.

RESULTS

Effects of Antioxidants on IL-1β Synthesis

In a first screening, several compounds were tested for capacity to inhibit the production of IL-1β in LPS-stimulated human peripheral blood mononuclear cell (PBM) cultures. Tetrahydropapaveroline (THP), a tetrahydroisoquinoline derivative, was found to be a potent inhibitor of IL-1β production (IC_{50} about 1.5 μM, FIGURE 1). The compound decreased intracellular IL-1β as well as cytokine in the culture medium. Other compounds structurally related to THP, 10,11-dihydroxyapor-phine (DHA) and norapomorphine, were also tested and found to inhibit IL-1 production efficiently (TABLE 1). The S(+) and R(−) stereoisomers of DHA were equipotent in this assay, showing separation from dopamine agonist activity; only the R(−) form is a dopamine agonist.

In view of reports that butylated hydroxyanisole (BHA), N-acetylcysteine, and probucol inhibit the production of TNFα and IL-1β in mouse macrophages,[26-30] various antioxidants were tested for capacity to inhibit the production of IL-1β in LPS-activated human PBM. Several moderately lipophilic antioxidants, including butylated hydroxyanisole (BHA) and nordihydroguaiaretic acid (NDGA), were found to be potent inhibitors of IL-1β production (IC_{50} 4 μM or lower, TABLE 1). NDGA is an inhibitor of 5-lipoxygenase, as well as of lipid peroxidation. However, another redox 5-lipoxygenase inhibitor, Zileuton, did not affect IL-1β formation, suggesting that 5-lipoxygenase products are not involved in the signal transduction system leading to cytokine production in LPS-activated monocytes. The antimalarial

TABLE 1. Antioxidants Vary Widely in Potency as Inhibitors of Cytokine Formation

High Activity	(IC_{50} μM)
Butylated hydroxyanisole (BHA)	2.9
Tetrahydropapaveroline (THP)	1.0
Apomorphine	2.6
Norapomorphine	1.6
Nordihydroguaiaauretic acid (NDGA)	1.3
Mepacrine	3.0
Low Activity (insignificant inhibition in the range 50–200 μM)	
Ascorbic acid	
α-Tocopherol	
Mannitol	
Trolox	
Butylated hydroxytoluene (BHT)	
Quercetin	
N,N′-Diphenyl-p-phenylene diamine	
Zileuton (5-lipoxygenase inhibitor)	

drug and phospholipase inhibitor mepacrine was also an effective inhibitor of cytokine production.

In contrast, the more hydrophilic antioxidants tested, ascorbic acid and trolox, had no effect on IL-1β production in concentrations up to 200 μM (TABLE 1). Mannitol, a hydroxyl radical scavenger, was inactive at 100 μM concentration. The same was true of the physiological lipophilic antioxidant α-tocopherol, as well as some classical antioxidants—butylated hydroxytoluene (BHT), quercetin, and N,N′-diphenyl-p-phenylene diamine. N-Acetylcysteine had some inhibitory effect (IC_{50} 42 mM), but this was much lower than that of several lipophilic antioxidants (TABLE 1).

The question arose whether the inhibitory effect of THP is selective for the signaling pathway initiated by LPS or applies also to other highly effective inducers, such as silica and Staphylococcus aureus Cowan I (Pansorbin). As shown in FIGURE 2, THP was equally potent in the inhibition of IL-1β production with all inducers tested. The drug also inhibited IL-1β production using a weaker inducer, Zymosan. These observations show that THP can inhibit the production of IL-1β by human

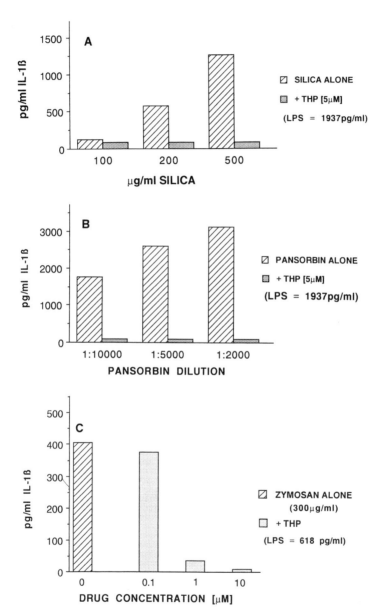

FIGURE 2. Tetrahydropapaveroline (THP, 1 to 5 μM) is a potent inhibitor of the production of IL-1β in human PBM induced by silica, pansorbin (*Staphylococcus* Cowan 1), and zymosan.[35]

PBM stimulated with several inducers. Similar observations were made with other antioxidants (not shown).

Effects on TNFα and IL-6 Production

THP, 10,11-dihydroxyaporphine, and NDGA were further tested for effects on the production of TNFα and IL-6 by LPS-stimulated human PBM. All three compounds were found to be approximately equipotent as inhibitors of the production of the three cytokines (TABLE 2, FIGURE 3). A nonspecific effect on protein synthesis was excluded: THP did not decrease the incorporation of ^{3}H leucine into monocytes (FIGURE 4) or U-937 promonocytic cells (TABLE 2) at concentrations up to 50 μM. The other agents tested required more than 20-fold greater concentrations to inhibit protein synthesis than cytokine production (TABLE 2).

Cell Type Selectivity and Irreversibility of the Inhibitory Effect

To ascertain whether this effect is exerted in all cell types, human dermal fibroblasts (HFF) and fibroblast-type cells from synovial tissue of patients with rheumatoid arthritis were studied. In these cells, IL-1 induces the production of IL-6. As shown in FIGURE 5, THP, BHA, 10,11-dihydroxyaporphine (apomorphine), and norapomorphine, in concentrations higher than are required to inhibit totally the production of IL-6 in PBM, had no significant effect on IL-6 production in synovial tissue fibroblasts and HFF.[35] Thus antioxidant-mediated inhibition of cytokine production does not occur in all cell types.

THP was also used to analyze the reversibility of the inhibitory effect. Adherent PBM were cultured with LPS and THP for two hours and repeatedly washed. Fresh medium containing the same amount of LPS was added, and the cultures were incubated overnight. Duplicate cultures were maintained with LPS and THP for the same period without washing. As shown in FIGURE 6, removal of the drug did not reverse its inhibitory effect. Thus, the inhibition of IL-1β production by THP appears to be irreversible, at least during the 18 hours studied.

In Vivo Effects

Some of the compounds in TABLE 1 were selected for analysis of *in vivo* effects on cytokine production. Two different assays were used, as described in Methods. In the first assay, IL-1β production was measured using elicited peritoneal cells from mice, four hours after LPS challenge. The cytokine was measured in lysates of cells directly

TABLE 2. Inhibition of Cytokine Production by Some Antioxidants: Comparative Effect on IL-1β, TNF-α, and IL-6

	IC$_{50}$ μM			
Agent	IL-1β	TNF-α	IL-6	Protein[a] Synthesis
Tetrahydropapaveroline	1.5	1.2	1.2	> 50
Apomorphine	2.6	2.2	1.8	47
NDGA	0.9	2.8	2.8	38

[a]^{3}H-Leu incorporation by U-937, after 4 hours incubation.

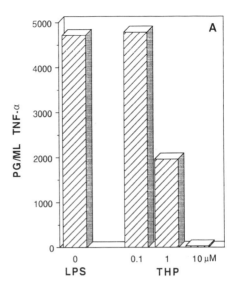

FIGURE 3. Dose-dependent inhibition by tetrahydropapaveroline (THP) of the production of TNFα and of IL-6 by human peripheral blood mononuclear cells activated by LPS. Cytokines in the supernatant were assayed.[35]

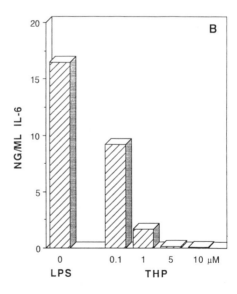

recovered from the peritoneal cavity (cell-associated IL-1β), as well as in the supernatants of cells after overnight culture (released IL-1β). Mice were pretreated with two doses of either THP or 10,11-dihydroxyaporphine (apomorphine, 50 mg/kg per dose) before LPS challenge (15 μg/mouse). A third dose of compound was administered two hours later. Both compounds suppressed the production of IL-1β by 53 to 86% (TABLE 3).

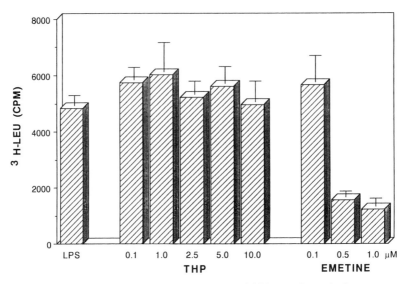

FIGURE 4. THP, up to 10 μM concentration, does not inhibit protein synthesis, as measured by ³H-Leu incorporation into human peripheral blood monocytes (4-h assay). Emetine used as a positive control was active at 0.5 μM concentration.

In the second assay, TNFα and IL-1β were measured in serum following a lethal challenge with LPS (200 μg/mouse). Levels of TNFα in circulating blood peak 1½ hours and those of IL-1β 4 hours after LPS injection. Subcutaneous administration of a single dose of apomorphine (100 mg/kg), given 30 minutes before challenge, inhibited TNFα production by 95%. Before IL-1β peak level, mice were given a

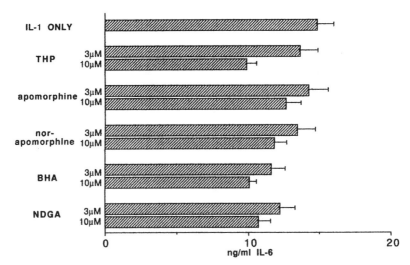

FIGURE 5. Lack of effect of antioxidants on the production of IL-6 in human fibroblast-type synovial cells induced by IL-1β.

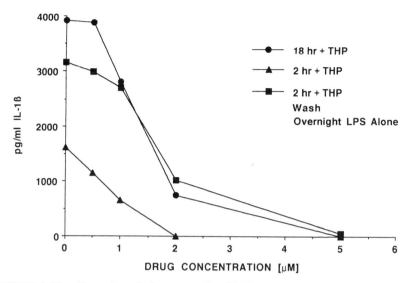

FIGURE 6. The effects of tetrahydropapaveroline (THP) on the production of IL-1β by LPS activated human PBM. Treatment with THP for 2 hours, washing cells, and culturing in the presence of LPS inhibits IL-1β production as effectively as having the drug present during all 18 hours of culture.[35]

second dose of apomorphine (50 mg/kg), 2 hours after LPS and 2 hours before bleeding. This treatment reduced the circulating levels of IL-1β by 88% (FIGURE 7). Thus, *in vivo* cytokine production is strongly inhibited by THP and by apomorphine.

DISCUSSION

We have found that several antioxidants are potent inhibitors of the production of TNFα, IL-1β, and IL-6 in LPS-stimulated human PBM. The same concentrations

TABLE 3. In vivo Activity of Some IL-1 Synthesis Inhibitors on LPS-induced IL-1β Production by Elicited Mice Peritoneal Cells

Agent	Route	Dose (mg/kg)	No. Mice	ng/ml ± SD (% Inhibition) IL-1β			
				Lysates		Supernatants	
THP	sc	Control	5	183 ± 75		217 ± 87	
	sc	50 × 30	5	85 ± 38	(53)	80 ± 42	(63)
	po	Control	4	792 ± 124		866 ± 246	
	po	100 × 3	4	382 ± 67	(52)	447 ± 69	(49)
Apomorphine	sc	Control	4	574 ± 152		622 ± 163	
	sc	50 × 3	4	112 ± 30	(81)	87 ± 20	(86)
	po	Control	4	215 ± 33		202 ± 24	
	po	50 × 3	4	92 ± 63	(58)	98 ± 59	(52)
Norapomorphine	sc	Control	4	574 ± 152		622 ± 163	
	sc	50 × 3	4	179 ± 44	(69)	163 ± 49	(74)
	po	Control	4	526 ± 101		611 ± 47	
	po	50 × 3	4	29 ± 27	(95)	92 ± 47	(85)

of antioxidants were equally effective in the inhibition of cytokine production in PBM irrespective of the stimulus (LPS, staphylococci, silica, and zymosan). Effects of antioxidants are not due to overall inhibition of protein synthesis and are gene selective. As reported separately at this meeting, the antioxidants do not affect transcription of the β-actin and c-jun genes,[34] and actually increase the production of

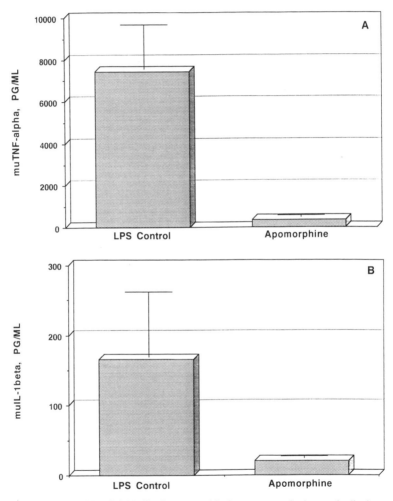

FIGURE 7. Apomorphine (10,11-dihydroxyaporphine) treatment of mice markedly decreases levels of TNFα and of IL-1β in the circulation of mice challenged with LPS.[35] See Methods for technical details.

the interleukin-1 receptor antagonist, as well as of lysozyme and of lysosomal enzymes in PBM.[37] Inhibition of cytokine production occurs at the level of transcription, and may be related to their observed inhibition of the activation of the transcription factors NFκB and AP-1.[34]

The effects of the antioxidants are also cell-type selective. Antioxidants that are potent inhibitors of IL-6 production in PBM do not inhibit production of the same cytokine in dermal or synovial fibroblasts. The mechanisms stimulating IL-6 production are diverse,[25] and presumably the transcription complexes used in fibroblasts are less susceptible to redox regulation than those in PBM. Other cell types should be studied, but our findings raise the possibility that selected antioxidants may be able to suppress the formation of proinflammatory cytokines in cells of the monocyte-macrophage lineage without having major effects in other cell types which could lead to unwanted side effects.

There is considerable variability in the potency of antioxidants as inhibitors of cytokine production. A tetrahydroisoquinoline, THP, and two compounds with some structural relationship to THP, 10,11-dihydroxyaporphine (apomorphine) and norapomorphine, were among the most potent inhibitors. Since both stereoisomers of dihydroxyaporphine were equipotent as inhibitors of cytokine production, there was separation of this activity from dopamine agonist activity.

Two classical antioxidants BHA and NDGA were also strong inhibitors of cytokine production. NDGA is an inhibitor of 5-lipoxygenase and of lipid peroxidation. However, zileuton, used in concentrations that inhibit 5-lipoxygenase activity, had no effect on cytokine production. This suggests that the antioxidant activity of NDGA, rather than its 5-lipoxygenase inhibitory activity, explains its effect on cytokine production. The common feature of the structurally diverse compounds with high activity listed in TABLE 1 is their capacity to function as antioxidants and their moderate lipophilicity.

The water-soluble antioxidants studied, ascorbic acid and Trolox, were inactive, suggesting that the antioxidants have to function in a lipid environment. However, this must be a specialized microenvironment within target cells. The physiological membrane antioxidant α-tocopherol was ineffective as an inhibitor of cytokine production, as were several classical antioxidants listed in TABLE 1 (butylated hydroxytoluene, quercetin, *N,N'*diphenyl-*p*-phenylene diamine). Further work is necessary to define structure-activity relationships of inhibitors of cytokine production, the intracellular compartment in which they are active, and the mechanism by which they block the activation of transcription factors.

Some of the compounds active in cultured cells also show activity *in vivo*. THP and dihydroxyaporphine were shown to inhibit strongly the production of TNFα and IL-1β in mice challenged with LPS. The antioxidants and mode of administration were not optimized, but the findings are encouraging. They are consistent with reports that 2-octadecylascorbic acid reduces mortality in a mouse model of endotoxemia[31] and that the 21-aminosteroid tirilazad mesylate, which has antioxidant activity,[32] mitigates clinical manifestations of endotoxemia in neonatal calves.[33]

The data presented in this paper show that the genes for TNFα, IL-1β, and IL-6 function as a casette, being coordinately expressed when monocytes are stimulated by LPS or staphylococci. This expression is inhibited by some antioxidants. Remarkably, we have found that the same antioxidants augment the expression of the IL-1ra gene and IL-1ra production in cultures of PBM.[37] Some long-acting antirheumatic drugs accelerate differentiation of monocytic lineage cells, thereby decreasing IL-1β formation, and augment IL-1ra production.[38] It has been postulated that a balance between the production of proinflammatory cytokines, such as TNFα and IL-1β, and of IL-1ra, plays an important role in determining the course of rheumatoid arthritis.[2] The same may be true of the arthritis associated with Lyme disease, caused by the bacterium *Borrelia burgdorferi*. Patients with high concentrations of IL-1ra and low concentrations of IL-1β in synovial fluid had rapid resolution of attacks of arthritis, whereas patients with the reverse pattern of cytokine concentrations had long intervals to recovery.[39] Using drugs to manipulate the balance of production of cytokines and IL-1ra in such a way as to have antiinflammatory effects is a novel therapeutic strategy.

REFERENCES

1. BEUTLER, B., Ed. 1992. Tumor Necrosis Factors: the Molecules and Their Emerging Role in Medicine. Raven Press. New York, N.Y.
2. AREND, W. P. & J.-M. DAYER. 1990. Cytokines and cytokine inhibitors or antagonists in rheumatoid arthritis. Arthritis Rheum. 33: 305–315.
3. DINARELLO, C. A. 1991. Interleukin-1 and interleukin-1 antagonism. Blood 77: 1627–1652.
4. BEVILACQUA, M. P., J. S. POBER, M. E. WHELLER, R. S. COTRAN & M. A. GIMBRONE. 1985. Interleukin-1 acts on cultured human vascular endothelium to increase the adhesion of polymorphonuclear leukocytes, monocytes, and related leukocyte cell lines. J. Clin. Invest. 76: 2003–2011.
5. DAYER, J.-M., B. DE ROCHEMONTEIX, B. BURNERS, S. DEMCZUK & C. A. DINARELLO. 1986. Human recombinant interleukin-1 stimulates collagenase and prostaglandin E_2 production by human synovial cells. J. Clin. Invest. 77: 645–648.
6. ROSSI, V., F. BREVARIO, P. GHEZZI, E. DEJANA & A. MANTOVANI. 1985. Prostaglandin induced in vascular endothelial cells by interleukin-1. Science 229: 174–176.
7. SCHNYDER, J., T. PAYNE & C. A. DINARELLO. 1987. Human monocyte or recombinant interleukin-1's are specific for the secretion of a metalloproteinase from chondrocytes. J. Immunol. 138: 496–503.
8. MACDONALD, B. R. & M. GOWAN. 1992. Cytokines and bone. Br. J. Rheumatol. 31: 149–155.
9. TAKAI, Y., G. G. WONG, S. C. CLARK, S. J. BURAKOFF & S. H. HERRMANN. 1988. B cell stimulatory factor-2 is involved in the differentiation of cytotoxic T lymphocytes. J. Immunol. 140: 508–512.
10. NAWATA, Y., E. M. EUGUI, S. W. LEE & A. C. ALLISON. 1989. IL-6 is the principal factor produced by synovia of patients with rheumatoid arthritis that induces B-lymphocytes to secrete immunoglobulin. Ann. N.Y. Acad. Sci. 557: 230–239.
11. GASTON, J. S. H., S. STROBER, J. J. SOLVERA, D. GANDOUR, N. LANE, D. SCHURMAN, R. T. HOPPE, R. C. CHIN, E. M. EUGUI, J. H. VAUGHAN & A. C. ALLISON. 1988. Dissection of the mechanisms of immune injury in rheumatoid arthritis using total lymphoid irradiation. Arthritis Rheum. 31: 21–30.
12. NARDELLA, F. A., J. M. DAYER, M. ROELKE, S. M. KROME & M. MANNIK. 1983. Self-associating IgG rheumatoid factors stimulate monocytes to release prostaglandins and mononuclear cell factors that stimulate collagenase and prostaglandin production by synovial cells. Rheumatol. Int. 3: 183–186.
13. ISHIMI, Y., C. MIYAURA, C. H. JIN, T. AKATSU, E. ABE, Y. NAKAMURA, A. YAMAGUCHI, S. YOSHIKI, T. MATSUDA, T. HIRANO, T. RISHIMOTO & T. SUDA. 1990. IL-6 is produced by osteoblasts and induces bone resorption. J. Immunol. 145: 3297–3303.
14. BRENNAN, F. M., D. CHANTRY, A. JACKSON, R. MAINI & M. FELDMANN. 1989. Inhibitory effect of TNFα antibodies on synovial cell interleukin-1 production in rheumatoid arthritis. Lancet 2: 244–247.
15. BERTIN, P. B., J. S. KENNEY, M. R. WELCH, H. B. LINDSLEY, R. TREVES & A. C. ALLISON. 1992. IL-1 inhibitors block IL-6 and IL-8 secretion by fragments of human rheumatoid arthritis synovium. Arthritis Rheum. 35(Suppl.): C189.
16. ELLIOTT, M. J., R. N. MAINI, M. FELDMANN, R. O. WILLIAMS, F. M. BRENNAN & C. Q. CHU. 1993. Treatment of rheumatoid arthritis with chimeric monoclonal antibodies to TNFα: safety, clinical efficacy and control of the acute-phase response. J. Cell. Biochem. 17B(Suppl.): 145.
17. LEBSACK, M. E., C. C. PAUL, D. C. BLOEDOW, F. X. BURCH, M. A. SACK, W. CHASE & M. A. CATALANO. 1991. Subcutaneous IL-1 receptor antagonist in patients with rheumatoid arthritis. Arthritis Rheum. 34(9, Suppl.): S45.
18. FONG, Y., K. J. TRACEY, L. L. MOLDAWER, D. G. HESSE, K. B. MANOGUE, J. S. KENNEY, A. T. LEE, G. C. KUO, A. C. ALLISON, S. F. LOWRY & A. CERAMI. 1989. Antibodies to

cachectin/tumor necrosis factor reduce interleukin-1β and interleukin-6 appearance during lethal bacteremia. J. Exp. Med. **170:** 1627–1633.

19. FISCHER, E., M. A. MARANO, K. VAN ZEE, C. S. ROCK, A. S. HAWES, W. A. THOMPSON, L. DE FORGE, J. S. KENNEY, D. G. REMICK, D. C. BLAEDOW, R. C. THOMPSON, S. F. LOWRY & L. L. MOLDAWER. 1992. Interleukin-1 receptor blockade improves survival and hemodynamic performance in *Escherichia coli* septic shock, but fails to alter host responses to sublethal endotoxemia. J. Clin. Invest. **89:** 1551–1557.

20. SCHREK, R., P. RIEBER & P. A. BAUERLE. 1991. Reactive oxygen intermediates as apparently widely used messengers in the activation of NFκB transcription factor and HIV-1. EMBO J. **10:** 2247–2258.

21. ISRAEL, N., M.-A. GOUGERAT-POCIDALO, F. AILLET & J.-L. VIRELIZIER. 1992. Redox status influences constitutive or induced NFκB translocation and HIV long terminal repeat activity in human T and monocytic cell lines. J. Immunol. **149:** 3386–3393.

22. DEVARY, Y., R. A. GOTTLIEB, L. F. LAU & M. KARIN. 1991. Rapid and preferential activation of the *c-jun* gene during the mammalian UV response. Mol. Cell. Biol. **11:** 2804–2811.

23. DATTA, R., D. E. HALLAHAN, S. M. KHARBANDA, E. RUBIN, M. L. SHERMAN, E. HUBERMAN, R. R. WEICHSELBAUM & D. W. KUFF. 1992. Involvement of reactive oxygen intermediates in the induction of c-jun gene transcription by ionizing radiation. Biochemistry **31:** 8300–8306.

24. SHAKHOV, A. N., M. A. COLLART, P. VASSALI, S. A. NEDOSPASOV & C. V. JONGENEAL. 1990. Kappa B-type enhancers are involved in lipopolysaccharide-mediated transcriptional activation of the tumor necrosis factor alpha gene in primary macrophages. J. Exp. Med. **171:** 35–47.

25. HIRANO, T., S. AKIRA, T. TASA & J. KISHIMOTO. 1990. Biological and clinical aspects of interleukin-6. Immunol. Today **11:** 443–449.

26. CHAUDHRI, G. & J. A. CLARK. 1989. Reactive oxygen species facilitate the *in vitro* and *in vivo* lipopolysaccharide-induced release of tumor necrosis factor. J. Immunol. **143:** 1290–1294.

27. PERISTERIS, P., B. D. CLARK, S. GATTI, R. FAGGIONI, A. MANTOVANI, M. MENGOZZI, S. F. ORENCOLE, M. SIRONI & P. GHEZZI. 1992. *N*-Acetylcysteine and glutathione as inhibitors of tumor necrosis factor production. Cell Immunol. **140:** 390–399.

28. KU, G., N. S. DOHERTY, L. F. SCHMIDT, R. L. JACKSON & R. J. DIVERSTEIN. 1990. *Ex vivo* lipopolysaccharide-induced interleukin-1 secretion from murine peritoneal macrophages inhibited by probucol, a hypocholesterolemic agent with antioxidant properties. FASEB J. **4:** 1645–1653.

29. AKESON, A. L., C. W. WOODS, L. B. MOSHER, C. E. THOMAS & R. L. JACKSON. 1991. Inhibition of IL-1β expression in THP-1 cells by probucol and tocopherol. Atherosclerosis **86:** 261–270.

30. ROCHE, Y., M. FAY & M. A. GOUGEROT-POCIDALO. 1987. Effects of quinolones on interleukin-1 production *in vitro* by human monocytes. Immunopharmacology **13:** 99–109.

31. NONAKA, A., T. MANABE & T. TOBE. 1990. Effect of a new synthetic free radical scavenger, 2-octadecyl ascorbic acid, on the mortality in mouse endotoxemia. Life Sci. **47:** 1933–1939.

32. BRAUGHLER, J. M., J. F. PREGENZER, R. L. CHASE, *et al.* 1987. Novel 21-aminosteroids as potent inhibitors of iron-dependent lipid peroxidation. J. Biol. Chem. **262:** 10438–10440.

33. ROSE, M. L. & S. D. SEMRAD. 1992. Clinical efficacy of tirilazad mesylate for treatment of endotoxemia in neonatal calves. Am. J. Vet. Res. **53:** 2305–2310.

34. ILNICKA, M., S. W. LEE & E. M. EUGUI. Antioxidants inhibit activation of transcription factors and cytokine gene transcription in monocytes. Ann. N.Y. Acad. Sci. (This volume.)

35. EUGUI, E. M., B. DELUSTRO, S. ROUHAFZA, M. ILNICKA, S. W. LEE, R. WILHELM & A. C. ALLISON. Some antioxidants inhibit, in a coordinate fashion, the production of TNFα, IL-1β and IL-6 by human peripheral blood mononuclear cells. Int. Immunol. (Submitted.)

36. KENNEY, J. S., M. P. MASADA, E. M. EUGUI, B. DE LUSTRO, M. A. MULKINS & A. C. ALLISON. 1987. Monoclonal antibodies to human interleukin-1β: inhibition of biological activity. J. Immunol. **138:** 4236–4242.
37. WATERS, R. V. & A. C. ALLISON. Some long-acting antirheumatic drugs and antioxidants induce differentiation of macrophage lineage cells and augment expression of the IL-1 receptor antagonist IL-1ra. Ann. N.Y. Acad. Sci. (This volume.)
38. ALLISON, A. C. & R. V. WATERS. Long-acting anti-rheumatic drugs induce differentiation of cells of the monocyte-macrophage lineage and alter the expression of cytokines and IL-1 receptor antagonist. Agents Actions. (In press.)
39. MILLER, L. C., E. A. LYNCH, S. ISA, J. W. LOGAN, C. A. DINARELLO & A. STEELE. 1993. Balance of synovial fluid IL-1β and IL-1 receptor antagonist and recovery from Lyme arthritis. Lancet **341:** 146.

Mycophenolic Acid and Some Antioxidants Induce Differentiation of Monocytic Lineage Cells and Augment Production of the IL-1 Receptor Antagonist

RUTH V. WATERS, DONNA WEBSTER, AND
ANTHONY C. ALLISON[a]

Syntex Discovery Research
3401 Hillview Avenue
Palo Alto, California 94304

INTRODUCTION

Rapidly acting antiinflammatory agents include glucocorticoids and cyclooxygenase inhibitors, which decrease pain and inflammation within days of the onset of treatment. In contrast, treatment of patients with rheumatoid arthritis (RA) for three months or longer with long-acting antirheumatic drugs such as gold salts (aurothiomalate and auranofin), chloroquine, and hydroxychloriquine is required before pain and joint swelling are alleviated.

One interpretation of the long treatment period required before such long-acting antirheumatic drugs show efficacy is that they are acting on a population of cells that is turning over relatively slowly. We have proposed that a primary target of long-acting drugs is cells of monocyte-macrophage lineage, the central cell type in the pathogenesis of chronic inflammation, including that in the synovial tissue of patients with rheumatoid arthritis.[1] These cells have been shown by *in situ* hybridization and immunocytochemistry to be the only producers in rheumatoid synovial tissue of the proinflammatory and catabolic mediators IL-1β[2,3] and TNFα.[4] Substantial evidence that TNFα and IL-1 participate in the pathogenesis of rheumatoid arthritis has accumulated.[1,5,6] TNFα and IL-1 induce the expression on endothelial cells of adhesion molecules involved in leukocyte recruitment; they induce the production by synovial fibroblasts of PGE$_2$; and they induce production of neutral metalloproteinases which contribute to degradation of cartilage and bone.

Cells of the macrophage lineage produce not only the proinflammatory cytokines TNFα, and IL-1β, but also an antiinflammatory 23K protein which binds to IL-1 receptors and functions as an antagonist.[5] This IL-1 receptor antagonist (IL-1ra), originally described in the supernatants of human monocytes adherent to IgG and in the urine of patients with myelomonocytic leukemia or fever, has been cloned and expressed, and the promoter for the IL-1ra gene characterized.[7] Administration of recombinant IL-1ra *in vitro* and in experimental animal models has been shown to inhibit effects of IL-1, including autocrine IL-1 release,[8] synovial cell PGE$_2$ production, bone resorption, chondrocyte collagenase production, cartilage proteoglycan

[a] Present address: 2513 Hastings Drive, Belmont, CA 94002.

release, and leukocyte migration into inflamed joints.[9,10] Based on activity in animal models, the IL-1ra is currently in clinical trials for the treatment of rheumatoid arthritis.[9]

Drugs acting on monocytic lineage cells to decrease the production of TNFα and IL-1β and augment production of IL-1ra could have antirheumatic activity. Recent published studies show that IL-1 and IL-1ra production in monocytes and macrophages is differentially regulated at both transcriptional and posttranscriptional levels.[11–14] Changing the balance of production of these two opposing molecules could therefore significantly alter the progression of chronic inflammation. Differentiation of monocytes into macrophages is accompanied by restriction of their capacity to produce IL-1 as well as acquisition of the capacity to produce the IL-1ra.[15,16] As monocytes differentiate *in vitro,* they constitutively produce IL-1ra protein, the levels

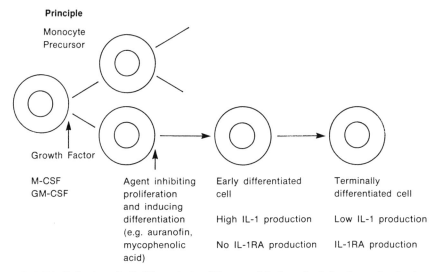

Principle

Monocyte Precursor			
Growth Factor			
M-CSF GM-CSF	Agent inhibiting proliferation and inducing differentiation (e.g. auranofin, mycophenolic acid)	Early differentiated cell High IL-1 production No IL-1RA production	Terminally differentiated cell Low IL-1 production IL-1RA production

FIGURE 1. Induction of cell differentiation. Diagram of the hypothesis for the mode of action of long-acting antirheumatic agents. An agent that inhibits proliferation of monocyte precursors and accelerates the differentiation of monocytes will eventually deplete the pool of precursors and early differentiated cells, thereby decreasing IL-1 production and augmenting IL-1ra production. This may be manifested as a slow-acting antirheumatic effect.

of which are enhanced by the continuous presence of GM-CSF.[16] Mature alveolar macrophages and synovial macrophages, cultured and stimulated under the same conditions, produce less IL-1 and more IL-1ra than peripheral blood monocytes do.[10,17–19]

These considerations led to our proposal[20] that some long-acting antirheumatic drugs might exert their activity by (1) inhibiting the proliferation of monocyte precursors in the bone marrow, thereby reducing recruitment into the inflamed synovium, and (2) accelerating the differentiation of recruited monocytes into macrophages with restricted capacity to produce proinflammatory cytokines and augmented capacity to produce IL-1ra (FIGURE 1). To test this hypothesis, we have examined the effects of established drugs (auranofin, gold sodium thiomalate, and chloroquine) on the proliferation and differentiation of human monocytic precursor cell lines arrested at different stages of development.[20] The HL60 cell line[21] is the counterpart of bipotential precursors in bone marrow which when stimulated with GM-CSF produce granulocyte-monocyte (GM) colonies. The U937 cell line[22] is a committed monocyte precursor arrested at the promonocytic stage. We found that clinically attainable concentrations of gold salts and of chloroquine inhibit proliferation and induce differentiation of these precursor cells by multiparameter analysis.[20] In addition, auronofin and chloroquine were found to induce differentiation of human peripheral blood monocytes in culture as measured by enzymatic markers. Induced differentiation of human peripheral blood monocytes in culture induction by these antirheumatic compounds was accompanied by increased production of IL-1ra.[20] The ability of these well-known antirheumatic drugs to increase the ratio of IL-1ra to IL-1 production in differentiating human monocytes validated our proposal that induction of differentiation may be a mechanism of antirheumatic action. Experiments were then performed to ascertain whether newer drugs with novel profiles of activity exert similar effects.

Mycophenolate mofetil, a prodrug of mycophenolic acid (MPA), is an immunosuppressive agent which depletes dGTP in T- and B-lymphocytes and thereby prevents proliferation.[23] MPA also depletes GTP in monocytes.[24] MPA and other inhibitors of inosine monophosphate dehydrogenase have been reported to be not only antiproliferative, but to induce differentiation of cells belonging to several lineages.[25-27] As reported here, MPA was found to inhibit proliferation and induce differentiation of human monocyte-macrophage lineage cells and significantly augment IL-1ra production in cultures of human peripheral blood monocytes.

Antioxidants have long been known to have antiinflammatory actions. Investigations from our laboratory have shown that some antioxidants inhibit, in a coordinate fashion, the production of TNFα, IL-1β, and IL-6 by human peripheral blood mononuclear cells (PBM).[28] We now report that these antioxidants can also accelerate differentiation and the production of IL-1ra by PBM.

MATERIALS AND METHODS

Monocyte Precursor Cell Lines

Human HL-60 promyelocytic[21] and U937 promonocytic[22] cells were obtained from American Type Culture Collection, Rockville, Md., and grown in RPMI-1640 medium containing 10% FCS, 2 mM glutamine, 100 μg/ml streptomycin, 100 U/ml penicillin, and 50 μg/ml gentamycin. For differentiation assays, cells in log phase growth were plated at a density of 0.2 million per square centimeter in Costar 96-well culture plates, and cultured in 5% CO_2 for 5 days at 37°C with and without mycophenolic acid (Ajinomoto Corporation, Osaka, Japan). Four replicate wells were tested per concentration. DMSO used to solubilize the test agents was present in a final concentration of 0.5%. After supernatant collection on the last day of culture, washed cell pellets were lysed with 0.05% triton-x 100 and the lysates used for enzymatic analysis.

Antiproliferative effects of MPA were determined from live cell counts (Trypan blue dye exclusion) on days 2 and 5 of culture. Differentiation was assessed by measuring of levels of mature monocyte/macrophage enzymatic markers. Supernatant lysozyme production was assessed using the Osserman Lysoplate method,[29] with hen egg white lysozyme standards. Lysosomal acid hydrolases were measured using standard spectrophotometric assays of the hydrolysis of PNP-substrates. Total cell protein was measured using BCA stain (Pierce ImmunoTechnology, Rockford, Ill.).

Human Peripheral Blood Monocyte Cultures

Ficoll-hypaque purified human peripheral blood mononuclear cells were seeded in 96-well culture plates at 1.4 million per square centimeter (0.4 million cells/well) and allowed to adhere for 1.5 h at 37°C in RPMI-1640 complete medium lacking serum. The nonadherent cells were washed off with phosphate-buffered saline lacking Ca^{2+} and Mg^{2+} at room temperature. The adherence-purified monocytes were cultured for 8 days in RPMI-1640 complete medium containing 5% FCS. Test agents were added to quadruplicate culture wells per test concentration one day following initiation of culture. Supernatants were harvested daily for analysis of IL-1ra and acid phosphatase levels. After supernatant removal, fresh medium was added back in addition to the test agents, which had been prepared on the first day of culture. Cell lysates were prepared of the washed adherent cultures on days 4 and 7 following drug addition by 2 successive freeze-thaw cycles of the cells in 100 μl of the complete culture medium plus 5% FCS.

Cell lysate lysosomal enzymes and total cell protein were measured as above. Immunoreactive IL-1ra protein levels were measured using a specific sandwich ELISA following standard techniques.[30] Goat IgG antihuman recombinant IL-1ra (R+D Systems, Minneapolis, Minn.) was used for the solid-phase coating antibody, and a polyclonal rabbit antibody to IL-1ra which was raised in our laboratory was used for the solution-phase antibody. The ELISA was developed using the goat antirabbit IgG-peroxidase conjugate system, and had a sensitivity of 0.1 ng/ml. Recombinant human IL-1ra (R+D Systems) was used as the standard.

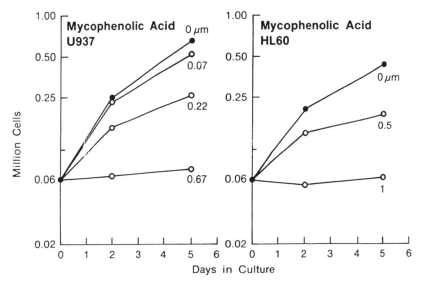

FIGURE 2. Dose-dependent antiproliferative effects of mycophenolic acid in cultures of human promyelocytes (HL-60) and promonocytes (U937).

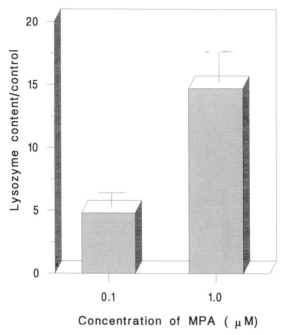

FIGURE 3. Mycophenolic acid induces a dose-dependent increase in supernatant lysozyme output on day 5 by cultured U937 cells. Control value is 53 ± 5 ng/million live cells. $n = 4$ replicates per treatment group. Results represent stimulation index = experimental divided by control.

OBSERVATIONS

Mycophenolic Acid Inhibits Proliferation of Monocyte Precursor Cell Lines and Induces Differentiation

As shown in FIGURE 2, MPA in a dose-related way inhibits the proliferation of HL60 and U937 monocyte precursor cells with IC_{50} values in the submicromolar range. The potency of MPA is comparable to that reported for auranofin in U937 cells. At antiproliferative concentrations MPA also induces differentiation of these cells assessed by standard enzymatic markers. FIGURE 3 shows a significant ($p \leq 0.02$) dose-dependent increase of 5- to 15-fold in supernatant lysozyme output by 5-day U937 cell cultures at 0.1 μM and 1 μM respectively. FIGURE 4 shows induction of approximately 2-fold increases in intracellular lysosomal enzyme content of 5-day cultures of U937 cells treated with MPA at 0.1 μM, a concentration that is ~50% antiproliferative.

Mycophenolic Acid Induces Monocyte Differentiation and IL-1ra Production

Long-acting antirheumatic drugs (auranofin and chloroquine) have been shown to augment the production of IL-1ra by cultured human monocytes.[20] MPA was tested for the ability to induce differentiation and IL-1ra production in cultures of human adherent monocytes. Results with 6 separate donors show variation in response in terms of the maximal stimulatory concentration and absolute magnitude of stimulation of the various parameters of differentiation and IL-1ra induction. In 5 of 7 assays, MPA treatment in the clinically relevant range of 0.1 to 10 μM significantly augmented parameters of differentiation, including IL-1ra production on days 4–7 of drug treatment with a bell-shaped dose-response curve. The most frequent maximal response was seen at 1 μM. FIGURE 5 summarizes results for a typical donor. In general, a larger percent increase in IL-1ra was found in the lysate rather than supernatant, as has been observed with GM-CSF induction of IL-1ra in *in vitro* derived human macrophages.[16] The total combined IL-1ra production

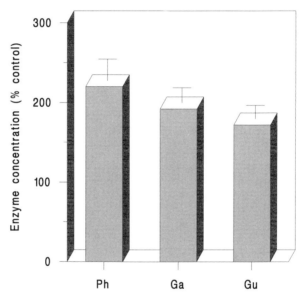

FIGURE 4. Mycophenolic acid, 0.1 μM, significantly increases the concentration of lysosomal acid hydrolases in day-5 U937 cell cultures. Control values for enzyme activity expressed as nmol PNP produced per 0.2 million cells are as follows: acid phosphatase (Ph) 10.5 ± 2.1, β-*N*-acetylglucosaminidase (Ga) 110.1 ± 17.1, β-glucuronidase (Gu) 4.6 ± 1.3. $n = 4$ replicates per treatment group.

(supernatant plus lysate) for 1 μM MPA averaged approximately 200% of control on day 7 following drug treatment. One of the eight donors showed IL-1ra increases of 4-fold magnitude (data not shown).

Antioxidants Augment IL-1ra Production and Differentiation Markers

Several antioxidants were found to augment significantly the production of IL-1ra by cultured PBM. A representative example is butylated hydroxyanisole (BHA). As shown in FIGURE 6, the concentration of BHA increasing the production of IL-1ra (1 μM) is the same as the concentration that inhibits, in a coordinate

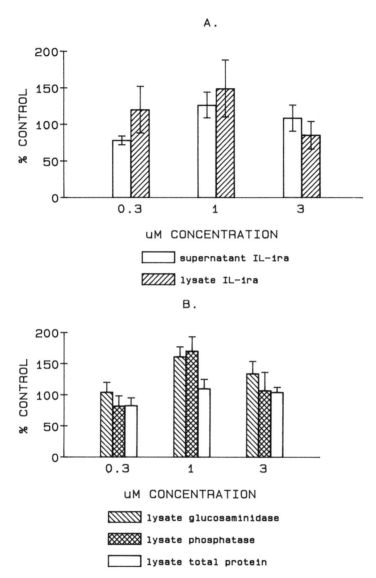

FIGURE 5. Mycophenolic acid, 1 μM, significantly augments the production of (A) IL-1ra and (B) intracellular lysosomal enzymes of human monocytes cultured with drug for 7 days. Control values are as follows: supernatant IL-1ra 160 ± 84 pg/culture, lysate IL-1ra 110 ± 25 pg/culture. Control values for enzyme activity expressed as nmol PNP produced per culture lysate are as follows: acid phosphatase 96.0 ± 9.4, glucosaminidase 233 ± 34.6. Total protein for control cultures is 18.7 ± 3.1 μg.

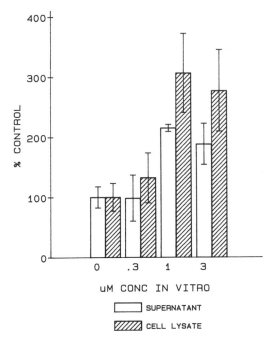

FIGURE 6. Butylated hydroxy-anisole, 1–3 μM, significantly augments the production of IL-1ra by 7 day cultures of human peripheral blood monocytes. Control values (pg immunoreactive IL-1ra/culture) on day 6 following drug treatment are as follows: supernatant 136 pg, lysate 65 pg. $n = 4$ microcultures per treatment.

fashion, the formation of TNFα, IL-1β, and IL-6 in PBM.[28] BHA also markedly increased the concentration of lysosomal enzymes in cultured PBM (FIGURE 7), suggesting that increased IL-1ra production is associated with accelerated differentiation towards macrophages. Propyl gallate was active at a higher concentration, with a 2-fold IL-1ra increase seen at 10–20 μM (data not shown). Not all tested antioxidants showed IL-1ra induction capability. For example, Zileuton (12 μM) was inactive when tested at concentrations known to inhibit 5-lipoxygenase (data not shown). MK886, which inhibits translocation of 5-lipoxygenase, had no demonstrable effect on IL-1ra formation (tested at 1 μM, data not shown).

DISCUSSION

Described here are results of studies to evaluate the effects of some antiinflammatory agents, including mycophenolic acid and some small molecular weight antioxidant molecules, on differentiation and IL-1ra production by human *in vitro* derived macrophages, a model for differentiated tissue macrophages. The capacity of cells of the monocyte-macrophage lineage to produce IL-1β and IL-1ra is known to be correlated with their degree of differentiation.[15–16] Maximal production of IL-1β is observed in monocytes; as they differentiate *in vitro*[15,16] and *in vivo*,[17,18,19] their capacity to produce IL-1β decreases while production of IL-1ra increases. Drug-induced acceleration of the differentiation of monocyte-macrophage lineage cells could therefore modify the balance of proinflammatory cytokine versus cytokine antagonist production in such a way as to exert long-acting antiinflammatory effects.

Observations from our laboratory already reported show that the long-acting antirheumatic drugs auranofin, and chloroquine inhibit the proliferation of human monocytic precursor cell lines and induce differentiation.[20] Mycophenolic acid has similar effects, which are potent (0.1–1 μM) and affect the great majority of cells in the population, as shown by the acquisition of mature macrophage surface markers in HL-60 cells.[20] While these cell lines provide convenient experimental models, the question arises whether their normal human counterparts respond to the drugs in a similar manner. Our observations are consistent with reports of Hamilton and Williams[31,32] on effects of antirheumatic drugs on colony formation by hematopoietic cells. Thus, the responses of the cell lines can be taken as representative of what happens to untransformed cells and may happen *in vivo.* Induction of differentiation in cultured human monocytes by reference long-acting agents (auranofin and chloroquine) was compared with that of the cell lines. The concentrations of long-acting drugs effective on the cell lines were found to be very similar to those effective on their normal human peripheral blood monocyte counterparts.[20]

As already reported, long-acting antirheumatic drugs not only induce PBM differentiation but also augment IL-1ra production.[20] The one- to twofold augmentation of IL-1ra reported may not seem large enough to exert significant biologic effects, but combined with decreased IL-1β production could over time tip the balance from proinflammatory to antiinflammatory activity. It should be remembered that the absolute amounts of IL-1ra versus IL-1β in inflammatory situations differ markedly, with IL-1ra concentrations as much as 100-fold greater than IL-1β.[9] Therefore a small fold increase in the IL-1ra would cause a large increase in total amounts of IL-1ra compared with those of IL-1β. It is known that while IL-1β and IL-1ra share amino acid sequences and are probably derived from the same precur-

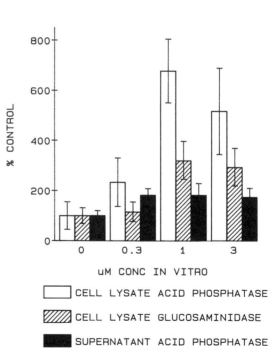

FIGURE 7. Butylated hydroxyanisole, 1–3 μM, significantly increases the activity of intracellular lysosomal enzymes in 7-day cultures of human peripheral blood monocytes. Control values for nmol PNP hydrolyzed per microwell culture are as follows: lysate acid phosphatase 0.71, lysate glucosaminidase 4.17, supernatant acid phosphatase 1.6. $n = 4$ microcultures per treatment.

sor, their expression is differentially regulated.[11–14] Some inducers, such as adherent IgG, preferentially stimulate IL-1ra formation,[9] and IL-4 suppresses the formation of IL-1β while augmenting IL-1ra expression both *in vitro*[33] and *in vivo*.[34] In addition, TGF-β, while inhibiting IL-1 production, stimulates IL-1ra production by human monocytes.[35] Long-acting antirheumatic drugs, by accelerating differentiation of monocytes to macrophages with restricted capacity to secrete IL-1β and stimulating IL-1ra production, could exert antiinflammatory effects via this mechanism. Since IL-1 contributes to cartilage and bone degradation, the drugs might also slow the rate of joint erosion and have disease-modifying effects.

Mycophenolate mofetil has shown clinical utility in patients with RA.[36] The immunosuppressive effect of the drug would be expected to exert therapeutic benefit within one month of treatment. However, the condition of patients continued to improve for three months following the onset of treatment, suggesting that the active component, mycophenolic acid (MPA), has long-acting antirheumatic activity. The observations now presented, showing induced differentiation of human cells of the monocyte-macrophage lineage, and augmented expression of the IL-1 receptor antagonist, are consistent with that mode of action. In Lyme disease, a chronic inflammatory response to the bacterium *Borrelia burgdorferi* produces a disease resembling RA. Lyme disease patients with high concentrations of IL-1β and low concentrations of IL-1ra synovial had long attacks of arthritis, whereas attacks resolved more rapidly in patients with high IL-1ra and low IL-1β in synovial fluid.[37] If mycophenolate mofetil can alter the ratio of IL-1ra to IL-1 in rheumatoid synovia, it might prevent cartilage and bone erosion. Systematic clinical studies are required to ascertain whether that is the case.

Since both TNFα and IL-1β are major mediators of inflammation, as well as of cartilage and bone erosion, we wished to develop small molecules that can inhibit the production of these cytokines while augmenting production of the IL-1 receptor antagonist. Some antioxidants can inhibit the activation of transcription factors and expression of the genes encoding TNFα, IL-1β, and IL-6 in human PBM.[28] As now reported, some of the same antioxidants augment production of IL-1ra by PBM. This is a novel antiinflammatory profile which would be expected to be useful in septic shock and in diseases with inflammatory pathogenesis. Thus antioxidants that alter the balance of production of proinflammatory cytokines and IL-1ra may prove to be useful long-acting antiinflammatory drugs.

ACKNOWLEDGMENTS

We are indebted to J. Kenney and M. Welch for collaboration in the development of immunoassays for cytokines and IL-1ra.

REFERENCES

1. ALLISON, A. C. 1988. Immunopathogenetic mechanisms of arthritis and modes of action of antirheumatic therapies. *In* Immunopathogenetic Mechanisms of Arthritis. J. Goodacre & W. C. Dick, Eds.: 211–245. MTP Press. Boston, Mass.
2. FIRESTEIN, G. S., J. M. ALVARO-GARCIA & R. MAKI. 1990. Quantitative analysis of cytokine gene expression in rheumatoid arthritis. J. Immunol. **144:** 3347–3353.
3. DELEURAN, B. W., C. Q. CHU, M. FIELD, F. M. BRENNAN, P. KATSIKIS, M. FELDMAN & R. MAINI. 1992. Localization of interleukin-1 alpha, type 1 interleukin-1 receptor and interleukin receptor antagonist in the synovial membrane and cartilage/pannus junction in rheumatoid arthritis. Br. J. Rheumatol. **31:** 801–809.

4. CHU, C. Q., M. FIELD, M. FELDMANN & R. N. MAINI. 1990. Localization of tumor necrosis factor in the synovial tissue and cartilage/pannus junction in rheumatoid arthritis. Arthritis Rheum. **34**: 1125–1132.
5. AREND, W. P. & J.-M. DAYER. 1990. Cytokines and cytokine inhibitors or antagonists in rheumatoid arthritis. Arthritis Rheum. **33**: 305–315.
6. FELDMANN, M., F. M. BRENNAN, D. CHANTRY, C. HAWORTH, M. TURNER, P. KATSIKIS, M. LONDEI, E. ABNEY, G. BUCHAN & K. BARRETT. 1991. Cytokine assays: role in evaluation of the pathogenesis of autoimmunity. Immunol. Rev. **199**: 105–123.
7. SMITH, M. F., JR., D. EIDLEN, M. T. BREWER, S. P. EISENBERG, W. P. AREND & A. GUTIERREZ-HARTMANN. 1992. Human IL-1 receptor antagonist promoter: cell type–specific activity and identification of regulatory regions. J. Immunol. **149**: 2000–2007.
8. CONTI, P., C. FELICIANI, R. C. BARBACANE, M. R. PANARA, M. REALE, F. C. PLACIDO, D. N. SAUDER, R. A. DEMPSEY & P. AMERIO. 1992. Inhibition of interleukin-1 beta rRNA expression and interleukin-1 alpha and beta secretion by a specific human recombinant interleukin-1 receptor antagonist in human peripheral blood mononuclear cells. Immunology **77**: 245–250.
9. DINARELLO, C. A. & R. C. THOMPSON. 1991. Blocking IL-1: interleukin-1 receptor antagonist *in vivo* and *in vitro*. Immunol. Today **12**: 404–410.
10. SMITH, R. J., J. E. CHIN, L. M. SAM & J. M. JUSTIN. 1991. Biologic effects of an interleukin-1 receptor antagonist protein on interleukin-1-stimulated cartilage erosion and chondrocyte responsiveness. Arthritis Rheum. **34**: 78–83.
11. AREND, W. P., M. F. SMITH, R. W. JANSON & F. G. JOSLIN. 1991. IL-1 receptor antagonist and IL-1β production in human monocytes are regulated differently. J. Immunol. **147**: 1530–1536.
12. POUTSIAKA, D. D., B. D. CLARK, E. VANNIER & C. A. DINARELLO. 1991. Production of interleukin-1 receptor antagonist and interleukin-1β by peripheral blood mononuclear cells is differentially regulated. Blood **78**: 1275–1281.
13. KLINE, J. N., M. M. MONICK & G. W. HUNNINGHAKE. 1992. IL-1 receptor antagonist release is regulated differently in human alveolar macrophages than in monocytes. J. Appl. Physiol. **73**: 1686–1692.
14. MOORE, S. A., R. M. STRIETER, M. W. ROLFE, T. J. STANDIFORD, M. D. BURKICK & S. L. KUNKEL. 1992. Expression and regulation of human alveolar macrophage-derived interleukin-1 receptor antagonist. Am. J. Respir. Cell. Mol. Biol. **6**: 569–575.
15. ROUX-LOMBARD, P., C. MODOUX & J.-M. DAYER. 1989. Production of interleukin-1 (IL-1) and a specific IL-1 inhibitor during human monocyte-macrophage differentiation: influence of GM-CSF. Cytokine **1**: 45–51.
16. JANSON, R. W., K. R. HANCE & W. P. AREND. 1991. The production of IL-1 receptor antagonist by human in-vitro derived macrophages: the effects of LPS and GM-CSF. J. Immunol. **147**: 4218–4223.
17. WEVERS, M. D., S. I. RENNARD, A. J. HANCE, P. B. BITTERMAN & R. G. CRYSTAL. 1984. Normal human alveolar macrophages obtained by bronchoalveolar lavage have a limited capacity to release interleukin-1. J. Clin. Invest. **74**: 2208–2218.
18. DANIS, V. A., L. M. MARCH, D. S. NELSON & P. M. BROOKS. 1987. Interleukin-1 secretion by peripheral blood monocytes and synovial macrophages from patients with rheumatoid arthritis. J. Rheumatol. **14**: 33–39.
19. GALVE-DE ROCHEMONTEIX, B., L. P. NICOD, A. F. JUNOD & J.-M. DAYER. 1990. Characterization of a specific 20-25 kD interleukin-1 inhibitor from cultured human lung macrophages. Am. J. Respir. Cell Mol. Biol. **3**: 355–361.
20. ALLISON, A. C. & R. V. WATERS. Long-acting anti-rheumatic drugs induce differentiation of cells of the monocyte-macrophage lineage and alter the expression of cytokines and IL-1 receptor antagonist. Agents Actions. (In press.)
21. GALLAGHER, R., S. COLLINS, J. TRIJILLO, K. MCCREDIE, M. AHEARN, S. TSAI, R. METZGAR, G. AULAKH, R. TING, F. RUCETTI & R. GALLO. 1979. Characterization of the continuous, differentiating myeloid cell line (HL60) from a patient with acute promyelocytic leukemia. Blood **54**: 713–733.
22. SUNDSTROM, C. & K. NILSSON. 1976. Establishment and characterization of a human histiocytic lymphoma cell line (U937). Int. J. Cancer **17**: 565–577.

23. ALLISON, A. C. 1992. Approaches to the design of immunosuppressive agents. *In* The Molecular Biology of Immunosuppression. A. W. Thomson, Ed.: 181–209. Wiley. New York, N.Y.

24. SOKOLOSKI, J. A., G. C. BLAIR & A. C. SARTORELLI. 1986. Alterations in glycoprotein synthesis and guanosine triphosphate levels associated with the differentiation of HL60 leukemia cells produced by inhibitors in inosine 5'-phosphate dehydrogenase. Cancer Res. **46:** 2314–2319.

25. KNIGHT, R. D., J. MAGNUM, D. L. LUCAS, D. A. COONEY, E. C. KHAN & D. G. WRIGHT. 1987. Inosine monophosphate dehydrogenase and myeloid cell maturation. Blood **69:** 634–639.

26. YU, J., V. LEMAS, T. PAGE, J. D. CONNER & A. YU. 1989. Induction of erythroid differentiation in K562 cells by inhibitors of inosine monophosphate dehydrogenase. Cancer Res. **49:** 5555–5560.

27. KIGUCHI, K., F. R. COLBERT, C. HENNING-CHULA & E. HUBERMAN. 1990. Induction of cell differentiation by inhibitors of IMP dehydrogenase expression and activity. Cell Growth Differ. **1:** 259–270.

28. EUGUI, E. M., B. DE LUSTRO, S. ROUHAFZA, M. ILNICKA, S. W. LEE, R. WILHELM & A. C. ALLISON. Some antioxidants inhibit, in a co-ordinate fashion, the production of TNFα, IL-1β and IL-6 by human peripheral blood mononuclear cells. Int. Immunol. (Submitted.)

29. NERURKAR, L. S. 1991. Lysozyme. *In* Methods for Studying Mononuclear Phagocytes. D. O. Adams, P. J. Edelson & H. Koren, Eds.: 667–683. Academic Press. New York, N.Y.

30. KENNEY, J. S., M. P. MASADA & A. C. ALLISON. 1990. Development of quantitative two-site ELISAs for soluble proteins. *In* Laboratory Methods in Immunology. H. Zola, Ed.: 231–240. CRC Press. Boca Raton, Fla.

31. HAMILTON, J. A. & N. WILLIAMS. 1985. *In vitro* inhibition of myelopoiesis by gold salts and D-penicillamine. J. Rheumatol. **12:** 892–896.

32. HAMILTON, J. A. & N. WILLIAMS. 1987. Effects of auranofin and other antirheumatic drugs on human myelopoiesis *in vitro.* J. Rheumatol. **14:** 216–220.

33. VANNIER, E., L. C. MILLER & C. A. DINARELLO. 1992. Coordinated anti-inflammatory effects of interleukin 4: interleukin 4 suppresses interleukin-1 production but up-regulates gene expression and synthesis of IL-1 receptor antagonist. Proc. Natl. Acad. Sci. USA **89:** 4076–4080.

34. WONG, H. L., G. L. COSTA, M. T. LOTZE & S. M. WAHL. 1992. IL-4 up-regulates expression of IL-1 receptor antagonists by human peripheral blood monocytes in vitro and in vivo. FASEB J. **1992:** A2055.

35. TURNER, M. D., D. CHANTRY, A. KATSIKIS, A. BERGER, F. M. BRENNAN & M. FELDMAN. 1991. Induction of the interleukin 1 receptor antagonist protein by transforming growth factor β. Eur. J. Immunol. **21:** 1635–1639.

36. SCHIFF, M. H., R. GOLDBLUM & M. M. C. REES. 1988. 2-Morpholinoethyl mycophenolic acid (ME-MPA) in the treatment of refractory rheumatoid arthritis. Arthritis Rheum. **33:** s155.

37. MILLER, L. C., E. A. LYNCH, S. ISA, J. W. LOGAN, C. A. DINARELLO & A. C. STEERE. 1993. Balance of synovial fluid IL-1β and IL-1 receptor antagonist and recovery from Lyme arthritis. Lancet **341:** 146–148.

Cyclooxygenase Gene Expression in Inflammation and Angiogenesis[a]

TIMOTHY HLA, ARI RISTIMÄKI, SUSAN APPLEBY,
AND JAVIER G. BARRIOCANAL

Department of Molecular Biology
Holland Laboratory
American Red Cross
15601 Crabbs Branch Way
Rockville, Maryland 20855

PROSTANOIDS IN INFLAMMATION AND ANGIOGENESIS

Prostaglandins and thromboxanes, collectively known as prostanoids (PGs), are produced by biologic oxidation of arachidonic acid.[1] PGs are synthesized and secreted by a wide variety of cells only when stimulated by a multitude of cell perturbations, ranging from mechanical to chemical stimuli.[1] Once released, PGs act as autocrine or paracrine factors to regulate the functions of various differentiated cells. The ubiquitous presence of PG-metabolizing enzymes makes these mediators unstable and their actions short-lived.[1] In addition, prostacyclin and thromboxanes are intrinsically unstable and are spontaneously hydrolyzed into inactive metabolites. Due to the short half-lives of PGs in general, the levels and activities of PG synthetic enzymes determine the bioactivity of PGs within tissues.[1]

Chronic inflammatory diseases are characterized by increased mononuclear cell infiltration, enhanced stromal cell proliferation, and exaggerated angiogenesis.[2] Exaggerated angiogenesis is thought to be necessary for the exponential phase of disease progression.[3] Thus, inflammation and angiogenesis are intrinsically coupled during many pathological processes such as rheumatoid arthritis.[2]

Angiogenesis is initiated primarily by the vascular endothelial cell (EC). While the normal vascular endothelium is quiescent *in vivo,* various stimuli can "activate" the EC to migrate, proliferate, and differentiate into new capillaries.[3] *In vitro* assays have been developed to study the phenomena of growth,[4] migration,[5] and differentiation[6] of EC, and, based on these assays, numerous mediators that modulate endothelial cell behavior have been identified. Angiogenic mediators have been classified into two distinct groups depending on their ability to stimulate the growth of endothelial cells. Thus, the mitogenic factors include the heparin-binding fibroblast growth factors (FGFs), acidic and basic FGF (FGF-1 and -2), transforming growth factor-α (TGF-α), and vascular endothelial cell growth factor (VEGF).[7] The nonmitogenic factors include the polypeptide cytokines interleukin-1 (IL-1), tumor necrosis factor (TNFα), transforming growth factor-β (TGF-β), as well as the nonpeptide mediators prostaglandin E_1 (PGE$_1$), PGE$_2$ and 1-monobutyrin.[7] The cytokines IL-1, TNFα, and TGF-β inhibit the growth of EC and promote a phenotypic change into a migratory, fibroblast-like phenotype.[8] While PGE$_1$ and PGE$_2$ are recognized as potent inducers of angiogenesis *in vivo,*[9] their role in the modulation of endothelial cell behavior is not known.

[a]This work is supported by National Institutes of Health grants DK45659 and HL49094 to TH.

197

Increased synthesis of PGs is associated with many types of inflammation. For example, inflamed synovium of rheumatoid arthritis produces increased levels of prostaglandin E_2.[10] Secondly, mediators of inflammation such as cytokines induce increased prostanoid synthesis. Thus, the cytokines IL-1 and TNF induce PG synthesis in fibroblasts, smooth muscle, and endothelial cells.[11] Thirdly, and perhaps most importantly, inhibitors of PG synthesis are potent antiinflammatory agents.[12] The role of PGs in angiogenesis, a critical component of chronic inflammatory diseases, is poorly understood. Angiogenesis assays *in vivo,* which utilize the chick embryo chorioallantois membrane as well as the rabbit cornea, have identified PGE_1 and PGE_2 as potent inducers of angiogenesis.[9] Furthermore, tumor-induced angiogenesis and growth-factor-induced angiogenesis *in vivo* are blocked by nonsteroidal antiinflammatory drugs,[13] and it is generally accepted that the inflammatory response serves to exaggerate angiogenesis *in vivo.*

ENZYMES OF PROSTANOID BIOSYNTHESIS

The cellular phospholipase A_2 family of enzymes initiates the first step in PG biosynthesis by catalyzing the release of arachidonic acid from the membrane fatty acids.[1] Both secreted and cytosolic forms of phospholipase A_2 have been characterized, and the cDNAs for these enzymes were cloned.[14] The recently isolated cytosolic form may be important in agonist-mediated release of arachidonic acid.[15] In addition, the expression of the cytosolic phospholipase A_2 appears to be regulated by inflammatory mediators such as IL-1α in fibroblasts.[16]

Once released, the arachidonic acid (AA) is oxidized by the cyclooxygenase (Cox) activity to PGG_2 and reduced by the peroxidase activity of the same enzyme to PGH_2.[1] The Cox enzyme irreversibly inactivates after a limited amount of catalysis, presumably due to a reactive free-radical intermediate generated during the arachidonic acid oxidation step.[1] The self-inactivated enzyme is more susceptible to proteolysis *in vitro,* and presumably is rapidly degraded under physiological conditions.[17] Thus the level of Cox expression is modulated by a variety of extracellular hormones and cytokines in a variety of differentiated cells (reviewed in Reference 18). After Cox has converted AA to PGH_2, it is then catalyzed by tissue-specific isomerases to biologically active PGs. For example, platelets and monocytes express the thromboxane synthase gene and hence synthesize thromboxane A_2 via the Cox pathway. While the Cox enzyme is expressed by almost all cells, differentiated cells express the PG isomerase enzymes in a tissue-specific fashion. Thus, differentiated cells of the monocytic lineage express thromboxane synthase, prostaglandin E synthase, and prostacyclin synthase whereas vascular endothelial cells express prostacyclin and prostaglandin E synthase predominantly, resulting in the tissue-specific synthesis of different PG profiles.[1] The molecular basis of the tissue-specific expression of the PG isomerases is poorly understood.

CYCLOOXYGENASE-1 AND -2 ISOENZYMES

The cDNA for Cox-1 was first isolated from ovine seminal vesicles, a tissue that is highly enriched in the Cox enzyme.[19,20] The enzyme of 576 amino acids is encoded by transcripts of 3 and 5 kb. The smaller transcript was sequenced completely and was shown to possess a small 5'-untranslated region (UTR), a 1.8-kb open reading frame, and a 1.1 kb 3'-UTR.[19,20] The molecular nature of the 5-kb mRNA species is not known. The human and murine genomic sequences encoding the Cox-1 mRNA has been characterized, and the open reading frame (ORF) is encoded by 11 exons spanning approximately 22 kb.[21,22] Site-directed mutagenesis analysis of the ovine Cox-1 cDNA has been conducted, and the mutant enzymes have been expressed in Cos cells for enzymatic analysis.[23,24] Using this approach, axial and distal heme-ligated histidine residues, the active-site tyrosine, and the N-linked glycosylation sites were identified.[23,24] Furthermore, the role of the aspirin-modified serine residue in the competitive inhibition of the substrate binding was confirmed.[23,24]

Rosen *et al.*, using low-stringency hybridization with Cox-1 probes, were the first to predict the existence of the Cox-2 gene.[25] However, investigators that were in the process of cloning novel immediate-early genes in chick embryo fibroblasts[26] and murine fibroblasts[27] fortuitously isolated the Cox-2 cDNAs. This is consistent with the observation that an early response of cellular activation by growth factors, cytokines, tumor promoters, and viruses is the enhanced production of PGs.[1] Thus, the Cox-2 gene appears to encode an early, activation-dependent isoform of the Cox enzyme. At the amino acid level, the Cox-1 and -2 polypeptides share approximately 60% sequence identity.[26–28] The Cox-2 enzyme is encoded by a transcript of approximately 4.5 kb in size. While the genomic organization of the Cox-2 gene is very similar to that of the Cox-1 gene, the size (approximately 8 kb) is considerably smaller.[29]

We have isolated the cDNA clones for both Cox-1 and -2 from human umbilical vein endothelial cells (HUVEC).[28] At the deduced amino acid level, the Cox-1 and -2 polypeptides are 61% identical. The alignment of the two polypeptides is shown in FIGURE 1. The putative N-terminal signal peptide region appears to be shorter in Cox-2. However, two N-terminal N-linked glycosylation sites, the axial and distal heme-ligating histidines, active-site tyrosine, and aspirin-modified serine are conserved. In addition, both polypeptides end with the sequence STEL, a sequence that is reminiscent of the endoplasmic reticulum retention sequence KDEL. At the C-terminal portion of the Cox-2 polypeptide, a unique 18 amino acid insertion containing a putative N-linked glycosylation site is found. The 3'-UTR of the Cox-2 transcript is estimated to be 2.5 kb in size. The human Cox-2 cDNA contains at least 12 copies of the AUUUA, "Shaw-Kamen" motif which was implicated in the rapid degradation of many cytokine and oncogene mRNAs.[30] In addition, the ORF of the Cox-2 cDNA is less stable than the Cox-1 ORF in transfected Cos cells,[28] suggesting that RNA instability motifs exist in both the ORF and the 3'-UTR and that they may be involved in the posttranscriptional regulation of the Cox-2 gene expression.

Transfection of either Cox-1 or -2 cDNAs into Cos cells results in the elaboration of Cox activity which was inhibited by both indomethacin and ibuprofen.[28] Meade *et al.* reported recently on the differential sensitivity of murine Cox-1 and -2 to nonsteroidal antiinflammatory drugs (NSAIDs).[31] It was found that some NSAIDs such as flurbiprofen, ibuprofen, meclofenamic acid, and docosahexaenoic acid were equipotent at inhibiting both isotypes of Cox, whereas piroxicam, indomethacin, and sulindac sulfide were better Cox-1 inhibitors.[31] Interestingly, 6-methoxy-2-naphthyl acetic acid, the active metabolite of nabumetone, exhibited significant selectivity against Cox-2.[31] These data suggest that it may be possible to develop selective inhibitors of the Cox isoenzymes. This is particularly important because of the multifunctional roles that Cox products are involved in in many organ systems. For example, in the treatment of rheumatoid arthritis (RA), it is highly desirable to inhibit the Cox enzyme in the inflamed synovium selectively but not the normal PG synthesis in the upper gastrointestinal tract (see below). In contrast to Cox-1, aspirin-treated Cox-2 enzyme exhibited a stimulated partial oxygenase activity, resulting in the production of 15-HETE and 13-HODE via the oxidation of arachi-

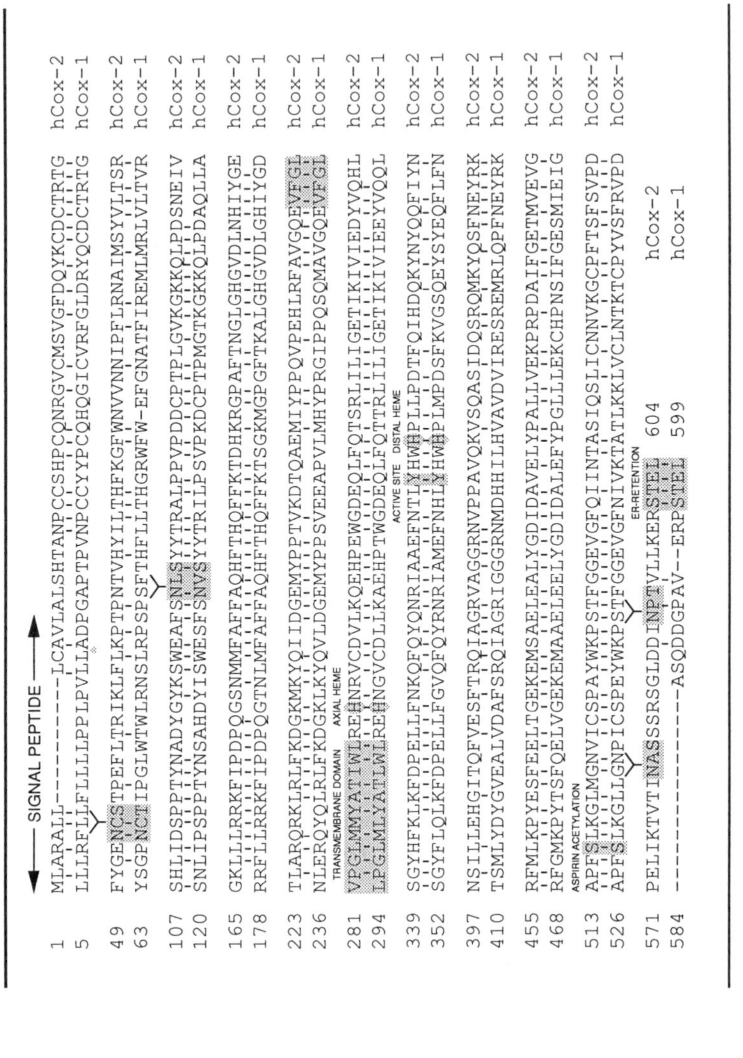

```
        ├──── SIGNAL PEPTIDE ────▶

  1     MLARALL-------LCAVLALSHTANPCCSHPCQNRGVCMSVGFDQYKCDCTRTG        hCox-2
  5     LLLRFLLFLLLLPPVLLÄDPGAPTPVNPCCYYPCQHQGICVRFGLDRYQCDCTRTG       hCox-1

 49     FYGENCSTPEFLTRIKLFLKPTPNTVHYILTHFKGFWNVNNIPFLRNAIMSYVLTSR      hCox-2
 63     YSGPNCTIPGLWTWLRNSLRPSPSFTHFLLTHGRWFW-EFGNATFIREMLMRLVLTVR     hCox-1

107     SHLIDSPPTYNADYGYKSWEAFSNLSYYTRALPPVPDDCPTPLGVKGKKQLPDSNEIV     hCox-2
120     SNLIPSPPTYNSAHDYISWESFSNVSYYTRILPSVPKDCPTPMGTKGKKQLPDAQLLA     hCox-1

165     GKLLLRRKFIPDPQGSNMMFAFFAQHFTHQFFKTDHKRGPAFTNGLGHGVDLNHIYGE     hCox-2
178     RRFLLRRKFIPDPQGTNLMFAFFAQHFTHQFFKTSGKMGPGFTKALGHGVDLGHIYGD     hCox-1

223     TLARQRKLRLFKDGKMKYQIIDGEMYPPTVKDTQAEMIYPPQVPEHLRFAVGQEVFGI     hCox-2
236     NLERQYQLRLFKDGKLKYQVLDGEMYPPSVEEAPVLMHYPRGIPPQSQMAVGQEVFGI     hCox-1
        TRANSMEMBRANE DOMAIN    AXIAL HEME

281     VPGLMMYATIWLREHNRVCDVLKQEHPEWGDEQLFQTSRLILIGETIKIVIEDYVQHL     hCox-2
294     LPGLMLYATIWLREHNGVCDLLKAEHPTWGDEQLFQTTRLILIGETIKIVIEEYVQQL     hCox-1
                                       ACTIVE SITE   DISTAL HEME

339     SGYHFKLKFDPELLFNKQFQYQNRIAAEFNTLYHWHPLLPDTFQIHDQKYNYQQFIYN     hCox-2
352     SGYFLQLKFDPELLFGVQFQYRNRIAMEFNHLYHWHPLMPDSFKVGSQSYSYEQFLFN     hCox-1

397     NSILLEHGITQFVESTTRQIAGRVAGGRNVPPAVQKVSQASIDQSRQMKYQSFNEYRK     hCox-2
410     TSMLYDYGVEALVDAFSRQIAGRIGGGRNMDHHILHVAVDVIRESREMRLQPFNEYRK     hCox-1

455     RFMLKPYESFEELTGEKEMSAELEALYGDIDAVELYPALLVEKPRPDAIFGETMVEVG     hCox-2
468     RFGMKPYTSFQELVGEKEMAAELEELYGDIDALEFYPGLLLEKCHPNSIFGESMIEIG     hCox-1
        ASPIRIN ACETYLATION

513     APFSLKGLMGNVICSPAYWKPSTFGGEVGFQIINTASIQSLICNNVKGCPFTSFSVPD     hCox-2
526     APFSLKGLLGNPICSPEYWKPSTFGGEVGFNIVKTATLKKLVCLNTKTCPYVSFRVPD     hCox-1
                                                    ER-RETENTION

571     PELIKTVTINASSSRSGLDDINPTVLLKERSTEL    604                      hCox-2
584     --------ASQDDGPAV-ERPSTEL             599                      hCox-1
```

FIGURE 1. Sequence comparison between the human Cox-1 and -2 polypeptides. Salient features are indicated as shown: Y = potential N-linked glycosylation site.

donic acid and linoleic acid, respectively.[31,32] This is particularly interesting because these hydroperoxy and hydroxy metabolites possess potent growth-modulatory activities.[33] Whether these metabolites are formed under physiological conditions, i.e., from self-inactivated Cox-2 enzyme, is not known.

REGULATION OF CYCLOOXYGENASE ISOENZYME EXPRESSION *IN VITRO* AND *IN VIVO*

The Cox-1 gene is expressed ubiquitously *in vivo* and *in vitro*. In contrast, the Cox-2 gene is expressed at very low levels in quiescent cells and in normal tissues *in vivo* (Hla, T., unpublished data). Numerous studies have focussed on the regulation of expression of Cox-1 and -2 mRNAs in cells in tissue culture (reviewed in Reference 18). We have studied the regulation of the Cox isozyme gene expression in HUVEC. These cells require FGF-1 for optimal growth *in vitro*.[4] However, the cytokine IL-1 and the tumor promoter phorbol myristic acetate (PMA) arrest the FGF-induced proliferation and induce phenotypic change.[8,34,35] Quiescent HUVEC that were deprived of FGF-1 expressed a sevenfold higher level of Cox-1 mRNA compared to the FGF-treated, proliferating cells.[36] The cells contained concomitant higher levels of Cox-1 protein and synthesized more prostacyclin in response to exogenous arachidonic acid. The doses of FGF-1 that are optimal for inducing the proliferation of HUVEC also maximally suppressed the Cox-1 mRNA, suggesting that the two processes may be linked.[36] These data suggested that proliferating endothelial cells may down regulate Cox-1 gene expression and that Cox-1 gene expression may be maximal under the conditions of endothelial cell quiescence.[36] In contrast, FGF-1 induces the Cox-2 transcript rapidly and transiently. As shown in FIGURE 2, treatment of quiescent HUVEC with 10 ng/ml of FGF-1 and heparin results in the immediate induction of the Cox-2 transcript whereas the Cox-1 transcript levels were suppressed by 24 h. Thus, in endothelial cells, the Cox isozyme gene expression appears to be differentially regulated by FGF-1, a potent growth factor and an inducer of angiogenesis. The phorbol ester PMA induces both Cox-1 and -2 mRNAs; however, the effect of PMA on the Cox-2 induction is highly significant. Within 4 h following the addition of PMA, the levels of Cox-2 mRNA are induced approximately 30-fold whereas Cox-1 mRNA levels rise threefold in 24 h.[28] Similar effect is seen with the cytokine IL-1 (Ristimaki and Hla, unpublished data). The induction of Cox-2 gene is an immediate-early response because it occurs in the presence of cycloheximide, an inhibitor of protein synthesis. Indeed, cycloheximide enhances the induction, resulting in the phenomenon referred to as "superinduction." This is presumably related to the ability of cycloheximide to inhibit the degradation of the Cox-2 transcript. In monocytes, the Cox-2 gene is induced as an immediate-early gene by lipopolysaccharide (LPS), a potent monocyte activator.[28] In contrast, the Cox-1 gene is expressed in quiescent conditions and is not further stimulated by LPS.[28] These *in vitro* data indicate that the Cox-2 gene is rapidly induced by many growth factors, cytokines, tumor promoters, and LPS. The Cox-1 gene, in contrast, appears to be maximally expressed under conditions that favor cellular quiescence. The mechanism of induction may involve activation at the transcriptional and/or posttranscriptional levels. Detailed understanding of the critical steps involved in the induction of the Cox-2 gene may reveal potentially novel steps of pharmacological intervention.

In order to determine the *in vivo* relevance of the induction of Cox enzyme isoforms in the development of a chronic inflammatory disease, we have investigated the expression of Cox isotypes in synovial tissue sections from patients with RA and osteoathritis (OA) as well as in the rat adjuvant and streptococcal cell wall (SCW) induced arthritis models.[37] RA is an aggressive chronic inflammatory disease that is characterized by a prominent angiogenic component in the affected joints.[38] In contrast, OA is less inflammatory and less angiogenic and, hence, less destructive.[38] Enhanced synthesis of PGE_2 in the RA synovium may directly contribute to juxtaarticular bone resorption, angiogenesis, and hyperplasia.[38] To characterize the expression of Cox in RA, immunohistochemical analysis was conducted using a polyclonal Cox antibody.[39] Enhanced staining of immunoreactive Cox antigen was observed in the angiogenic and inflamed RA tissues. Blood vessels, infiltrating monocytes, and the synovial fibroblasts were the cells that expressed the highest

FGF-1 Treatment

H_2O 0 2 4 10 24 hours

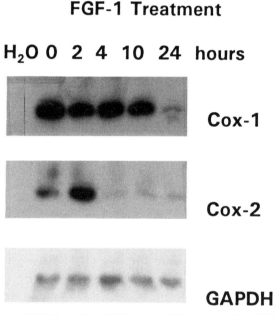

FIGURE 2. Effect of FGF-1 on the mRNA levels of Cox-1 and -2 in HUVEC. Quisecent HUVEC were treated with 10 ng/ml of FGF-1 in the presence of 5 μ/ml of heparin, total RNA was isolated at indicated times, and the levels of Cox-1, -2 and glyceraldehyde 3-phosphate dehydrogenase (GAPDH) mRNAs were determined by reverse transcriptase–polymerase chain reaction procedures (RT-PCR).[36] H_2O = minus RNA control for the PCR.

amounts of the immunoreactive Cox antigen.[37] Statistically significant increases in the Cox immunoreactivity was observed in the RA synovium compared to the OA tissue. In the rat models of experimental arthritis, the induction and exaggerated expression of the Cox immunoreactivity was observed and correlated with the development of the inflammatory arthritic disease. These studies indicated that the extent and intensity of the Cox expression within the inflammatory site correlated with the progression of the disease.[37] Since the completion of these studies, the Cox-2 gene was discovered and the differential regulation of the gene expression of Cox isoenzymes was described *in vitro*. Using a quantitative radioimmunoprecipitation procedure to resolve the Cox-1 and -2 polypeptides, we investigated the *de novo* synthesis of these two isoenzymes in tissue explants from RA patients. The Cox-1 polypeptide was preferentially synthesized in quiescent tissues; whereas treatment with either PMA or IL-1 induced preferentially the synthesis of Cox-2 polypeptide. Interestingly, the induction was blocked completely by pretreatment of the tissue explants with physiological doses of the antiinflammatory steroid dexamethasone (dex).[40] These data strongly suggested that the Cox-2 is induced by proinflammatory mediators and suppressed by antiinflammatory steroids in the inflamed, hyperplastic synovial tissues. The effects of IL-1, PMA, and dex at the levels of the Cox-2 mRNA were studied in the early passage RA synovial fibroblasts. Similar to the induction patterns of Cox-2 protein synthesis, IL-1 and PMA selectively induced the Cox-2 transcript to high levels and the induction was suppressed by dex.[40] The mechanism of induction and the dex suppression is not known but may involve the transcriptional effects of cytokine- and PMA-activated *trans*-factor action and/or posttranscriptional modulation of the Cox-2 mRNA stability. Indeed, sequence analysis of the 5'-flanking region of the human Cox-2 gene indicated the presence of several NFκB motifs, which are known to be cytokine and PMA-responsive *cis*-acting elements. Thus, exaggerated induction of the Cox-2 isotype within the inflammatory tissues may be an important molecular event in the pathogenesis of RA. How the enhanced Cox-2 induction and the imbalance of the two Cox isotypes contribute to the highly inflamed, hyperplastic, and angiogenic state is not well understood. It is highly likely that the products of the Cox pathway, namely PGs, hydroxylated fatty acids, and peroxides, are involved in the uncontrolled evolution of the inflammatory disease into a highly angiogenic and destructive state.

REFERENCES

1. NEEDLEMAN, P., J. TURK, B. A. JACSHICK, A. R. MORRISON & J. B. LEFKOWITH. 1986. Annu. Rev. Biochem. **55:** 69–102.
2. ROBBINS, S. L., R. S. COTRAN & V. KUMAR. 1984. Pathological Basis of Disease. 3rd edit.: 40–70. Saunders. New York, N.Y.
3. FOLKMAN, J. 1985. Adv. Cancer Res. **43:** 175–203.
4. MACIAG, T., G. A. HOOVER, M. B. STEMERMAN & R. WEINSTEIN. 1981. J. Cell Biol. **91:** 420–426.
5. TERRANOVA, V. P., R. DIFLORIO, R. M. LYALL, S. HIC, R. FRIESEL & T. MACIAG. 1985. J. Cell Biol. **101:** 2330–2334.
6. FOLKMAN, J. & C. C. HAUDENSCHILD. 1980. Nature **288:** 551–556.
7. FOLKMAN, J. & M. KLAGSBRUN. 1987. Science **235:** 442–447.
8. NORIOKA, K., M. HARA, A. KATANI, T. HIROSE, M. HARIGAI, K. SUZUKI, M. KAWAKAMI, H. TABATA, M. KAWAGOE & H. NAKAMURA. 1987. Biochem. Biophys. Res. Commun. **145:** 969–975.
9. ZICHE, M., J. JONES & P. M. GULLINO. 1982. J. Natl. Cancer Inst. **69:** 475–482.
10. ROBINSON, D. R., A. H. J. TASHIJIAN & L. LEVINE. 1975. J. Clin. Invest. **56:** 1181–1188.
11. RISTIMÄKI, A. & L. VIINIKKA. 1992. Prostaglandins Leukotrienes Essent. Fatty Acids **47:** 93–99.
12. GOLDSTEIN, I. M. 1988. *In* Inflammation: Basic Principles and Clinical Correlates. Gallin *et al.,* Eds.: 935–946. Raven Press. New York, N.Y.
13. PETERSON, H. 1983. Invasion Metastasis **3:** 151–159.
14. SMITH, W. L. 1989. Biochem. J. **259:** 315–324.
15. LIN, L., A. LIN & J. KNOPF. 1992. Proc. Natl. Acad. Sci. USA **89:** 6147–6151.
16. LIN, L., A. LIN & D. L. DEWITT. 1992. J. Biol. Chem. **267:** 23451–23454.
17. CHEN, Y. P., M. J. BIENKOWSKI & L. J. MARNETT. 1987. J. Biol. Chem. **262:** 16892–16899.
18. DEWITT, D. 1991. Biochim. Biophys. Acta **1083:** 121–134.
19. DEWITT, D. & W. L. SMITH. 1988. Proc. Natl. Acad. Sci. USA **85:** 1412–1416.
20. MERLIE, J. P., D. FAGAN, J. MUDD & P. NEEDLEMAN. 1988. J. Biol. Chem. **263:** 3550–3553.

21. YOKOYAMA, C. & T. TANABE. 1989. Biochem. Biophys. Res. Commun. **165:** 888–894.
22. KRAEMER, S. A., E. A. MEADE & D. L. DEWITT. 1992. Arch. Biochem. Biophys. **293:** 391–400.
23. SHIMOKAWA, T. & W. L. SMITH. 1991. J. Biol. Chem. **266:** 6168–6173.
24. SMITH, W. L. 1992. Am. J. Physiol. **263**(32): F181–191.
25. ROSEN, G. D., T. M. BIRKENMEIER, A. RAZ & M. J. HOLTZMAN. 1989. Biochem. Biophys. Res. Commun. **164:** 1358–1365.
26. XIE, W., J. G. CHIPMAN, D. L. ROBERTSON, R. L. ERIKSON & D. L. SIMMONS. 1991. Proc. Natl. Acad. Sci. USA **88:** 2692–2696.
27. KUJUBU, D. A., B. S. FLETCHER, B. C. VARNUM, R. W. LIM & H. R. HERSCHMAN. 1991. J. Biol. Chem. **266:** 12866–12872.
28. HLA, T. & K. NEILSON. 1992. Proc. Natl. Acad. Sci. USA **89:** 7384–7388.
29. FLETCHER, B. S., D. A. KUJUBU, D. M. PERRIN & H. R. HERSCHMAN. 1992. J. Biol. Chem. **267:** 4338–4344.
30. SHAW, G. & R. KAMEN. 1986. Cell **46:** 659–667.
31. MEADE, E. A., W. L. SMITH & D. L. DEWITT. 1993. J. Biol. Chem. **268:** 6610–6614.
32. HOLTZMAN, M. J., J. TURK & L. P. SHORNICK. 1992. J. Biol. Chem. **267:** 21438–21445.
33. GLASGOW, W. C., C. A. AFSHARI, J. C. BARRETT & T. E. ELING. 1992. J. Biol. Chem. **267:** 10771–10779.
34. MONTESANO, R., L. ORCI & P. VASSALLI. 1985. J. Cell. Physiol. **122:** 424–434.
35. MONTESANO, R. & L. ORCI. 1985. Cell **42:** 469–477.
36. HLA, T. & T. MACIAG. 1991. J. Biol. Chem. **266:** 24059–24063.
37. SANO, H., T. HLA, J. MAIER, L. CROFFORD, J. CASE, T. MACIAG & R. L. WILDER. 1992. J. Clin. Invest. **89:** 97–108.
38. HARRIS, E. D. 1990. N. Engl. J. Med. **322:** 1277–1289.
39. HLA, T., M. P. FARRELL, A. KUMAR & J. M. BAILEY. 1986. Prostaglandins **6:** 829–865.
40. CROFFORD, L. J., R. L. WILDER, A. RISTIMAKI, E. F. REMMERS, H. R. EPPS & T. HLA. (Submitted for publication.)

Preclinical and Clinical Activity
of Zileuton and A-78773

R. L. BELL, C. LANNI, P. E. MALO, D. W. BROOKS,
A. O. STEWART, R. HANSEN, P. RUBIN,
AND G. W. CARTER

Immunosciences Research Area
D-47K, AP9
Abbott Park, Illinois 60064

INTRODUCTION

5-Lipoxygenase inhibitors, such as zileuton, have been suggested to be a novel therapeutic approach to the management of several important inflammatory diseases.[3] Early human trials with zileuton have demonstrated that the molecule selectively prevents the production of leukotrienes in the blood when assayed *ex vivo*,[7] in rectal dialysates from ulcerative colitis patients,[8] and in nasal washings after allergen challenge.[9] More recently, zileuton has shown promise in ulcerative colitis and asthma.[4–6]

Recently, we described some of the biochemistry and pharmacology of A-78773, a 5-lipoxygenase inhibitor structurally related to zileuton with enhanced potency and improved pharmacokinetic profile.[7] Zileuton and A-78773 have been further characterized biochemically in lung cells, lung fragments, and trachea contraction assays. In addition, the relative potency of the two molecules was examined in arachidonic acid–induced ear edema, inflammatory cell influx, and edema in the rat and in a guinea pig bronchospasm model.

METHODS

RBL-1 Cell Lysate 5-Lipoxygenase Inhibitor Potency

Adherent rat basophilic leukemia (RBL-1) cells (2H3 subline) were harvested by trypsinization, suspended (3.0×10^7 cells/ml) in BES-PIPES buffer pH 6.8, and lysed by sonication. The lysate was centrifuged at $20,000 \times g$ for 20 minutes, and the supernatant containing 5-lipoxygenase activity stored frozen until used. Enzyme assays were performed as described by Carter *et al.*[1]

Myeloperoxidase Inhibition

Myeloperoxidase was obtained from the $40,000 \times g$ supernatant of sonicates of frozen human PMNL. The effect of zileuton on myeloperoxidase activity of these preparations was determined by quantitating enzyme activity as follows: 50 μl of cell supernatants (2×10^6/ml); 25 μl 0.15 M sodium phosphate buffer pH 6.2; 50 μl substrate consisting of 6 mM *o*-dianisidine (SIGMA, St. Louis, Mo.) and 0.02% v/v hydrogen peroxide (Fisher, Itasca, Ill.) were incubated in a 96-well microtiter plate and distilled water added up to 250 μl. The microtiter plate was incubated at ambient temperature for 5–15 minutes, and the reaction stopped by the addition of 50 μl of 0.5% sodium azide. Reaction product formed was quantitated by reading the absorbance at 450 or 490 nm.

Neutrophil Degranulation

Degranulation of human PMNLs by f-Met-Leu-Phe was detected by measuring release of the azurophilic granule enzyme N-acetyglucosaminidase. N-Acetylglucosaminidase levels in the cell free supernatants were determined by incubating 25 μl cell free supernatant and 200 μl substrate solution consisting of 1.4 mg/ml p-nitrophenyl-N-acetylglucosamine in buffer consisting of 0.15 M sodium citrate 0.05% bovine serum albumin (Pentex, West Haven, Conn.) overnight at room temperature. The enzyme reaction was stopped by addition of 20 μl of 2 N sodium hydroxide, and product formation quantitated by reading absorbance at 405 nm.

Human Whole Blood Eicosanoid Production

The production of LTB_4 and TXB_2 from ionophore-stimulated whole blood was assessed as described by Carter et al.[1] 12-HETE and 15-HETE were measured by radioimmunoassay using kits supplied by Advanced Magnetics (Cambridge, Mass.).

Arachidonic Acid–Induced Mouse Ear Edema Model

A modification of the methods described by Young et al.[10] and Opas et al.[11] was used. Briefly, a 10-μl aliquot of an acetone solution of 2.5% arachidonic acid (AA) was applied to both the inner and outer surfaces of the right ears of male mice weighing 20–30 g. The left ears received a like treatment of acetone vehicle. One hour later, the mice were sacrificed with CO_2 and a 7-mm section removed from the ears with a biopsy punch. These sections were immediately weighed for wet weight determinations. Test compounds or vehicle was orally gavaged 15 minutes prior to the AA application. Edema was calculated as the percent increase in ear weight of the AA-treated ear compared to the contralateral acetone-treated ear.

Agonist and Antigen-Induced Contraction of Guinea Pig Tracheal Smooth Muscle or Human Bronchial Strips In Vitro

Adult male albino Hartley strain guinea pigs (250–300 g; Charles River Laboratories, Portage, Mich.) were immunized using a modification of the procedure of Herxheimer.[12] Tracheal spirals were connected via silk suture to force displacement transducers (Harvard Instruments, South Natick, Mass.) for recording isometric contractions. The tissue baths and buffer were maintained at 37°C and constantly gassed with O_2/CO_2 (95:5). After equilibration, the tissues were treated with potassium chloride (KCl, 40 mM) to determine viability and reactivity and to provide a basis for normalizing subsequent contractions. Only tissues exhibiting a maximum contraction to KCl of at least 0.5 g were used. Spirals were then washed twice with fresh buffer and permitted to return to basal tone. Thirty minutes prior to commencement of the concentration-response curve to OA, Zileuton (3, 10 μM) or DMSO vehicle was added to the appropriate baths. The addition of DMSO to the trachea did produce some baseline relaxation, which was subtracted prior to the commencement of the antigen concentration-response curve. Zileuton did not change the relaxation caused by DMSO. Ten minutes prior to OA challenge, meclofenamic acid (1 μM) and mepyramine (10 μM) were added to the baths in order to eliminate the effects of arachidonate cyclooxygenase products and histamine.

Measurement of In Vivo Pulmonary Mechanics

Guinea pigs (male Hartley, 350–750 g) were anesthetized with an intraperitoneal (ip) injection of pentobarbital (20–24 mg/kg) and urethane (1.6 g/kg). Following induction of anesthesia, the trachea was surgically exposed and intubated with an endotracheal tube. Animals were permitted to breathe room air spontaneously. The jugular vein was cannulated for the delivery of drugs and solutions. Body temperature was monitored rectally, and the animal was warmed during the experiment using a heated table. Prior to oral dosing, animals were fasted for 12–18 hours. Animals were dosed two hours prior to anesthesia. To study the mechanical properties of the lungs and airways, airflow rate (ml/s), tidal volume (ml/breath), and transpulmonary pressure (cm water) were recorded simultaneously by previously published methods.[13] Dynamic lung compliance (C_{dyn}), an indicator of small peripheral airway function, was derived from the recorded changes in tidal volume and transpulmonary pressure.

After an equilibration period of 10–15 minutes, the animal was pretreated with intravenous meclofenamic acid (2 mg/kg) and mepyramine (4 mg/kg) 10 minutes prior to aerosol ovalbumin challenge (5 mg/ml, 30 s exposure). Aerosols were delivered by a calibrated Monaghan Ultrasonic Nebulizer (Model 675), coupled to a Harvard small animal respirator. The stroke volume was adjusted to deliver 10 ml/kg, with a rate of 60 breaths per minute. Lung mechanics were measured every 30 seconds for 25 minutes after OA challenge.

Statistical Methods

Percentage inhibition was computed by comparing individual values in treatment groups to the mean value of the control group. Statistical significance was determined using one-way analysis of variance and Duncan's multiple range test. Linear regression was used to estimate IC_{50} and ED_{50} values.

BIOCHEMICAL POTENCY AND SELECTIVITY OF A-78773 AND ZILEUTON

Inhibition of leukotriene formation *in vitro* can be accomplished with several types of inhibitors. A number of inhibitors have been described that apparently act as inhibitors of the release of arachidonate as substrate for the 5-lipoxygenase,[14,15] although many of these lack specificity and potency. Several laboratories have also described compounds that inhibit the activation of the 5-lipoxygenase in intact cells[16–18] via interaction with the 5-lipoxygenase activating protein (FLAP). Zileuton and A-78773 appear to act as active site inhibitors. The inhibition seen with these molecules is readily reversible[1] and as shown in FIGURE 1 for zileuton is also dependent on substrate concentration. A-78773 gave similar results yielding an IC_{50} of 34 nM with 6 μM arachidonic acid as substrate. Both compounds were found to be selective inhibitors of the 5-lipoxygenase in comparison with their activity against other arachidonate-metabolizing enzymes. As shown in FIGURE 2, zileuton was approximately 40- to 100-fold more potent against human whole blood LTB_4 biosynthesis than against whole blood cyclooxygenase or 12-lipoxygenase product formation in the same samples.

In addition, zileuton was tested against human neutrophil myeloperoxidase. At concentrations 200-fold higher than its IC_{50} against 5-lipoxygenase (100 μM), the compound did not inhibit this enzyme. In contrast NDGA, a nonspecific antioxidant, inhibited myeloperoxidase with an IC_{50} of 4 μM.

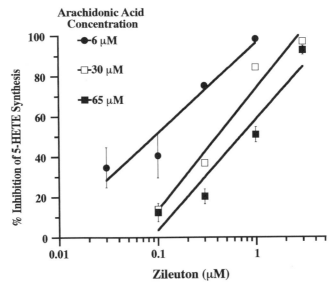

FIGURE 1. Inhibition of 5-HETE formation in RBL lysates by zileuton. 5-HETE inhibition was assessed as described by Carter *et al.*[1] Zileuton inhibited the formation of 5-HETE at 6, 30, and 65 μM arachidonic acid. The IC_{50}s calculated from the curves shown with (95% confidence limits) were 92 nM (50–140), 400 nM (300–500), and 670 nM (500–900) respectively at those three substrate concentrations.

INHIBITION OF LEUKOTRIENE FORMATION
IN LUNG CELLS AND LUNG FRAGMENTS

The presumed cell source of LTB_4 in human whole blood is the neutrophil. In order to examine the possibility of cell-specific 5-lipoxygenase inhibition, cells from guinea pig lung were prepared[19] and stimulated with ionophore A 23187 or passively sensitized and challenged with antigen. Guinea pig lung cells were first prepared as a monodisperse preparation containing eosinophils, mononuclear cells, and mast cells. This preparation was further purified by elutriation into purified cells. As shown in TABLE 1, zileuton inhibited ionophore-induced LTB_4 production from the lung monodisperse cells, as in the purified mast cells, eosinophils, and mononuclear cells

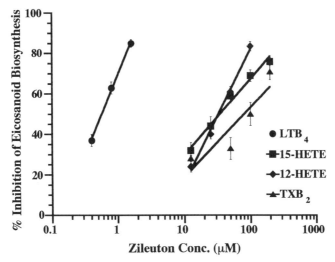

FIGURE 2. Effect of zileuton on the biosynthesis of eicosanoids in ionophore-stimulated human whole blood. Human whole blood was challenged as described.[2] LTB_4 and TXB_2 were measured by enzyme-immunoassay and 12- and 15-HETE by radioimmunoassay. The IC_{50}'s and 95% confidence limits for inhibition of LTB_4, TXB_2, 12-HETE and 15-HETE were 0.74 μM (0.59–0.84), 84 μM (61–120), 32 μM (27–36), and 30 μM (23–37), respectively.

with similar potency. A-78773 was also effective, but at concentrations 25- to 80-fold lower. Interestingly, the potency of zileuton was similar with antigen challenge or ionophore challenge. Rat peritoneal mast cells were also prepared and similar data obtained. In one set of experiments, human lung was obtained and again similar data for each compound were obtained with the monodisperse cell preparation. Thus, in several cell types, the ratio of the potency of the two compounds was quite similar, indicating no significant differences in the susceptibility of the 5-lipoxygenases in the various cells to inhibition.

Rat mast cells and the monodisperse cell preparation from guinea pig lung released significant amounts of histamine in concert with the leukotriene release

TABLE 1. Inhibition of LTB_4 Release from Various Cell Types by Zileuton and A-78773

Cell Population/Stimulus	Zileuton IC_{50} $(\mu M)^a$	A-78773 IC_{50} $(\mu M)^a$
Guinea pig monodisperse/ionophore[b]	0.8	0.020
Guinea pig monodisperse/ovalbumin[c]	1.2	0.039
Guinea pig mast cells/ionophore[b]	1.6	0.041
Guinea pig eosinophils/ionophore[b]	1.4	0.035
Guinea pig mononuclear cells/ionophore[b]	1.1	0.023
Rat peritoneal mast cells/ionophore[b]	0.8	0.019
Human monodisperse/ionophore[b]	1.0	0.025

[a]Results shown are means of several experiments performed in triplicate.
[b]10.0 $\mu g/ml$ ionophore (A 23187).
[c]0.1 $\mu g/ml$ ovalbumin.

TABLE 2. Inhibition of LTB_4 Release from Chopped Lung by A-78773 and Zileuton

Species	A-78773 IC_{50} $(\mu M)^a$	Zileuton IC_{50} $(\mu M)^a$
Human	0.030	0.4
Rhesus monkey	0.060	0.6
Guinea pig	0.230	3.2

^{a}Results shown are means of triplicate determinations.

described above. In both cell preparations, no inhibition of histamine release was seen with zileuton, even at very high concentrations (100 μM).

Lung fragments from several species have been shown to be capable of leukotriene formation following calcium ionophore stimulation.[20] A-78773 and zileuton were potent inhibitors of LTB_4 formation in stimulated lung fragments from human, rhesus, and guinea pig lung (TABLE 2). A-78773 was 10- to 15-fold more potent than zileuton in all three preparations. Both compounds were less potent in inhibiting LTB_4 formation by guinea pig lung fragments than against leukotriene formation by lung preparations from either human or monkey. Similar to the isolated cell data, zileuton did not affect histamine release in lung fragments from any of the three species at concentrations 100-fold above the IC_{50} for inhibition of leukotriene biosynthesis.

INHIBITION OF LEUKOTRIENE-MEDIATED BRONCHOSPASM

The earliest published biological effect of leukotrienes was in bronchial smooth muscle contraction.[21] Sensitized guinea pig tissues have been used extensively as a model of the response of human tissue to antigen. Zileuton effectively inhibits the contraction of guinea pig trachea to antigen in the presence of an antihistamine. As shown in FIGURE 3, 3 μM zileuton was slightly inhibitory, but 10 μM of the compound gave nearly complete inhibition of the contraction. Zileuton showed no bronchodilation of tissues challenged with acetylcholine, PGD_2, or U-44060, a thromboxane mimetic (data not shown).

Antigen challenged guinea pigs respond with decreases in lung function that are leukotriene and histamine dependent.[23] In the presence of mepyramine to block histamine effects, zileuton completely blocks compliance changes induced by aerosolized antigen in sensitized animals.[22] As shown in FIGURE 4, an oral dose of zileuton (24 mg/kg) completely inhibited bronchospasm. The ED_{50} calculated from dose-response studies was 12 mg/kg.[22] These data are consistent with the pulmonary effects recently seen for zileuton in man.[5,6]

INHIBITION OF LEUKOTRIENE-MEDIATED INFLAMMATION

Leukotrienes have been proposed to be important in inflammatory reactions in a variety of animal models, although data with specific inhibitors or antagonists are somewhat limited. Zileuton was previously reported to have some activity in inhibiting the edema elicited by topical application of arachidonic acid to the ears of mice.[1] The compound was active as an oral agent at concentrations above 30 mg/kg. As shown in FIGURE 5, A-78773 was approximately 10-fold more potent than zileuton as an inhibitor of edema in this model. The compound was also more potent in inhibiting the formation of LTC_4 in the ear giving 58% inhibition at 1 mg/kg orally. Greater than 50% inhibition of leukotriene biosynthesis in the ear appears to be required for significant effects on the edematous response.

A few animal models are available that show leukotriene-dependent inflammatory cell influx.[1,24,25] In all studies thus far, leukotrienes appear to be only one of several mediators responsible for cell influx. One such model is the Arthus reaction in the rat pleural cavity.[1] As described for zileuton previously,[1] the compound inhibited inflammatory cell influx into the pleural cavity. The inhibition seen was only partial, however, plateauing around 60% (56% at 30 mg/kg). Like zileuton, A-78773 also inhibited the increase of fluid in the cavity albeit again only partially (36% at 30 mg/kg). The antiinflammatory effects of the two compounds appear to be leukotriene related and not nonspecific inhibition of neutrophil function, since in other studies, zileuton did not inhibit degranulation of human neutrophils stimulated with fMLP (data not shown).

These data indicate that in this model, the inflammatory response is only partially leukotriene dependent. Interestingly, inhibition of leukotrienes in the pleural exudates needed to be >85% before statistically significant effects were seen in exudate volume or inflammatory cell influx. Nonetheless, these data clearly show that there is a leukotriene component to both inflammatory responses. In addition, A-78773 was again shown to be a more potent inhibitor than zileuton with greater efficacy at lower doses.

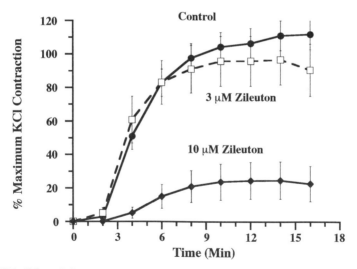

FIGURE 3. Effect of zileuton on antigen-induced contraction of guinea pig trachea. The effect of two concentrations of zileuton on the contraction of isolated guinea pig trachea induced by a single concentration of ovalbumin. Tissues received both 10 μM mepyramine and 10 μM meclofenamic acid 10 minutes prior to ovalbumain challenge and zileuton 30 minutes prior to ovalbumin challenge. Significance values were determined by the mean population of differences in conjunction with an *f* and *t* test. At 10 μM, zileuton significantly inhibited the contraction induced by ovalbumin.

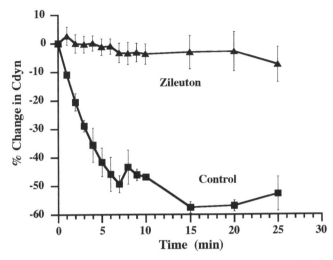

FIGURE 4. The effect of zileuton on antigen-induced bronchospasm in sensitized guinea pigs. Zileuton was dosed orally two hours prior to aerosol-antigen challenge of anesthetized guinea pigs. Guinea pigs were pretreated with mepyramine and melofenamic acid. C_{dyn} changes were measured as described by Malo et al.[22]

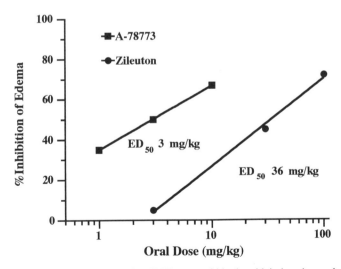

FIGURE 5. The effect of zileuton and A-78773 on arachidonic acid–induced ear edema in the mouse. Compounds were given orally 15 minutes prior to the topical application of arachidonic acid to the ear of mice. Edema was calculated as the wet-weight difference between treated and nontreated ears. The control group was 20 animals, and treatment groups were 10 animals each.

EARLY CLINICAL RESULTS WITH A-78773

Zileuton has an oral half-life in man of 2.3 hours.[3] As reported previously, A-78773 is considerably longer lived in monkeys than zileuton.[2] This was also found to be the case in man, where an oral elimination half-life was found to be 5.9 hours (Abbott Laboratories, unpublished observations). This longer half-life, combined with the greater potency of A-78773, translated into significantly longer inhibition of leukotriene production in man as assessed by *ex vivo* LTB_4 formation. As shown in FIGURE 6, A-78773 at a single 100-mg dose gave more complete and sustained inhibition of LTB_4 in whole blood than a single 800-mg dose of zileuton. In addition complete inhibition of LTB_4 was seen for several hours after a single dose. Thus, A-78773 when compared to zileuton is a more potent and longer-acting 5-lipoxygenase inhibitor in man.

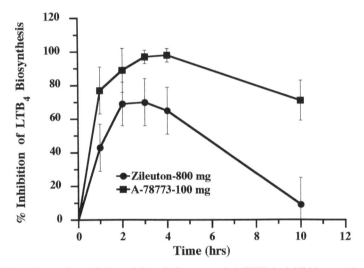

FIGURE 6. Comparison of the activity of zileuton and A-78773 in inhibiting *ex vivo* LTB_4 formation in human volunteers. Zileuton and A-78773 were given orally at the doses shown, and blood drawn and challenged with the calcium ionophore A23187 at the times indicated.

CONCLUSION

As described above, zileuton has shown considerable promise in the treatment of asthma and ulcerative colitis. The biochemical and pharmacological studies done with the compound indicate that it is a selective direct inhibitor of 5-lipoxygenase and that this inhibition appears to be the mechanism responsible for its activity in inflammatory and allergic responses in animals and man. A-78773 was compared to zileuton and in all cases was found to be a more potent 5-lipoxygenase inhibitor. Consistent with its potency, it proved to be effective in animal models of inflammation and bronchoconstriction at lower oral doses than zileuton. Finally, A-78773 gave longer and more complete inhibition of leukotriene formation in man at doses significantly lower than those used for zileuton. These data would predict that A-78773 should have superior clinical efficacy compared to zileuton.

SUMMARY

The importance of leukotrienes as mediators of inflammation and bronchoconstriction was examined with two recently described 5-lipoxygenase inhibitors, zileuton and A-78773.[1,2] Preclinical evaluation of these two molecules indicates that they are potent, selective, direct, reversible inhibitors of 5-lipoxygenase with activity in a variety of purified cells and in more complex biological systems such as whole blood, lung fragments, and tracheal tissues. In various animals models of inflammation and allergy, the molecules inhibited edema, inflammatory cell influx, and bronchospasm. These observations are consistent with the recent clinical success of zileuton in treating asthma and inflammatory bowel disease.[3-6] In all preclinical systems tested thus far, A-78773 is more potent and longer acting than zileuton, indicating that the molecule could be even more effective in the clinic than zileuton and that both molecules are useful tools in defining the role of leukotrienes in preclinical and clinical settings.

ACKNOWLEDGMENTS

The authors acknowledge the technical support of T. Shaughnessy, E. Otis, J. Bouska, S. Majest, C. Goodfellow, D. Wilcox, W. Hinz, and Y. Wiley. We especially thank Dr. Frank Graziano for the generous use of his laboratory and help with preparing lung cell suspensions. We also thank A. Niemi for assistance in preparing the manuscript.

REFERENCES

 1. CARTER, G. W., et al. 1991. 5-Lipoxygenase inhibitory activity of zileuton. J. Pharmacol. Exp. Ther. **256:** 929–937.
 2. BELL, R. L., D. W. BROOKS, P. R. YOUNG, C. LANNI, A. O. STEWART, J. BOUSKA, P. E. MALO & G. W. CARTER. 1993. A-78773: a selective, potent 5-lipoxygenase inhibitor. J. Lipid Mediators **6:** 259–264.
 3. RUBIN, P., et al. 1991. Pharmacokinetics, safety, and ability to diminish leukotriene synthesis by zileuton, an inhibitor of 5-lipoxygenase. Agents Actions Suppl. Prog. Inflammation Ther. **35:** 103–116.
 4. COLLAWN, C., et al. 1992. Phase II study of the safety and efficacy of a 5-lipoxygenase inhibitor in patients with ulcerative colitis. Am. J. Gastroenterol. **87:** 342–346.
 5. ISRAEL, E., et al. 1990. The effects of a 5-lipoxygenase inhibitor on asthma induced by cold, dry air. N. Engl. J. Med. **323:** 1740–1744.
 6. ISRAEL, E., et al. 1992. 5-Lipoxygenase inhibition by zileuton causes acute bronchodilation in asthma. Am. Rev. Respir. Dis. **145:** A16.
 7. SIROIS, P., et al. 1991. Effect of zileuton on the 5-lipoxygenase activity of human whole blood ex vivo. Agents Actions **34:** 117–120.
 8. LAURSEN, L. S., et al. 1990. Selective 5-lipoxygenase inhibition in ulcerative colitis. Lancet **335:** 683–685.
 9. KNAPP, H. 1990. Reduced allergen-induced nasal congestion and leukotriene synthesis with an orally active 5-lipoxygenase inhibitor. N. Engl. J. Med. **323:** 1745–1748.
10. YOUNG, J. M., D. A. SPIRES, C. J. BEDORD, B. WAGNER, S. J. BALLARON & L. M.

DeYoung. 1984. The mouse ear inflammatory response to topical arachidonic acid. J. Invest. Dermatol. **82:** 367–371.
11. Opas, E. E., R. J. Bonney & J. L. Humes. 1985. Prostaglandin and leukotriene synthesis in mouse ears inflamed by arachidonic acid. J. Invest. Dermatol. **84:** 253–256.
12. Herxheimer, H. 1952. Repeatable microshocks of constant strength in guinea pig anaphylaxis. J. Physiol. **117:** 251.
13. Malo, P. E., M. A. Wasserman & R. L. Griffin. 1982. The effects of lidocaine and hexamethonium on prostaglandin F_2 alpha and histamine-induced bronchoconstriction in normal and *Ascaris*-sensitive dogs. Drug Dev. Res. **2:** 567.
14. Marshall, L. A., B. Bolognese, W. Yuan & M. Gelb. 1991. Phosphate phospholipid analogs inhibit human phospholipase A_2. Agents Actions **34:** 106–109.
15. Mayer, R. & L. Marshall. 1993. New insights on mammalian phospholipase A_2(s); comparison of arachidonoyl-selective and -nonselective enzymes. FASEB J. **7:** 339–348.
16. Wong, A., S. M. Hwang, M. N. Cook & G. Ko. 1988. Interactions of 5-lipoxygenase with membranes: studies on the association of soluble enzyme with membranes and alterations in enzyme activity. Biochemistry **27:** 6763.
17. Rouzer, C. A., A. W. Ford-Hutchinson, E. Morton, J. W. Gillard, H. Rycut, R. Fortin, J. Y. Gauthier, J. Rodkey, R. Rosen, I. S. Sigal, C. D. Strader & J. F. Evans. 1990. MK866, a potent and specific leukotriene biosynthesis inhibitor blocks and reverses the membrane association of 5-lipoxygenase in ionophore challenged leukocytes. J. Biol. Chem. **265:** 1436–1436.
18. Miller, D. K., J. W. Gillard, P. J. Vicker, S. Sadowski, C. Levelle, J. Mancine, P. Charleson, R. Dixon & A. W. Ford-Hutchinson. 1990. Identification and isolation of a membrane protein necessary for leukotriene production. Nature. **343:** 278.
19. Undem, B. J., F. Gree, T. Warner, C. K. Buckner & F. M. Graziano. 1985. A procedure for isolation and partial purification of guinea pig lung mast cells. J. Immunol. Methods **81:** 187.
20. Kusner, F. J., R. L. Maks, D. Ahany & R. Krell. 1989. Inhibition by REV-5901 of leukotriene release from guinea pig and human lung tissue in vitro. Biochem. Pharmacol. **38:** 4183–4189.
21. Kellaway, C. H. & E. R. Trethewie. 1940. The liberation of a slow reacting smooth muscle–stimulating substance in anaphylaxis. Q. J. Exp. Physiol. **30:** 121.
22. Malo, P. E., R. L. Bell, T. K. Shaughnessy, J. Bouska, J. B. Summers, D. W. Brooks & G. W. Carter. The 5-lipoxygenase inhibitory activity of zileuton in models of antigen-induced airway anaphylaxis. Pulmonary Pharmacol. (In press.)
23. Kallos, P. & L. Kallos. 1984. Experimental asthma in guinea-pigs revisited. Int. Arch. Allergy Appl. Immunol. **73:** 77.
24. Brady, H. R., R. Persson, B. J. Ballermann, B. M. Brenner & C. N. Serhan. 1990. Leukotrienes stimulate neutrophil adhesion to mesangial cells: modulation with lipoxins. Am. J. Physiol. **134:** 285.
25. Errasfa, M. & F. Russo-Marie. 1988. Characterization of a polyacylamide gel–induced granuloma in mice: involvement of arachidonate metabolites. Agents Actions **24:** 123.

The Use of Brequinar Sodium for Transplantation[a]

DONALD V. CRAMER,[b] FRANCES A. CHAPMAN, AND
LEONARD MAKOWKA

Transplantation Biology Research Laboratory
Department of Surgery
Cedars-Sinai Medical Center
Los Angeles, California

INTRODUCTION

Organ transplantation has become an important and effective medical therapy, largely as the result of the development of immunosuppressive agents to control the rejection reaction. Cyclosporin A (CsA) is the most potent of these immunosuppressive agents, and it is highly effective for preventing the rejection of allografts in a variety of experimental and clinical settings. For most organ systems, the first year allograft survival rates approach 80–85%, a level of success that makes organ transplantation a preferred treatment strategy for many chronic diseases. In the future, however, the continued development of organ transplantation will be shaped by at least three issues that have emerged with the recent maturation of this medical specialty. The first is the need to develop new immunosuppressive techniques that will provide more effective control of graft rejection, especially xenograft rejection, without exacerbating the problems of toxic side effects or susceptibility to infection. The second is pressure to broaden the application of transplantation as a treatment modality to include patients, such as those presensitized to potential donors, that are not currently considered to be good candidates for transplantation. The third is the necessity of the use of organs from other species (xenografts) to provide a solution to an acute and growing shortage of human donor organs.

Current immunosuppressive protocols rely heavily of the use of CsA as the principal immunosuppressive agent for preventing graft rejection.[1,2] CsA is extremely effective for preventing allograft rejection, primarily due to its activity in inhibiting early T lymphocyte activation. The drug is generally considered to be ineffective for preventing the rejection of allografts in sensitized recipients or xenografts, probably as the result of the importance of humoral immune responses in mediating these types of rejection reactions. The rejection of xenografts, for example, differs from that of allografts in that the rejection process is mediated by preformed or newly induced antidonor antibody production and/or complement activation. CsA has a minimal ability to prevent antibody production and cannot provide effective protection from immune responses that are mediated by B lymphocytes. Accordingly, we expect that in the future there will be a high priority placed on the development of new immunosuppressive drugs that can be used in combination with current CsA-based immunosuppressive protocols. Drugs that are synergistic

[a]The work presented in this paper was supported by grants from the DuPont Merck Pharmaceutical Company, Wilmington, Delaware.

[b]Address correspondence to: Transplantation Biology Research Laboratory, Suite 250N, 150 North Robertson Boulevard, Beverly Hills, California 90211.

216

when used in combination with CsA and effective against B lymphocyte–mediated reactions have the potential to broaden the immunosuppressive control of humoral and cellular immune responses while reducing adverse side effects of the individual drugs.

Brequinar sodium (BQR) is an antimetabolite that exhibits a number of pharmacologic and immunosuppressive characteristics that are highly desirable for use in the development of new immunosuppressive protocols. The following is a description of unique features of the activity of Brequinar sodium that suggest that this new drug may have an important role addressing some of the issues of immunosuppression that currently limit the clinical application of transplantation.

PHARMACOLOGIC CHARACTERISTICS OF BREQUINAR SODIUM

Brequinar sodium exhibits a number of pharmacologic characteristics that are desirable for use in a clinical setting. The drug inhibits pyrimidine biosynthesis and was originally developed and tested as an anticancer agent. As with many antineoplastic compounds, BQR is very effective for inhibiting *in vivo* and *in vitro* immune responses. BQR acts to noncompetitively inhibit the activity of the enzyme dihydroorotate dehydrogenase (DHO-DH).[3,4] This disruption of the *de novo* pyrimidine pathway results in the depletion of the nucleotide precursors (UTP and CTP) necessary for the synthesis of RNA and DNA. Lymphocytes cannot utilize the pyrimidine salvage pathway for pyrimidine biosynthesis and are highly sensitive to *de novo* inhibition of DNA and RNA synthesis by BQR during the active, proliferative phases of an immune response. Once the effectiveness of BQR for preventing normal immune responses was established, we extended these experiments to the *in vivo* rejection of vascularized allografts. During the early stages of the experimental work, a series of studies were conducted to characterize the pharmacologic characteristics of the drug that are important for its potential use in organ transplantation.

Brequinar sodium is a water soluble drug with excellent bioavailability. Following oral administration in humans, the drug exhibits a peak plasma level in 2 to 4 hours with a greater than 90% bioavailability. The drug circulates in the peripheral blood tightly bound to serum proteins with a half-life of approximately 15 hours in humans and 17 hours in rats. Once the drug is absorbed, it is distributed rapidly to peripheral organs, including the liver and kidney.[5] The areas under the curve (AUC) for plasma levels of the drug increase linearly with the dose of the drug, and the plasma clearance is 19.2 ± 7.7 ml/min per mm^2.[6] The extended half-life and the low plasma clearance allow for the use of the drug at intervals of 24 to 48 hours. As described below, the use of BQR in rodents is most effective when it is administered as a single dose three times weekly.

While the metabolism of the drug is not been clearly defined, radioactive labeling of the parent compound has suggested that approximately 20 to 30% of the drug is eliminated in the urine and approximately 60% in the feces, presumably due to biliary excretion. The predominance of nonrenal routes of excretion is an advantage as the primary toxic effects of CsA are the kidney, and the use of BQR should not exacerbate the adverse effects of CsA treatment.

The high level of bioavailability, the relative ease with which the compound can be administered, and the prolonged half-life are all features of the pharmacokinetics of BQR that make the compound attractive for use in a clinical setting. In addition to these characteristics, the levels of the compound in the blood can be directly measured using high-pressure liquid chromatography. This allows for a relatively simple method of measuring the levels of the drug. The drug levels can then be compared to the level of suppression of lymphocyte function or nucleotide levels. The inhibition of a specific enzyme, dihydroorotate dehydrogenase, offers the potential of correlating plasma levels of the drug with the depletion of pyrimidine nucleotides in the target lymphocytes.[7]

IMMUNOSUPPRESSIVE ACTIVITY

There are several features of the immunosuppressive activity of Brequinar that may be useful when included in the development of new immunosuppressive protocols. BQR is effective as a primary immunosuppressive agent for preventing allograft rejection, the activity of the drug is directed at proliferating cells so that both T and B cell mediated responses are inhibited, and BQR exhibits a high level of synergism when used in combination with CsA and other new immunosuppressive drugs, including FK 506 and Rapamycin. The synergism with other immunosuppressive drugs and the inhibition of humoral immune responses are prominent features of the activity of BQR in a variety of experimental models, particularly the rejection of xenografts and allografts in previously sensitized recipients.

Primary Suppression of Allograft and Xenograft Rejection

Brequinar has been demonstrated to be an effective primary immunosuppressive drug. Administration of the drug alone is capable of inducing long-term allograft and xenograft survival in rodents and closely related species.[8] The effectiveness of BQR in preventing allograft and xenograft rejection, two very different forms of graft rejection, is unique. The allograft reaction is primarily mediated by a T cell dominated cellular immune response.[9,10] CsA and FK 506 are two macrolide antibiotics that are highly effective for preventing allograft rejection, a consequence of their ability to prevent the early events of T cell activation. In contrast to allografts, the rejection of xenografts is characterized by the involvement of humoral immune responses, including antidonor antibody, either preformed or induced after transplantation, and the activation of complement.[11-13] The use of immunosuppressive regimens that are primarily directed at the suppression of T cell mediated responses, such as CsA and FK 506, has proven to be ineffective for preventing this type of xenograft rejection.[14-17] As described below, BQR is effective for preventing both of these reactions, perhaps as the result of an effective antiproliferative effect on both activated T and B cells.

Allografts

The use of BQR as a primary immunosuppressive agent is characterized by effective inhibition of rejection in several models of vascularized allografts in rodents.[18] The prolonged plasma half-life has led to the use of treatment protocols in which BQR can be effectively administered every other day. Treatment of LEW rat recipients of ACI strain hearts, livers, or kidneys with increasing amounts of BQR is associated with significant prolongation of graft survival. As with many primary immunosuppressive agents, there is evidence of differences in the ability of BQR to prolong graft survival for different organ systems. In the case of the heart, the length of allograft survival is a function of the continued treatment of the recipient.

Treatment for periods of up to 90 days does not induce tolerance to the cardiac grafts, and withdrawal of the drug results in a loss of the graft to rejection in several days to a few weeks.[19] In contrast, treatment with the drug for 30 days is sufficient to induce a permanent, donor-specific tolerance in the majority of recipients of kidney and liver allografts. The differences in the ease of induction of tolerance for these types of allografts is also associated with an increased sensitivity of the recipients to the toxic effects of the drug. This suggests that there may be differences in the metabolism of the drug, depending upon the nature of the organ graft.

Xenografts

The hamster-to-rat heart xenograft is an example of an accelerated xenograft reaction. The rejection of the hamster heart is mediated by IgM antibody produced within three to four days in response to placement of the graft. Brequinar is capable of suppressing this xenograft reaction and is the most effective single agent for prolonging survival for this type of xenograft.[20] The survival of the heart grafts correlates closely with a suppression of antidonor antibody production. The antidonor antibody levels remain low during the period of graft survival and become elevated immediately prior to rejection of the graft.

Sensitized Allografts

The ability of BQR to prevent the rejection of xenografts and the correlation with the suppression of antibody production led us to examine the ability of this compound to prevent the rejection of allografts in sensitized recipients. In patients on waiting list for kidney grafts, there are many individuals who have become sensitized to a large number of potential donors, primarily because of repeated blood transfusions prior to transplantation. These patients have circulating antidonor antibodies and are more likely to mount aggressive rejection reactions that are resistant to CsA treatment. In rats, a comparable model for this form of allograft reactivity can be established by donor skin grafting of recipients one week prior to heart transplantation.[21] Sensitization of the recipient accelerates the rejection of heart allografts in the ACI-to-LEW combination from 7 days to 2 days posttransplantation. Brequinar is more effective than either CsA or cyclophosphamide (CyP) in preventing the accelerated rejection of the grafts and antidonor antibody production associated with graft rejection.[22] Treatment with BQR during sensitization, after placement of the challenge heart graft, or during both periods significantly prolongs graft survival. Although the most effective treatment is during the response to both skin and heart grafts, treatment beginning at transplantation, even in the presence of preformed antidonor antibody, is effective for preventing graft rejection.

Cellular and Humoral Immunosuppression

The experimental studies of BQR have clearly demonstrated that one of the important features of the immunosuppressive activity of the drug is its ability to prevent humoral immune responses. The antiproliferative activity of the drug, however, is also effective for preventing T lymphocyte–mediated immune responses. This can be most easily demonstrated *in vitro* where BQR can be shown to be capable of efficient inhibition of a wide variety of cellular immune responses, including alloantigen and mitogen-induced proliferative responses,[23] and *in vivo* suppression of graft-versus-host and contact sensitivity (DTH) responses.[24]

While BQR is more effective than CsA for preventing the type of rejection reactions that are mediated by antibody, it is clear that CsA alone has an important effect on preventing graft rejection in sensitized recipients. The combination of the two drugs (see below) is much more effective than either used alone. It is appropriate, therefore, to assume that BQR has an effect on both T and B cell–mediated responses and that the use of BQR in combination with CsA (and the closely related FK 506) will be particularly effective because of an extensive overlap in the functional activities of the two drugs.

BQR AND COMBINATION IMMUNOSUPPRESSIVE THERAPY

One of the most striking features of the immunosuppressive activity of Brequinar sodium is its ability to synergistically interact with a number of other agents to prevent allograft and xenograft rejection. Cyclosporin A, and the closely-related FK 506, act early in the lymphokine-mediated activation phase of the rejection reaction. BQR, by virtue of its antiproliferative effect, acts later after activation has led to the proliferation of T and B lymphocytes in response to the foreign allograft or xenograft. The use of BQR in combination with either CsA or FK 506 is highly synergistic, and a substantial reduction in the amount of both agents can be made without interfering with the effectiveness of the immunosuppressive activity.[16,17,25]

The synergistic effect of the use of BQR and CsA in combination is apparently more pronounced for preventing the rejection of xenografts (hamster-to-rat) than allografts. The effectiveness of these two drugs when used together to prevent allograft and xenograft rejection can be expressed mathematically as a combination index.[26] The interaction of CsA and BQR displays a moderate level of synergism for rat cardiac allografts and a striking synergism for hamster-to-rat heart xenografts (FIGURE 1). The ability of these two immunosuppressive agents to provide for almost permanent xenograft survival in this species combination is unique. Although survival in excess of 100 days has been reported previously for the hamster-to-rat donor/recipient combination,[27,28] these results are based upon the use of total lymphoid irradiation, a technique that would have limited clinical application. The use of CsA in combination with an antimetabolite, such as BQR, is a more traditional form of immunosuppression and should prove to be a safe and effective combination for use in patients.

The synergistic activity seen with the combination therapy with BQR and CsA is also observed with other immunosuppressive drugs. BQR displays the same synergistic activity with FK 506, a new immunosuppressive drug that shares a close functional relationship with CsA.[16] The combination of BQR and CsA with Rapamycin is also very effective for prolonging heart allograft survival.[29] Each of these three drugs acts via different biochemical pathways, and the use of these three drugs in combination demonstrates that each is capable of adding to the immunosuppressive synergism. CsA and Rapamycin in combination at subtherapeutic doses are synergistic, and the addition of BQR results in additional synergistic activity. One very interesting facet of the use of BQR in combination therapy is the observation that two antimetabolite drugs, BQR and Mycophenolate mofetil (RS-61443, mycophenolic acid) can interact positively to enhance allograft survival.[30] Mycophenolate mofetil acts by inhibiting the synthesis of purine, rather than pyrimidine, nucleotides. When used in combination, the two drugs induce prolonged cardiac allograft survival in rats (> 100 days) without evidence of adverse side effects.

We have recently examined the potential for BQR and CsA drug interactions in our experimental transplant models. We had observed evidence of increased plasma levels of BQR and adverse side effects in some of the higher dosage levels with the combination of BQR and CsA. Accordingly, we included measurements of BQR and CsA levels in our detailed studies of the synergistic effect of these two drugs when used in combination. LEW recipients of ACI heart grafts were treated with low doses of BQR and/or CsA, and 24 hour drug trough levels were established at 2 weeks posttransplantation[25] (TABLE 1). Increasing the level of CsA administration was associated with consistently higher levels of BQR when compared to the groups treated with BQR alone. There was no apparent effect of BQR on CsA levels. These

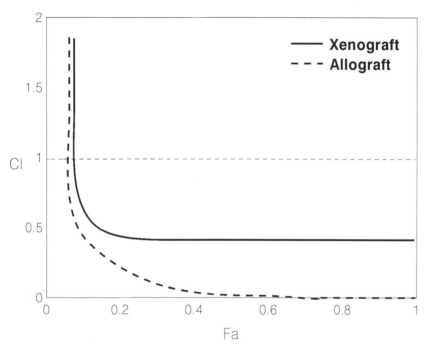

FIGURE 1. Synergistic activity exhibited by a combination of BQR and CsA for cardiac allografts and xenografts. Combination index (CI) of less than 1 is an indication of synergism.

results suggest that CsA and BQR share a common metabolic pathway, such as the mitochondrial cytochrome oxidase system.

The large number of new immunosuppressive drugs and the experimental evidence that many of them may exhibit synergistic activity indicate the tremendous potential for the application of multidrug therapy in organ transplantation. Many of the agents currently in development exhibit different mechanisms of action, allowing for the selective use of drug combinations for different clinical applications. The effectiveness of BQR when used with many different drugs is an illustration of how a mix of drugs in different combinations might be very effective for preventing specific types of immune responses. This is an area of investigation in transplantation that has a great potential for simultaneously improving graft survival and reducing the drug-related toxic side effects associated with treatment of rejection.

THERAPEUTIC MONITORING OF IMMUNOSUPPRESSIVE ACTIVITY

The ability to measure BQR levels directly and their effect on lymphocyte function may be an important component of developing clinically useful monitoring techniques. Once BQR has been administered, the drug levels can be measured using a reverse phase high-pressure liquid chromatography (HPLC) assay.[31] We have used this assay procedure to examine the relationship between drug levels and functional immunosuppressive activity in an attempt to define a "therapeutic window" that would allow for optimal graft survival without toxic side effects for the recipient.

TABLE 1. BQR and CsA Levels Seen in Treated Cardiac Allograft (ACI to LEW) Recipients

Treatment Group	n	Survival MST ± 1 SD	BQR (ng/mL)	CsA (ng/mL)
None	7	6.6 ± 0.2	—	—
BQR 3 mg/kg per 3 × wk	6	10.4 ± 0.5	1.6 ± 0.3	—
BQR 1.5 mg/kg per 3 × wk	6	8.3 ± 1.9	0.65 ± 23	—
CsA 5 mg/kg per day	6	20.1 ± 5.2	—	395 ± 322
CsA 2.5 mg/kg per day	6	16.3 ± 5.3	—	591 ± 293
BQR 3 mg/kg per 3 × wk CsA 5 mg/kg per day	6	32.0 ± 2.0	2.78 ± 0.48[a]	493 ± 532
BQR 3 mg/kg per 3 × wk CsA 2.5 mg/kg per day	6	31.0 ± 5.7	2.03 ± 0.84[a]	406 ± 380
BQR 1.5 mg/kg per 3 × wk CsA 2.5 mg/kg per day	6	29.0 ± 1.5	1.53 ± 0.5[a]	886 ± 332

[a] $p < 0.01$.

The relationship between BQR blood levels and rejection was first evaluated in a heart xenograft model.[17] LEW recipients of Golden Syrian hamster hearts were treated with 4 mg/kg per day of BQR beginning one day before transplantation and continuing for a period of 14 days. The dosage was then reduced to 3 mg/kg per day until rejection. In the untreated control group, the xenografts were rejected as expected at 4 days posttransplantation. In the BQR-treated animals, the median graft survival was 26.5 days. There was no significant difference in the BQR blood levels when the recipients with functioning grafts were compared to animals that rejected their grafts. This apparent lack of a correlation of the 24-hour trough levels for BQR and prolongation of graft survival was also seen in studies performed in Cynomolgus monkeys. Administration of 4 mg/kg BQR three times weekly is associated with a significant prolongation of graft survival to 20 days when compared to 8 days in the untreated controls ($p < 0.02$).[32] These results would suggest that the peak levels, rather than 24-hour trough levels, may be more important for establishing the blood level of drug required to induce optimal graft survival.

Despite the apparent lack of correlation between 24-hour trough levels and graft survival, our data would suggest that BQR blood levels may be an accurate indicator of recipient toxicity. When BQR was maintained at 3 mg/kg per day and CsA increased to 15 mg/kg in the cardiac xenograft recipients, the animals exhibited signs of toxicity and exhibited elevations in mean BQR blood level to 16.1 ± 9.0 μg/ml.[7] As described earlier, this increase in BQR plasma levels may reflect an overlap in the metabolism of BQR and CsA. Similarly, allograft studies in rats have shown that doses of BQR that are well tolerated in the recipients of heterotopic heart grafts may cause significant adverse side effects for the recipients of the orthotopic kidney and liver grafts.[18] When BQR is delivered at 24 mg/kg 3 × per week, cardiac graft survival without evidence of recipient toxicity is seen for a minimum of 6 weeks. This dose produces substantial toxicity in the recipients of kidney allografts with BQR blood levels of 33.7 ± 7.13 μg/ml at the time of death.

DRUG-RELATED SIDE EFFECTS

Brequinar sodium is an antimetabolite that interferes with cell proliferation. Inhibition of the enzyme dihydroorotate dehydrogenase disrupts pyrimidine biosynthesis and prevents DNA and RNA synthesis. When used in experimental animals, the toxic effects of the drug have been primarily in tissues with rapid cell turnover, such as the bone marrow, gastrointestinal tract, and lymphoid system.[18,33,34] These side effects are consistent for a variety of different species, although substantial differences in the sensitivity of individual species to the drug are observed. The dog appears to be most sensitive to the toxic effects of BQR, and evidence of gastrointestinal toxicity and bone marrow suppression can be seen with maximum tolerated doses that are less than 10% of those seen with rodents. The miniature pig is intermediate in its sensitivity to the drug. Monkeys and humans appear to be less sensitive to the effects of BQR, and the maximum tolerated doses of the drug are similar to those seen in rodents.[35]

The development of BQR as an antineoplastic drug was associated with clinical and pharmacokinetic trials in humans to establish safety levels for clinical trials.[6,36,37] The side effects observed in patients are the same as those observed in experimental animals. The primary dose-limiting toxicities have been thrombocytopenia, dermatitis, and mucositis.[6] Other dose-related effects included diarrhea, leukopenia, and granulocytopenia. Once the adverse side effects have appeared, the noncompetitive nature of the enzyme inhibition provides the opportunity to reduce or withdraw treatment with the drug with rapid reversal of the drug-related effects.

CONCLUSIONS

Our primary preclinical model for examining the efficacy of BQR for preventing allograft and xenograft rejection has been in rodents and closely related species. While it is difficult to estimate the direct application of these data for the immunosuppressive efficacy of BQR in humans, our experience in a number of experimental systems has demonstrated that (1) BQR is an effective primary immunosuppressive agent for the prevention of the rejection of vascularized allografts and xenografts, (2) BQR displays a marked synergism when used *in vivo* in combination with a variety of immunosuppressive drugs, including cyclosporine, (3) BQR actively suppresses T and B lymphocyte–mediated immune responses, particularly IgM and IgG antibody production, and is highly effective for preventing those rejection reactions that are dependent upon humoral immune responses, (4) BQR can disrupt an ongoing rejection reaction and provide for highly effective rescue of rejecting allografts, (5) the pharmacokinetics of BQR allow for consistent, predictable oral administration, and (6) standard laboratory measurements of the plasma levels of the drug and *in vitro* measurements of the immunosuppressive activity provide the opportunity to develop simple and effective monitoring techniques for use of the drug in patients. We believe that this combination of pharmacologic and immunosuppressive features will be important advantages for the use of this agent in the development of more effective and safe immunosuppressive protocols for organ transplantation.

REFERENCES

1. WHITE, D. J. G. & R. Y. CALNE. 1982. The use of cyclosporin A immunosuppression in organ grafting. Immunol. Rev. **65:** 115–131.
2. KAHAN, B. D. 1989. Cyclosporine. N. Engl. J. Med. **321:** 1725–1738.
3. CHEN, S-F., R. RUBEN & D. DEXTER. 1986. Mechanism of action of the novel anticancer agent 6-fluoro-2-(2′-fluoro-1,1′-biphenyl-4-yl)-3-methyl-4-quinolinecarboxylic acid sodium salt (NSC 368390): inhibition of de novo pyrimidine nucleotide biosynthesis. Cancer Res. **46:** 5014–5019.
4. CHEN, S-F., L. M. PAPP, R. J. ARDECKY, G. V. RAO, D. P. HESSON, M. FORBES & D. L. DEXTER. 1990. Structure-activity relationship of quinoline carboxylic acids: a new class of inhibitors of dihydroorotate dehydrogenase. Biochem. Pharmacol. **40:** 709–714.
5. SHEN, H-S., S-F. CHEN, D. BEHRENS, C. WHITNEY, D. DEXTER & M. FORBES. 1988. Distribution of the novel anticancer drug candidate Brequinar sodium (Du 785, NSC 368390) into normal and tumor tissues of nude mice bearing human colon carcinoma xenografts. Cancer Chemother. Pharmacol. **22:** 183–186.
6. ARTEAGA, C. L., T. BROWN & J. KUHM. 1989. Phase I clinical and pharmacokinetic evaluation of Brequinar sodium. Cancer Res. **49:** 4648.
7. EIRAS-HREHA, G. 1993. Brequinar sodium: monitoring immunosuppressive activity. Transplant. Proc. **25**(Suppl. 2): 32–36.
8. MAKOWKA, L. & D. V. CRAMER. Brequinar sodium: mode of action and effects on graft rejection. *In* Immunosuppressive Drugs: Developments in Anti-Rejection Therapy. A. W. Thomson & T. E. Starzl, Eds. Edward Arnold. Kent. (In press.)
9. COLVIN, R. B. 1990. Cellular and molecular mechanisms of allograft rejection. Annu. Rev. Med. **41:** 361–375.
10. BRADLEY, J. A. & E. M. BOLTON. 1992. The T-cell requirements for allograft rejection. Transplant. Rev. **6:** 115–129.
11. PLATT, J. L., G. M. VERCELLOTTI, A. P. DALMASSO, A. J. MATAS, R. M. BOLMAN, J. S. NAJARIAN & F. H. BACH. 1990. Transplantation of discordant xenografts: a review of progress. Immunol. Today **11:** 450–455.
12. AUCHINCLOSS, H., JR. 1988. Xenogeneic transplantation: a review. Transplantation **46:** 1–20.
13. PAUL, L. C. 1991. Mechanism of humoral xenograft rejection. *In* Xenotransplantation. The Transplantation of Organs and Tissues between Species. D. K. C. Cooper, E. Kemp, K. Reemtsma & D. J. G. White, Eds.: 47–67. Springer-Verlag. Berlin, Germany.
14. NAKAJIMA, K., K. SAKAMOTO, T. OCHIAI, M. NAGATA, T. ASANO & K. ISONO. 1988. Prolongation of cardiac xenograft survival in rats treated with 15-deoxyspergualin alone and in combination with FK506. Transplantation **45:** 1146–1148.
15. HASAN, R., J. B. VAN DEN BOGAERDE, J. WALLWORK & D. J. G. WHITE. 1992. Evidence that long-term survival of concordant xenografts is achieved by inhibition of antispecies antibody production. Transplantation **54:** 408–413.

16. MURASE, N., T. E. STARZL, A. J. DEMETRIS, L. A. VALDIVIA, M. TANABE, D. V. CRAMER & L. MAKOWKA. 1993. Hamster-to-rat heart and liver xenotransplantation with FK 506 plus antiproliferative drugs. Transplantation **55:** 701–708.

17. COSENZA, C., P. J. TUSO, F. A. CHAPMAN, Y. D. MIDDLETON, D. V. CRAMER, G. D. WU & L. MAKOWKA. 1993. Prolonged xenograft survival following combination therapy with Brequinar sodium and cyclosporine. Transplant. Proc. **25**(Suppl. 2): 59–60.

18. CRAMER, D. V., F. A. CHAPMAN, B. D. JAFFEE, E. A. JONES, M. KNOOP, G. HREHA-EIRAS & L. MAKOWKA. 1992. The effect of a new immunosuppressive drug, Brequinar sodium, on heart, liver, and kidney allograft rejection in the rat. Transplantation **53:** 303–308.

19. CRAMER, D. V., F. A. CHAPMAN, B. D. JAFFEE & L. MAKOWKA. 1993. Inhibition of the pyrimidine biosynthetic pathway with S-8660, an analogue of Brequinar sodium, prolongs cardiac allograft survival in rats. J. Heart Lung Transplant. **12:** 140–146.

20. CRAMER, D. V., F. A. CHAPMAN, B. D. JAFFEE, I. ZAJAC, G. HREHA-EIRAS, C. YASUNAGA, G.-D. WU & L. MAKOWKA. 1992. The prolongation of concordant hamster-to-rat cardiac xenografts by Brequinar sodium. Transplantation **54:** 403–408.

21. HANCOCK, W. W., R. DISTEFANO, P. BRAUN, R. T. SCHWEIZER, N. L. TILNEY & J. W. KUPIEC-WEGLINSKI. 1990. Cyclosporine and anti-interleukin 2 receptor monoclonal antibody therapy suppress accelerated rejection of rat cardiac allografts through different effector mechanisms. Transplantation **49:** 416–421.

22. YASUNAGA, C., D. V. CRAMER, F. A. CHAPMAN, H. K. WANG, M. BARNETT, G.-D. WU & L. MAKOWKA. The prevention of accelerated cardiac allograft rejection in sensitized recipients following treatment with Brequinar sodium. Transplantation. (In press.)

23. EIRAS-HREHA, G., D. V. CRAMER, E. CAJULIS, C. COSENZA, L. MILLS, K. HOUGH, M. FRANKLAND, F. A. CHAPMAN, H. K. WANG, I. ZAJAC, R. HARRIS, E. JONES, B. D. JAFFEE & L. MAKOWKA. 1993. Correlation of the *in vitro* and *in vivo* immunosuppressive activity of Brequinar sodium. Transplant. Proc. **25:** 708–709.

24. JAFFEE, B. D. 1993. The unique immunosuppressive activity of Brequinar sodium. Transplant. Proc. **25**(Suppl. 2): 19–22.

25. COSENZA, C. A., D. V. CRAMER, G. EIRAS-HREHA, E. CAJULIS, H. K. WANG & L. MAKOWKA. Brequinar sodium and cyclosporine are synergistic when used in combination to prevent allograft rejection in the rat. Transplantation. (In press.)

26. CHOU, T-C. & P. TALALAY. 1984. Quantitative analysis of dose effect relationships: the combined effects of multiple drugs or enzyme inhibitors. Adv. Enzyme Regul. **22:** 27.

27. STEINBRÜCHEL, D. A., H. H. T. MADSEN, B. NIELSEN, E. KEMP, S. LARSEN & C. KOCH. 1991. The effect of combined treatment with total lymphoid irradiation cyclosporin A, and anti-CD4 monoclonal antibodies in a hamster-to rat heart transplantation model. Transplant. Proc. **23:** 579–580.

28. KNECHTLE, S. J., E. C. HALPERIN & R. R. BOLLINGER. 1987. Xenograft survival in two species combinations using total-lymphoid irradiation and cyclosporine. Transplantation **43:** 173–175.

29. STEPKOWSKI, S. M. & B. D. KAHAN. 1993. The synergistic activity of the triple combination: cyclosporine, rapamycin, and Brequinar. Transplant. Proc. **25**(Suppl. 2): 29–31.

30. HULLETT, D. A. & H. W. SOLLINGER. 1993. Mycophenolate mofetil and Brequinar sodium: new immunosuppressive agents. Transplant. Proc. **25**(Suppl. 2): 45–47.

31. PETERS, G. J., E. LAURENSSE, A. LEYVA & H. M. PINEDO. 1987. A sensitive, nonradiometric assay for dihydroorotic acid dehydrogenase using anion-exchange high-performance liquid chromatography. Anal. Biochem. **161:** 32–38.

32. MAKOWKA, L., D. TIXIER, A. CHAUX, D. HILL, P. O'NEILL, G. EIRAS-HREHA, G. D. WU, K. HOUGH, E. CAJULIS, I. ZAJAC, B. D. JAFFEE, F. A. CHAPMAN & D. V. CRAMER. 1993. The use of Brequinar sodium for preventing cardiac allograft rejection in primates. Transplant. Proc. **25** (Suppl. 2): 48–53.

33. PETERS, G. J., J. C. NADAL, E. J. LAURENSSE, E. DE KANT & H. M. PINEDO. 1990. Retention of in vivo antipyrimidine effects of Brequinar sodium (DUP-785; NSC 368390) in murine liver, bone marrow and colon cancer. Biochem. Pharmacol. **39:** 135–144.

34. LOVELESS, S. E. & R. H. NEUBAUER. 1986. Antimetastatic activity of DUP-785: a novel anticancer agent. Proc. Am. Assoc. Cancer Res. **27:** 276.

35. EIRAS-HREHA, G., D. V. CRAMER, E. CAJULIS, D. HILL, M. FRANKLAND, K. HOUGH, L. MILLS, B. NICHOLSON, F. A. CHAPMAN, B. D. JAFFEE, I. ZAJAC & L. MAKOWKA. 1993. Individual and species differences in the *in vitro* sensitivity to Brequinar sodium. Transplant. Proc. **25**(Suppl. 2): 61–64.
36. PETERS, G. J., G. SCHWARTSMANN, J. C. NADAL, E. LAURENSSE, C. J. VAN GROENINGEN, W. J. F. VAN DER VIJGH & H. M. PINEDO. 1990. In vivo inhibition of the pyrimidine de novo enzyme dihydroorotic acid dehydrogenase by Brequinar sodium (DUP-785; NSC 368390) in mice and patients. Cancer Res. **50**: 4644–4649.
37. SCHWARTSMANN, G., P. DODION, J. B. VERMORKEN, W. W. TEN BOKKEL HUININK, G. JOGGI, B. WINOGRAD, H. GALL, G. SIMONETTI, W. J. VAN DER VIJGH, M. B. VAN HENNIK, N. CRESPEIGNE & H. M. PINEDO. 1990. Phase I study with Brequinar sodium (NSC 368390) in patients with solid malignancies. Cancer Chemother. Pharmacol. **25**: 345–351.

Cytidine Potentiates the Inhibitory Effect of Brequinar Sodium on Xeno-MLR, Antibody Production, and Concordant Hamster to Rat Cardiac Xenograft Survival[a]

JACKY WOO,[b] LUIS A. VALDIVIA, FAN PAN,
SUSANNA CELLI, JOHN J. FUNG,
AND ANGUS W. THOMSON

Pittsburgh Transplant Institute and
Department of Surgery
University of Pittsburgh
Pittsburgh, Pennsylvania 15213

INTRODUCTION

Traditional immunosuppressive therapies have had limited success in preventing the rejection of experimental organ xenografts. Thus, drugs such as cyclosporine A (CsA) and FK 506, which are highly effective in inhibiting the predominantly cellular responses that are responsible for allograft rejection, fail to prolong the survival of concordant hamster-to-rat cardiac xenografts beyond 3–4 days.[1,2] In this model, antibody and complement have been shown to be the primary mediators of graft rejection.[3–5] Debilitating therapies, such as combination of CsA with total lymphoid irradiation and monoclonal anti-CD4 antibody, however, can permit the survival of hamster-to-rat xenografts for several months, but this approach has very limited clinical application. The combination of cyclophosphamide (Cy) with CsA or FK 506 (but not Cy alone) can lead to prolonged (> 100 day) cardiac xenograft survival, with associated suppression of anti–hamster antibody production,[5] but may also lead to serious morbidity, due to infection consequent upon excessive immunosuppression.

Recently, a new immunosuppressive drug, brequinar sodium (BQR), which inhibits *de novo* pyrimidine biosynthesis and, consequently, both DNA and RNA synthesis,[6–8] has been shown by Cramer *et al.* to prolong hamster-to-rat heterotopic cardiac xenograft survival (to a median of 26.5 days) and to suppress anti–donor species IgM levels in the rat when administered as the sole immunosuppressant.[9] Studies in our laboratory, using the same model, have shown a less pronounced effect of BQR on xenograft survival. We have also shown, however, that the antilymphocytic activity of BQR against both T- and B-cells can be potentiated *in vitro* by the pyrimidine nucleoside cytidine.[10,11] In view of these findings, we sought to determine the influence of BQR alone, or with cytidine, on xeno–mixed lymphocyte reactivity

[a]This work was supported by project grant No. DK 29961 from the National Institutes of Health, Bethesda, Md.
[b]Correspondence Address: Department of Surgery, E1554 Biomedical Science Tower, University of Pittsburgh, Pittsburgh, Pa. 15213.

(MLR) and IgM antibody production *in vitro* and on hamster to rat cardiac xenograft survival.

MATERIALS AND METHODS

Animals

Adult LEW (RT1[1]) rats (10-12 weeks of age) and Syrian Golden hamsters were purchased from Charles River Laboratories. All animals were certified virus free, and the colony was monitored regularly for accidental contamination with infectious diseases. The animals were housed in microisolator cages in isolated animal facilities and fed rodent laboratory chow (Purina Mills, Inc., St. Louis, Mo.) and tap water *ad libitum.*

Reagents

Brequinar sodium (DuPont Merck Pharmaceutical Company, Wilmington, Del.) was kindly provided by Dr. L. Makowka, Department of Surgery, Cedars-Sinai Medical Center, Los Angeles, Calif. For addition to cell cultures, it was dissolved fresh in filter-sterilized isotonic saline at 1 μg/ml and diluted to working concentrations with RPMI-1640 (Gibco, Grand Island, N.Y.), supplemented with 2 mM glutamine, 50 u/ml penicillin G sodium, 50 mg/ml streptomycin sulfate, 25 mM Hepes, and 10% heat-inactivated fetal bovine serum (FBS) (Gibco). The nucleosides cytidine and uridine were purchased from Sigma Chemical Co., St. Louis, Mo, dissolved in sterile saline, and diluted in RPMI-1640 with 10% FBS.

Recombinant (r) human IL-6 was purchased from Research & Diagnostics Systems, Inc., Minneapolis, Minn., and was reconstituted with phosphate-buffered saline (PBS) containing 0.1% w/v bovine serum albumin (BSA) at 1 μg/ml. The rIL-6 was diluted to the required concentrations in RPMI-1640 with 10% FBS and was used in concentrations ranging from 0.05–3.2 ng/ml.

Mixed Lymphocyte Reaction

The sensitivity of rat/hamster xenogeneic mixed lymphocyte responses to inhibition with BQR was tested by incubation of purified rat and hamster lymph node lymphocytes with increasing concentrations of the drug. A total of 2×10^5 rat lymphocytes/well were cultured with 2.85×10^5 irradiated hamster lymph node lymphocytes for 5 days in 5% CO_2 at 37°C. The culture medium consisted of RPMI 1640 medium (Gibco) containing 5% heat-inactivated ACI rat serum, 2 mM L-glutamine, 1×10^{-5} M 2-mercaptoethanol, 100 U/ml penicillin, and 100 μg/ml streptomycin. Twenty-four hours prior to harvesting, the cultures were pulsed with 1 μCi of [3H]-thymidine. The cultures were harvested onto glass fiber discs, and the level of thymidine incorporation was measured by counting in a beta-plate scintillation counter (Pharmacia, Gaithersburg, Md.). The results are expressed as counts per minute (cpm).

B-Cell Line

The SKW 6.4 cell line is a human IL-6-dependent, IgM-secreting, B-cell line. Cells were purchased from the American Type Culture Collection (ATCC, Rockville, Md.) and maintained in RPMI 1640, supplemented with 10% (v/v) heat-inactivated FBS (Gibco) at 37°C and in humidified atmosphere of 5% CO_2 in air. They were grown in suspension in 75-cm^2 vented culture flasks (Costar, Cambridge, Mass.) and were split weekly to maintain a density of $< 10^5$ cells/ml. To determine the effect of BQR on IL-6-induced IgM production, 10^4 cells were cultured in duplicate in 200 μl of culture medium in round-bottom, 96-well tissue culture plates (Corning, N.Y.). Recombinant IL-6, BQR, cytidine, or uridine was added at the beginning of the culture, and plates were incubated at 37°C in 5% CO_2 in air for 72 h. After incubation, the plates were centrifuged and 100 μl supernatant was collected and stored at -70°C until analysis.

Measurement of IgM

IgM secreted in culture supernatants was measured using a sandwich enzyme linked immunosorbent assay (ELISA). Briefly, 96-well flat-bottom microtiter ELISA plates were precoated with 100 μl/well of sodium carbonate buffer, pH 9.6, containing 10 μg/ml of μ chain–specific goat anti–human IgM antibody (Sigma). The plates were incubated at 4°C overnight and then washed three times with PBS containing 0.05% Tween 20. After blocking of nonspecific binding by incubating the plate with 200 μl of PBS containing 1% BSA for 30 min, samples to be assayed (100 μl) were added and the plate was incubated at room temperature for 2 h. The plates were then washed four times with PBS and incubated for an additional 3 h at room temperature with 100 μl/well of a 10^{-4} dilution of a peroxidase-conjugated goat anti–human IgM antibody (Sigma). The plates were then washed again, and 200 μl/well of a 2 mg/ml solution of *o*-phenilenediamine dihydrochloride (Sigma) in citrate-phosphate buffer, pH 5.4, was added. The reaction was stopped by addition of H_2O_2 (0.03% v/v). Absorption at 490 nm was measured with an ELISA plate reader (MR5000, Dynatech), and the values were compared to those of known human IgM standards run simultaneously with the unknown samples.

Heterotopic Cardiac Xenografts

The donor hamsters and recipient rats were anesthetized with methoxyfluorance inhalation. Intraabdominal heterotopic cardiac xenografting was performed by using a modification (4) of the technique originally described by Ono and Lindsey.[12] Operative times ranged from 30 to 40 min, with a success rate of approximately 95%. The grafts were evaluated daily for function by abdominal palpation, and all grafts were removed for examination on the day of cessation of heartbeat. The hearts were fixed in 10% buffered formalin for 24 h before processing and staining with hematoxylin and eosin.

Complement-Dependent Cytotoxicity Assay (CDC)

Complement fixing lymphocytotoxic antibodies were measured in the recipient rat sera by a standard 2-step microcytotoxicity test, using target cells prepared from hamster cervical lymph nodes. After washing and isolation, the cells were resuspended at a concentration of 5×10^6/ml. Duplicate samples of 1 μl of various dilutions of serum samples and 1 μl of lymphocyte suspensions were placed into 72-well tissue-typing trays (Robbins Scientific, Sunnyvale, Calif.). After incubation for 30 min at room temperature, 2 μl of baby rabbit complement diluted 10 times

(Cedarlane Laboratories Ltd., Hornby, Ontario) were added to each well with reincubation for another 30 min at 37°C in 95% O_2, 5% CO_2. Five μl of 0.4% trypan blue was added to each well for staining. The lymphocytotoxic antibody titer was defined as the highest serum dilution with more than 25% cell lysis. Normal hamster serum served as a negative control.

RESULTS

Inhibition of Xeno MLR

Strong proliferative responses of rat lymph node lymphocytes in response to irradiated hamster cells were observed in 5-day mixed lymphocyte cultures (TABLE 1). Addition of BQR at the start of the culture period resulted in a dose-related inhibition of ^{3}HTdR incorporation, with an IC_{50} of 1 μg/ml; almost 90% inhibition of DNA synthesis was achieved with 5 μg/ml BQR. Cytidine potentiated the inhibitory effect of BQR, but only at concentrations of 0.5 μg/ml BQR or above. When BQR and cytidine were added at the start of cultures, 90% inhibition of the MLR was achieved with 1 μg/ml BQR. Cytidine alone (0.1 mM) had no significant effect on the xeno MLR.

Inhibition of In Vitro IgM Production

As shown in TABLE 2, addition of IL-6 to the B-cell line SKW6.4 resulted, at 72 h, in a cytokine dose-dependent increase in IgM production. BQR at 0.1 μg/ml effectively reduced IgM production, at all concentrations of IL-6 tested. The suppression of IgM production by BQR was not due to its inhibitory effect on cellular proliferation, as BQR did not suppress spontaneous proliferation of SKW6.4 cells (data not shown). Since BQR is known to mediate its effect through inhibition of the generation of pyrimidine nucleosides, the effect of addition of exogenous nucleotides on the inhibitory effect of BQR was examined. While addition of exogenous uridine (0.1 mM) at the start of cultures reversed the inhibitory effect of BQR on IL-6-induced IgM production, the addition of cytidine (0.1 mM) augmented the capacity of BQR (0.3–0.5 μg/ml) to suppress antibody production (TABLE 2). Cytidine alone had little effect on IgM production, except for a minor inhibitory action at higher IL-6 concentrations.

TABLE 1. Inhibition of the Xeno-MLR by BQR Alone or in Combination with Cytidine

BQR Conc. (μg/ml)	cpm ($\times 10^{-3}$)	
	BQR	BQR + Cytidine (0.1 mM)
0	50.03 ± 13.8 (untreated control)	36.87 ± 5.76 (cytidine control)
0.05	43.62 ± 9.93 (12.8)[a]	44.00 ± 11.56 (0)[b]
0.1	41.76 ± 8.09 (16.6)	35.17 ± 6.18 (4.6)
0.5	37.44 ± 18.29 (25.2)	21.95 ± 0.94 (40.5)
1	24.53 ± 3.04 (51.0)	4.50 ± 0.62 (87.8)
5	5.88 ± 1.17 (88.2)	0.95 ± 0.15 (87.5)

[a] % reduction compared with untreated control.
[b] % reduction compared with cytidine control.

TABLE 2. Effect of BQR and Cytidine on IL-6-Induced IgM Production

IL-6 (ng/ml)	BQR (µg/ml)	IgM (ng/ml)	
		BQR	BQR + Cytidine (0.1 µM)
0.2	0	48.45	46.06
	0.1	32.72 (32.5)[a]	13.18 (71.4)[b]
	0.5	13.44 (72.3)	3.80 (91.8)
0.8	0	61.84	63.88
	0.1	20.98 (66.1)	15.77 (75.3)
	0.5	15.02 (75.7)	5.26 (91.8)
3.2	0	90.47	70.29
	0.1	29.96 (66.9)	13.99 (80.1)
	0.5	11.36 (87.5)	3.72 (94.7)

[a] % reduction compared with appropriate untreated control.
[b] % reduction compared with cytidine-treated control.

Prolongation of Xenograft Survival

Since BQR proved very effective in suppressing IgM production, and to determine the effects of BQR and cytidine on xenograft survival, rats receiving heterotopic hamster cardiac transplants were treated with either agent alone or with the two drugs in combination. The effects of treatment on graft survival is shown in FIGURE 1.

The median survival time (MST) of heterotopic hamster cardiac xenografts in the Lew rat was 3.0 ± 0.0 days. Treatment of graft recipients with BQR alone (3 mg/kg per day) resulted in an MST of 5.8 ± 0.7 days. MST was significantly prolonged to 17.5 ± 14.1 days, however ($p < 0.05$ Wilcoxon Signed Rank Test), when BQR was combined with cytidine. Cytidine administration alone did not affect xenograft survival (data not shown).

Antihamster Responses of Xenografted Rats

The influence of treatment of graft recipients with BQR and cytidine on the capacity of lymph node lymphocytes to respond to xenoantigen was determined by mixed lymphocyte culture. As shown in FIGURE 2, the *ex vivo* responses of xenografted rat lymphocytes (obtained 4 days after transplant) to xenoantigens expressed on hamster lymphocytes was unaffected by treatment of the rats with BQR alone or in combination with cytidine. Sera obtained from the xenografted rats at various times after transplant and at the time of graft rejection were titrated against hamster lymphocytes in a complement-dependent cytotoxicity (CDC) assay. The results are shown in FIGURE 3. BQR treatment alone significantly reduced CDC antibody titers measured at the time of xenograft rejection. No further significant reduction in CDC titer was detected in animals given both BQR and cytidine; in animals whose grafts survived beyond one week, antibody titers continued to rise. Beyond four weeks, similar titers were observed in the drug combination group to those found at the time of graft rejection in untreated, transplanted controls.

DISCUSSION

The results reported in this study show that BQR plus cytidine is more effective than BQR alone in the prevention of concordant cardiac xenograft rejection. The

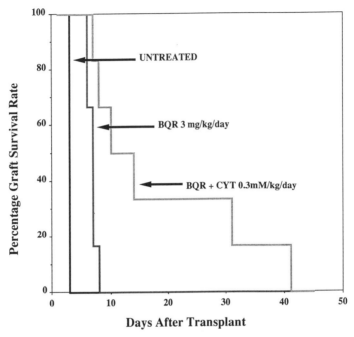

FIGURE 1. The influence of BQR and BQR + cytidine on hamster cardiac xenograft survival in the Lewis rat.

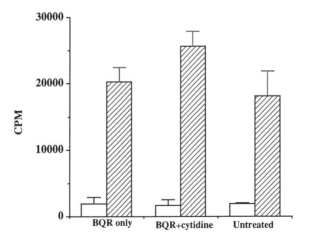

FIGURE 2. Xeno-MLR responses of lymph node lymphocytes from Lewis rats transplanted 4 days previously with hamster hearts and treated with BQR or BQR+ cytidine.

MST of grafts in BQR-treated recipients in this report is shorter than that reported recently by Cramer *et al.*[9] The BQR + cytidine combination had little *in vivo* toxicity, despite prolonged treatment, and the body weight of the treated animals continued to increase throughout the study period (data not shown). In order to investigate the mechanism of prolonged graft survival in the drug combination group, lymph node lymphocytes were isolated and the reactivity of recipient's lymphocytes to hamster cells was determined by MLR. Despite an effect of BQR in inhibiting MLR *in vitro,* the *in vivo* treatment of transplanted animals with BQR with or without cytidine did not affect the xenoreactivity of Lewis rat lymphocytes. This discrepancy may be due to the relatively short half-life of BQR *in vivo.* Rapid clearance of BQR would clearly lead to the disappearance of its inhibitory effect in the *in vitro* MLR cultures. Earlier study has shown that culture of BQR-treated L1210 cells in fresh medium results in recovery of dihydroorotic dehydrogenase after 24 h.[6]

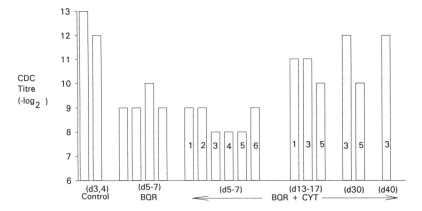

FIGURE 3. Complement-dependent cytotoxicity (CDC) titers of sera obtained from Lewis rats at the time (d = days) of hamster cardiac xenograft rejection. Figures in columns refer to individual rats treated with BQR + cytidine.

The *in vitro* experiments also demonstrated that BQR alone or with cytidine was very effective in controlling IgM production in IL-6-stimulated human SKW6.4 B cell lines. This effect may have contributed to the prolonged heart survival. Although BQR alone and BQR plus cytidine were both effective in controlling antihamster cytotoxic antibody production, no further reduction in antibodies by supplementation with cytidine was observed. Thus, although the beneficial effect of combining BQR and cytidine *in vivo* is unclear, difficulties in interpretation of their effects may have arisen as a result of the rapid *in vivo* clearance rate of the drug and the stringency of the (xenograft) model employed.

REFERENCES

1.   VAN DEN BOGAERDE, J., R. ASPINALL, M.-W. WANG, N. CARY, S. LIM, L. WRIGHT & D. WHITE. 1991. Induction of long-term survival of hamster heart xenografts in rats. Transplantation **52:** 15–20.

2. GUDAS, V. M., P. G. CARMICHAEL & R. E. MORRIS. 1989. Comparison of the immunosuppressive and toxic effects of FK 506 and cyclosporin in xenograft recipients. Transplant. Proc. **21:** 1072.

3. FISCHEL, R. J., R. M. BELMAN III, J. L. PLATT, J. S. NAJARIAN, F. H. BACH & A. J. MATAS. 1990. Removal of IgM anti-endothelial antibodies results in prolonged cardiac xenograft survival. Transplant. Proc. **22:** 1077.

4. HENRY, M. L., L. K. HAN, C. G. OROSZ & R. M. FERGUSON. 1990. Modification of xenograft hyperacute rejection via xenoantibody depletion. Transplant. Proc. **22:** 1081.

5. HASAN R., J. B. VAN DEN BOGAERDE, J. WALLWORK & D. J. G. WHITE. 1992. Evidence that long-term survival of concordant xenografts is achieved by inhibition of antispecies antibody production. Transplantation **54:** 408.

6. PETERS, G. J., S. L. SHARMA, G. LAURENSSE & H. M. PINEDO. 1987. Inhibition of pyrimidine de novo synthesis by DUP-785 (NSC 368390). Invest. New Drugs **5:** 235.

7. PETERS, G. J., G. SCHWARTSMANN, J. C. NADAL, et al. 1990. In vivo inhibition of the pyrimidine de novo enzyme dihydroorotic acid dehydrogenase by brequinar sodium (DUP-785; NSC 368390) in mice and patients. Cancer Res. **50:** 4644.

8. CHEN, S.-F., R. L. RUBEN & D. L. DEXTER. 1986. Mechanism of action of the novel anticancer agent 6-fluoro-2-(2'-fluoro-1,1'-biphenyl-4-yl)-3-methyl-4-quinoline-carboxylic acid sodium salt (NSC 368390): inhibition of de novo pyrimidine nucleotide biosynthesis. Cancer Res. **46:** 5014.

9. CRAMER, D. V., F. A. CHAPMAN, B. D. JAFFEE, et al. 1992. The prolongation of concordant hamster-to-rat cardiac xenografts by brequinar sodium. Transplantation **54:** 403.

10. THOMSON, A. W., J. WOO, B. LEMSTER, S. TODO, J. J. FUNG & T. E. STARZL. 1993. Potentiation of the antilymphocytic activity of brequinar sodium for murine lymphocytes by exogenous cytidine. Transplant. Proc. **25:** 704.

11. WOO, J., B. LEMSTER, K. TAMURA, T. E. STARZL & A. W. THOMSON. 1993. The antilymphocytic activity of brequinar sodium and its potentiation by cytidine: effects on lymphocyte proliferation and cytokine production. Transplantation **56:** 374.

12. ONO, K. & E. S. LINDSEY. 1969. Improved technique of heart transplantation in rats. J. Thoracic Cardiovasc. Surg. **57:** 225.

Efficacy of FK506 in Renal Transplantation

SHIRO TAKAHARA

Department of Urology
Osaka University Hospital
Yamadaoka 2-2
Suita-City
Osaka, Japan 565

FK506 is estimated to be a more potent immunosuppressive agent than cyclosporine (CyA). Its strong immunosuppressive activity was shown *in vitro, in vivo,* and in experimental organ transplantation with much smaller doses than those of CyA. In clinical liver transplantation, FK506 was superior in suppressing rejection and CyA-resistant rejection.[1]

Its effectiveness in renal transplantation was also demonstrated in studies from a Pittsburgh group and a Japanese group.[2,3] The major adverse effects of FK506 were renal impairment,[4] hyperglycemia,[5] hyperkalemia, cardiac symptoms, and abdominal distention. The present study indicated that the incidence of adverse effects of FK506 would be decreased if the dosage were adjusted by monitoring the blood level of FK506.

PATIENTS AND METHODS

The Early Phase II Study

Thirty-seven primary renal transplant patients were enrolled in this study (TABLE 1). All recipients were 16 years of age or older and had ABO blood matching. They were negative in the T-cell cross-match test.

FK506 (0.075 mg/kg) was given every 12 hours intravenously over 4 hours for 3 consecutive days after revascularization, followed by 0.15 mg/kg orally every 12 hours (FIGURE 1). The daily dose of FK506 was adjusted depending on the patient's clinical status or the severity of the acute rejection. Prednisolone was used as a concomitant immunosuppressive agent in accordance with the protocol.

The Late Phase II Study

Seventy primary renal transplant patients were enrolled in this study (TABLE 1). Inclusion criteria of the transplant recipients were the same as those of the early phase II study.

An oral dose of FK506, 0.15 mg/kg per day every 12 hours, was initially administered for 2 days before transplantation; 0.1 mg/kg per day of the drug was given intravenously for 3 consecutive days after revascularization (FIGURE 1). The oral dose was adjusted to maintain the drug whole blood trough level at 20 ng/ml for 10 days after transplantation and 15 ng/ml from 11 to 90 days. The dose was adjusted when rejection or adverse events were observed.

Assay Method of FK506 Blood Level

Blood level of FK506 was measured by the double antibody enzyme-linked immunosorbent assay (ELISA) (see FIGURE 2). Both plasma and whole blood samples were obtained simultaneously for the early phase II study, and only whole blood samples were used for the late phase II study.

Heparinized whole blood was centrifuged at room temperature ranging from 20–25°C, and supernatant plasma was obtained. The blood samples were extracted by dichloromethane. These samples were processed by the ELISA method. The detection limit was 0.5 ng/ml in whole blood and 0.05 ng/ml in plasma. The variations of both intra- and interassay coefficients were less than 20%.

RESULTS

Classification of Patients

In the early phase II study, one patient was excluded due to unsuitable entry criteria (ABO mismatch) and one patient dropped out because of a dose schedule

TABLE 1. Recipient and Donor Characteristics

		Early Phase II ($n = 37$)	Late Phase II ($n = 70$)
Donor	Living-related	31	39
	Cadaver	6 (16.2%)	31 (44.3%)
Age	Donor	55.3 ± 7.6	50.2 ± 12.0
	Recipient	31.6 ± 8.4	36.9 ± 8.9
HLA	Mismatched ABDR antigens	1.8 ± 1.0	1.8 ± 1.2
PRA	0%	31 (83.8%)	55 (78.6%)
	0–10%	4	12
	>10%	0	3
ATN	Yes	5 (13.5%)	24 (34.3%)

violation. In the late phase II study, one patient was withdrawn from the study due to violation of concomitant drug regulation. In the early phase II study, 26 (74.3%) completed the 12-week treatment with FK506, and 12 (34.3%) changed the regimen under the protocol because of adverse effects or the onset of acute rejection. In the late phase II study, 55 (79.7%) completed it and 14 (20.3%) changed the regimen within 12 weeks.

The reasons of discontinuation of FK506 were nephrotoxicity (30.4%), rejection (17.4%), rejection + nephrotoxicity (8.7%), cardiac symptoms (13.0%), infection (13.0%), hyperglycemia (8.7%), pancreatitis (4.3%), and rupture of aneurysm (4.3%).

Patient and Graft Survival

In the early phase II study, all 37 renal transplant patients, including 12 who switched to different regimens from the original one, were alive, and all renal grafts were functioning at the end of the 12-week treatment. In the late phase II study, the

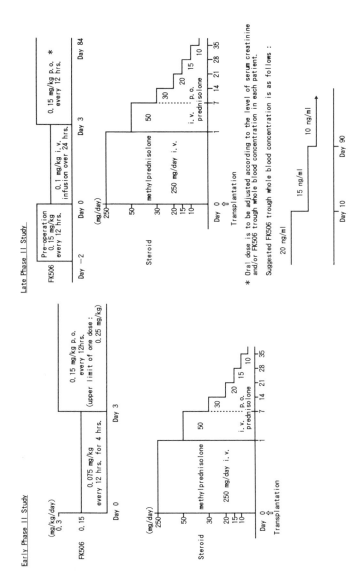

FIGURE 1. Treatment schedule of FK506 and steroids.

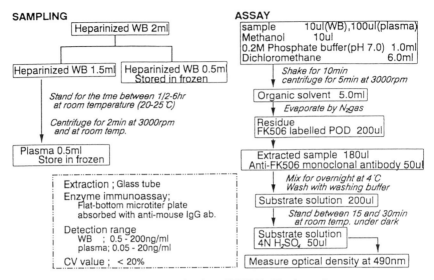

FIGURE 2. Determination of FK506 in blood samples.

patient survival rate at 3 months after transplantation was 95.7%. All grafts from living donors were functioning at the end of the treatment. The total graft survival rate at 3 months was 94.2%.

Efficacy of FK506

Acute rejection was observed in 16 patients (45.7%) of the early phase II study and 25 cases (36.2%) of the late phase II study. Steroid-resistant rejection episodes were observed in 5 of the 16 patients (31.3%) in the early phase II study and in 15 of the 25 patients (60.0%) in the late phase II study.

Safety of FK506

Major adverse events in the early phase II study were renal impairment (44.4%), abdominal distention (30.6%), cardiac symptoms (27.8%), hyperkalemia (27.8%), tremor (27.8%), hyperglycemia (25.0%), and headache (19.4%) (TABLE 2).

Major adverse events in the late phase II study were renal impairment (27.1%), abdominal distention (14.3%), cardiac symptoms (18.6%), hyperkalemia (25.7%), tremor (10.0%), hyperglycemia (31.4%), and headache (5.7%) (TABLE 2). There were no life-threatening adverse events.

In the early phase II study, insulin-dependent hyperglycemia occurred in 7 patients within 3 months after transplantation. However, insulin therapy was required in only 5 patients between 4 and 6 months, and in 2 patients between 7 and 12 months. In the late phase II study, 17 of the 22 hyperglycemic patients required insulin therapy, but insulin therapy was withdrawn in 12 of them within 5 months.

Renal impairment was diagnosed by the findings of tubular lesion with vacuolization or calcification and vascular lesion of the arteriole in graft biopsy specimens.

Renal impairment was observed in 16 patients of the early phase II study and 19 patients of the late phase II study. In the late phase II study, complete recovery of renal function was observed in 7 of the 19 patients. The dosage of FK506 was reduced in 5 of them and was discontinued in 1.

Infections were observed in 30.6% of the early phase II study and 22.9% of the late phase II study. The incidence of CMV virus infection was high. One patient died of CMV infection, and one died of meningitis and sepsis caused by *Staphylococcus aureus*. One patient who died of rupture of mycotic aneurysm had aurinary tract infection caused by *Candida* from the cadaveric donor. All patients with infections except for these three recovered.

Monitoring of FK506 Blood Concentration

Plasma Separation

The effect of temperature of whole blood incubation and plasma separation on distribution of FK506 in human blood was investigated (FIGURE 3). When the

TABLE 2. Adverse Effects

	Number of Patients (%)			
Symptom	Late Phase II Study (n = 70)		Early Phase II Study (n = 36)	
Tremor	7 (10.0)		10 (27.8)	
Headache	4 (5.7)		7 (19.4)	
Numbness	2 (2.9)	14	1 (2.8)	15
Peripheral sensory abnormality	1 (1.4)	(20.0)		(41.7)
Agitation—unconsciousness			1 (2.8)	
Disorientation			1 (2.8)	
Chest pain	7 (10.0)		5 (13.9)	
Abnormal ECG	4 (5.7)		2 (5.6)	
Chest discomfort	2 (2.9)		2 (5.6)	
Distressed feeling of chest	1 (1.4)	13		10
Palpitation	1 (1.4)	(18.6)	2 (5.6)	(27.8)
Decreased cardiac function	1 (1.4)			
Decreased ejection fraction			1 (2.8)	
Tachycardia at exercise			1 (2.8)	
Abdominal distention	10 (14.3)		11 (30.6)	
Nausea—vomiting	6 (8.6)		4 (11.1)	
Diarrhea	4 (5.7)	14	1 (2.8)	17
Abdominal pain	1 (1.4)	(20.0)		(47.2)
Gastric ulcer			2 (5.6)	
Renal impairment	19 (27.1)		16 (44.4)	
Polyuria			2 (5.6)	
Hyperglycemia	22 (31.4)		9 (25.0)	
Acute pancreatitis	1 (1.4)		1 (2.8)	
Hot flush	9 (12.9)		2 (5.6)	
Facial hot flush	1 (1.4)			
Pruritus	2 (2.9)			
Alopecia	1 (1.4)			
Gingival papilloma	1 (1.4)			

temperature ranged between 1–25°C at the time of equilibration centrifugation, there was a minimal change of the plasma concentration of FK506, whereas in the temperature range between 30–37°C, the plasma concentration increased markedly. The ratio of the plasma concentrations between 25°C and 37°C was 2.2 at 20 ng/ml of whole blood spiked with FK506 and was 2.5 at 200 ng/ml.

Pharmacokinetics

The concentration of FK506 after intravenous administration of 0.075 mg/kg over 4 hours ($n = 10$) declined rapidly in the initial phase, and then slowly reached the distribution equilibrium (FIGURE 4). The half-life of FK506 ranged from 4.27–18.8 (mean 8.04 ± 4.87) hours for the whole blood and 3.77–12.4 (mean 6.86 ± 2.91) hours for the plasma. $AUC_{(0-12\,h)}$ (area under the blood concentration–time curve) was 300–758 (mean 481 ± 129) ng × h/ml for the whole blood and

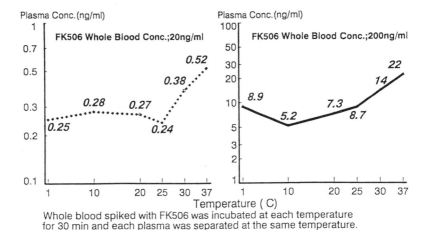

Whole blood spiked with FK506 was incubated at each temperature for 30 min and each plasma was separated at the same temperature.

FIGURE 3. Effect of temperature of whole blood incubation and plasma separation on distribution of FK506 in human blood.

8.02–73.1 (mean 20.0 ± 19.5) ng × h/ml for the plasma. Twelve patients were examined for pharmacokinetics of FK506 given at 0.15 mg/kg orally. FK506 was absorbed quickly after administration and reached peak concentration within 2 hours in approximately two-thirds of the patients. $AUC_{(0-12\,h)}$ was 95.1–743 (mean 249 ± 180) ng × h/ml for the whole blood and 1.67–13.3 (mean 5.94 ± 3.39) ng × h/ml for the plasma.

Correlation between Acute Rejection or Adverse Events and FK506 Blood Level

We examined the correlation between acute rejection or adverse events and the FK506 trough level. In the early phase II study, the mean whole blood trough level (BTL) in patients with adverse effects was 23.2 ± 9.7 ng/ml and the mean plasma trough level (PTL) was 0.69 ± 0.46 ng/ml. The BTL in patients with adverse effects was higher than those in the control group who had no episodes ($p < 0.01$). The PTL

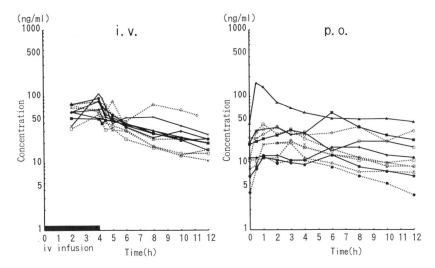

FIGURE 4. Pharmacokinetics of FK506 (whole blood concentration).

between both groups showed significant difference ($p < 0.05$). Similarly, the BTL in patients with renal impairment was 23.9 ± 7.9 ng/ml and the PTL was 0.64 ± 0.43 ng/ml. The BTL in patients with renal impairment was statistically higher than that in patients with acute rejection ($p < 0.01$). There was no significant difference in PTL between both groups.

FIGURE 5 shows the average trough levels up to the onset of each episode in patients with acute rejection or side effects. The trough levels in the whole blood in patients with side effects showed continuously high levels of > 20 ng/ml, which were

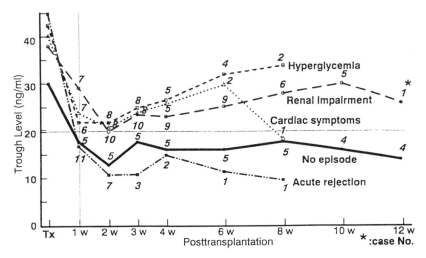

FIGURE 5. Mean FK506 whole blood trough level up to onset of episode (rejection/adverse effects) (early phase II study).

significantly higher than that in patients with no episode. The trough level in the whole blood in patients with acute rejection was less than 15 ng/ml which was lower than that in patients with no episode.

The trough levels in the plasma did not show any significant difference between both groups.

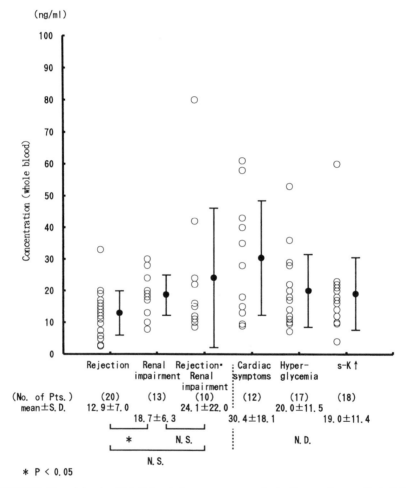

FIGURE 6. Trough levels within 5 days before appearance of rejection or adverse effects (late phase II study).

In the late phase II study, the BTL in patients with rejection was 12.9 ± 7.0 ng/ml and the BTL in those with renal impairment was 18.7 ± 6.3 ng/ml (FIGURE 6). This difference was statistically significant ($p < 0.05$). In patients with cardiac symptoms, hyperglycemia, and hyperkalemia, the trough levels were 30.4 ± 18.1 ng/ml, 20.0 ± 11.5 ng/ml, and 19.0 ± 11.4 ng/ml, respectively (FIGURE 6).

DISCUSSION

The present early[3,5] and late[6] phase II studies produced valuable data on the efficacy, safety, optimal therapeutic dose, and blood level of FK506 in patients undergoing kidney transplantation.

In particular, a higher reproducibility was indicated in blood level monitoring by whole blood samples than by plasma samples. This monitoring method was achieved by the liquid phase method using dichloromethane. The method is different from the column extraction method available in the United States. It is known that the liquid phase extraction method is better for analysis recovery than the column extraction method.

It is concluded that the drug concentration of FK506 is better monitored with whole blood than with plasma because of the following reasons: (1) the distribution of FK506 to the plasma is temperature dependent, (2) the concentration of FK506 is prominently lower in the plasma than in the whole blood, (3) the fluctuation of the drug concentration is more prominent in the plasma than in the whole blood. Our recent blood level monitoring of FK506 was performed with whole blood samples.

We also succeeded in reducing the dosage of prednisolone in more than half of the patients to less than 10 mg/day at 4 months after transplantation.

To decrease the rate of adverse events, the blood level of FK506 should be at the lowest level. The purpose of our studies was to determine an optimal protocol of FK506 in renal transplantation by monitoring FK506 blood level.

In the early phase II study, the dosage of FK506 was principally adjusted to maintain certain whole blood trough levels depending on the rejection episode or adverse events.

In the late phase II study, FK506 dosage was adjusted to the optimal trough level (FIGURE 1). The results of this study were compared with those of the early phase II study.

There was no obvious difference in graft and patient survival rates between these two studies. However, the incidence of acute rejection within 3 months after transplantation was lower in the late phase II study (36.2%) than in the early phase II study (45.7%). We also observed that the mean trough level of FK506 within 5 days before a rejection episode was 12.9 ± 7.0 ng/ml, which was lower than the minimum optimal level (15 ng/ml) of the late phase II study.

As for adverse effects of FK506, the incidence of renal impairment, abdominal distention, and cardiac symptoms decreased more in the *late phase II study* than in the *late phase II study.*

However, the incidence of hyperglycemia increased in the late phase II study. Hyperglycemia was frequently observed (31.4%) in spite of the dose adjustment of FK506. In some cases of hyperglycemia, insulin therapy was unnecessary for several months with reduction of the dosage of FK506 by blood level monitoring. Further studies are necessary to detect the diabetogenicity and to prevent it.

In conclusion, this multicenter study of FK506 therapy showed that a good graft function and lower adverse events could be achieved by monitoring the FK506 trough level in the whole blood.

REFERENCES

1. STARZL, T. E., S. TODO, J. FUNG, A. J. DEMETRIUS, R. VENKATARAMANAN & A. JAIN. 1989. FK506 for human liver, kidney and pancreas transplantation. Lancet 2: 1000–1004.
2. STARZL, T. E., J. FUNG, M. JORDAN, R. SHAPIRO, A. TZAKIS, J. MCCAULEY, J. JOHNSTON, Y.

IWAKI, A. JAIN, M. ALESSIANI & S. TODO. 1990. Kidney transplantation under FK506. JAMA **264:** 63–67.
3. Japanese FK506 Study Group. 1992. Japanese study of kidney transplantation. 1. Results of early phase II study. Transplant Int. **5:** S524–S528.
4. RANDHAWA, P. S., R. SHAPIRO, M. L. JORDAN, T. E. STARZL & A. J. DEMETRIS. 1993. The histopathological changes associated with allograft rejection and drug toxicity in renal transplant recipients maintained on FK506. Am. J. Surg. Pathol. **17:** 60–68.
5. Japanese FK506 Study Group. 1992. Japanese study of FK506 on kidney transplantation. 2. Follow-up study of FK506-treated patients. Transplant Int. **5:** S552–S555, 1992.
6. Japanese FK506 Study Group. 1993. Japanese study of FK506 on kidney transplantation: results of late phase II study. Transplant. Proc. **25:** 649–654.

Incidence of CD4$^+$ IL-2Rα$^+$ and CD4$^+$ CD45RA$^+$ T-Cells in Progressive Multiple Sclerosis and the Influence of Short-Term (3 Months) FK 506 Therapy

ANGUS W. THOMSON,[a] JACKY WOO, BONNIE LEMSTER,
WILLIAM IRISH, LINDA L. HUANG, PATRICIA B. CARROLL,
HORATIO R. RILO, KAREEM ABU-ELMAGD,
AND BENJAMIN EIDELMAN[b]

Departments of Surgery and Neurology[b]
University of Pittsburgh Medical Center
Pittsburgh, Pennsylvania 15213

Multiple sclerosis (MS) is postulated to be a T-cell-mediated autoimmune disease associated with abnormalities in immune regulation.[1–3] A number of changes in the subset distribution of peripheral blood T-cells has been observed in MS, and many of these resemble the alterations seen in other autoimmune disorders, such as systemic lupus erythematosus.[1–3] The CD4$^+$ T (helper) cell population can be subdivided into two mutually exclusive subsets,[4] CD45RO$^+$ (CD29$^+$) inducers of help for B-cell antibody production and (CD45RA$^+$ = 2H4$^+$) inducers of suppressor CD8$^+$ T-cells. A selective loss of circulating suppressor-inducer T-cells has been reported in progressive MS.[5]

Clinical trials with the potent inhibitor of CD4$^+$ T-cell activation cyclosporine A (CsA) in MS have not yielded substantial positive results.[6] This may be due to failure of CsA to pass the blood-brain barrier or to resistance of chronically stimulated T-cells to the drug. FK 506 is a powerful new immunosuppressant with a similar though not identical molecular action to CsA.[7] FK 506 is considerably more potent than CsA and, unlike the latter drug, has the capacity to reverse cellular rejection of organ allografts.[8] It also inhibits the development of experimental allergic encephalomyelitis—a disease that mimics MS in laboratory animals.[9] Recently, a trial of FK 506 in progressive MS has begun at the University of Pittsburgh Medical Center (UPMC). Here we report early (3-month follow-up) observations both on activated CD4$^+$ T-cells and regulatory CD4$^+$ T-cell subsets in peripheral blood of these FK 506–treated subjects.

PATIENTS AND METHODS

Fifteen patients (8 male, 7 female; age range 27–56 years; median 43 years) with clinically confirmed MS were studied during outpatient visits to the UPMC. Progressive MS was indicated by a decline of at least one grade on the Kurzke disability status scale or ambulation index during the preceding nine months, without periods

---

[a]Correspondence to: University of Pittsburgh Medical Center, W1544 Biomedical Science Tower, Terrace and Lothrop Streets, Pittsburgh, Pennsylvania 15213.

of improvement. The pretreatment Kurtzke scores ranged from 5.5–7.5, and the ambulation index range was 2.0–8.0. No patients had received steroids for at least one month, or immunosuppressive drugs for at least one year, at the time of blood sampling. The minimum follow-up time on FK 506 treatment was 91 days (range: 91–234 days; median 143 days). Blood was drawn before start of treatment, at 7, 14, 21, and 28 days and monthly thereafter.

FLOW CYTOMETRY

Monoclonal antibodies used in flow cytometric analysis of patients' peripheral blood mononuclear cells or those obtained from healthy adults included phycoery-thrin (PE) conjugated anti-CD4, PE-conjugated anti-CD8, and FITC-conjugated anti-CD25 (IL-2Rα-chain), and were diluted 1/10 in Hanks' balanced salt solution (HBSS) with 1% BSA and 0.1% NaN_3. PE-conjugated mouse IgG and FITC-conjugated mouse IgG were used as isotypic controls. These antibodies were purchased from Dako, Carpinteria, Calif. To determine the proportion of 2H4+ cells within the CD4+ cell population, a kit containing FITC-conjugated T4 and RD1-conjugated anti-2H4 was purchased from Coulter Immunology, Hialeah, Fla. The antibodies were diluted 1/10 in the HBSS/1% BSA/0.1 NaN_3 buffer. Cells isolated from blood samples were incubated with diluted antibodies for 30 min at 4°C. After incubation, cells were washed twice with buffer and were fixed in 1% paraformalde-hyde until analysis by flow cytometry. Five thousand gated cells were counted using a FACSTAR flow cytometer, and results were expressed as percentage positive cells.

FUNCTIONAL STUDIES

Responses of peripheral blood lymphocytes to recombinant (r) human (h) IL-2 (Gibco, Grand Island, N.Y.; 30 units/ml) and concanavalin A (Con A; Sigma; 5 μg/ml) were measured. Cells (2×10^5 well) were cultured in round-bottomed, 96-well microculture plates in 200 μl of RPMI-1640 (Gibco) containing 10% heat-inactivated fetal bovine serum for 72 h. ^{3}HTdR was added at 48 h, and cells were harvested onto glass fiber discs before counting in a liquid scintillation counter. Results are expressed as counts per minute (cpm).

STATISTICAL ANALYSES

Rate of change in (1) incidence of positively staining cells or (2) cpm were determined for each patient using simple logistic regression and simple linear regression respectively.[10,11] These rates were summarized using weighted analysis[12] and expressed on the logit (incidence) or natural logarithmic scales (cpm), respectively. The Wilcoxon Sign Rank test, a nonparametric equivalent to the paired "t"-test was used to compare pre- and post- (3 months) FK 506 values, while the Wilcoxon Rank Sum test was used to compare pre–FK 506 values and those obtained from normal volunteers.

RESULTS AND DISCUSSION

The mean incidence of CD4+ peripheral blood lymphocytes and the mean CD4:CD8 ratio in the 15 MS patients before treatment with FK 506 were 48.1 ± 7.4% and 1.77 ± 0.44, respectively. At 3 months after the start of FK 506 treatment, these values were reduced to 42.3 ± 8.5% and 1.45 ± 0.32, respectively. The reduction in CD4:CD8 ratio compared to the pretreatment value was statistically significant ($p = 0.013$). As shown in FIGURE 1, there was also a significant reduction ($p < 0.001$) in CD4+ IL-2Rα+ T-cells and a concomitant, though not statistically significant, elevation in the mean incidence of suppressor-inducer CD4+ 2H4+ T cells compared to pretreatment values. The significant relation between the incidences of IL-2Rα+ and 2H4+ cells in blood samples obtained from the 15 MS

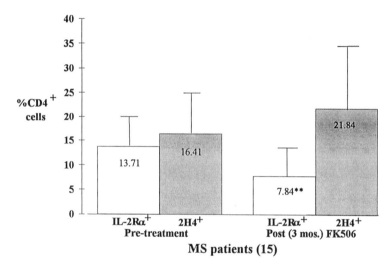

FIGURE 1. The incidences of IL-2Rα+ CD4+ and 2H4+ CD4+ T-cells determined by two-color flow cytometry in peripheral blood of 15 patients with progressive MS before and 3 months after start of FK 506 treatment. Results are means + 1 standard deviation. **,$p < 0.001$ compared to pretreatment value.

patients at various times before or after the start of FK 506 treatment (65 samples) is shown in FIGURE 2. The proliferative responses of FK 506–treated patients' lymphocytes either to rh IL-2 or to Con A did not differ significantly from pretreatment levels (data not shown).

TABLE 1 shows the mean rate of change in immunological parameters in the 15 patients studied, in relation to time on FK 506. In this analysis, all time points for which data were available (duration of follow-up 91–234 days) were taken into account. Significant ($p < 0.05$) negative rates of change with time on FK 506 were observed for CD4, CD4:CD8, CD4 IL-2Rα, CD8 IL-2Rα, and the response to Con A. In contrast, the rate of change in CD4+2H4+ cells was positively correlated ($p < 0.05$) with time on FK 506.

Previous studies have shown that activated T-cells are increased in the peripheral blood of patients with progressive MS.[13] In the present study, pretreatment levels of

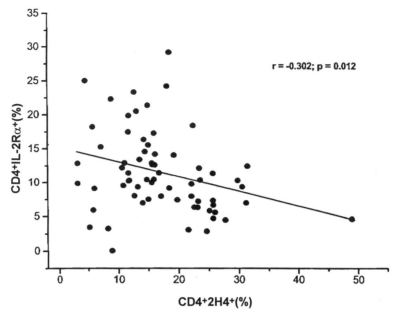

FIGURE 2. Relationship between IL-2Rα⁺ and 2H4⁺ cells in a total of 65 blood samples obtained from 15 MS patients before and at various times after the start of FK 506 treatment (median follow-up time, 143 days).

activated (IL-2Rα⁺) CD4⁺ cells (13.7 ± 6.3%) were significantly elevated above normal values for healthy adults (9.3 ± 2.1%; $p < 0.025$), but were reduced significantly 3 months after start of FK 506 treatment. This *in vivo* effect of the drug is consistent with its known capacity to inhibit CD4⁺ T-cell activation and cytokine production *in vitro*.[7] To our knowledge, this is the first time that a reduction in blood

TABLE 1. Immunological Parameters Affected by Time on FK 506 (15 MS patients; minimum follow-up 3 months)

Parameter	Average Rate of Change (Bw)	s.e.$_w$[e]	95% Confidence Limits	
			Lower	Upper
CD4⁺ cells	−0.0129[b]	0.0035	−0.0197	−0.0060[a]
CD8⁺ cells	0.0009[b]	0.0005	−0.0000	0.0018 NS
CD4:CD8 ratio	−0.0026[d]	0.0012	−0.0049	−0.0004[a] ↓
CD4⁺ IL-2Rα⁺ cells	−0.0063[b]	0.0022	−0.0106	−0.0020[a] ↓
CD8⁺ IL-2Rα⁺ cells	−0.0048[b]	0.0022	−0.0092	−0.0005[a] ↓
CD4⁺ 2H4⁺ cells	0.0055[b]	0.0025	0.0005	0.0104[a] ↑
IL-2 response	0.0025[c]	0.0017	−0.0008	0.0058 NS
Con A response	−0.0068[c]	0.0026	−0.0118	−0.0017[a] ↓

[a] $p < 0.05$.
[b] Rate of change in incidence expressed on the logit scale.
[c] Rate of change in counts/min expressed on the natural logarithmic scale.
[d] Rate of change expressed on the linear scale.
[e] Standard error of weighted average.

levels of activated T-cells has been demonstrated in nontransplant patients treated with FK 506. It has been argued previously that levels of CD4+ 2H4+ (suppressor-inducer) T-cells in MS may correlate positively with T-cell suppression and with inhibition of T-cell and B-cell clones reactive with elements of the central nervous system.[5] Our preliminary results suggest that FK 506 inhibits CD4+ T-cell activation in progressive MS and that there is an increase in suppressor-inducer cells that is related to time on FK 506 therapy. At present, it is too early to determine whether the drug significantly affects the course of the disease or whether these changes in nonspecific immunological parameters are related to change in function of lymphocytes or other cells responsible for the immunologically mediated neurological lesions in MS.

REFERENCES

1. HAFLER, D. A. & H. L. WEINER. 1989. MS: a CNS and systemic autoimmune disease. Immunol. Today **10:** 104–107.
2. HINTZEN, R. Q., C. H. POLMAN, C. J. LUCAS & R. A. W. VAN LIER. 1992. Multiple sclerosis: immunological findings and possible implications for therapy. J. Neuroimmunol. **39:** 1–10.
3. MARTIN, R., H. F. MCFARLAND & D. E. MCFARLIN. 1992. Immunological aspects of demyelinating diseases. Annu. Rev. Immunol. **10:** 153–87.
4. MORIMOTO, C., E. L. REINHERZ, Y. BOREL & S. F. SCHLOSSMAN. 1983. Direct demonstration of the human suppressor inducer subset by anti-T cell antibodies. J. Immunol. **130:** 157–161.
5. MORIMOTO, C., D. A. HAFLER, H. L. WEINER, N. L. LETVIN, M. HAGAN, J. DALEY & S. F. SCHLOSSMAN. 1987. Selective loss of suppressor-inducer T-cell subset in progressive multiple sclerosis N. Engl. J. Med. **316:** 67–72.
6. TINDALL, R. S. A. 1992. Immunointervention with cyclosporin A in autoimmune neurological disorders. J. Autoimmunity **5**(Suppl. A): 301–303.
7. THOMSON, A. W. 1989. FK 506—how much potential? Immunol. Today **10:** 6–9.
8. STARZL, T. E., A. W. THOMSON, S. TODO & J. J. FUNG, Eds. 1991. Proceedings of the First International Congress on FK 506. Transplant Proc. **23:** 2709–3380.
9. INAMURA, N., M. HAHIMOTO, K. NAKAHARA, Y. NAKAJIMA, M. NISHIO, H. AOKI, I. YAMAGUCH & M. KOHSAKA. 1988. Immunosuppressive effect of FK 506 on experimental allergic encephalomyelitis in rats. Int. J. Immunopharmacol. **10:** 991–995.
10. COLLETT, D. 1991. Modelling Binary Data: 277. Chapman and Hall. London, England.
11. MONTGOMERY, D. C. 1981. Introduction to Linear Regression Analysis. Wiley. New York, N.Y.
12. MATTHEWS, J. N. S. 1993. A refinement to the analysis of serial data using summary measures. Stat. Med. **12:** 27–37.
13. HAFLER, D. A., D. A. FOX, S. E. MANNING, S. F. SCHLOSSMAN, E. L. REINHERZ & H. L. WEINER. 1985. In vivo activated T lymphocytes in the peripheral blood and cerebrospinal fluid of patients with multiple sclerosis. N. Engl. J. Med. **312:** 1405–1411.

FK 506 Inhibits Cytokine Gene and Adhesion Molecule Expression in Psoriatic Skin Lesions[a]

B. LEMSTER, H. R. RILO, P. B. CARROLL,
M. A. NALESNIK, AND A. W. THOMSON[b]

Departments of Surgery, Pathology, and
Molecular Genetics and Biochemistry
University of Pittsburgh
Pittsburgh, Pennsylvania 15213

Psoriasis is a genetically determined, cutaneous inflammatory disorder, characterized by epidermal keratinocyte hyperproliferation and is thought to involve dysregulation of the skin immune system.[1-3] The dermal infiltrate consists mainly of T lymphocytes (predominantly CD4+) and macrophages. There is also an increase in the number of antigen-presenting cells (APC; including Langerhans cells) capable of activating autologous T-cells. Cell lines established from lesional psoriatic skin are predominantly CDw29+ (helper-inducer) T-cells,[4] and these T-cell clones demonstrate autoreactivity[4,5] towards autologous epidermal cells or peripheral blood mononuclear cells.[5]

There is also evidence of the up regulation in affected skin of a variety of cytokines that stimulate endothelial cell adhesiveness for lymphocytes. These include interleukin-1 (IL-1), tumor necrosis factor-α (TNF-α), interferon-γ (IFN-γ), and IL-4. Epidermal keratinocytes (especially when injured) have been shown to secrete IL-1, IL-3, IL-6, IL-7, IL-8, IL-10, granulocyte-macrophage colony stimulating factor, other cell growth factors, and TNF-α.[6] With the exception of IL-10, which down regulates cutaneous inflammation, these cytokines have proinflammatory properties. IL-1 and TNF-α up regulate intercellular adhesion molecule-1 (ICAM-1) and endothelial-leucocyte adhesion molecule-1 (ELAM-1; E-selectin) on vascular endothelium. Moreover, skin-homing, infiltrating T-cells may produce IFN-γ, which can induce ICAM-1 expression on keratinocytes and is therefore likely to promote leucocyte exocytosis into the epidermis. Antigen-dependent, skin APC-T-cell interactions that amplify and perpetuate the immune response may then ensue.

The immune suppressant cyclosporine A (CsA) inhibits selectively CD4+ T-cell activation and cytokine production and is highly effective when administered systemically, in the treatment of psoriasis.[7] Among its reported effects on lesional skin are inhibition of adhesion molecule expression on vascular endothelium and marked reductions in the inflammatory T-cell infiltrate. FK 506 is a new immunosuppressant, with a similar but not identical molecular action to CsA.[8-10] FK 506, however, is considerably more potent than CsA[9] and is effective both in the prevention and the reversal of clinical organ allograft rejection.[11] It may also exhibit fewer side effects than CsA. Recently, it has been reported that FK 506 is effective in the treatment of

[a] This work was supported in part by a grant from the United Scleroderma Foundation.
[b] Author to whom correspondence should be addressed at: University of Pittsburgh Medical Center, W1544 Biomedical Science Tower, Terrace and Lothrop Streets, Pittsburgh, Pennsylvania 15213.

severe recalcitrant, chronic plaque psoriasis.[12] We have therefore examined the influence of FK 506 on cytokine gene and adhesion molecule expression in psoriatic skin with the aim of defining its effects on these components of the cutaneous inflammatory response.

MATERIALS AND METHODS

Patients

A total of 11 patients (6 male, 5 female) aged 29–53 years (mean 38.7 years) with severe, chronic, recalcitrant, plaque-forming psoriasis were studied. All treatments for psoriasis, except for bland emollients, were stopped 2 weeks prior to FK 506 therapy. Patients received 0.1–0.3 mg/kg per day FK 506 (Fujisawa Pharmaceutical Company, Osaka, Japan); plasma trough drug levels at the time of follow-up biopsy ranged from 0.3–1.5 ng/ml (mean 1.0 ng/ml).

Biopsies

Five-millimeter punch biopsies were taken under local anesthesia (lidocaine) from lesional skin immediately before the start of FK 506 and at various intervals thereafter. Tissue was mounted in OCT (Miles Inc., Elkhart, Ind.), snap frozen on dry ice, and stored at −70°C. Normal skin specimens from healthy adults were also examined for comparison. Conventional histological examination was performed on hematoxylin and eosin stained 5 μm sections.

Immunohistochemistry

Two-micron-thick cryostat sections were fixed in acetone for 5 min, air dried, then incubated for 1 h at room temperature with predetermined optimal dilutions of primary mouse IgG monoclonal antibodies directed against human ICAM-1 (1:100; Gen Trak Inc., Plymouth Meeting, Pa.) or E-selectin (1:75; BioSource International, Camarillo, Calif.). The sections were then incubated for 30 min with biotin-conjugated horse anti–mouse IgG (1:200; Vector Lab. Inc., Burlingame, Calif.) in 4% v/v normal human serum in Dulbecco's phosphate-buffered saline (PBS). They were then treated for 30 min with avidin biotin complex peroxidase (ABC-P) (1:200; Vector Lab. Inc.) in PBS, and the color reaction was developed for 6 min, using a peroxidase chromogen kit (AEC; Biomedia Corp., Foster City, Calif.). Controls included the omission of primary antibody and the use of an irrelevant antibody isotype control. Sections were counterstained lightly with hematoxylin. Stained cells in coded sections were examined at ×400 magnification in a minimum of five sequential grid fields.

Detection of Cytokine mRNA Using the Polymerase Chain Reaction

Total cellular RNA was isolated from approx. 300 mg of frozen lesional or normal skin, using a modification of the acid guanidinium thiocyanate/phenol/chloroform extraction procedure.[13] The frozen tissue was homogenized in RNAzol B

(Biotecx Labs., Inc., Houston, Tex.) with a Polytron (Brinkman Instruments Co. Inc., Westbury, N.Y.), and RNA was stored at $-70°C$. The RNA concentration was determined spectrophotometrically. First strand cDNA was synthesized from total RNA (1 µg) using reverse transcriptase and oligo-dT primers. Oligonucleotides used were synthesized at the University of Pittsburgh DNA synthesis facility. Aliquots of the cDNA were used with specific primers for 30–40 cycles of PCR amplification (DNA Thermal Cycler; Perkin-Elmer, Cetus Norwalk, Conn.) on the same samples, with synthetic primers for β-actin as control. PCR products were analyzed by electrophoresis on 2.0% agarose gels and visualized by ethidium bromide staining.

RESULTS

Clinical Response

A marked improvement in psoriasis was observed in all patients within 4 weeks of the start of FK 506 therapy. Histological examination revealed a diminution in the inflammatory cell infiltrate, with progressive loss of elongated rete pegs and a return towards a fully formed stratum corneum.

Cytokine Gene Expression

Samples from five patients before start of pretreatment and from two patients whose skin had cleared in response to FK 506 therapy were analyzed for cytokine message by PCR. The results are shown in FIGURE 1. Cytokines analyzed included IL-2, IL-4, IL-6, IL-8, IL-10, IFN-γ, and TNF-α, with β-actin as a control. Patient samples studied both pre- and posttreatment showed no detectable IL-2 or IL-4 message. IL-6 was detected in a majority (4/5) of pretreatment samples, but only very weakly in one of the posttreatment biopsies. Three of the five pretreatment patients showed IL-8 message, but this was not detected in skin that had cleared in response to FK 506. IL-10 was detected in all samples; it was noted however, that the signal for this cytokine was especially strong in one of the posttreatment biopsies. IFN-γ was detected in 5/5 pretreatment biopsies, but in neither of the patients on FK 506. TNF-α was detected in all patients with active disease and was also expressed in the patients on treatment.

Adhesion Molecule Expression

In active disease, both the dermis and epidermis showed a pronounced lympho-cytic infiltrate, comprising both CD4+ (predominantly) and CD8+ cells. Isolated IL-2R+ mononuclear cells were evident, particularly in the upper dermis, but were very scant in number compared with either CD4+ or CD8+ cells (data not shown). Intense staining for ICAM-1 and E-selectin (FIGURE 2) on blood vessels and on a minor proportion of MNC was also evident. Weak expression of ICAM-1 was observed on vascular endothelium in normal skin. In FK 506–treated patients in remission, there was a marked reduction in ICAM-1 and E-selectin staining on capillary endothelium and in the number of MNC that were positive for these epitopes (FIGURE 2).

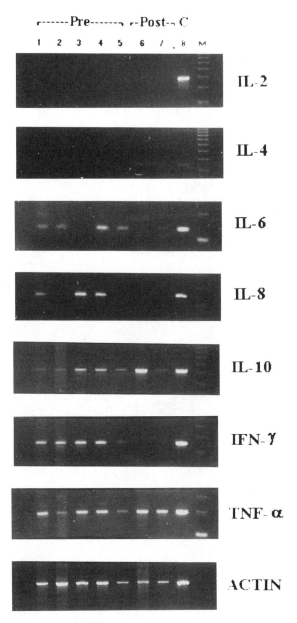

FIGURE 1. The influence of FK 506 treatment on cytokine gene expression pre- and posttreatment in lesional skin of psoriasis patients determined by polymerase chain reaction (PCR). Each lane represents one patient sample, with the positive control (c) in lane 8 being a sample of PBL from a normal individual stimulated with Con A for 20 h.

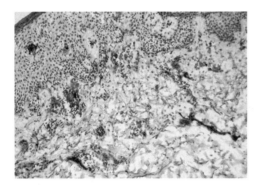

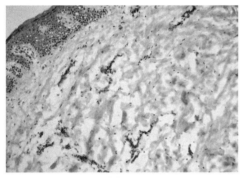

FIGURE 2. ABC-P staining for adhesion molecules in lesional psoriatic skin. **A** (top): Strong ICAM-1 (CD54) expression, predominantly on dermal capillary endothelium prior to FK 506 treatment. **B:** Marked reduction in ICAM-1 staining, with a return towards normal skin architecture after 6 weeks FK 506 treatment.**C:** E-selectin expression on capillary vessels before start of FK 506 administration. **D:** Diminished E-selectin staining 6 weeks after start of treatment. ×220. Reduced to 40%.

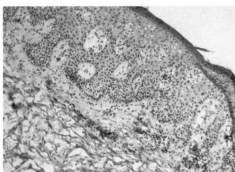

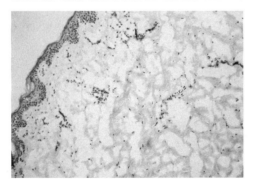

DISCUSSION

FK 506 is a macrocyclic lactone (MW 822 daltons) which, although structurally distinct from the cyclic peptide CsA (MW 1202 daltons), inhibits signal transduction in CD4[+] T-cells by similar molecular mechanisms.[14] Each drug binds selectively to members of distinct families of ubiquitous, cytosolic receptors, or immunophilins— the FK 506 binding proteins (FKBPs; predominant member FKBP12) or the cyclophilins (predominant member cyclophilin A), respectively. Inhibition by the drug-immunophilin complex of the phosphatase activity of calcineurin is thought to be associated with inhibition of dephosphorylation and translocation to the nucleus of the preformed cytoplasmic component of the nuclear gene transcription regulatory factor of activated T-cells, NF-AT-1.[15,16] This effect results in the blockade of IL-2 gene transcription. The *in vitro* production by T-cells of other cytokines, including IL-4, IFN-γ, and granulocyte-macrophage colony stimulating factor, is also suppressed.

From the preliminary data we have obtained, inhibition of the production by activated CD4[+] T-cells and other cells of a variety of cytokines (including IL-6, IL-8, and IFN-γ) is the most plausible explanation for the reductions in leukocyte accumulation, adhesion molecule expression, and keratinocyte hyperplasia seen with disease resolution in response to FK 506 administration. The absence of IL-2 message in patients with active disease is somewhat surprising; IL-2, however, is expressed early in the T-cell activation process and its message may be weak or nondetectable as later events occur. Moreover, our present and earlier results have shown very few IL-2R[+] cells in psoriatic lesions.[17] IL-6, a growth factor for keratinocytes, has been shown to be secreted by epidermal keratinocytes,[6] and this is probably a source of this cytokine in active disease. Similarly, it has been proposed that keratinocytes may influence inflammatory events by secretion both of TNF-α and the neutrophil and T-cell chemoattractant IL-8.[18] Like CsA,[19] FK 506 may have an indirect effect on keratinocyte cytokine production by inhibiting T-cell activation and secondary keratinocyte activation. Persistence of TNF-α, which is produced by macrophages/dendrocytes in papillary dermis in addition to activated keratinocytes, may account in part for the persistent (though substantially reduced) expression of ICAM-1 and E-selectin on the microvascular endothelium in the FK 506–treated subjects. The absence of IFN-γ message in biopsy samples from patients whose skin had been cleared by FK 506 indicates that the suppression of production of this cytokine may have had a major influence on adhesion molecule expression on blood vessels in affected skin. IL-10 is a cytokine that down regulates activation of the immune response and is found in several cell types in addition to T-cells.[20] Although the precise cell source(s) of IL-10 message was not identified, IL-10 signal was found in both pre- and posttreatment biopsies. It is possible that the complex immunoregulatory effects of FK 506 in psoriasis may be partially mediated by this cytokine.

ACKNOWLEDGMENTS

We thank Ms. Beverley Gambrell for expert technical assistance.

REFERENCES

1. VALDIMARSSON, H., B. S. BAKER, I. JONSDOTTIR & I. FRY. 1986. Psoriasis: a disease of abnormal keratinocyte proliferation induced by T lymphocytes. Immunol. Today. **7:** 256–259.

2. Bos, J. D. 1988. The pathomechanisms of psoriasis: the skin immune system and cyclosporin. Br. J. Dermatol. **118:** 141–155.
3. Nickoloff, B. J. & C. E. M. Griffiths. 1990. Lymphocyte trafficking in psoriasis: a new perspective emphasizing the dermal dendrocyte with active dermal recruitment mediated via endothelial cells followed by intraepidermal T-cell activation. J. Invest. Dermatol. **95:** 35S–37S.
4. Nikaein, A., C. Phillips, S. C. Gilbert, D. Savino, A. Silverman, M. J. Stone & A. Menter. 1991. Characterization of skin-infiltrating lymphocytes in patients with psoriasis. J. Invest. Dermatol. **96:** 3–9.
5. Cooper, K. D. 1990. Psoriasis: leukocytes and cytokines. *In* Immunodermatology. D. N. Sauder, Ed. **8:** 737–745. Dermatologic Clinics. City, State.
6. Schwarz, T. & T. E. Luger. 1992. Pharmacology of cytokines in the skin. *In* Pharmacology of the Skin. H. Mahktar, Ed.: 283–313. CRC Press. Boca Raton, Fla.
7. Ellis, C. N., M. S. Fradin, J. M. Messana, *et al.* 1991. Cyclosporine for plaque-type psoriasis: results of a multidose, double-blind trial. N. Engl. J. Med. **324:** 277–284.
8. Kino, T., H. Hatanaka, S. Miyata, *et al.* 1987. FK 506, a novel immunosuppressant isolated from a *Streptomyces.* II. Immunosuppressive effect of FK 506 *in vitro.* J. Antibiot. **40:** 1256–1265.
9. Thomson, A. W. 1989. FK 506. How much potential? Immunol. Today. **10:** 6–9.
10. Schreiber, S. L. & G. R. Crabtree. 1992. The mechanism of action of cyclosporin A and FK 506. Immunol. Today. **13:** 136–142.
11. Starzl, T. E., J. J. Fung, R. Venkataramanan, S. Todo, A. J. Demetris & A. Jain. 1989. FK 506 for liver, kidney and pancreas transplantation. Lancet **ii:** 1000–1004.
12. Jegasothy, B. V., C. D. Ackerman, S. Todo, J. J. Fung, K. Abu-Elmagd & T. E. Starzl. 1992. Tacrolimus (FK 506)—a new therapeutic agent for severe recalcitrant psoriasis. Arch. Dermatol. **128:** 781–785.
13. Chomczynski, P. & N. Sacchi. 1987. Single-step method of RNA isolation by acid guanidinium thiocyanate-phenol-chloroform extraction. Anal. Biochem. **162:** 156–159.
14. Sigal, N. H. & F. J. Dumont. 1992. Cyclosporin A, FK 506, and rapamycin: pharmacologic probes of lymphocyte signal transduction. Annu. Rev. Immunol. **10:** 519–560.
15. Liu, J., J. D. Farmer, W. S. Lane, J. Friedman, L. Weissman & S. L. Schreiber. 1991. Calcineurin is a common target of cyclophilin-cyclosporin A and FKBP-FK 506 complexes. Cell. **66:** 807–815.
16. Flanagan, W. M., B. Corthesy, R. J. Bram & G. R. Crabtree. 1991. Nuclear association of a T-cell transcription factor blocked by FK 506 and cyclosporin A. Nature **352:** 803–807.
17. Horrocks, C., A. D. Ormerod, J. I. Duncan & A. W. Thomson. 1989. The influence of systemic cyclosporin A on interleukin-2 and epidermal growth factor receptor expression in psoriatic skin lesions. Clin. Exp. Immunol **78:** 166.
18. Nickoloff, B. J., G. D. Karabin, J. N. W. N. Barker, *et al.* 1991. Localization of IL-8 and its inducer TNF-α in psoriasis. Am. J. Pathol. **138:** 129–140.
19. Wong, R. L., C. M. Winslow & K. D. Cooper. 1993. The mechanisms of action of cyclosporin A in the treatment of psoriasis. Immunol. Today **14:** 69–74.
20. Zlotnik, A. & K. W. Moore. 1991. Interleukin 10. Cytokine **3:** 366–371.

Inhibitory Effect of FK 506 on Autoimmune Thyroid Disease in the PVG Rat

K. TAMURA,[a,d] J. WOO,[a] N. MURASE,[a] M. NALESNIK,[b]
AND A. W. THOMSON[a,c,e]

[a]Department of Surgery
[b]Department of Pathology
[c]Department of Molecular Genetics and Biochemistry
University of Pittsburgh
Pittsburgh, Pennsylvania

[d]Product Development Laboratories
Fujisawa Pharmaceutical Co., Ltd.
Osaka, Japan

In the autoimmune disease Hashimoto's thyroiditis, the patient produces autoantibodies and sensitized T-cells specific for thyroid antigens. The immune response is characterized by intense infiltration of the thyroid gland by lymphocytes, plasma cells, and macrophages, which form lymphocytic follicles and germinal centers. Autoantibodies are produced to a variety of thyroid proteins, including thyroglobulin (TG) and thyroid peroxidase, resulting in impaired uptake of iodine and reduced production of thyroid hormones (hypothyroidism).[1]

Experimental autoimmune thyroiditis (EAT) can be induced in susceptible strains of mice or rats by immunization with TG in complete Freund's adjuvant or by neonatal thymectomy and further T-cell depletion using sublethal irradiation.[2] The latter manipulations are thought to remove a specific immunoregulatory cell subset. Immunohistochemical findings in the thyroids of these animals are similar to those of Hashimoto's thyroiditis; the animals develop T_{DTH} cells directed against TG and anti-TG autoantibodies and there is biochemical evidence of thyroid dysfunction. T-cell clones specific for TG can be isolated from EAT animals and can induce the disease in normal individuals. Thus, there is substantial evidence for defective T-cell immunoregulation in EAT. Hassman et al. showed that administration of the T-cell suppressant cyclosporine A (CsA) during disease induction reduced the histological grade of thyroiditis and circulating autoantibody levels.[3]

The macrocyclic lactone FK 506 is a powerful new immunosuppressive agent with a similar molecular action to CsA.[4] It is however, considerably more potent than CsA. FK 506 inhibits selectively the activation of CD4+ T (helper) cells and the expression of genes encoding interleukin-2 (IL-2), interferon-γ (IFN-γ), and other cytokines.[5] Early studies with FK 506 in clinical organ transplantation indicate that it can both prevent and reverse allograft rejection. Moreover, it may exhibit greater steroid-sparing activity and fewer side effects than CsA.[6] FK 506 may therefore have considerable potential for the treatment of those autoimmune disorders[7] in which

[e]Author to whom correspondence should be addressed at: Department of Surgery, University of Pittsburgh, W1544 Biomedical Science Tower, Terrace and Lothrop Streets, Pittsburgh, Pa. 15213.

T-cells are believed to play a central role. In this study, we have examined the capacity of FK 506 to inhibit the development of EAT when administered after the detection of circulating anti-TG autoantibodies. We have also examined the effect of FK 506 on thyroid-infiltrating cells, and both major histocompatibility complex (MHC) class II antigen and adhesion molecule expression within the affected tissue.

MATERIALS AND METHODS

Autoimmune thyroiditis was induced in groups of 9 female PVG/c rats according to the method of Penhale et al.[2] and as shown in FIGURE 1. FK 506 (Fujisawa Pharmaceutical Co., Ltd.; preparation for animal use containing HCO-60 and D mannitol) was suspended (3 mg/ml) in saline and administered intramuscularly (0.5 mg/kg per day for 3 weeks from week 15). Serum anti-TG antibody was measured by enzyme-linked immunosorbent assay (ELISA).[8] The degree of disease activity in thyroid glands was assessed histologically, using the following scale: 0 = normal appearance; 1 = occasional foci of lymphocyte infiltration; 2 = multiple discrete foci; 3 = diffuse thyroiditis; and 4 = diffuse thyroiditis with follicular obliteration. A portion of each thyroid was snap frozen in OCT (Miles Inc., Elkhart, Ind.), and 6 μm sections were cut and stored at −80°. Immunohistological analyses of cell surface antigen expression were performed using primary mouse monoclonal antibodies (mAb) (TABLE 1) and the avidin-biotin complex (ABC) immunoperoxidase technique. AffiniPure F(ab')$_2$ rat anti–mouse IgG (1:500, Jackson Immunoresearch Lab., Inc., West Grove, Pa.) and Vectastain Elite ABC kit (Vector Lab., Inc., Burlingame, Calif.) were used to develop the immunoperoxidase reaction.

RESULTS

Serum anti-TG autoantibody levels (OD 490 units) in normal, disease control, and FK 506–treated rats at 19 weeks were 0.16 ± 0.03, 1.53 ± 0.08, and 0.80 ± 0.83, respectively. The change in anti-TG antibody levels pre and posttreatment in the FK 506–treated group compared with the disease control group was statistically signifi-

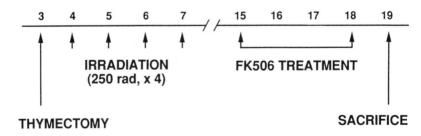

FIGURE 1. Protocol for the induction of autoimmune thyroiditis and FK 506 treatment in female PVG/c rats. The model is based on that described originally by Penhale et al.[2]

TABLE 1. Monoclonal Antibodies Used for Immunohistochemical Analysis of Thyroids

Antibody	Cluster of Differentiation	Dilution (Reciprocal)	Source	Specificity
OX19	CD5	100	Sera-Lab[a]	Thymocytes, T lymphocyte
TCR-αβ chains	—	100	Sera-Lab	α/β T cell receptor
W3/25	CD4	100	Sera-Lab	Th, thymocytes, subset of macrophage
OX-8	CD8	200	Sera-Lab	Ts/c, thymocytes, NK cells
ED1	—	50	Serotec[b]	macrophages, monocyte
OX-6	—	1000	Sera-Lab	MHC class II (Ia)
ART 18	CD25	20	Sera-Lab	Interleukin-2 receptor (α-chain)
ICAM-1	CD54	50	Seikayaku Corp.[c]	Intercellular adhesion molecule-1
LFA-1α	CD11a	50	Seikayaku Corp.	Lymphocyte function associated antigen-1α
LFA-1β	CD18	50	Seikayaku Corp.	Lymphocyte function associated antigen-1β

[a]Sera-Lab Sussex, England.
[b]Serotec Co., Oxford, England.
[c]Seikayaku Corp., Tokyo, Japan.

cant ($p < 0.05$, Wilcoxon rank sum test). There was a significant difference in the severity of lymphocytic thyroiditis between animals in the disease control group and those treated with FK 506 (FIGURE 2). The mean disease severity for the disease control and FK 506–treated groups was 2.33 ± 1.33 and 1.11 ± 0.57, respectively ($p < 0.05$ using the Wilcoxon rank sum test). The majority of FK 506–treated animals showed preservation of comparatively normal thyroid follicular architecture (FIGURE 3).

The results of immunohistochemical analyses of thyroid tissue obtained from normal female PVG/c rats, untreated disease control rats, and FK 506-treated animals are summarized in TABLE 2. T-cell-specific mAbs directed against T-cell receptor α/β (TCRα/β) or CD5 stained only a minority of the thyroid-infiltrating mononuclear cells (MNC) in untreated disease controls. Many of the leukocytes were CD4$^+$ (T-cells and macrophages), and MHC class II$^+$ cells (macrophages and dendritic cells) were also numerous. B-cells (OX-33$^+$) were not detected. Although CD8$^+$ cells (T-cells and NK cells) were present, they were less numerous than the CD4$^+$ cells. CD25$^+$ (IL-2Rα$^+$) MNC were few in number. The dendritic morphology of the numerous MHC class II$^+$ cells, together with the comparative prominence of CD4$^+$ MNC and relative scarcity of ED1$^+$ cells (macrophages), points to a high incidence of dendritic cells within the inflammatory infiltrate. Only a minor proportion of the remaining follicular epithelial cell profiles in untreated disease control rats were MHC class II$^+$. Similarly, ICAM-1 was expressed on infiltrating MNC and occasionally on thyroid epithelium and vascular endothelium. In some instances, apparent ICAM-1 staining on thyrocytes may have been due to staining of closely adjacent endothelial cells. Lymphocyte function associated antigen-β (LFA-1β) but not LFA-1α was detected on a small proportion of infiltrating MNC. FK 506 administration markedly reduced staining for all markers on MHC. Intercellular adhesion molecule-1 (ICAM-1) expression on vascular endothelium and staining of OX-6 on thyrocytes was also reduced, by treatment with the immunosuppressant.

DISCUSSION

The capacity of a 3-week course of FK 506 to decrease the severity of autoimmune thyroid disease in rats and our accompanying immunohistochemical studies are consistent with and extend previous observations on the effects of CsA in this experimental model.[3] The inhibition of cell infiltration and follicular destruction

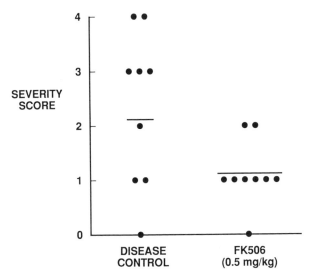

FIGURE 2. Histological assessment of the severity of thyroiditis in individual disease control and FK 506–treated PVG/c rats. Vertical bars indicate mean values.

within the thyroid by FK 506 was accompanied by reductions in T-cells and LFA-1β+ cells and in MHC class II+ dendritic cells. Both dendritic cells and macrophages have been reported previously to be numerous both in human and experimental autoimmune thyroid disease.[9,10] MHC class II antigen and ICAM-1 staining on follicular cells was also reduced by FK 506.

There is evidence that thyrocytes can be activated by cytokines [including IFN-γ and tumor necrosis factor-α (TNF-α)] to express MHC class II antigens and ICAM-1[11–13] and to liberate IL-1 and IL-6[14]—all properties of antigen-presenting cells. The capacity of FK 506 to interfere *in vitro* with cytokine secretion by T_{H1} cells[5] is in agreement with the substantially reduced recruitment of MHC class II+ dendritic cells and with down regulation of MHC class II and ICAM-1 expression on potential cellular targets of host inflammatory cells. It has recently been reported that MNC infiltrates in Hashimoto's thyroiditis are LFA-1 (CD11a) positive, while

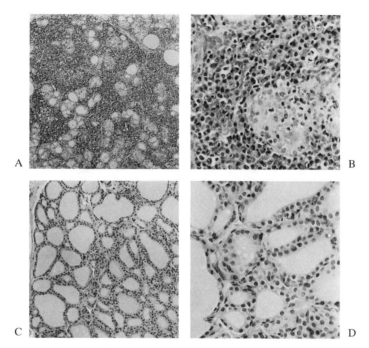

FIGURE 3. Compared with the histological appearance of the thyroid in an untreated disease control animal (a, b), the thyroid of an FK 506–treated rat (c, d) shows substantial reduction in the lymphocytic infiltrate. Hematoxylin & eosin. (a, c) × 125; (b, d) × 500. Whole figure reduced to 75%.

ICAM-1 is present on thyrocytes.[13,15] Significantly, Bagnasco *et al.* also found MHC class II+ thyrocytes in almost all patients with autoimmune thyroid disease.[15]

Adhesion-dependent cytotoxic mechanisms are very likely to be involved in organ-specific autoimmunity. Our demonstration that FK 506 reduces CD4+ CD8+,

TABLE 2. Influence of FK 506 on Thyroid-Infiltrating Cells, MHC Class II Antigen, and Adhesion Molecule Expression[a]

Cell Surface Antigen	Normal	Disease Control	FK 506 treated
CD5	−	+	±
TCR-αβ	−	+	±
CD4	−	+++	±
CD8	−	++	±
CD25 (IL-2-Receptor)	−	±	−
ED1 (macrophage)	−	+	−
MHC-class II (OX-6)	−	+++	−
ICAM-1	±	++	±
LFA-1α	−	−	−
LFA-1β	−	+	−

[a]The areas occupied by stained cells were scored as follows: +++, >30%; ++, 15–30%; +, 2.5–15%; ±, <2.5%; −, 0%.

MHC class II$^+$, ICAM-1$^+$, and LFA-1β^+ cells in EAT is consistent with an immuno-suppressive effect mediated via interference with interactions between infiltrating cytotoxic T-cells and other recruited inflammatory leukocytes and target epithelial cells. The most plausible explanation for this effect is interference with production of adherence-promoting cytokines, such as IFN-γ and TNF-α.

REFERENCES

1. WEETMAN, A. P. 1990. Thyroid autoimmune disease. *In* Werner and Ingbar's The Thyroid. L. E. Braverman & R. D. Utiger, Eds.: 1295–1310. J. B. Lippincott Co., Philadelphia, Pa.
2. PENHALE, W. J., A. FARMER & W. J. IRVINE. 1975. Thyroiditis in T cell–depleted rats: influence of strain, radiation dose, adjuvants and antilymphocyte serum. Clin. Exp. Immunol. **21:** 362–375.
3. HASSMAN, R. A., C. DIEGUEZ, D. P. RENNIE, A. P. WEETMAN, R. HALL & A. M. MCGREGOR. 1985. The influence of cyclosporin A on the induction of experimental autoimmune thyroid disease in the PVG/c rat. Clin. Exp. Immunol. **59:** 10–16.
4. THOMSON, A. W. 1990. FK 506: profile of an important new immunosuppressant. Transplant. Rev. **4:** 1–13.
5. TOCCI, M. J., D. A. MATKOVICH, K. A. COLLIER, *et al.* 1989. FK 506 selectively inhibits expression of early T cell activation genes. J. Immunol. **143:** 718–726.
6. STARZL, T. E., J. FUNG, R. VENKATARAMANAN, S. TODO, A. J. DEMETRIS & A. JAIN. 1989. FK 506 for liver, kidney and pancreas transplantation. Lancet **ii:** 1000–1004.
7. THOMSON, A. W. & T. E. STARZL. 1992. FK 506 and autoimmune disease: perspective and prospects. Autoimmunity **12:** 303–313.
8. VOLLER, A., D. E. BIDWELL & C. L. BUREK. 1980. An enzyme-linked immunoabsorbent assay (ELISA) for antibodies to thyroglobulin. Proc. Soc. Exp. Biol. Med. **163:** 402–405.
9. COHEN, S. B., C. D. DIJKSTRA & A. P. WEETMAN. 1988. Sequential analysis of experimental autoimmune thyroiditis induced by neonatal thymectomy in the Buffalo strain rat. Cell Immunol. **114:** 126–136.
10. KABEL, P. J., H. A. M. VOORBIJ, M. DE HAAN, R. D. VAN DER GAAG & H. A. DREXHAGE. 1988. Intrathyroidal dendritic cells. J. Clin. Endocrinol. Metab. **66:** 199–207.
11. TODD, I., R. PUJOL-BORRELL, L. J. HAMMOND, G. F. BOTTAZZO & M. FELDMANN. 1985. Interferon-γ induces HLA-DR expression by thyroid epithelium. Clin. Exp. Immunol. **61:** 265–273.
12. TOLOSA, E., C. ROURA, M. MARTI, A. BELFIORE & R. PUJOL-BORRELL. 1992. Induction of intercellular adhesion molecule-1 but not of lymphocyte function-associated antigen-3 in thyroid follicular cells. J. Autoimmunity **5:** 119–135.
13. WEETMAN, A. P., S. COHEN, M. W. MAGKOBA & L. K. BARYSIEWICZ. 1989. Expression of an intercellular adhesion molecule ICAM-1, by human thyroid cells. J. Endocrinol. **122:** 185–191.
14. GRUBECK-LOEBENSTEIN, B., G. BUCHAN, D. CHANTRY, H. KASSAL, M. LONDEI, K. PIRICH & K. BARRETT. 1989. Analysis of intrathyroidal cytokine production in thyroid autoimmune disease: thyroid follicular cells produce interleukin-1 and interleukin-6. Clin. Exp. Immunol. **77:** 324–330.
15. BAGNASCO, M., A. CARETTO, D. OLIVE, B. PEDINI, G. W. CANONICA & C. BETTERLE. 1991. Expression of intercellular adhesion molecule-1 (ICAM-1) on thyroid epithelial cells in Hashimoto's thyroiditis but not in Graves' disease or papillary thyroid cancer. Clin. Exp. Immunol. **83:** 309–313.

Deoxyspergualin

Mode of Action and Clinical Trials

SEIICHI SUZUKI[a]

Department of Surgical Research
National Cardiovascular Center
5-7-1, Fujishiro-dai, Suita
Osaka 565, Japan

INTRODUCTION

Deoxyspergualin (DSG) has been reported to have a strong immunosuppressive effect on cardiac allograft in rats[1,2] and kidney transplantation in dogs[3,4] and Japanese monkeys.[5] The various *in vivo* studies, such as heart transplantation in rats,[2] allostimulation in mice,[6] and graft-versus-host disease in rats,[7] demonstrated that DSG specifically inhibits the differentiation and proliferation of cytotoxic T cells. The drug was also shown to suppress antibody production from B cells.[8,9] Differently from ciclosporine or FK506, the production of IL-1 and IL-2 from macrophages and T cells, respectively, was not inhibited in DSG-treated rats.[10] At an intracellular level, the drug was suggested to inhibit the polyamine biosynthetic pathway[11] as well as DNA polymerase alpha activity.[12]

Due to these unique immunosuppressive effects of the drug, DSG pulse therapy was highly effective on acute graft rejection in rat heart transplantation[2] and canine kidney transplantation.[13] DSG also prolonged the survival of cardiac xenograft in a hamster-to-rat combination.[14]

From August 1988 to March 1989, an early phase II clinical study was performed for recurrent graft rejections in 30 renal recipients.[15] The overall remission rate was 79% in 34 episodes of rejection, including accelerated, acute, and chronic rejections. Adverse reactions such as facial numbness, gastrointestinal disorders, leukocytopenia, and thrombocytopenia were noted, but all these events were mild and temporary. On the basis of this pilot study, a late phase II clinical study was carried out to find an optimal dose and treatment period of the drug.[16] As a result, doses of 3 to 5 mg/kg per day were judged to be recommendable, and the 7 days was evaluated as a suitable duration of treatment.

In this paper, we will discuss mechanisms of action of DSG based on our experimental studies using rat heart transplantation, and will present a novel clinical trial of the drug for discontinuation of corticosteroid in the recipients after kidney transplantation.

IMMUNOSUPPRESSIVE MECHANISMS OF DSG IN ALLOGRAFTED RATS

Using the model of heterotopic heart transplantation in rats, recipients were intraperitoneally injected with DSG at a dose of 5 mg/kg per day for 15 days from the

---

[a]Present affiliation: Department of Experimental Surgery and Bioengineering, National Children's Medical Research Center, 3-35-31, Taishi-do, Setagaya-ku, Tokyo 154, Japan.

onset day of rejection.[2] This treatment successfully reversed the rejection. Furthermore, it is demonstrated that immunological unresponsiveness could be achieved to a greater degree by initiating the administration of DSG from the onset day of graft rejection rather than by initiating it from the day of grafting. In addition, the adoptive transfer of immunological unresponsiveness succeeded in rats receiving spleen cells from syngeneic recipients with permanently surviving grafts. In the spleen cells of recipients 7 to 10 days following DSG treatment, there was also evidence of suppressor cells, although the activity of these cells was not strong enough to induce unresponsiveness. These results suggest that DSG selectively inhibits donor-specific expanded lymphocyte clones at the onset of rejection, and that suppressor cells, spared by DSG, increase their activities in a time-related manner and participate in the maintenance of immunological unresponsiveness. It is also reported in mice that DSG therapy was effective for recipients with ongoing graft-versus-host disease, and the surviving recipients acquired immunological unresponsiveness that could be adoptively transferred to secondary recipients by administration of their lymph node cells.[17,18]

However, no graft prolongation was observed in allografted rats receiving serum from unresponsiveness-induced recipients.[2]

Due to its unique immunosuppressive effects mentioned above, the concurrent administration of DSG with pretransplant immunization of donor antigens was considered to lead to the induction of immunological unresponsiveness. To verify this hypothesis, we administered donor spleen cells into recipients twice at a 2-week interval and then injected DSG for 5 days starting on the day of the secondary cell injection. The donor hearts were transplanted to the recipients 7 days after the initiation of secondary cell transfusion. Unresponsiveness was effectively induced by this combined pretransplant therapy.[19] In addition, the induced unresponsiveness was specific to immunized antigen before transplantation.

In the next study, we purified T cells from spleen cells in the recipients (primary recipients) with long-surviving grafts, and transferred these cells to the syngeneic rats (secondary recipients) grafted with specific or nonspecific donor hearts. T cells were obtained by passing the splenocytes through a Cytofrac-MT column (Asahi Medical Co., Tokyo). In the passed cells, T cell population was 85.4 ± 7.4%, and B cell population was 0.7 ± 0.2%. Although suppressor T cells were not detected in the primary recipients one month after grafting, they were observed from 2 months after transplantation. The suppressor T cells acted antigen nonspecifically and antigen specifically 2 and 3 months, respectively, after grafting. It was also demonstrated that the suppressor T cells acquired specificity against antigens that had been recognized by the nonspecific suppressor T cells. From these results, we concluded that long-term graft survival was mediated by the additional effect of DSG and nonspecific suppressor T cells during early phase after grafting and thereafter by that of both nonspecific and specific suppressor T cells. Around 3 months after grafting, immunological unresponsiveness may be maintained mainly by antigen-specific suppressor T cells.[20]

IMMUNOSUPPRESSIVE MECHANISMS OF DSG IN XENOGRAFTED RATS

As DSG strongly inhibits the differentiation and proliferation of antibody-producing cells, the administration of DSG into xenografted recipients in a hamster-to-rat combination was remarkably effective in prolonging graft survival.[14,21,22] B cell population was significantly increased in the spleen cells, but not in the peripheral lymphocytes, of the control recipients 3 days after xenografting.[22] Therefore, splenectomy on the day of grafting significantly delayed antibody formation to the donor, resulting in prolongation of graft survival.[14] In addition, xenograft rejection and specific antibody production were observed to be almost completely inhibited during the term of DSG administration in combination with splenectomy.[14] Of interest is that IgM production was not suppressed by DSG alone, but was remarkably inhibited by splenectomy. In the recipient treated with DSG and splenectomy, cardiac arrest occurred 2 to 10 day after termination of DSG administration, with a lower titer of IgG and IgM than in the control.[14] These suggest that the xenograft rejection might be induced not only by antibody-mediated immunity but by other mechanisms, including at least in part antibody-depent cell responses.

CLINICAL TRIAL OF DSG FOR STEROID WITHDRAWAL

DSG has been shown to strongly inhibit differentiation and proliferation of both cytotoxic T cells and antibody-producing cells in various experimental models of organ transplantation as described above. On the basis of these extensive animal studies, the first clinical trial was started on August 1989 in renal patients with various types of graft rejection, resulting in excellent recovery from acute rejection. On the other hand, we have been trying to use DSG for induction therapy of immunosuppression in combination with other drugs. The purpose of this therapy was to withdraw steroid during the maintenance phase of immunosuppression. Since 1990 we have been applying this protocol to renal recipients with low numbers of incompatible donor HLA antigens and well-functioning grafts.

Immunosuppressive Protocol for Steroid Withdrawal

Immunosuppression is performed based on the following schedule. Cyclosporine orally administered at a daily dose of 10 mg/kg, and the dose is adjusted to maintain its trough level ranging between 100 and 150 ng/ml in whole blood. Mizoribine is orally given at 2 mg/kg per day. Three courses of intravenous administration of DSG are conducted at a dose of 5 mg/kg per day from day 3 to 9, day 21 to 25, and day 35 to 39 after grafting. Methylprednisolone is injected iv at 500 mg during the operation procedure. Prednisolone is started at 50 mg on the day of transplantation, and daily tapered by 10 mg until 3 days after grafting when its dose is 20 mg. This dosage is continued until 2 weeks, 15 mg for the next week, and 10 mg for the following two weeks. The patients satisfying the criteria for steroid withdrawal are further reduced on the prednisolone to 5 mg from 5 weeks after grafting, and then to 2.5 mg from 7 weeks. Usually, nine to 10 weeks after transplantation in these patients, the administration of prednisolone is discontinued, and they are maintained with cyclosporine and mizoribine. When acute rejection occurred, recipients are treated with DSG in combination with methylprednisolone or without it as mentioned previously.[15,16]

Criteria for Steroid Withdrawal

The criteria are as follows. The recipients received first kidney grafts, with an excellent graft function (less than 2.0 mg/dl of serum creatinine level), and without any rejection episode or with only one episode of mild rejection during their clinical course.

TABLE 1. Results of Quadruple Immunosuppression

Final Dose of PLS (mg)	Number of Patients
0	8
5	2
10	7
15	2[a]

[a]Two patients lost their grafts due to recurrent rejection.

Outcomes of the Recipients Treated with the Protocol

The protocol using quadruple immunosuppression was applied to 19 recipients, of which 13 patients received cadaver kidneys and 6 received living related ones. As shown in TABLE 1, 8 recipients were completely discontinued on prednisolone, 2 were reduced to 5 mg, and 7 were continued at 10 mg. Two recipients lost their grafts.

The numbers of incompatible donor HLA antigens in the recipients are demonstrated in TABLES 2 and 3. These numbers were low both in patients with cadaver grafts and in those with living grafts. CR60 and CR73 frequently encountered severe graft rejection and finally lost their graft function, and CR65 and CR70 showed their serum creatinine level over 2.0 mg/dl. These 4 cases were judged to be out of criteria for steroid withdrawal. CR62 suffered from steroid withdrawal symptom 2 weeks after its discontinuation, and was readministered 5 mg of prednisolone. Acute rejection occurred in CR72 and LR35 after withdrawal or reduction of prednisolone. However, these patients have been maintaining graft function well after readministration of prednisolone at 10 mg.

TABLES 4 and 5 show recent creatinine levels in the recipients with functioning grafts. All steroid-free recipients were observed to have an excellent graft function

TABLE 2. Recipients Treated with Quadruple Immunosuppressants using CsA, PLS, MZ, and DSG—Cadaver Grafts

Recipient	Donor	HLA-Mismatch A,B	DR	Final Dose of PLS (mg)	Misc.
CR58(42y,F)	18y,M	1	0	0	
CR59(47y,M)	34y,M	0	0	0	
CR60(43y,F)	59y,M	2	0	15	Graft loss[a] (8 mths.)
CR61(22y,F)	51y,M	0	0	0	
CR62(59y,M)	60y,F	2	0	5	Withdrawal sym.[b]
CR64(42y,M)	20y,M	1	1	5	
CR65(36y,M)	73y,M	1	0	10	Cr > 2.0
CR66(16y,M)	19y,M	2	1	0	
CR69(37y,M)	17y,F	1	1	0	
CR70(44y,M)	61y,F	1	0	10	Cr > 2.0
CR71(49y,F)	70y,M	1	0	0	
CR72(23y,F)	58y,F	0	0	2.5 ≫ ≫ 10[c]	Rejection
CR73(23y,F)	56y,F	2	1	15	Graft loss[a] (4 mths.)

[a]Due to recurrent rejection.
[b]General fatigue, loss of appetite, and articulator pain.
[c]After administration of PLS at 2.5 mg/day for 83 days.

TABLE 3. Recipients Treated with Quadruple Immunosuppressants Using CsA, PLS, MZ, and DSG—Living Grafts

Recipient	Donor	HLA-Mismatch A,B	DR	Final Dose of PLS (mg)	Misc.
LR35(22y,M)	Father(50y)	1	1	$0 \gg \gg 10^a$	Rejection
LR36(27y,M)	Father(57y)	1	1	10	
LR37(33y,F)	Mother(57y)	1	1	0	
LR38(26y,M)	Mother(52y)	1	1	10	
LR39(35y,M)	Mother(61y)	1	1	0	
LR40(38y,F)	Mother(58y)	0	0	10	

[a]Due to rejection 5 months after withdrawal of PLS. All recipients were one-haplotype identical to their donors.

TABLE 4. Serum Creatinine Level in the Recipients with Functioning Graft (Cadaveric Grafts)

Recipients	Months on Steroid Free	Months after Grafting	Present Cr Level
CR-58	2.1	32.0	1.0 mg/dl
CR-59	2.0	31.5	1.9
CR-61	2.0	30.7	1.3
CR-62		27.0	1.3
CR-64		24.5	1.8
CR-65		22.7	2.0
CR-66	8.7	22.3	1.4
CR-69	2.4	18.7	1.2
CR-70		17.7	2.4
CR-71	11.3	15.0	1.6
CR-72		11.5	1.7
			(March 31, 1993)

TABLE 5. Serum Creatinine Level in the Recipients with Functioning Graft (Living Grafts)

Recipients	Months on Steroid Free	Months after Grafting	Present Cr Level
LR-35		19.0	2.0 mg/dl
LR-36		14.0	1.8
LR-37	8.0	11.5	0.9
LR-38		10.3	1.9
LR-39	2.9	9.5	1.4
LR-40		8.3	1.9
			(March 31, 1993)

9.5 to 32 months after grafting. In addition, five patients were withdrawn from the steroid 2 to 3 months after grafting, and 3 were withdrawn 8 to 11.3 months after transplantation.

Adverse Reactions

Adverse reactions such as facial numbness, leukocytopenia, and thrombocytopenia were observed, but these reactions were much more mild than those observed in graft rejection patients treated with DSG.

Summary

Corticosteroids are commonly used in combination with cyclosporine in clinical kidney recipients, and administered indefinitely to many patients. Long-term administration of steroids is associated with a number of serious side effects including hypertension, obesity, hyperlipidemia, diabetes mellitus, cataract, osteoporosis, infection, moon face, and so on. A disturbance of growth is also a serious problem in pediatric patients. It is therefore desirable to discontinue the administration of steroid in renal allograft patients.

For the withdrawal of steroid, it is quite important to thoroughly inhibit the recipient immune responses during the induction phase of immunosuppression without any serious adverse effect, that the patient may not retain immunological memories against donor antigens for a long period. Thus, we have been performing extensive immunosuppressive therapy using quadruple drugs, that is, DSG, cyclosporine, mizoribine, and prednisolone, during the early stage after kidney transplantation for withdrawal of prednisolone during the maintenance stage. Up to now, 19 recipients were treated with this protocol. In these patients, 8 were completely discontinued on the steroid and have been maintaining excellent graft function 9.2 to 32 months after transplantation, and 2 were reduced on the steroid to 5 mg. The present protocol may contribute greatly toward the quality of life in renal recipients.

REFERENCES

1. SUZUKI, S., M. KANASHIRO, H. AMEMIYA. 1987. Effect of a new immunosuppressant, 15-deoxyspergualin, on heterotopic rat heart transplantation, in comparison with cyclosporine. Transplantation 44: 483–487.
2. SUZUKI, S., M. KANASHIRO, H. WATANABE & H. AMEMIYA. 1988. Therapeutic effect of 15-deoxyspergualin on acute graft rejection detected by 31P nuclear magnetic resonance spectroscopy, and its effect on rat heart transplantation. Transplantation 46: 669–672.
3. AMEMIYA, H., S. SUZUKI, S. NIIYA, K. FUKAO, N. YAMANAKA & J. ITO. 1989. A new immunosuppressive agent, 15-deoxyspergualin, in dog renal allografting. Transplant. Proc. 21: 3468–3470.
4. AMEMIYA, H., S. SUZUKI, H. MANABE, K. FUKAO, Y. IWASAKI, K. DOHI, K. ISONO, K. ORITA & N. YAMANABE. 1988. 15-Deoxyspergualin as an immunosuppressive agent in dogs. Transplant. Proc. 20: 229–232.
5. SUZUKI, S. & H. AMEMIYA. 1990. 15-Deoxyspergualin—a novel immunosuppressant: experimental studies and clinical trials. Transplant. Immunol. Lett. 7: 17–19.
6. NISHIMURA, K. & T. TOKUNAGA. 1989. Mechanism of action of 15-deoxyspergualin. I. Suppressive effect on the induction of alloreactive secondary cytotoxic T lymphocytes in vivo and in vitro. Immunology 68: 66–71.

7. NEMOTO, K., M. HAYASHI, F. ABE, T. TAKITA & T. TAKEUCHI. 1991. Deoxyspergualin in lethal murine graft-versus-host disease. Transplantation **51:** 712–715.

8. NEMOTO, K., M. HAYASHI, F. ABE, T. NAKAMURA, M. ISHIZUKA & H. UMEZAWA. 1987. Immunosuppressive activities of 15-deoxyspergualin in animals. J. Antibiot, Tokyo **40:** 561–562.

9. MAKINO, M., M. FUJIWARA, T. AOYAGI & H. UMEZAWA. 1987. Immunosuppressive activities of deoxyspergualin. II. The effect on the antibody responses. Immunopharmacology **14:** 115–122.

10. NEMOTO, K., F. ABE, T. NAKAMURA, M. ISHIZUKA, T. TAKEUCHI & H. UMEZAWA. 1987. Blastogenic responses and the release of interleukin 1 and 2 by spleen cells obtained from rat skin allograft recipients administered with 15-deoxyspergualin. J. Antibiot. Tokyo **40:** 1062–1064.

11. HIBASAMI, H., T. TSUKADA, R. SUZUKI, K. TAKANO, S. TAKAJI, T. TAKEUCHI, S. SHIR-AKURA, T. MURATA & K. NAKASHIMA. 1991. 15-Deoxyspergualin, an antiproliferative agent for human and mouse leukemia cells shows inhibitory effects on the synthetic pathway of polyamines. Anticancer Res. **11:** 325–330.

12. MULLER, W. E. G., N. WEISSMANN, A. MAIDHOF, M. BACHMANN & H. C. SCHRODER. 1987. Deoxyspergualin, a potent antitumor agent: further studies on the cytobiological mode of action. J. Antibiot. Tokyo **40:** 1028–1035.

13. ITOH, J., T. TAKEUCHI, S. SUZUKI & H. AMEMIYA. 1988. Reversal of acute rejection episodes by deoxyspergualin (NKT-01) in dogs receiving renal allografts. J. Antibiot. Tokyo **41:** 1503–1505.

14. SUZUKI, S., H. NISHIMORI, H. OHDAN, S. NIIYA & H. AMEMIYA. Prolongation of cardiac xenograft survival in hamster-to-rat combination by recipient treatment with deoxymethylspergualin. Transplantation. (In press.)

15. AMEMIYA, H., S. SUZUKI, K. OTA, K. TAKAHASHI, T. SONODA, M. ISHIBASHI, R. OMOTO, I. KOYAMA, K. DOHI, Y. FUKUDA & K. FUKAO. 1990. A novel rescue drug, 15-deoxyspergualin. First clinical trials for recurrent graft rejection in renal recipients. Transplantation **49:** 337–343.

16. AMEMIYA, H. Deoxyspergualin: clinical trials in renal graft rejection. 1993. Ann. N.Y. Acad. Sci. **685:** 196–201.

17. NEMOTO, K., M. HAYASHI, H. FUJII, J. ITO, T. NAKAMURA, T. TAKEUCHI & H. UMEZAWA. 1987. Effect of 15-deoxyspergualin on graft-versus-host disease in mice. Transplant. Proc. **19:** 3985–3986.

18. NEMOTO, K., Y. SUGAWARA, T. MAE, M. HAYASHI, F. ABE, A. FUJII & T. TAKEUCHI. 1991. Immunological unresponsiveness by deoxyspergualin in therapy in mice undergoing lethal graft-versus-host disease, and successful adoptive transfer of unresponsiveness. Transplant. Proc. **23:** 862–863.

19. SHIMATANI, K., S. SUZUKI, R. HAYASHI & H. AMEMIYA. 1989. Prolongation of cardiac allograft survival in rats by recipient pretreatment with donor spleen cells and 15-deoxyspergualin. Transplantation. **48:** 895–897.

20. HIROSE, K. 1993. Induction of transplantation unresponsiveness by deoxyspergualin and the role of suppressor T cells for its maintenance in heart-allografted rats. Jpn J. Transplant. (Abstr. English.) **28:** 400–408.

21. SUZUKI, S., H. NISHIMORI, R. HAYASHI, D. QUINONEZ & H. AMEMIYA. 1992. Prolonged survival of cardiac allografts and xenografts in rat-to-rat and hamster-to-rat transplantation by treatment with deoxyspergualin. Transplant. Proc. **24:** 1638–1639.

22. SUZUKI, S., H. NISHIMORI, K. KIDO, S. ARITA, H. TASHIRO, H. OHDAN, D. QUINONES & H. AMEMIYA. 1993. Continuous administration of methyldeoxyspergualin prolongs xenograft survival in hamster-to-rat cardiac transplantation. Transplant Proc. **25:** 430–431.

Combination of Immunosuppressive Drugs for Organ Transplantation

TAKENORI OCHIAI, YOSHIO GUNJI, MATSUO NAGATA,
AND KAICHI ISONO

Department of Surgery
School of Medicine
Chiba University
1-8-1 Inohana, Chuo-ku
Chiba 260, Japan

INTRODUCTION

Success in the clinical introduction of cyclosporine (CYA) and the subsequent discovery of FK506 (FK) have stimulated the development of new immunosuppressive agents. Rapamycin (RAP) and RS-61443 (RS), thereafter, have received attention as new immunosuppressive agents. In the development of a new immunosuppressive agent, evaluation of both immunosuppressive activity and toxicity is essential. Regarding CYA, nephrotoxicity might be an obstacle that prevents the ultimate goal of its use as an immunosuppressive agent in organ transplantation in spite of its prominent immunosuppressive potency.[1]

FK and RAP have been recognized as more potent immunosuppressive drugs as compared to CYA.[2-5] During the several years since the first publication about FK, it has been used in a large number of humans initially in Pittsburgh, and both positive and negative effects have been reported.[6] Taking into account the effectiveness and toxicity of FK observed in our experimental studies and in clinical cases, FK still leaves us short of a final goal in terms of an immunosuppressant in organ transplantation. RAP also showed side effects in experimental studies at Cambridge and our laboratory.

Most of the available immunosuppressive agents belong to the category of either antimetabolites (RS, Azathioprine), inhibitors of T cell function (CYA, FK, RAP), or anti–T cell antibody (ALG, OKT-3) (TABLE 1). Recently, the monoclonal antibody against adhesion molecules is interesting as an immunosuppressant in organ transplantation, since the mechanisms of antibody inhibiting rejection are different from the drugs available now. The remarkable inhibitory effect of anti-ICAM-1 and anti-LFA-1 antibodies on rejection was clearly demonstrated in the mouse;[7] however, it was less effective in the rat. Therefore, combination treatment of the antibody with preexisting drugs was performed in allografting of the rat.

At the present time, although a variety of immunosuppressants are available, none of them are perfect. In an attempt to find the most effective and safest use of the immunosuppressive drugs, combination use of the agents has been attempted in experimental organ allografting. In this article, we focus our experimental results of the combined use of novel immunosuppressive agents.

POTENCY AND SIDE EFFECTS OF NOVEL IMMUNOSUPPRESSANTS

FK506

FK was first found to be a more potent immunosuppressive agent as compared with CYA in *in vitro* studies.[2] Subsequent experiments with organ allografting in the rat and dog demonstrated that FK was immunosuppressive at a lower dose than CYA,[3,8] and that the optimal serum trough levels of FK for inhibition of allograft rejection were a hundred times lower than CYA.[9,10]

One of the most important features of FK as compared with CYA was that lymphocytes infiltrating in the graft at the time of acute rejection disappeared with rescue treatment with FK and the rejection was reversed.[9]

On the other hand, FK showed drug toxicities both in animals and human.[11] The renal recipient dog receiving FK lost appetite and developed deathly malaise. Histological studies showed nephrotoxicity of degeneration and vacuolation in the tubular cells of the renal allograft of the dog receiving FK.[12,13] Vascular changes were frequently found in the renal recipient dog. They were observed mainly at the heart vessels of the dog receiving nonimmunosuppressive doses of FK, but they were less frequent in the dog receiving an immunosuppressive dose. Thus, vascular toxicity was inversely proportional to the dose, but malaise and nephrotoxicity were dose

TABLE 1. Immunosuppressive Agents in Organ Transplantation

1. Antimetabolite
Azathioprine, Methotrexate, Mizoribine, RS-61443
2. Antibiotic
Cyclosporine, FK 506, Rapamycin, 15-Deoxyspergualin
3. Antibody
ALG, OKT-3, Anti-ICAM-1 antibody, Anti-LFA-1 antibody

dependent. There was a dilemma in that the sufficient immunosuppressive dose induced malaise and nephrotoxicity, and the reduced dose treatment induced vascular toxicity.

On the basis of our experimental data, we hypothesized that vascular changes are induced not only by toxic effects of FK itself but also by immune responses of the host due to insufficient immunosuppression in the transplant recipient, and that sufficient immunosuppression by a combination treatment of FK at a lower dose with a different immunosuppressant could bring about inhibition of rejection to prolong recipient survival times, and suppression of the immune-response-related vascular toxicity. On this hypotheses, we attempted to show the effect of combination treatment on inhibition both of rejection and side effects in experimental organ allografting and xenografting.

Rapamycin

RAP was initially found to be potent against *Candida albicans* and active against several murine tumor models.[14,15] As both RAP and FK are macrolides and structurally related, RAP was investigated to determine if it has immunosuppressive qualities like FK in organ transplantation. Calne, Moris, and our laboratory have reported potent immunosuppressive activity of RAP in cardiac allografting of the rat; however, RAP was toxic in renal allografting of the dog.[4,5,16] The serum amylase level of the renal recipient dog elevated after administration of RAP. More than half of the dogs receiving RAP at 0.3 mg/kg only once a week developed deathly malaise. Autopsy showed that the main histological lesion was vasculitis in the intestinal tract. Since the vasculitis was a major concern as a side effect of FK, pathological features of vasculitis in renal recipient dogs are compared between FK and RAP (TABLE 2). Fibrinoid necrosis in the vascular wall is the most remarkable finding in RAP treatment. Similarly to FK, vascular changes by RAP are inversely proportional to the dose.

EFFECTS OF COMBINATION ON REJECTION

FK with CYA

Canine renal allografting was mainly used for the evaluation of combination treatment in our study. It was performed using female beagle dogs 8 months old and weighing 8 to 10 kg (Hazleton research Products, Kalamazoo, Mich.) throughout the

TABLE 2. Pathological Features of Vasculitis in Renal-Recipient Dogs

	Immunosuppressants	
Pathological Features	FK506 0.32 mg/kg per day	RAP 0.3 mg/kg per wk
Hypertrophy of the wall (edema, fibrosis)	+	+
Cell infiltration	+	+ +
Fibrinoid necrosis	+	+ + +
Organs involved	Heart	Gastrointestinal tract

experiment. Single kidneys were exchanged between 2 unrelated dogs and transplanted to the iliac fossa of the recipient. The contralateral kidney was then removed, and the survival time was compared between the treatment groups for evaluation of the combination effect.

The result of combination treatment of FK with CYA in renal allografting of the dog is shown in FIGURE 1. The oral formula of FK (Fujisawa Pharmaceutical Co., Osaka, Japan) was packed in a gelatin capsule and administered once a day. CYA (Sandoz Co., Basel, Switzerland) was given orally once a day.

The median survival time was 15.5 days in renal recipient dogs without immunosuppressants (group 3). All 5 recipients survived for more than 140 days when treated with FK at 1.0 mg/kg (group 6) and were finally sacrificed with well-functioning grafts. Treatment with FK at 0.32 mg/kg (group 5) or CsA at 2.5 mg/kg (group 4) did not affect the recipients' survival (17.5 and 13.0 days, respectively). Combined treatment with FK and CsA (group 7) at the same doses as single treatment prolonged survival significantly (37.0 days; $p < 0.01$). Two of these 5 recipients survived for 2 months and were sacrificed on day 60 posttransplant with well-functioning grafts.

On the other hand, when FK at 0.32 mg/kg was combined with pred at 0.5 mg/kg (group 8), no favorable effect on survival was seen (19.5 days). In contrast to our results, Todo et al. reported synergism of FK and steroid.[17]

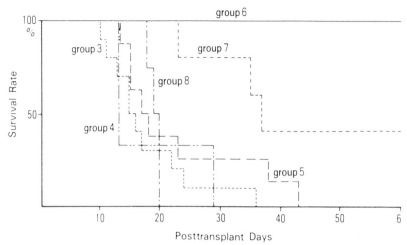

FIGURE 1. Combination of FK with CYA or prednisolone. Survival rates of renal-recipient dogs receiving various kinds of immunosuppressive treatments. Group 3: no immunosuppressant ($n = 10$; median survival time 15.5 days). Group 4: CsA 2.5 mg/kg per day ($n = 3$; 13.0 days). Group 5: FK 0.32 mg/kg per day ($n = 8$; 17.5 days). Group 6: FK 1.0 mg/kg per day ($n = 5$; >140 days). Group 7: FK 0.32 + CsA 2.5 mg/kg per day ($n = 5$; 37.0 days). Group 8: FK 0.32 + pred 0.5 mg/kg per day ($n = 4$; 19.5 days). Statistical difference; group 3 vs. group 7: <0.01; and group 3 vs. group 4, group 3 vs. group 5, group 3 vs. group 8: not significant.

FK with RAP

The effect of combination treatment of FK with RAP is shown in FIGURE 2. Twenty mg of RAPA (Wyeth-Syerst Research, Princeton, N.J.) was prepared for use by dissolving in 0.2 ml of *N,N*-dimethylacetamide and mixing with 0.1 ml of Polysorbate-80 and adjusting to a final volume of 1.0 ml with polyethylene glycol-400, NF. RAPA was given to the recipient by the intramuscular route. FK at 0.08 mg/kg

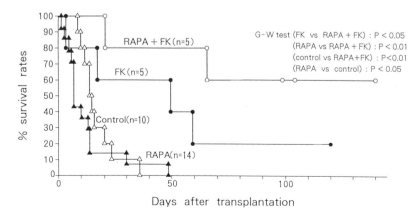

FIGURE 2. Combination of FK with RAP. FK: 0.08 mg/kg per day im, RAP/0.3 mg/kg per week im, FK vs. FK + RAP; $p < 0.05$, RAP vs. FK + RAP; $p < 0.01$. Control vs. FK + RAP; $p < 0.01$. p value was calculated by G-W test.

per day im prolonged recipients' survival times as compared to the control ($p < 0.05$). An additional treatment with an ineffective dose of RAP significantly prolonged survival times as compared to FK treatment alone ($p < 0.05$).

FK with RS

The effect of combination treatment of FK with RS is shown in FIGURE 3. RS was supplied in powder form by Syntex Inc. Palo Alto, Calif. A suspension of RS in carboxymethyl cellulose vehicle (100 mg/ml) was prepared and given to the recipient orally. Combination of FK at 0.32 mg/kg per day per oral with RS at 10 mg/kg per day, po was effective on prolongation of survival times ($p < 0.05$).

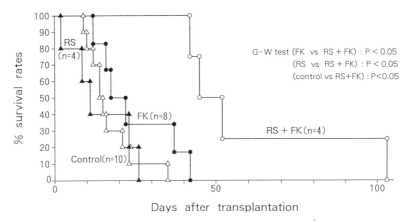

FIGURE 3. Combination of FK with RS. FK; 0.32 mg/kg per day po, RS; 10 mg/kg per day po. FK vs. FK + RS; $p < 0.05$. RS vs. FK + RS; $p < 0.05$. Control vs. FK + RS; $p < 0.05$ by G-W test.

FK with 15-Deoxyspergualin

The effect of FK in combination with 15-Deoxyspergualin (DSG) was studied in segmental pancreas allografting in the pancreatectomized dog. Nonimmunosuppressed control dogs died at 12.0 days. FK at 0.1 or 0.2 mg/kg per day im did slightly prolong recipient survival but not statistically significantly. FK at 0.3 mg/kg per day im killed all the recipients due to malaise. Combination of FK at 0.1 mg/kg per day with DSG at 0.3 mg/kg per day iv prolonged the survival significantly ($p < 0.02$) (TABLE 3).

RAP with CYA

Combination of RAP with CYA is shown in FIGURE 4. Weekly injection of RAP at a dose of 0.3 mg/kg was immunosuppressive but toxic in the renal recipient dog. In combination with a nonimmunosuppressive dose of CYA at 2.5 mg/kg per day, the recipient survived significantly longer.

TABLE 3. Effect of FK in Combination with 15-Deoxyspergualin in Pancreas Allografting of the Dog[a]

	Drugs	No. of Dogs	Survival days (Mean + SD)	
	—	5	12.0 + 4.8	
FK	0.1	7	14.3 + 6.9	NS
(im)	0.2	4	20.5 + 8.3	NS
	0.3	5[a]	30.8 +21.3	<0.05
FK	0.1			
+		3	44.7 + 3.8	<0.02
DSG	0.3			

[a]All dogs died of emaciation.

RAP with RS

RAP at 0.3 mg/kg per week im was combined with RS at 10 mg/kg per day po in renal allografting in the dog. The group of dogs receiving the combination treatment survived longer than the control dogs (FIGURE 5).

EFFECTS OF COMBINATION ON SIDE EFFECTS

Vasculitis

As the vascular toxicity was related to non-immunosuppressive doses of FK or RAP, sufficient immunosuppression was given to the renal recipient dog by the combination treatment and the occurrence of vasculitis was studied. In the experiment of FIGURE 1, the frequency of vasculitis was compared among the treatment groups (TABLE 4). Vascular changes were not found in the nontransplant dogs receiving FK alone at 0.32 mg/kg or 1.0 mg/kg for 14 days (groups 1 and 2). All the heart specimens taken from 5 renal recipient dogs receiving 0.32 mg/kg of FK and

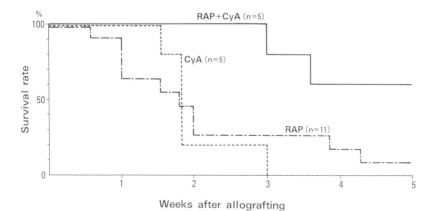

FIGURE 4. Combination of RAP with CYA. RAP; 0.3 mg/kg per twice a week im. CYA; 2.5 mg/kg per day, po. RAP vs. RAP + DYA; $p < 0.01$. CYA vs. RAP + CYA; $p < 0.05$.

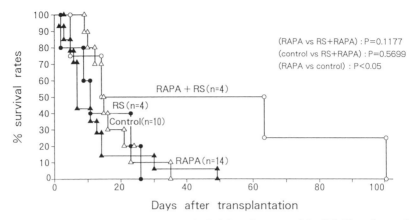

FIGURE 5. Combination of RAP with RS. RAP; 0.3 mg/kg per week im. RS; 10 mg/kg per day po. RAP vs. RAP + RS; $p = 0.12$. RS vs. RAP + RS; $p = 0.26$. Control vs. RAP + RS $p < 0.05$.

dying of rejection between 13 and 43 days posttransplant showed small round cell infiltrations in the vascular wall (group 5) (FIGURE 2). Similar vascular changes were also found in the renal recipient dogs without any immunosuppression (group 3) (FIGURES 3 and 4) and in those receiving CsA treatment at 2.5 mg/kg (group 4) (FIGURE 5). On the other hand, only 1 out of 5 recipients receiving FK at 1.0 mg/kg for as long as 140 days or more showed marginal changes of wall thickening (group 6). Additional treatment with CsA at 2.5 mg/kg together with FK at 0.32 mg/kg reduced the frequency of the vascular changes significantly (group 7, $p < 0.01$); only one showed a mild change of fibrinoid necrosis in the vessel wall, but cell infiltration was not seen.

The addition of Pred to FK failed to prevent the occurrence of vascular changes (group 8).

In the experiment using RAP, the frequency of vasculitis was 63.6% in the

TABLE 4. Frequency of Vascular Changes in the Heart of Renal-Recipient Dogs[a]

Group	Treatment (mg/kg)	Lengths of FK Treatment (days)	No. Dogs Examined	No. Dogs Dying of Rejection	No. Dogs Showing Vascular Changes
Nontransplant dog:					
1	FK 0.32	14	5	0	0
2	FK 1.0	14	3	0	0
Renal-transplant dog:					
3	None	0	4	4	2
4	CsA 2.5	0	3	3	3
5	FK 0.32	13–43	5	5	5
6	FK 1.0	144–173	5	0	1
7	FK 0.32 + CsA 2.5	23–60	5	3	1
8	FK 0.32 + Pred 0.5	18–20	4	4	2

[a]Statistical difference of frequency of vascular changes: group 5 vs 6, $p < 0.01$; group 5 vs. 7, $p < 0.01$.

TABLE 5. Effect of Combination Treatment on the Frequency of Vasculitis[a]

	No. of Dogs	Heart	Gastrointestinal
Nontransplant			
RAP	3	0	1 (33.3%)
Renal transplant			
RAP	11	1 (9.1%)	7 (63.6%)
RAP + CYA	5	0	0
RAP + FK	5	0	0
RAP + RS	4	1 (25.0%)	0

[a]RAP, 0.3 mg/kg per wk; CYA, 2.5 mg/kg per day; RS, 10 mg/kg per day.

renal-recipient dog receiving RAP alone, but when CYA, FA, or RS was combined, the frequency of vasculitis decreased, similarly to the case of FK (TABLE 5).

Serum Amylase Levels

Elevation of serum amylase levels was one of the abnormal results in the renal-recipient dog receiving RAP, although the pathological meaning has not been clear. When other immunosuppressants were combined with RAP, elevation of serum amylase levels was inhibited (FIGURE 6).

The renal-recipient dogs receiving FK or RAP lost appetite and developed deathly malaise; however, in the dogs receiving the same dose of FK or RAP with other immunosuppressants, decrease in body weight was not so severe. Thus, the combination treatment is effective in reduction of side effects.

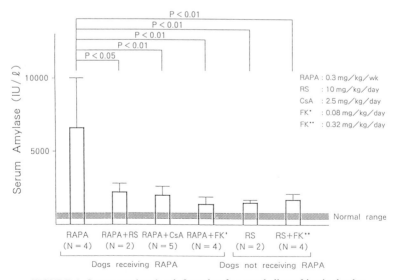

FIGURE 6. Serum amylase levels 2 weeks after renal allografting in the dog.

XENOTRANSPLANTATION

Xenogenic transplantation has been believed to be more difficult to achieve than allogenic transplantation, mainly because of the strength and complexity of rejection. The relatively little progress made in this area must be due to a lack of understanding of the rejection mechanism as well as a dearth of effective immunosuppressants. After introduction of FK506, the effect on xenograft rejection was studied using a skin and cardiac transplantation model from the hamster to the rat or from the mouse to the rat. In the mouse-rat combination, treatment with FK prolonged skin graft survival times significantly, but failed to prolong heart xenograft survival times.[18,19] In the hamster-rat combination, again, FK506 prolonged skin xenograft survival times, but it failed to prolong heart xenograft survival.[20] FK506 enhanced the prolongation of survival times when used in combination with 15-Deoxyspergualin. The effect of FK506 on vascularized organ xenografting was compared with that of cyclosporine or 15-Deoxyspergualin. T cell specific immunosuppressive agents such

TABLE 6. Effects of Anti-ICAM-1 and Anti-LFA-1 on Cardiac Allografts in Rats[a]

Anti-ICAM-1[b]	Anti-LFA-1[b]	CyA[c]	n	Graft Survival (days)	MST + SD	p[d]
0	0	0	10	6(×10)	6.0 + 0.0	NS
1.5	0	0	6	6(×5),7	6.3 + 0.5	NS
5.0	0	0	5	(2),(4)(×3),(5)		
1.5	1.5	0	4	6(×3),8	6.5 + 0.8	NS
0	0	3.2	9	6 (×6),7(×3)	6.3 + 0.5	NS
0.5	0	3.2	20	15,20,21,(×2), 24,25,26,31,33, 34,35(×2),37, >100(×6)	>49.5 + 34.4	.01
0	1.5	3.2	6	28, >100(×5)	>88.0 + 29.4	.01

[a]Parentheses indicate that the patient died before rejection occurred.
[b]Anti-ICAM-1 and anti-LFA-1 were continuously given to the recipients intraperitoneally using miniosmotic pump (model 2ML2, Alza) for 7 days.
[c]CyA was given subcutaneously for 11 days after grafting.
[d]Significance was determined by the Mann-Whitney U test.

as FK506 and Cyclosporine seemed to be insufficient for suppression of xenograft rejection. On the other hand, Valdivia et al. reported long-term survival of hepatic xenograft recipients in a hamster-rat combination.[21] FK506 was more effective than cyclosporine in their system, but it worked only in the liver and not in heart xenotransplant.

MONOCLONAL ANTIBODIES AGAINST ADHESION MOLECULES

Allograft rejection of vascularized organs is mostly mediated by T cells and initially requires the binding of antigen-presenting cells (APCs) of the graft to the T-helper cells of the recipient. ICAM-1, a surface glycopotein in the immunoglobulin superfamily, is induced on the cell membrane of endothelial cells and macrophages and activated by various lymphokines, including interleukin 1, tumor necrosis factor, and -interferon. LFA-1, which is a member of the integrin family, is expressed on T lymphocytes but not regulated by lymphokines. *In vitro* studies have demonstrated that cell surface adhesion molecules, including ICAM-1 and LFA-1, are important not only for adhesion of the cells, but also as factors for interaction between APCs of the graft and T-helper cells of the recipient, as well as for antigen recognition by the T cell receptor.[22,23]

Adhesion of lymphocytes to endothelial cells is also important for the entry of lymphocytes into the graft during the allograft rejection, and the level of ICAM-1 on the endothelial cells is elevated in the rejecting graft. From these observations, it is expected that adhesion molecules play important roles in allograft rejection, and rejection could be suppressed by monoclonal antibodies against adhesion molecules. We have observed that monoclonal anti-ICAM-1 antibody and monoclonal anti-LFA-1 antibody completely suppress mixed lymphocyte culture in rats.

Isobe *et al.* reported that anti-ICAM-1 prolonged survival times of vascularized heart allografts in the mouse.[7] We studied the effect of anti-ICAM-1 and anti-LFA-1 on cardiac allografting of the rat.[24] As shown in TABLE 6, monotherapy or combined therapy of anti-ICAM-1 and/or anti-LFA-1 did not have any effect on prolongation of graft survival times; however, in combination with a low dose of CYA at 3.2 mg/kg, significant prolongation of graft survival times were observed. Similar results were obtained by Cosimi *et al.*, who reported that renal allograft survival times of the cynomolgus monkey were prolonged by anti-ICAM-1 antibody treatment with CYA.[25]

In application to humans, anti-ICAM-1 and anti-LFA-1 would be used with other immunosuppressants that have different modes of action in suppression of rejection.

SUMMARY

Several novel immunosuppressive agents have been developed in recent years. They exhibited not only remarkable immunosuppressive potency but also side effects. They are still short of the final goal in terms of immunosuppression for organ transplantation. Combination treatment is more effective and safer to use, and it will prevail in the future.

REFERENCES

1. INAMURA, N., K. NAKAHARA, T. KINO, T. GOTO, H. AOKI, I. YAMAGUCHI, M. KOHSAKA, & T. OCHIAI. 1988. Prolongation of skin allograft survival in rats by a novel immunosuppressive agent, FK506. Transplantation **45**: 206–209.
2. KINO, T., H. HATANAKA, S. MIYATA, N. INAMURA, M. NISHIYAMA, T. YAJIMA, T. GOTO, M. OKUHARA, M. KOHSAKA, H. AOKI & T. OCHIAI. 1987. FK506, a novel immunosuppressant isolated from a streptomyces. II. Immunosuppressive effect of FK506 in vitro. J. Antibiot. **40**(9): 1256–1265.
3. OCHIAI, T., K. NAKAJIMA, M. NAGATA, S. HORI, T. ASANO & K. ISONO. 1987. Studies of the induction and maintenance of long-term graft acceptance by treatment with FK506 in heterotopic cardiac allotransplantation in rats. Transplantation **44**(6): 734–738.
4. CALNE, R. Y., D. ST. J. COLLIER & S. LIM. 1989. Rapamycin for immunosuppression in organ allografting. Lancet **2**: 227.
5. OCHIAI, T., Y. GUNJI, M. NAGATA, T. ASANO & K. ISONO. Effects of rapamycin in experimental organ allografting. Transplantation **56**(1): 15–19.
6. STARZL, T. E., S. TODO, J. FUNG, A. J. DEMETRIS, R. VENKATARAMMAN & A. JAIN. 1989. FK506 for liver, kidney, and pancreas transplantation. Lancet **ii**: 1000–1004.
7. ISOBE, M., H. YAGITA, KO. OKUMURA & A. IHARA. 1992. Specific acceptance of cardiac allograft after treatment with antibodies to ICAM-1 and LFA-1. Reports: 1125–1127.

8. OCHIAI, T., M. NAGATA, K. NAKAJIMA, T. SUZUKI, K. SAKAMOTO, K. ENOMOTO, Y. GUNJI, T. UEMATSU, T. GOTO, S. HORI, T. KENMOCHI, T. NAKAGOURI, T. ASANO, K. ISONO, K. HAMAGUCHI, H. TSUCHIDA, K. NAKAHARA, N. INAMURA & T. GOTO. 1987. Studies of the effects of FK506 on renal allografting in the beagle dog. Transplantation 44(6): 729–733.

9. OCHIAI, T., Y. GUNJI, K. SAKAMOTO, T. SUZUKI, N. ISEGAWA, T. ASANO & K. ISONO. 1989. Optimal serum trough levels of FK506 in renal allotransplantation of the beagle dog. Transplantation 48: 189–193.

10. JAIN, A. B., J. J. FUNG, A. G. TZAKIS, R. VENKATARAMANAN, K. ABU-ELMAGD, M. ALESSIANI, J. REYES, W. IRISH, V. WARTHY, S. MEHTA, S. MEHTA, S. TODO & T. E. STARZL. 1991. Comparative study of cyclosporine and Fk506 dosage requirements in adult and pediatric orthotopic liver transplant patients. Transplant. Proc. 23(6): 2763–2766.

11. FUNG, J. J., M. ALESSIANI, K. ABU-ELMAGD, S. TODO, R. SHAPIRO, A. TZAKIS, D. VAN THIEL, J. ARMITAGE, A. JAIN, J. MCCAULEY, R. SELBY & T. E. STARZL. 1991. Adverse effects associated with the use of FK506. Transplant. Proc. 23(6): 3105–3108.

12. OCHIAI, T., K. SAKAMOTO, Y. GUNJI, K. HAMAGUCHI, N. ISEGAWA, T. SUZUKI, H. SHIMADA, H. HAYASHI, A. YASUMOTO, T. ASANO & K. ISONO. 1989. Effects of combination treatment with FK506 and cyclosporine on survival time and vascular changes in renal-allograft-recipient dogs. Transplantation 48: 193–197.

13. SEHGAL, S. N., H. BAKER & C. VEZINA. 1975. Rapamycin (AY-22,989), a new antifungal antibiotic. II. Fermentation, isolation and characterization. J. Antibiot. 28: 727–732.

14. ENG, C. P., S. N. SEHGAL & C. VEZINA. 1984. Activity of Rapamycin against transplanted tumors. J. Antibiot. 37: 1231–1237.

15. MORRIS, R. E. & B. M. MEISER. 1989. Identification of a new pharmacologic action for an old compound. Med. Sci. Res. 17: 609–610.

16. TODO, S., Y. UEDA, J. A. DEMETRIS, O. IMVENTARZA, M. NALESNIK, R. VENKATARAMANAN, L. MAKOWKA & T. E. STARZL. 1988. Immunosuppression of canine, monkey, and baboon allografts by FK506: with special reference to synergism with other drugs and to tolerance induction. Surgery 104(2): 239–249.

17. OCHIAI, T., M. NAGATA, K. NAKAJIMA, K. ISONO, N. INAMURA & K. NAKAHARA. 1987. Effects of FK-506 on xenotransplantation of the heart and skin in a mouse-rat combination. Transplant. Proc. 19(Suppl. 6): 84–86.

18. NAKAJIMA, K., K. SAKAMOTO, T. OCHIAI, M. NAGATA, T. ASANO & K. ISONO. 1988. Prolongation of cardiac xenograft survival in rats treated with 15-deoxyspergualin alone and in combination with FK506. Transplantation 45(6): 1146–1148.

19. VALDIVIA, L. A., J. J. FUNG, A. J. DEMETRIS & T. E. STARZL. 1991. Differential survival of hamster-to-rat liver and cardiac xenografts under FK506 immunosuppression. Transplant. Proc. 23: 3269–3271.

20. SPRINGER, T. A. 1990. Adhesion receptors of the immune system. Nature 346(2): 425–434.

21. SEVENTER, G. A. V., Y. SHIMIZU, K. J. HORGAN & S. SHAW. 1990. The LFA-1 ligand ICAM-1 provides an important costimulatory signal for T cell receptor–mediated activation of resting T cells. J. Immunol. 144: 4579–4586.

22. KOMORI, A., M. NAGATA, T. OCHIAI, K. NAKAJIMA, S. HORI, T. ASANO, K. ISONO, T. TAMATANI & M. MIYASAKA. 1993. Role of ICAM-1 and LFA-1 in cardiac allograft rejection of the rat. Transplant. Proc. 25(1): 831–832.

23. COSIMI, A. B., D. CONTI, F. L. DELMONICO, F. I. PREFFER, S. L. WEE, R. ROTHLEIN, R. FAANES & R. B. COLVIN. 1990. In vivo effects of monoclonal antibody to ICAM-1 (CD54) in nonhuman primates with renal allografts. J. Immunol. 144: 4604–4612.

Immunosuppressant Combinations in Primate Cardiac Xenografts[a]

A Review

ROBERT P. McMANUS,[b] DANIEL P. O'HAIR,[b,e]
RICHARD KOMOROWSKI,[c] AND J. PAUL SCOTT[d]

[b]Department of Cardiothoracic Surgery
[c]Department of Pathology
[d]Department of Pediatrics
Medical College of Wisconsin
8700 West Wisconsin Avenue
Milwaukee, Wisconsin 53226
and
[d]The Blood Center of Southeastern Wisconsin

INTRODUCTION

The severe shortage of human donors for heart transplantation has renewed interest in xenografts as a potential source of donor organs.[1] Successful short-term cardiac xenotransplantation has been achieved both clinically and experimentally.[2,3] Long-term (>1 year) cardiac xenograft survival has been reported using toxic immunosuppression involving total lymphoid irradiation.[4]

In humans, long-term cardiac allograft survival is limited by the development of coronary vasculopathy.[5] Similar vascular pathologic changes have been observed in xenografts within months of transplantation.[6] Humoral rejection with progressive increases in antibody levels parallels progression of vascular pathologic changes in xenografts and limits long-term primate cardiac xenograft survival.[7] Vascular pathologic changes have been reported in xenografts, and their importance may increase as survival times increase.

This series, a review of 17 xenografts, represents experience with various immunosuppressive regimens used in primate cardiac xenotransplantation, parts of which have been reported earlier.[3,6,8] The effects of various clinically tolerable immunosuppressant combinations on primate cardiac xenograft survival and histopathology are presented.

METHODS

Transplants

All primates were fasted on the evening prior to operation but allowed water *ad libitum.* Animals were sedated with ketamine 10 mg/kg by intramuscular (im)

[a]This work was supported in part by American Heart Association grant no. 90-GA-09 and by VA Merit Review no. 5565-02P.
[e]Author to whom correspondence should be addressed at: Medical College of Wisconsin, Department of Surgery, 9200 W. Wisconsin Avenue, Milwaukee, Wisconsin 53226.

injection and received atropine 0.4 mg/kg im. Sodium pentobarbital was administered 15 mg/kg intravenously (iv), and the animals were intubated and supported on a volume cycled ventilator during operation.

Cynomolgous monkeys (*Macacca fascicularis*) weighing 3–5 kg served as donors for ABO matched, crossmatch negative, baboons (*Papio anubis*) weighing 10–15 kg. Heterotopic cardiac transplantation was performed in the neck of the baboon as previously described.[9] Graft function was monitored daily by visualization and palpation, and local EKG was performed if necessary. Graft biopsy was performed at 1, 2, 4, 8, and 12 weeks postoperatively in groups 3 and 4 with follow-up biopsy 1 week after rejection therapy. Graft survival was measured from transplant date to loss of graft pulse or signal.

Immunosuppression

Group 1 baboons received no immunosuppression. Group 2 baboons received CsA 15 mg/kg per day by intramuscular injection beginning 1 day prior to operation. Methylprednisolone sodium succinate (Solumedrol) 125 mg was given intravenously on day 0 and 1. Baboons then received methylprednisolone acetate (Depomedrol) 0.8 mg/kg per day im. Group 3 baboons received the same regimen as group 2 with the addition of azathioprine 4 mg/kg per day orally beginning 21 days preoperatively and continuing postoperatively until rejection. Group 4 had the same regimen as group 3 with the substitution of Mycopenolate Mofetil 70 mg/kg per day orally for azathioprine.

Episodes of rejection were defined as moderate or severe based on previously described criteria.[10] When present, rejection was treated initially with methylprednisolone sodium succinate (Solumedrol) 250 mg iv for 3 days followed by methylprednisolone acetate (Depomedrol) 2 mg/kg per day im for 4 days. Biopsy was repeated after this initial course. Persistent rejection was treated with antithymocyte globulin (ATG) (ATGAM, Upjohn) 10 mg/kg per day iv for 7 days.

Histopathology

Needle biopsy specimens and explanted xenografts were fixed in 10% formalin solution and subsequently stained with hematoxylin-phloxine-saffron. All slides were examined and graded blindly by a pathologist. The grading scale of the International Society for Heart Transplantation was used to assess mild, moderate, or severe rejection.[10] Sections through blood vessels were evaluated for the presence of endothelial swelling, perivascular inflammatory infiltrates, or intimal proliferation leading to occlusion.

RESULTS

Group 1 baboons (*n* = 4), who received no immunosuppression, had a mean survival of nine days (range 8–10 days). Rejection was usually complete within 24 hours of onset and always within 48 hours. Histologic examination of all specimens from this group showed dense mononuclear and polymorphonuclear cellular infiltrates, extensive myocyte necrosis, edema, interstitial hemmorhage, and vascular thrombosis consistent with severe mixed humoral and cellular rejection.

The addition of cyclosporine and steroids in group 2 prolonged survival to 77 days (range 16–200 days). Using this immunosuppressant combination, hearts undergoing early rejection showed a histologic picture of rejection similar to group 1. Those with longer survival demonstrated histological appearance consistent with repeated episodes of rejection with healing and gradual replacement of myocardium with connective tissue.[3]

In group 3, rejection surveillance was performed and treated as previously described.[8] Survival was prolonged to 94 days (range 3–392). Using this regimen of early detection and treatment of rejection, four of nine rejection episodes were reversed using high dose steroids. ATG 10 mg/kg per day intravenously reversed 2/4 episodes of steroid resistant rejection.[8] Despite rescue from cellular rejection, these grafts were later lost to humoral rejection.

In group 4, Mofetil was substituted for azathioprine and mean survival was 296 days (range 49–618). In this group, a biopsy at 618 days of survival showed a coronary artery free of intimal occlusive disease. Evidence of less severe coronary artery disease was found in only two biopsy specimens and consisted of moderate endothelial swelling. There was no evidence of coronary intimal proliferation in this group.

DISCUSSION

The continuing and progressive donor shortage has renewed interest in xenotransplantation. This review of 17 primate cardiac xenografts performed over a five year period has provided several key insights into the future of xenotransplantation and the drugs used to combat xenograft rejection. The importance of parenterally administered cyclosporine has been established in this model.[3] Xenograft rejection has been shown to be a reversible process using currently available agents.[8]

Cellular rejection may be controlled and in some cases reversed, but progressive increases in lymphocytotoxic antibody lead invariably to eventual graft loss. The importance of an endothelial cell directed antibody in cardiac xenograft rejection was first suggested in 1992.[11] In this study, the appearance of this specific antibody was a predictor of iminent terminal xenograft rejection. Mofetil clearly has antilymphocyte properties and may have strong B cell suppressor responses.[12] Mofetil has reduced the incidence and severity of graft coronary artery disease in a rat allograft model.[13] The mechanism of suppression of vascular pathologic changes in long-term primate cardiac xenografts by Mofetil is currently under investigation and may be related to the development of antibody directed at the vascular endothelial cell.

Vascular rejection, an important factor in long-term allograft survival, appears to have an increasing role in xenografts as survival increases. The development of immunosuppressant agents that delay or inhibit this phenomenon will have important implications in both allograft and xenograft heart transplantation. Long-term cardiac xenograft survival is possible using currently available immunosuppressive agents.

SUMMARY

ABO matched cynomolgous monkey to baboon heterotopic xenografts were performed using three different immunosuppressant regimens. Group 1 ($n = 4$) baboons, which did not receive immunosuppression, had a mean graft survival of 9 days. Group 2 ($n = 6$) received cyclosporine (CsA) and methylprednisolone acetate which prolonged graft survival to an average of 78 days. Group 3 ($n = 5$) received CsA, Pred, and azathioprine (Aza) as well as steroid pulses and antithymocyte globulin (ATG) for rejection episodes. Survival in this group averaged 94 days. In Group 4 ($n = 3$), the same regimen as group 3 was used; however, Mycophenolate Mofetil was substituted for Aza. This resulted in a mean survival of 296 days. Histologic examination of the coronary vasculature in baboons treated with Mofetil showed a reduction in vascular pathologic changes when compared to those treated with Aza. Long-term cardiac xenograft survival is possible using currently available immunosuppressive agents.

REFERENCES

1. MCMANUS, R. P., D. P. O'HAIR, et al. 1993. J. Heart Lung Transplant. **12**(2): 159–172.
2. BAILEY, L. L., S. L. NEHLSON-CANNARELLA, W. CONCEPCION, et al. 1985. JAMA **254**: 3321.
3. MICHLER, R. E., R. P. MCMANUS, C. R. SMITH, et al. 1987. Transplantation **44**(5): 632–636.
4. ROSLIN, M. S., R. F. TRANBOUGH, A. PANZA, et al. 1992. Transplantation **54**(6): 949–955.
5. GAO, S. Z., S. A. HUNT, J. S. SCHROEDER, et al. 1990. Semin. Thoracic Cardiovasc. Surg. **2**: 247.
6. MCMANUS, R. P., D. P. O'HAIR, J. B. HUNTER, et al. 1992. Transplant. Proc. **24**(2): 619–624.
7. FUZESI, L., P. PEPINO, C. L. BERGER, et al. 1989. Transplant. Proc. **21**: 537.
8. MCMANUS, R. P., T. KINNEY, R. KOMOROWSKI, et al. 1991. J. Heart Lung Transplant. **10**(4): 567–575.
9. MICHLER, R. E., R. P. MCMANUS, C. R. SMITH, et al. 1985. J. Med. Primatol. **14**: 357.
10. BILLINGHAM, M. E., N. R. CARY, M. E. HAMMOND, et al. 1990. J. Heart Lung Transplant. **9**(6): 587–593.
11. O'HAIR, D. P., R. P. MCMANUS, C. P. JOHNSON, et al. 1992. Transplant. Proc. **24**(2): 506–507.
12. PLATZ, K. P., H. W. SOLLINGER, D. A. HULLETT, et al. 1991. Transplantation **51**(1): 27–31.
13. MORRIS, R. E., J. WANG, J. R. BLUM, et al. 1991. Transplant. Proc. **23**(2) (Suppl. 2): 19–25.

Optimizing Combination Chemotherapy for Rheumatoid Arthritis

DANIEL E. FURST

Virginia Mason Research Center
Clinical Research Programs
1100 Ninth Avenue
Post Office Box 900, GB-CRP
Seattle, Washington 98111

Effective treatment of rheumatoid arthritis should be rational and should be based on a knowledge of rheumatoid arthritis, a knowledge of the patients who will receive therapy, and a knowledge of the clinical pharmacology of the drugs to be used. It is beyond the scope of this discussion to detail the pathogenesis and manifestations of rheumatoid arthritis. Instead, a general overview of rheumatoid arthritis's pathogenesis will be outlined. This will be followed by a brief discussion of the type of rheumatoid arthritis patient who is most likely to require, and receive, combination disease modifying antirheumatic drug (DMARD) therapy.[a]

Thereafter, the clinical pharmacology of a few of these drugs will be outlined, demonstrating their putative mechanisms of action, pharmacokinetics, and toxicity. Based on these data, some examples of a rational approach toward developing combination therapy for rheumatoid arthritis will be demonstrated. Because a number of combination DMARD trials have been carried out, the applicability of this rational approach can be "tested" by examining the results of some clinical trials of combination therapy that were actually carried out.

Because a complete description of this approach goes well beyond the limits of this symposium, examples will be used simply to demonstrate the possibilities inherent in such an approach.

PATHOGENESIS OF RHEUMATOID ARTHRITIS

Rheumatoid arthritis is characterized by inflammation of the joints and involvement of a number of other organs, including the eyes, lungs, heart, kidneys, muscles, skin, and peripheral nerves.[1] On a genetic background, it is thought that rheumatoid arthritis can be activated by environmental influences which then activate the immune system. Antigen processing cells metabolize the putative antigen and present the antigen to T cells in the context of MHC class II receptors. This results in T and B cell activation, cytokine release, and amplification of the immune response. Amplification leads to eicosanoid and enzyme release and neutrophil recruitment. The end point of this cascade is angiogenesis, synovitis, pannus formation, tissue destruction . . . and clinical disease.[1]

---

[a]In the context of the present discussion, DMARD will be defined as the following medications: organic gold therapy, hydroxychloroquine, D-penicillamine, methotrexate, sulfasalazine, and azathioprine; it does not include alkylating agents such as cyclophosphamide.

PATIENT POPULATION MOST APPROPRIATE FOR
COMBINATION DMARD THERAPY

DMARD studies to date have not stratified their patients on prognostic disease factors or disease severity factors. However, given the toxicities inherent in combination DMARD therapy, an approach using appropriate patient subsets would be most welcome.

Unfortunately the data defining the population with the most progressive disease are neither uniform nor complete. Despite this, future studies should strongly consider such subsetting. The following factors are likely to define patients with more severe disease: age, disease severity (poor functional status, extraarticular features, nodules, increasing numbers of swollen and tender joints), rheumatoid factor positivity, and elevated acute phase reactants.[2–5] HLA-D (MHC class II) genes may also be associated with increasing severity of disease. Several studies indicate that patients homozygous for variants of HLA-DR4 are susceptible to disease and, perhaps, more severe disease.[6–8]

EXAMPLES OF THE STATE OF KNOWLEDGE WITH RESPECT TO THE
CLINICAL PHARMACOLOGY OF DMARDs

Mechanisms of Action

Cyclosporin

During this symposium, the latest knowledge about cyclosporin A's mechanism of action has been carefully discussed, and need not be reiterated in detail here. At a relatively "macro" level, cyclosporin A inhibits the production of IL-2, inhibits IL-1-like activating factor, and inhibits IFN-gamma (leading to decreased expression of MHC products).[9]

Methotrexate

Methotrexate, through effects on dihydrofolate reductase, thymidelate synthetase, and amino imidazole carboxamide ribonucleoside transformylase (AICAR), has multiple mechanisms of action. These secondarily result in decreased LTB4, decreased polymorphonuclear adhesion, and decreased macrophage IL-1 secretion.[10,11]

Similar delineations for the mechanisms of action of D-penicillamine, sulfasalazine, azathioprine, and hydroxychloroquine can be made. TABLE 1 summarizes such a listing for each medication.[12] A "+" indicates that a listed mechanism of action is likely to apply to the drug in question. From TABLE 1, it is easy to see those DMARDs with overlapping mechanisms of action. Those drugs with the most overlapping mechanisms of action are least likely to be synergistic. It is obvious that the validity of TABLE 1 relies on the detail and certainty with which a given mechanism of action is known, and this table could potentially undergo a very large expansion. The usefulness of the table, however, must lie in a balance between reasonable certainty, specificity, and practicality. It will certainly benefit from later modifications, but is sufficient for purposes of demonstration at present.

Human Pharmacokinetics

As in the examples relating to mechanism of action, cyclosporin and methotrexate will be used to exemplify the kinetics used in the rational selection of combination DMARD therapy.

Cyclosporin A is a highly lipophilic compound with variable absorption (4–50%) and low protein binding. Interestingly, cyclosporin binds to high and low density lipoprotein, as opposed to albumin, which is common to most DMARDs. As a lipophilic drug, cyclosporin A is highly concentrated in the liver, pancreas, and adrenals; despite the lipophilic nature of the central nervous system (CNS), this drug does not cross the blood-brain barrier, so it does not concentrate in this organ. Cyclosporin A undergoes mostly biliary excretion, with renal excretion accounting for only 6% of the total. Cyclosporin's terminal half-life is 25–30 hours, thus clearly allowing once daily therapy. It is highly metabolized in the liver with a very high first-pass effect.[13]

Methotrexate, on the other hand, is generally well absorbed, with a bioavailability averaging 70%. It has a short terminal serum half-life of approximately 6 hours, although its half-life ranges from 2–24 hours. Like cyclosporin, this drug's protein

TABLE 1. Mechanism(s) of DMARDs (Combined Sources)

Inhibits:	SSZ	HCQ	CSA	Gold	DPA	MTX	AZA
SOD	+			+	SOD-like		
PMN Chemo	+					+	
DHFR	+					+	
IL-1		+	+			+	
IL-2			+	+			
Purines						+	+
Thymidine						+	+
B-cells	+			+	+	+	+
T-cells		+	+		+		+
Membranes	+						
Other	+			+	+		

binding is low about (50%) although, unlike cyclosporin, it is bound to albumin. Unlike cyclosporin, this drug undergoes intracellular metabolism, forming active polyglutamates.[13-15] Ten percent of methotrexate is metabolized to a mildly active 7-OH- metabolite. In contrast to cyclosporin, methotrexate is principally renally excreted, although some biliary excretion also occurs.[13,14]

In a manner similar to that utilized for mechanisms of action, a table of comparative pharmacokinetics can be constructed (TABLE 2).[12] With such a table, it is possible to examine drugs whose kinetics may interfere with each other. From TABLE 2, for example, one might predict metabolic interactions between sulfasalazine, hydroxychloroquine, cyclosporin, and, possibly, methotrexate. Likewise, methotrexate and cyclosporin both undergo biliary excretion in contrast with sulfasalazine, hydroxychloroquine, gold, and D-penicillamine, which are not known to be excreted through the biliary tract.

Toxicities

TABLE 3 displays some of the toxicities requiring discontinuation, distilled from 71 trials using DMARDs in rheumatoid arthritis. This table is modified from an

TABLE 2. Pharmacokinetics of DMARDs (Combined Sources)

	SSZ	HCQ	CSA	Gold	DPA	MTX
Bioavail. (%)	15/33	74	4/50	>95	40/70	70
Vol. of dist.		++++		++		
Prot. bind. (%)			20/70	>90		50
Liver metab.	++	++	++++		+/−	+
Renal excr.			+/−	++	++	++
Biliary excr.			++++			+
Fecal excr.	++		++		+	

article by Felson *et al.* published in 1990.[16] While this table only lists *some* of the side effects found when these DMARDs are used and, further, only lists the adverse incidents causing drug discontinuations ≥ 1%, it once more illustrates the principle. That is, using this approach, one can rationally design combination DMARD regimens without overlapping toxicity. From TABLE 3, it can be seen that it would not be appropriate to combine D-penicillamine and gold, as they are associated with the highest incidence of rash. Likewise, methotrexate, D-penicillamine, sulfasalazine, and gold sodium thiomalate all cause decreased white blood cell counts, thus making their combinations less rational than any one of those with either auranofin or hydroxychloroquine.

RATIONAL APPROACH TO DMARD COMBINATIONS

From the foregoing construct, one can examine the rationale for combining any two DMARDs, using the overlapping (or lack of overlap) in mechanism of action, pharmacokinetics, and toxicities as a guide. To examine the potential utility of such a construct, we will examine a few examples of DMARD combinations, and predict their outcome, were they to be tested in clinical trials. Then actual clinical trials with those combinations will be used to see how well the predictions worked.

TABLE 4 outlines the rationale for combinations of methotrexate with other DMARDs. A "+" indicates no overlap, while a "−" indicates probable negative

TABLE 3. Organ Specific Toxicities Requiring Dropout (%) (Only for Percentage > or Equal to 1%) A&R 33:1449, 1990—Metanalysis of 71 Trials

	Plac.	AF	HCQ/CQ	MTX	DPA	SSZ	GST
Fever	—	—	—	—	—	1.1	—
Rash	1.2	3.2	2.3	—	7.1	3.8	13.0
Stomatitis	—	—	—	2.6	—	—	1.8
Taste	—	—	—	—	2.5	—	—
Decr. WBC (no hct, plts)	—	—	—	1.0	1.0	1.1	1.5
Proteinuria (no ARF)	—	—	—	—	5.0	—	3.7
Eyes	—	—	0.7	—	—	—	—
GI tract	1.0	1.1	3.3	2.1	—	—	1.3
N/V	—	—	1.3	2.1	2.0	12.5	—
Diarrhea	—	3.9	—	—	—	—	—
Hepatic	—	—	—	10.3	—	1.6	—
"Other"	—	1.4	1.0	—	—	1.1	2.2

TABLE 4. Rationales for Combinations: Methotrexate[a]

	Mech.	pk	Toxicity
Hydroxychlor.	+	+	+
D-Penicillamine	+	+(k)	−(m)
Cyclosporin A	+	+	−(k)
Azathiporine	−(pur)	+	−(m)
Sulfasalazine	−(sod, dhfr)	+	−(r, h)
Gold	+	−(k)	−(st)

[a] − = antagonism/overlap; + = nonoverlap.

interactions. This table, it may be discerned, is a selective condensation of TABLES 1–3.

TABLE 4 would predict that a study using gold plus methotrexate would not show this combination to be better than either drug alone. This is because there are two probable negative interactions for this combination: pharmacokinetic, where both drugs are excreted principally through the kidneys; and toxic, where both cause stomatitis and leukopenia. A 335 patient, double-blind, parallel, 38-week, randomized study of auranofin (6 mg daily), methotrexate (7.5 mg weekly), or their combination was published in 1992.[17] Using the percent of patients with >50% improvement as an example of the responses, the following results were obtained: joint tenderness count: 33% vs. 38% vs. 39% for auranofin, methotrexate or their combination, respectively; median change in ESR (mm/h): −16 vs. −27 vs. vs. −21, respectively; discontinuations for adverse events: 14% vs. 15% vs. 21%, respectively. Clearly combination therapy was not better than auranofin or methotrexate, corroborating the prediction from TABLE 4.

A similar table could be constructed for combinations of azathioprine with other DMARDs. In that case one would predict that azathioprine and methotrexate would not be an appropriate combination to use. This is because both azathioprine and methotrexate will inhibit purine metabolism and both will have leukopenia as one of their principal toxicities. In this case kinetics would be complementary, as they do not overlap. The results of a 24-week, double-blind, parallel, randomized study of azathioprine vs. methotrexate vs. their combination supports this prediction.[18] Thirty percent response rates (chosen by the authors as significant response) were as follows: painful joint count: 44% vs. 55% vs. 61% for azathioprine, methotrexate, and their combination, respectively; swollen joint count: 44% vs. 66% vs. 58%, respectively; patient global response; 38% vs. 51% vs. 55%, respectively. The combination of these two drugs was never better than methotrexate alone, although it occasionally appeared superior to azathioprine alone.

TABLE 5. Inhibition (%) of PWM-Induced Blast Formation Using DMARDs with Chloroquine (5 mcg/ml)[a]

	Conc. (mcg/ml)	Alone	Plus CQ
Azathioprine	0.025	35%	30%
Cyclosporine	0.025	28%	90%[b]
D-Penicillamine	0.025	10%[b]	1%
Methotrexate	0.025	68%	50%

[a] Clin. Exp. Rheum. **8**: 455, 1990.
[b] $p < 0.025$.

This approach, it must be realized, is not infallible. This is not surprising as we certainly do not fully understand these drugs' mechanisms of action, kinetics, and toxicities. For example, it would have been predicted that D-penicillamine and hydroxychloroquine would make an effective combination, as there is no overlap in the mechanisms, kinetics, or toxicities. A two year, double-blind trial of hydroxychloroquine, penicillamine, or their combination, however, showed no synergy for the combination as compared to either drug alone. For example, the percent of patients with >50% improvement in their disease was 25% in their hydroxychloroquine-treated group, 11% in the D-penicillamine group, and 8% in the combination group. Likewise, discontinuations for toxicity were 6% for hydroxychloroquine, 19% for D-penicillamine, and 18% in the combination.[19] An *in vitro* study done in 1990 is of interest in this respect.[20] This study examined the effect of D-penicillamine, azathioprine, methotrexate, and cyclosporin (at concentrations achieved *in vivo*) upon pokeweed-mitogen-stimulated blast formation of monocytes (TABLE 5). The third column is the percent inhibition after the drug alone, while the fourth column is the percent inhibition when chloroquine is added. When one looks at the effect of adding chloroquine to D-penicillamine, one sees a *decrease* in inhibition. This would predict that the combination would not work.

SUMMARY

A potential approach toward rational decision making when using combinations of DMARDs has been presented. This approach combines knowledge of DMARD mechanisms of action, kinetics, and toxicities to look for "nonoverlapping" combinations. When using this approach to predict responses and comparing them to studies that have been done, some encouraging results were obtained. Nevertheless, as exemplified by the combination of D-penicillamine and hydroxychloroquine, this approach is not infallible. The use of refinements of such rational choices, however, should be continued in an effort to improve the chances of success and decrease the costs of testing drug combinations.

REFERENCES

1. ZVAIFLER, N. J. 1993. Etiology and pathogenesis of rheumatoid arthritis. *In* Arthritis and Allied Conditions. D. J. McCarty & W. J. Koopman, Eds. 12th Edit.: 723–736. Lea and Febiger. London, England.
2. LEIGH, J. P. & J. F. FRIES. 1991. Mortality pridictors among 263 patients with rheumatoid arthritis. J. Rheum. **18:** 1307–1312.
3. RASKER, J. J. & J. A. COSH. 1984. The natural history of rheumatoid arthritis: a fifteen year follow-up study. Clin. Rheum. **3:** 11–20.
4. ERHARDT, C. C., P. A. MUMFORD, P. J. W. VENABLES & D. MAINI. 1989. Factors predicting a poor life prognosis in rheumatoid arthritis: an eight year prospective study. Ann. Rheum. Dis. **48:** 7–13.
5. VAN DER HEIJDE, D. M. F. M., P. L. C. M. VAN RIEL, M. H. VAN RYSWYK & L. B. A. VAN DE PUTTE. 1988. Influence of prognostic features on the final outcome in rheumatoid arthritis: a review of the literature. Semin. Arthritis Rheum. **17:** 284–292.
6. SINGAL, D. P., D. GREEN, B. REID, D. D. GLADMAN & W. W. BUCHANAN. 1992. HLA-D region genes and rheumatoid arthritis (RA): importance of DR & DQ genes in conferring susceptibility to RA. Ann. Rheum. Dis. **51:** 23–28.
7. XAO, X., E. GAZIT, A. LIVNEH & P. STASTNY. 1991. Rheumatoid arthritis in Israeli Jews: shared sequences in the third hypervariable region of DRB1 alleles are associated with susceptibility. J. Rheum. **18:** 801–803.

8. WEYAND, C. M., K. C. HICOK, D. L. CONN & J. J. GORONZY. 1992. The influence of HLA-DRB1 genes on disease severity in rheumatoid arthritis. Ann. Intern. Med. 117: 801–806.
9. HARRISON, W. B. 1992. Cyclosporin. *In* Second-Line Agents in the Treatment of Rheumatic Diseases. J. S. Dixon & D. E. Furst, Eds.: 311–334. Marcel Dekker. New York, N.Y.
10. MATHERS, D. & A. S. RUSSELL. 1992. Methotrexate. *In* Second-Line Agents in the Treatment of Rheumatic Diseases. J. S. Dixon & D. E. Furst, Eds.: 287–310. Marcel Dekker. New York, N.Y.
11. CRONSTEIN, B. N., M. A. EBERLE, H. E. GRUBER & R. I. LEVIN. 1991. Proc. Acad. Sci. 88: 2441–2445.
12. DIXON, J. S. & D. E. FURST. 1992. *In* Second-Line Agents in the Treatment of Rheumatic Diseases. J. S. Dixon & D. E. Furst, Eds.: 181–362. Marcel Dekker. New York, N.Y.
13. HERMAN, R. A., J. HOFFMAN & D. E. FURST. 1989. Pharmacokinetics of low dose methotrexate. J. Pharm. Sci. 78: 165–171.
14. FURST, D. E., R. A. HERMAN, R. KOEHNKE, N. ERICKSON, L. HASH, C. E. RIGGS, A. PORRAS AND P. VENG-PEDERSON. 1990. The effect of aspirin and sulindac on methotrexate clearance. J. Pharm. Sci. 79: 782–786.
15. SONGSIRIDEJ, N. & D. E. FURST. 1991. Methotrexate, the rapidly acting drug. *In* Balliers Clinical Rheumatology. P. Brooks, Ed.: 575–595. Harcourt Brace. London, England.
16. FELSON, D. T., J. J. ANDERSON & R. F. MEENAN. 1990. The comparative efficacy and toxicity of second-line drugs in rheumatoid arthritis: results of two metaanalyses. Arthritis Rheum. 33: 1449–1461.
17. WILLIAMS, H. J., J. R. WARD, J. C. READING, R. H. BROOKS, D. O. CLEGG, J. L. SKOSEY, *et al.* 1992. Comparison of auranofin, methotrexate and the combination of both in the treatment of rheumatoid arthritis: a controlled trial. Arthritis Rheum. 35: 259–269.
18. WILLKENS, R. F., M. D. UROWITZ, D. M. STAHLEIN, R. J. R. MCKENDRY, JR., R. G. BERGER, J. H. BOX, *et al.* 1992. Comparison of azathioprine, methotrexate and the combination of both in the treatment of rheumatoid arthritis: a controlled clinical trial. Arthritis Rheum. 35: 849–856.
19. BUNCH, T. W., J. D. O'DUFFY, R. B. TOMPKINS & W. M. O'FALLON. 1984. Controlled trial of hydroxychloroquine and D-penicillamine singly and in combination in the treatment of rheumatoid arthritis. Arthritis Rheum. 27: 267–276.
20. DIJKMANS, B. A., *et al.* 1990. Synergistic and additive effects of disease modifying anti-rheumatic drugs combined with chloroquine on the mitogen-driven stimulation of mononuclear cells. Clin. Exp. Rheumatol. 8: 455–459.

Effects of Nonsteroidal Antiinflammatory Drugs on Bone Loss in Chronic Inflammatory Disease

MARJORIE K. JEFFCOAT,[a] MICHAEL S. REDDY,[a]
LARRY W. MORELAND,[b] AND WILLIAM J. KOOPMAN[b]

[a] University of Alabama School of Dentistry
[b] University of Alabama School of Medicine
1919 Seventh Avenue South
Birmingham, Alabama 35294-0007

INTRODUCTION

The effect of nonsteroidal antiinflammatory drugs on the progression of bone loss in chronic inflammatory diseases has long been controversial. Conventional wisdom states that nonsteroidal antiinflammatory drugs may provide symptomatic relief and reduction of inflammation but do not alter the course of bone loss. One of the challenges facing the clinical investigator studying the potential of such compounds as disease modifying drugs lies in the fact that the bone loss is generally slowly progressive in chronic inflammatory diseases. Furthermore, routine clinical evaluations, including the interpretation of routine unstandardized radiographs, are insensitive and nonquantitative. Thus, clinical trials utilizing such methods necessarily require the study of large numbers of subjects for long periods of time, if differences in disease progression between drug and placebo groups are to be detected.[1]

The purpose of this paper is threefold. First, quantitative digital subtraction radiography as implemented in our laboratory will be described. This quantitative radiographic technique is sufficiently sensitive to detect as little as 0.1 mm or 1.0 mg of bone loss using clinical radiographs. Second, the rationale for the use of nonsteroidal antiinflammatory drugs for the slowing of bone loss in periodontitis will be briefly reviewed. The efficacy of nonsteroidal antiinflammatory drugs in slowing bone loss has been assessed in several independent double-blind placebo-controlled clinical trials using digital subtraction radiography and has shown a significant decrease in the progression of bone loss associated with nonsteroidal antiinflammatory drug treatment. Third, the use of digital subtraction radiography to study the fate of bone erosions in patients with rheumatoid arthritis will be presented.

DIGITAL SUBTRACTION RADIOGRAPHY—PRINCIPLES AND VALIDATION

Accurate and precise quantification of bone loss is fundamental to the clinical assessment of the effectiveness of any chemotherapeutic agent in slowing bone loss. Simple interpretation of routine clinical radiographs has several limitations inherent to the radiographic technique. Unstandardized radiographs may vary in geometry, brightness, and contrast, challenging the investigators to detect small osseous changes that have occurred between radiographic examinations.[2] Furthermore, since routine radiographs represent a two-dimensional mapping of the three-dimensional anatomy, unchanging features may overlap the area of osseous change again challenging the investigator to actually detect the change.

Digital subtraction radiography utilizes computerized image processing to overcome many of these limitations.[3–7] Radiographs taken at different examination periods are digitized and aligned. Anatomic structures that have not changed between examinations are subtracted. The resultant subtraction image shows bone gain or bone loss as light or dark areas, respectively, against a neutral gray background. Thus, digital subtraction radiography is an image enhancement technique that facilitates detection of osseous change by eye. The image may be further processed by the use of pseudocolor[8,9] to indicate the location of bone loss in shades of red and bone gain in shades of green. Although the use of pseudocolor does not increase the amount of information in an image, the use of color coded subtraction images does significantly enhance the detection of small osseous changes, especially in the hands of inexperienced clinicians. Clinical interpretation of the subtraction is additionally aided by superimposing the area of change on the original radiograph.[10] Thus, the clinical investigator may locate the area of change and determine which bony site is affected.

Photographic subtraction radiography has been used to subtract overlying osseous structures from angiograms since the 1930s. Digital subtraction radiography utilizes a computer to manipulate the image and has the power to implement specialized image processing algorithms, making quantitative digital subtraction radiography practical today. Digital subtraction radiography has been in use in the study of bone loss due to periodontitis since the early 1980s,[3–5] and clinicians are able to detect as little as 5% loss of bone mineral as confirmed by I-125 absorptiometry from digital subtraction images.[5]

In order to successfully align and subtract radiographs taken at sequential examinations, the radiographs must have similar brightness, contrast, and angulation. Fortunately, the presence of an image processing computer makes it possible to implement algorithms to correct for variations in brightness and contrast without the use of a reference step wedge in each film.[11] The standardization of image geometry is equally important and may be accomplished by any one of three methods. The video feedback method[12] is suited to use for studies in both rheumatology and periodontology.[13] A fixed video camera and x-ray tube are used. The video camera captures a picture of the area of interest at the instant the radiograph is taken. This reference picture is saved to computer disk. At the time of the subsequent examination, the operator recalls the sorted reference image which appears on a monitor as a negative image. The camera captures a live picture of the region of interest, continuously subtracting the live image from the reference image. When the patient is realigned in the same position as in the original radiographs, the stored and live images will cancel resulting in a gray monitor screen, and the subsequent radiograph is exposed.

For the study of bone around teeth either of two additional methods may be used. The cephalostat method[14] exploits the fact that tooth geometry is relatively contrasting. The patient is placed in a head holder and the x-ray tube is fixed, so that only film tilt remains as a major source of variation in image geometry. Aphine warp algorithms[15] are then applied to correct for the planar component of geometric distortion. The stent method[5,16] is also applicable to intraoral radiography. In the stent method, the x-ray is physically coupled to the teeth and film using a custom made film holder fabricated in a dental laboratory.

The subtraction process is illustrated schematically in FIGURE 1. Once satisfactory radiographs are exposed, corrected for contrast, aligned, and subtracted, the subtraction image may be either interpreted or subjected to further processing for quantitative analysis of bone loss. Several laboratories have exploited the gray scale information in the subtraction image in order to measure the amount of bone change between examinations.[2,10,17-20] The units may be specially defined, or may be expressed in terms of mass or distance along a tooth root for periodontal applications.

In our laboratory, specialized computer software has been developed and validated which may be used to (1) isolate regions of bone loss or gain from the background image, (2) measure the area of change and calculate its equivalent mass by comparison with a reference wedge in the image, and (3) superimpose the area of change on the original radiograph to allow location of the area of bone loss or gain.[2,10,20]

The quantitative digital subtraction method has been validated *in vitro* and *in vivo*. Small chips of bone equivalent material (ranging in size from 1–39 mg) are

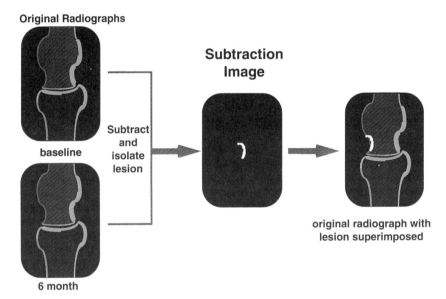

FIGURE 1. Schematic representation of digital subtraction radiography. Two radiographs taken at different examinations are aligned, digitized, and subtracted. Areas of bony change are isolated. The area of change is superimposed on the original radiograph.

placed in a skull, and a reference wedge is positioned between the teeth. A reference radiograph is taken. The chips are removed, and a second radiograph is exposed. The resultant radiographs are digitized, aligned, subtracted, and algorithms applied to permit calculation of the mass of the bone equivalent chip. FIGURE 2 shows the representative data from one such validation study. There was a high correlation between calculated and actual chip mass ($r^2 = 0.969$, $p < .01$, slope $- 0.96$, intercept $= -1.39$).

The subtraction method was also validated in terms of the investigators ability to detect small osseous lesions in periodontal and rheumatologic applications. Separate calibration studies have been performed for investigators experienced with periodontal bone loss and erosions due to rheumatoid arthritis. The results are summarized in TABLE 1. The sensitivity in detecting small osseous lesions too small to be detected by

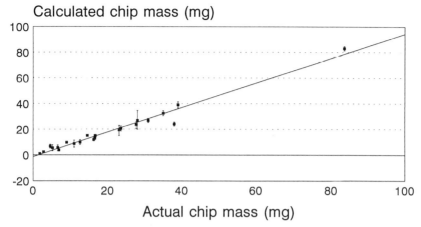

FIGURE 2. Validation of quantitative digital subtraction radiography. Note the excellent correlation between calculated and actual chip mass ($r^2 = 0.969$).

the unaided eye was 94% in the periodontal model[21] and 85% in the rheumatology model.[13] The specificity in ruling out lesions was 97% in the periodontal model and 100% in the rheumatology model.

These validation data indicate that the digital subtraction methodology is sufficiently sensitive and specific to permit use in clinical trials. The radiographs take approximately 10 minutes to expose, and image processing can be performed immediately or at the investigator's convenience.

EFFICACY OF NONSTEROIDAL ANTIINFLAMMATORY DRUGS ON THE PROGRESSION OF BONE LOSS IN PERIODONTITIS

Several lines of evidence have pointed to a role for nonsteroidal antiinflammatory drugs in the slowing of bone loss due to periodontitis. Periodontitis is a chronic inflammatory disease initiated by bacterial plaque and characterized by loss of bone and soft tissue supporting the teeth. Although the rate of bone loss may vary widely from patient to patient and over time, periodontitis can lead to tooth mobility, abscess, and tooth loss. In the early 1970s, investigators reported that inflamed gingiva from patients with periodontal diseases had significantly higher levels of

TABLE 1. Diagnostic Accuracy of Digital Subtraction Radiography

Periodontal applications	
Sensitivity	94%
Specificity	97%
Accuracy	96%
Rheumatologic applications	
Sensitivity	85%
Specificity	100%
Accuracy	92%

PGE_2 than in control patients.[22] When such gingiva are cultured, the media resorbs bone *in vitro,* and this bone loss may be blocked by indomethacin.[23] In a pioneering study, Offenbacher later demonstrated that patients undergoing active periodontal destruction had higher gingival crevicular fluid PGE_2 levels than either healthy patients or patients with quiescent periodontitis.[24,25]

Epidemiologic evidence also supported a potential role of nonsteroidal antiinflammatory drugs in slowing bone loss due to periodontitis.[26,27] Subjects who reported chronic nonsteroidal antiinflammatory drug intake had less severe bone loss than matched control patients. This finding was observed in spite of the clinical expectation that such patients as a groups might have limited manual dexterity and therefore perform imperfect plaque control, thereby increasing the severity of periodontitis.

Beginning in the early 1980s, placebo-controlled studies in animals also supported the efficacy of nonsteroidal antiinflammatory drugs in slowing bone loss due to periodontitis. This series of animal experiments reported by Williams *et al.* utilized a common experimental design and therefore provided an opportunity to compare

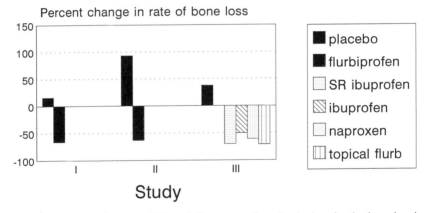

FIGURE 3. Efficacy of nonsteroidal antiinflammatory drugs in slowing alveolar bone loss in naturally occurring periodontitis in beagles. Change in rate of bone loss from pretreatment period through treatment period.

the efficacy of several nonsteroidal antiinflammatory drugs in beagle dogs.[28–34] In the absence of adequate plaque control, beagle dogs develop plaque, calculus, periodontal pockets, and alveolar bone loss that can eventually lead to tooth loss. Thus, the beagle dog with naturally occurring periodontitis provides an excellent model for the study of agents that may slow alveolar bone loss. In each experiment, all dogs were studied for a six-month pretreatment period. Analysis of the bone height around the teeth, determined from radiographs taken during the pretreatment period, permitted calculation of a pretreatment rate of bone loss. The animals were then randomly assigned to either a placebo or active treatment group and were treated for a 6–12 month period depending on the study. Thus, the rate of bone loss during the treatment period in each treatment group could be compared to baseline. The results of these studies are summarized in FIGURE 3. The nonsteroidal antiinflammatory agents flurbiprofen (0.2 mg/kg), slow release ibuprofen (4 mg kg), ibuprofen (4 mg/kg and 0.4 mg/kg), and naproxen (2.0 mg/kg for 1 month and 0.2 mg/kg for 6 months) significantly slowed the progression of bone loss relative to placebo in naturally occurring periodontal disease in beagles. This effect was not observed when indomethacin (1.0 mg/kg) was administered. Furthermore, gingival crevicular fluid levels of both PGE2 and thromboxane decreased from baseline with systemic ibuprofen, systemic naproxen, or topical flurbiprofen treatment.

Results using the monkey ligature model for induced periodontitis were also supportive of the concept. In this model, a ligature, usually of silk suture material, is tied around the teeth to promote plaque accumulation and speed periodontal destruction. Some laboratories also apply putative periodontopathic bacteria to the ligature to further enhance the rate of destruction. A slowing of the progression of periodontitis relative to placebo has been observed in studies using flurbiprofen[35] or meclofenamic acid.[36]

APPLICATION OF DIGITAL SUBTRACTION RADIOGRAPHY TO THE STUDY OF NONSTEROIDAL ANTIINFLAMMATORY DRUGS IN HUMAN CLINICAL TRIALS

As a direct result of the success of the animal studies, double-blind placebo-controlled randomized clinical trials began in the mid-1980s. Our laboratory has been performing such clinical trials using the digital subtraction technology. The major advantage of digital subtraction radiography is that it allows the investigator to determine whether or not drug administration is successful in a relatively short period of study. For patients with rapidly progressive or refractory disease, studies can be as short as 2–3 months. For more typical adult periodontitis patient studies are usually conducted for a minimum of 6 months. FIGURE 4 shows a representative set of radiographs and subtraction images from a patient treated with the nonsteroidal antiinflammatory drug flurbiprofen.

Moderately severe bone loss is evident at the start of the study. Following treatment with the nonsteroidal antiinflammatory drug flurbiprofen, the subtraction image revealed a small amount of bone gain in the base of the bony defect. Composite results from separate randomized double-blind studies using flurbiprofen, naproxen, and meclofenamic acid are shown in FIGURE 5.[21,37–39] All nonsteroidal antiinflammatory drugs had a significant effect on slowing the progression of periodontitis.

The efficacy of flurbiprofen over a longer time period has been documented by Williams *et al.*[40] This long-term double-blind placebo-controlled randomized clinical trial was initiated prior to the time that the digital subtraction technique was readily available and utilized an older radiographic measurement method that expressed bone loss as a percent of tooth root length. The overall results were similar to those obtained using digital subtraction radiography. That is, the progression of bone loss was reduced in the subject taking flurbiprofen, relative to the subjects taking placebo. Nonetheless, due to the lack of sensitivity of the older radiographic technique, the groups were not observed to be significantly different until 12 months of therapy. It is also interesting to note that chronic systemic administration of nonsteroidal antiinflammatory drugs for periodontitis poses many of the same compliance issues observed in other nonpainful chronic diseases. After months of therapy, compliance decreased and the progression of disease recurred. One possible approach to solving this problem could involve the use of daily topical rinses or toothpastes formulated with effective nonsteroidal antiinflammatory drugs as the active agent. Beagle studies have clearly demonstrated that topical flurbiprofen administration is effective in slowing bone loss in periodontitis.[32] The effectiveness of topical ibuprofen (8%) and topical meclofenamic acid (5%) has been compared to topical placebo in the monkey ligature model.[36] While 100% of the ligated sites experienced bone loss in the placebo treated group, only 67% of the topical ibuprofen treated sites and 44% of the topical meclofenamic acid group experienced bone loss during the study period.

DIGITAL SUBTRACTION RADIOGRAPHY
AND RHEUMATOID ARTHRITIS

The use of digital subtraction radiography for the detection of progressive erosions in patients with rheumatoid arthritis has been demonstrated in a proof of

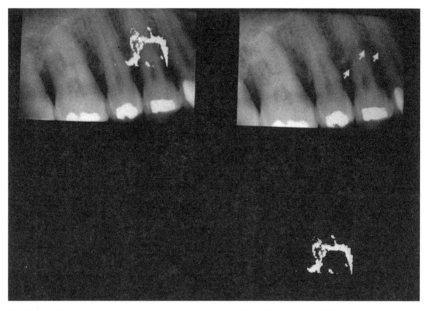

FIGURE 4. Progressive bone loss in adult periodontitis as demonstrated by digital subtraction radiography. **Upper left:** Original radiograph with superimposed area of bone loss detected by digital subtraction radiography (white area). On the computer monitor the area of loss is red. **Upper right:** Original radiograph. **Lower right:** Area of bone change detected with digital subtraction radiography.

principle study in an open label study of patients taking flurbiprofen.[13] FIGURE 6 shows the appearance of progressive erosion in a PIP joint. Progression of the lesion was not detectable by comparison of sequential radiographs; however, the subtraction technique clearly demonstrated a progressive lesion. It was interesting to note that in this population, the odds of experiencing a progressive erosion in a joint undergoing worsening clinical signs (increased tenderness or swelling) were 5.46 times that of joints with an unchanged or improved clinical status ($p < 0.05$). These preliminary data indicate that this methodology should be of value for future study of bone erosions in chronic inflammatory disease.

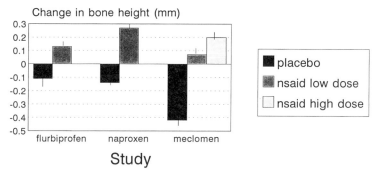

Change in bone height (mm)

flurbiprofen 50 mg bid, naproxen 500 mg bid, meclomen 50 mg or 100 mg bid

FIGURE 5. Efficacy of nonsteroidal antiinflammatory drugs in slowing alveolar bone loss in controlled clinical trials in patients. Bone loss measured by digital subtraction radiography.

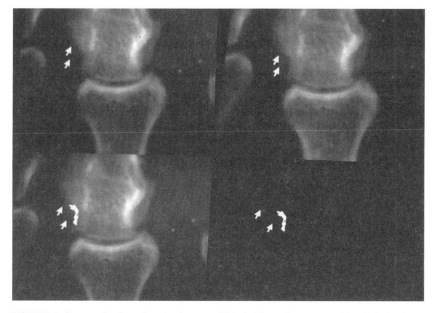

FIGURE 6. Progressive bone loss in rheumatoid arthritis as demonstrated by digital subtraction radiography. **Upper left:** Original radiograph **Upper right:** Radiograph following six months of flurbiprofen treatment. Radiographic changes between the examinations are not readily visible by eye. **Lower left:** Original radiograph with superimposed area of bone loss detected by digital subtraction radiography (white area). On the computer monitor the area of loss is red. **Lower right:** Area of bone change detected with digital subtraction radiography.

SUMMARY

Several controlled clinical trials have indicated that nonsteroidal antiinflammatory drugs may slow alveolar bone loss in periodontitis. Demonstration of this efficacy is dependent on the development of accurate, sensitive, and specific quantitative methods for the assessment of bony change, such as digital subtraction radiography. Further studies of such methodologies are required to more fully investigate the effect of nonsteroidal antiinflammatory drugs in rheumatoid arthritis.

REFERENCES

1. JEFFCOAT, M. K. 1992. The effect of experimental design parameters on the determination of sample size. J. Periodontal Res. **28:** 320–322.
2. JEFFCOAT, M. K. 1992. Radiographic methods for the detection of progressive alveolar bone loss. J. Periodontol. **63**(Suppl.): 367–372.
3. WEBBER, R. L., U. E. RUTTIMAN & H. G. GRONDAHL. 1982. X-Ray image subtraction as a basis for assessment of periodontal changes. J. Periodontal Res. **17:** 509–511.
4. GRONDAHL, H. G. & K. GRONDAHL. 1983. Subtraction radiography for the diagnosis of periodontal bone lesions. Oral Surg. Oral Med. Oral Pathol. **55:** 208–213.
5. HAUSMANN, E., L. CHRISTERSSON, R. DUNFORD, U. WIKESJO, J. PHYO & R. J. GENCO. 1985. Usefulness of subtraction radiography in the evaluation of periodontal therapy. J. Periodontol. **56:** 4–7.
6. BRÄGGER, U., L. PASQUALI, H. WEBER & K. S. KORNMAN. 1989. Computer-assisted densitometric image analysis (CADIA) for the assessment of alveolar bone density changes in furcations. J. Clin. Periodontol. **16:** 46–52.
7. JEFFCOAT, M. K., M. S. REDDY, R. VAN DEN BERG & E. BERTENS. 1992. Quantitative digital subtraction radiography for the assessment of peri-implant bone change. Clin. Oral Impl. Res. **3:** 22–27.
8. BRAEGGER, U. & L. PASQUALI. 1989. Color conversion of alveolar bone density changes in digital subtraction images. J. Clin. Periodontol. **16:** 209–214.
9. REDDY, M. S., J. M. BRUCH, M. K. JEFFCOAT & R. C. WILLIAMS. 1991. Contrast enhancement as an aid to interpretation in digital subtraction radiography. Oral Surg. Oral Med. Oral Rad. **71:** 763–769.
10. JEFFCOAT, M. K., M. S. REDDY & R. L. JEFFCOAT. 1990. A morphologically aided technique for quantitative subtraction of dental radiographic images. IEEE/EMBS **12:** 2068–2070.
11. RUTTIMANN, U. E., R. L. WEBBER & E. SCHMIDT. 1986. A robust digital method for film contrast correction in subtraction radiography. J. Periodontal Res. **21:** 486–495.
12. REDDY, M. S., R. L. WEBBER, R. VAN DEN BERG, R. WEEMS, F. VAN DER VEN & M. K. JEFFCOAT. 1991. A video feedback repositioning method for standardized dental radiographs. IEEE/EMBS **13:** 352–353.
13. MORELAND, L. W., M. S. REDDY, W. J. KOOPMAN, R. L. WEBBER, G. S. ALARCON & M. K. JEFFCOAT. 1992. Digital subtraction radiography for the assessment of bone changes in rheumatoid arthritis. J. Rheumatol. **19:** 1697–1703.
14. JEFFCOAT, M. K., M. S. REDDY, R. L. WEBBER, R. C. WILLIAMS, & U. RUTTIMANN. 1987. Extraoral control of geometry for digital subtraction radiography. J. Periodontal Res. **22:** 396–402.
15. JEFFCOAT, M. K., R. JEFFCOAT & R. C. WILLIAMS. 1984. A new method of the comparison of bone loss measurements on non-standardized radiographs. J. Periodontol Res. **19:** 434–440.
16. HAUSMANN, E., R. DUNFORD, U. WIKESJÖ, L. CHRISTERSSON & K. MCHENRY. 1986. Progression of untreated periodontitis as assessed by subtraction radiography. J. Periodontal Res. **21:** 716–721.
17. RUTTIMANN, U. E. & R. WEBBER. 1987. Volumetry of localized bone lesions by subtraction radiography. J. Periodontal Res. **22:** 215–216.

18. BRAEGGER, U., L. PASQUALI, H. WEBER & K. S. KORNMAN. 1989. Computer-assisted densitometric image analysis (CADIA) for the assessment of alveolar bone density changes in furcations. J. Clin. Periodontol. **16:** 46–52.

19. WEBBER, R. L., U. E. RUTTIMANN & T. J. HEAVEN. 1990. Calibration errors in digital subtraction radiography. J. Periodontal. Res. **25:** 268–275.

20. JEFFCOAT, M. K., M. S. REDDY, R. VAN DEN BERG & E. MARTENS. 1992. Quantitative digital subtraction radiography for the assessment of peri-implant bone change. Clin. Oral Implants Res. **3:** 22–27.

21. JEFFCOAT, M. K., R. PAGE, M. S. REDDY, A. WANNAWISUTE, P. WAITE, K. PALCANIS & R. COGEN. 1991. Use of digital radiography to demonstrate the potential of naproxen as an adjunct in the treatment of rapidly progressive periodontitis. J. Periodontal Res. **26:** 415–421.

22. GOODSON, J. M., F. E. DEWHIRST & A. BRUNETTI. 1974. Prostaglandin E2 levels and human periodontal disease. Prostaglandins **6:** 81–85.

23. GOLDHABER, P., L. RABADJIJJA, W. R. BEYER & A. KORNHAUSER. 1973. Bone resorption in tissue culture and its relevance to periodontal disease. J. Am. Dent. Assoc. **87:** 1027–1033.

24. OFFENBACHER, S., B. M. ODLE & T. E. VAN DYKE. 1986. The use of crevicular fluid prostaglandin E_2 levels as a predictor of Periodontal attachment loss. J. Periodontal Res. **21:** 101–112.

25. OFFENBACHER, S., B. M. ODLE, R. C. GRAY & T. E. VAN DYKE. 1984. Crevicular fluid prostaglandin E levels as a measure of the periodontal disease status of adult and juvenile periodontitis patients. J. Periodontal Res. **19:** 1–13.

26. FELDMAN, R. S., B. SZETO, H. H. CHAUNCEY & P. GOLDHABER. 1983. Non-steroidal anti-inflammatory drugs in the reduction of human alveolar bone loss. J. Clin. Periodontol. **10:** 131–136.

27. WAITE, I. M., C. A. SAXTON, A. YOUNG, B. J. WAGG & M. CORBETT. 1981. The periodontal status of subjects receiving non-steroidal anti-inflammatory drugs. J. Periodontal Res. **16:** 100–108.

28. WADE, W. G. & M. ADDY. 1989. In vitro activity of a chlorhexidine-containing mouthwash against subgingival bacteria. J. Periodontol. **60:** 521–525.

29. WILLIAMS, R. C., M. K. JEFFCOAT, M. L. KAPLAN, P. GOLDHABER, H. G. JOHNSON & W. J. WECHTER. 1985. Flurbiprofen: a potent inhibitor of alveolar bone loss in beagles. Science **227:** 640–642.

30. WILLIAMS, R. C., M. K. JEFFCOAT, T. H. HOWELL, C. M. HALL, H. G. JOHNSON, W. J. WECHTER & P. GOLDHABER. 1987. Indomethacin or flurbiprofen treatment of periodontitis in beagles: comparison of effect on bone loss. J. Periodontal Res. **22:** 403–407.

31. WILLIAMS, R. C., S. OFFENBACHER, M. K. JEFFCOAT, T. H. HOWELL, H. G. JOHNSON, C. M. HALL, W. J. WECHTER & P. GOLDHABER. 1988. Indomethacin or flurbiprofen treatment of periodontitis in beagles: effect on crevicular fluid arachidonic acid metabolites compared with effect on alveolar bone loss. J. Periodontal Res. **23:** 134–138.

32. WILLIAMS, R. C., M. K. JEFFCOAT, T. H. HOWELL, M. S. REDDY, H. G. JOHNSON, C. M. HALL & P. GOLDHABER. 1988. Topical flurbiprofen treatment of periodontitis in beagles. J. Periodontal Res. **23:** 166–169.

33. HOWELL, T. H., M. K. JEFFCOAT, P. GOLDHABER, M. S. REDDY, M. L. KAPLAN, H. G. JOHNSON, C. M. HALL & R. C. WILLIAMS. 1991. Inhibition of alveolar bone loss in beagles with the NSAID naproxen. J. Periodontal Res. **26:** 498–501.

34. WILLIAMS, R. C., M. K. JEFFCOAT, T. H. HOWELL, M. S. REDDY, H. G. JOHNSON, C. M. HALL & P. GOLDHABER. 1988. Ibuprofen: an inhibitor of alveolar bone resorption in beagles. J. Periodontal Res. **23:** 225–229.

35. OFFENBACHER, S., L. D. BRASWELL, A. S. LOOS, H. G. JOHNSON, C. M. HALL, H. McCLURE, J. L. ORKIN, E. A. STROBERT, M. D. GREEN & B. M. ODLE. 1987. Effects of flurbiprofen on the progression of periodontitis in *Macaca mulatta*. J. Periodontal Res. **22:** 473–481.

36. KORNMAN, K. S., R. F. BLODGETT, M. BRUNSVOLD & S. C. HOLT. 1990. Effects of topical applications of meclofenamic acid and ibuprofen on bone loss, subgingival microbiota

and gingival PMN response in the primate *Macaca fascicularis.* J. Periodontal Res. **25:** 300–307.

37. JEFFCOAT, M. K., R. C. WILLIAMS, M. S. REDDY, R. ENGLISH & P. GOLDHABER. 1988. Flurbiprofen treatment of human periodontitis: effect on alveolar bone height and metabolism. J. Periodontal Res. **23:** 381–385.

38. JEFFCOAT, M., R. PAGE, M. REDDY, R. COGEN, P. WAITE, K. PALCANIS, R. C. WILLIAMS & C. BASCH. 1989. Naproxen as an adjunct in the treatment of rapidly progressive periodontitis. J. Dent. Res. **68:** 999 (Abstr. no. 1055.)

39. REDDY, M. S., K. G. PALCANIS, M. L. BARNETT, S. HAIGH, C. H. CHARLES & M. K. JEFFCOAT. Efficacy of Meclofenamate Sodium in the treatment of rapidly progressive periodontitis. J. Clin. Periodontol. **9.** (In press.)

40. WILLIAMS, R. C., M. K. JEFFCOAT, T. H. HOWELL, A. ROLLA, D. STUBBS, K. W. TEOH, M. S. REDDY & P. GOLDHABER. 1989. Altering the progression of human alveolar bone loss with the non-steroidal anti-inflammatory drug flurbiprofen. J. Periodontol. **60:** 485–490.

Cyclooxygenase Inhibitors Vary Widely in Potency for Preventing Cytokine-Induced Bone Resorption

ANTHONY C. ALLISON,[a] RUEI-CHEN CHIN, AND
YVONNE CHENG

Syntex Discovery Research
3401 Hillview Avenue
Palo Alto, California 94304

INTRODUCTION

Periodontal disease is the major cause of tooth loss in adults living in industrialized countries. The gingival inflammatory response is elicited by bacteria in dental plaque, including *Actinobacillus actinomycetemcomitans, Porphyromonas gingivalis,* and *Eikenella corrodens*.[1] Lipopolysaccharides and other products of these bacteria induce the production of cytokines, including TNF-α and IL-1β by monocytes, IL-1α by oral epithelial cells, and IL-6 by many cell types. These cytokines can induce resorption of bone in culture, and together they have additive or synergistic effects.[2,3] Part of the role of IL-1 in osteoclastic bone resorption may be mediated by PGE_2 release.[4] As reviewed by Jeffcoat in this volume,[5] systemically administered cyclooxygenase inhibitors can decrease the rate of alveolar bone loss in experimental animals and humans with periodontal disease. Because these drugs produce gastrointestinal damage, attempts have been made to administer them as oral rinses or toothpastes. Topical application of flurbiprofen significantly retards bone loss associated with periodontitis in beagle dogs.[6] Effects of topical application of cyclooxygenase inhibitors on alveolar bone loss in the primate *Macaca fascicularis* have also been investigated.[7] For a cyclooxygenase inhibitor to be effective topically, it must be potent. The objective of our research was to identify a cyclooxygenase inhibitor with high potency in preventing cytokine-induced bone resorption as well as other properties compatible with topical use in humans with periodontal disease.

METHODS

Rat fetal long bones were labeled with radioactive calcium. Rats 18 days pregnant were injected subcutaneously with 300 μCi of ^{45}Ca in saline the day before the experiment. From the fetuses, radii and ulnas were recovered, pooled, and cartilaginous extremities removed. Organ cultures were established using randomly selected bone pairs in Linbro dishes with 0.5 ml BGJb (Gibco) medium containing 1 mg/ml bovine serum albumin. Cultures were incubated overnight at 37°C, medium discarded, and fresh medium containing 500 pg/ml recombinant human IL-1β (Immunex) added. Acidic forms of the drugs used were neutralized with 0.1 N NaOH to make a stock 10^{-2} M solution and diluted with BGJb to obtain concentrations in

[a] Present address: 2513 Hastings Drive, Belmont, California 94002.

the range 1 to 10,000 nanomolar. From the recovered media, aliquots (0.1 ml) were added to 10 ml Ready Safe in scintillation vials. At the end of the experiment, the pair of bones was transferred to a drain vial and 0.5 ml 0.1 N HCl added to extract ^{45}Ca for counting. The percentage of ^{45}Ca released per pair of bones was calculated from the cumulative CPM in the media divided by the total ^{45}Ca (in media and residual bone samples). IL-1β markedly increased ^{45}Ca release, and the potency of different cyclooxygenase inhibitors in preventing this effect of IL-1 was calculated (percent inhibition of IL-1-induced erosion). Immunoassays for PGE$_2$ in culture media were also performed. A minimum of five pairs of bones were used per group assay, and standard errors of arithmetic means were calculated.

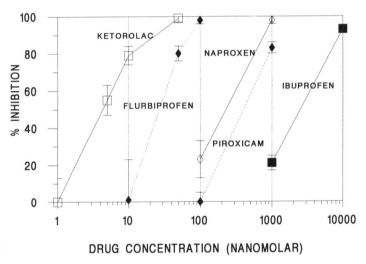

FIGURE 1. Dose-response curves showing the potency of different drugs tested as inhibitors of IL-1β-induced erosion of rat fetal long bones. Means ± standard errors of means are shown.

OBSERVATIONS

Comparative Potency of Cyclooxygenase Inhibitors in Preventing IL-1-induced Bone Erosion

Recombinant human IL-1α and IL-1β were found to be potent inducers of bone resorption in this system, as shown by release of ^{45}Ca into the culture medium. Other studies have demonstrated that IL-1 also augments release of PGE$_2$, proteoglycan, and collagen degradation products from bones in culture.[2] We found that cyclooxygenase inhibitors, added with IL-1β (500 pg/ml), were able to prevent completely the augmentation of bone erosion by the cytokine. However, cyclooxygenase inhibitors varied widely in potency in this assay (FIGURE 1, TABLE 1). The most effective was ketorolac (FIGURE 2), with an IC$_{50}$ in different assays in the range 4–6 nM. Ketorolac was consistently about 7 times as potent as flurbiprofen in preventing cytokine-induced bone resorption and 700 times as potent as ibuprofen. Other cyclooxygenase inhibitors tested were intermediate in potency. IL-1β also markedly stimulated PGE$_2$

TABLE 1. Effect of Cyclooxygenase Inhibitors on IL-1β-Induced Resorption of Rat Fetal Long Bones in Organ Culture

Compound	IC_{50} for Inhibition of Bone Resorption (nanomolar)	Relative Potency
Ketorolac	4	750
Fluribiprofen	28	107
Naproxen	300	10
Piroxicam	350	9
Ibuprofen	3000	1

production by the bone cultures, and again ketorolac was the most potent inhibitor of PGE_2 production (data not shown).

DISCUSSION

The remarkable and unexpected potency of ketorolac as an inhibitor of bone resorption is evident from our observations. The drug has other properties that make it particularly suitable for topical application in periodontal disease. Unlike most cyclooxygenase inhibitors, ketorolac is not irritant when applied to seromucous surfaces,[8] and it is well absorbed from such surfaces. Ketorolac is also a potent inhibitor of angiogenesis, the formation of new blood vessels in response to basic fibroblast growth factor and other inducers.[9] Periodontitis has a variable component of granulation tissue: new blood vessel formation associated with inflammation. The newly formed blood vessels are fragile and bleed when teeth are cleaned. Topically applied ketorolac should decrease the granulation-tissue-type response and gingival bleeding in periodontal disease.

The mechanism by which cyclooxygenase inhibitors block cytokine-induced bone erosion is not fully understood. Angiogenesis may be needed for expansion of bone-eroding surfaces. In fibroblasts and other connective tissue cells, IL-1 induces the production of PGE_2 and the expression of genes for metalloproteinases (prostromelysins, procollagenases) as well as serine proteinases (plasminogen activators).[10] If PGE_2 production is inhibited, there is no effect on expression of genes for neutral metalloproteinases, but expression of genes for plasminogen activators is prevented.[10] Plasminogen activators catalyze production from precursors of plasmin, a serine esterase with broad specificity that can initiate activation of metalloprotein-

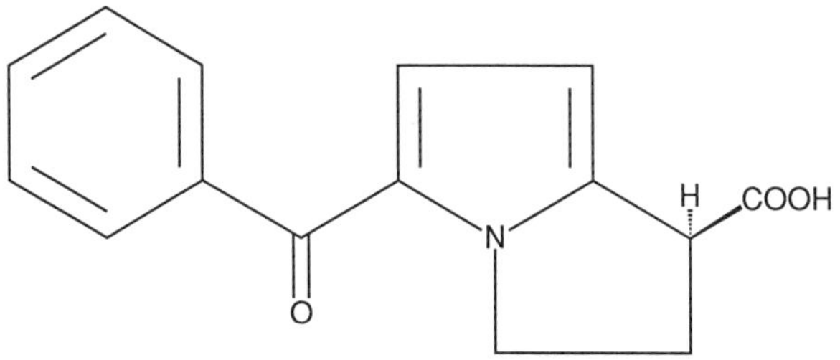

FIGURE 2. Structure of $(-)$ (S) ketorolac, the active enantiomer.

ases from inactive proenzymes. This may be one mechanism by which cyclooxygenase inhibitors retard the degradation of bone proteoglycan and collagen. Whatever the mechanism of action, topical ketorolac could be highly effective in preventing alveolar bone erosion in humans with periodontal disease.

REFERENCES

1. DRINK, J. L., A. C. R. TANNER, A. D. HAFFAJEE & S. S. SOCRANSKY. 1985. Gram negative species associated with active destructive periodontal lesions. J. Clin. Periodontol. **12:** 648–659.

2. MACDONALD, B. R. & M. GOWEN. 1992. Cytokines and bone. Br. J. Rheumatol. **31:** 149–155.

3. ISHIMI, Y., C. MIYAURA, C. H. JIN, T. AKATSU, E. ABE, Y. NAKAMURA, A. YAMAGUCHI, S. YOSHIKI, T. MATSUDA, T. HIRANO, T. KISHIMOTO & T. SUDA. 1990. IL-6 is produced by osteoblasts and induces bone resorption. J. Immunol. **145:** 3297–3303.

4. RICHARDS, D. & R. B. RUTHERFORD. 1988. The effects of interleukin 1 on collagenolytic activity and prostaglandin-E secretion by human periodontal-ligament and gingival fibroblasts. Arch. Oral Biol. **33:** 237–243.

5. JEFFCOAT, M. K., M. S. REDDY, L. W. MORELAND & W. J. KOOPMAN. Effects of nonsteroidal antiinflammatory drugs on bone loss in chronic inflammatory disease. Ann. N.Y. Acad. Sci. (This volume.)

6. WILLIAMS, R. C., M. K. JEFFCOAT, T. H. HOWELL, M. S. REDDY, H. G. JOHNSON, C. M. HALL & P. GOLDHABER. 1988. Topical flurbiprofen treatment of periodontitis in beagles. J. Periodont. Res. **23:** 166–169.

7. KORNMAN, K. S., R. F. BLODGETT, M. BRUNSVOLD & S. C. HOLT. 1990. Effects of topical applications of meclofenamic acid and ibuprofen on bone loss, subgingival microbiota and gingival PMN response in the primate *Macaca fascicularis*. J. Periodont. Res. **25:** 300–307.

8. ROOKS, W. H., II, P. J. MALONEY, L. D. SHOTT, M. E. SCHULER, H. SEVELIUS, A. M. STROSBERG, L. TANNENBAUM, A. J. TOMOLONIS, M. B. WALLACH, D. WATERBURY & J. P. YEE. 1985. The analgesic and anti-inflammatory profile of ketorolac and its tromethamine salt. Drugs. Exp. Clin. Res. **11:** 479–492.

9. KOWALSKI, J., H. H. KWAN, S. D. PRIONAS, A. C. ALLISON & L. F. FAJARDO. 1992. Characterization and applications of the disc angiogenesis system. Exp. Mol. Pathol. **56:** 1–19.

10. LEIZER, T., B. J. CLARRIS, P. E. ASH, J. VAN DAMME, J. SAKLATVALA & J. A. HAMILTON. 1987. Interleukin-1 beta and interleukin-1 alpha stimulate the plasminogen activator activity and prostaglandin E_2 levels of human synovial cells. Arthritis Rheum. **30:** 562–566.

Treatment of Autoimmune Uveitis

SCOTT M. WHITCUP AND ROBERT B. NUSSENBLATT

National Eye Institute
National Institutes of Health
Building 10, Room 10N 202
Bethesda, Maryland 20892

The uvea is the middle coat of the eye and consists of the choroid, ciliary body, and iris. Inflammation of the uveal tract is termed uveitis, although this term is now used to more generally describe intraocular inflammation involving not only the uvea, but other ocular tissues including the retina, vitreous, and sclera. Uveitis is often classified according to the anatomical site of the ocular inflammation, since the etiology of the disease is often unknown. In some cases, uveitis is caused by a known ocular infection. However, there are many noninfectious causes of intraocular inflammatory disease, and autoimmunity is felt to play a role in the pathogenesis in a number of these conditions. The study of uveitis offers a unique opportunity to visualize both clinical and pathologic manifestations of autoimmune inflammatory disease. Inflammatory sequellae such as vasculitis, vascular leakage, and inflammatory cell infiltration can be easily visualized and photographed. Similarly, the effects of antiinflammatory therapy on these disease manifestations can be directly observed to an extent not possible in other organs.

AUTOIMMUNITY AND UVEITIS

The concept that uveitis may be caused by antibodies directed against antigens in the eye was proposed in the early part of this century. Uhlenhuth demonstrated autoantibodies produced against the lens in 1903,[1] and Elschnig hypothesized on the possible pathogenic role of autoantigens in 1910.[2] Early attempts at inducing ocular inflammation in experimental animals by injecting uveal extracts were unsuccessful. However, in 1965 Wacker and Lipton showed that intradermal injections of retinal extracts could induce uveitis in guinea pigs.[3] Retinal S-antigen, also known as arrestin, was found in the photoreceptor outer segments and identified as the uveitogenic antigen.[4]

The retinal S-antigen has a molecular weight of about 50,000 daltons and has been found not only in the retina, but also in the pineal gland of some species. Subsequent studies showed that immunization with S-antigen at sites far from the eye could induce bilateral intraocular inflammation in a number of experimental animals including the mouse, rat, rabbit, guinea pig, and monkey.[5] Disease is first observed clinically about 10 to 14 days after immunization. Depending on the species of animal and dose of retinal antigen, animals develop vitritis, choroidal and retinal infiltrates, and retinal vasculitis (FIGURE 1). This animal model of intraocular inflammation is currently termed experimental autoimmune uveitis (EAU). Histologically, there is destruction of the photoreceptor layer and disruption of the retinal architecture with evidence of retinal infiltrates, hemorrhage, and vasculitis in severe disease (FIGURE 2). T lymphocytes have been shown to be the predominant inflammatory cell infiltrating the eye.[6] Subsequent studies demonstrated that CD4+ cells invade the eye in the initial phase of EAU, but that CD8+ cells predominate in the latter stages of the disease.[7] Macrophages also infiltrate eyes with EAU, and appear to be especially important for the development of disease in the mouse.[8] In addition, animal species with greater number of mast cells in the uveal tract appear more susceptible to developing EAU, suggesting a pathogenic role of mast cells in this disease.[9]

A number of other ocular antigens that induce uveitis when injected into animals have now been identified. Immunization with interphotoreceptor retinoid-binding protein (IRBP), opsin, and rhodopsin induces a disease similar to S-antigen-induced EAU,[10,11] and injection of an extract of the retinal pigment epithelium (RPE) has been shown to produce anterior uveitis and choroiditis.[12] Although these animal models of uveitis demonstrate that an immune response directed against ocular antigens can cause intraocular inflammation, what evidence suggests that this mechanism plays a role in human disease? The similarity of the clinical and pathological appearance of certain forms of human uveitis to EAU suggests that the pathophysiology of the conditions may be similar. There are, however, certain ocular inflammatory diseases where the evidence for an autoimmune etiology is more striking.

Sympathetic ophthalmia is a bilateral granulomatous uveitis that results from a penetrating ocular injury to one eye (the exciting eye), followed by inflammation in the contralateral eye (sympathizing eye). Disease in the contralateral eye occurs days to years following the initial injury.[13] Clinically, the disease is characterized by granulomatous inflammation in the anterior segment of the eye, moderate to severe vitritis, and choroidal infiltrates. Histologic findings include diffuse granulomatous uveal inflammation, sparing of the choriocapillaris, epithelioid cells containing

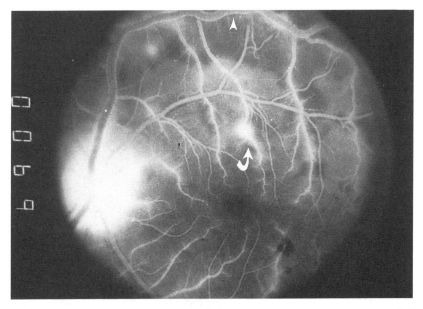

FIGURE 1. Fluorescein angiogram of a monkey with experimental autoimmune uveoretinitis following immunization with interphotoreceptor-retinoid binding protein. Angiogram demonstrates severe retinal vasculitis with staining of the blood vessel walls (arrowhead) and leakage of dye from the retinal vessels (arrow) and optic disc.

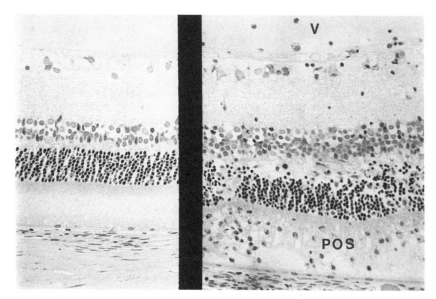

FIGURE 2. Photomicrograph showing normal mouse retina (left) and experimental autoimmune uveoretinitis (right). There is destruction of the photoreceptor outer segments (POS) with infiltration of inflammatory cells, retinal edema, and disruption of the retinal architecture. Inflammatory cells are also seen in the overlying vitreous (V).

phagocytosed uveal pigment, and Dalen-Fuchs nodules composed of collections of epithelioid cells lying between Bruch's membrane and the retinal pigment epithelium.[14,15] Chan and coworkers showed that CD4+ T cells infiltrated the choroid in a traumatized eye that was enucleated several months following an injury.[16] The contralateral sympathizing eye was ultimately removed and demonstrated predominantly CD8+ T cells in the chronic stage of the disease.

Sympathetic ophthalmia is both clinically and histologically very similar to EAU in the monkey.[11] In addition, Marak and colleagues showed that lymphocyte proliferation could be elicited from the peripheral blood lymphocytes from patients with sympathetic ophthalmia stimulated with retinal pigment epithelium and retinal antigen but not choroidal extract.[13] These data suggest that sympathetic ophthalmia may result from the release of previously sequestered retinal antigens following ocular injury. Bacteria that can enter the eye following ocular injury may act as an adjuvant to promote the development of the disease, and this may explain why the incidence of sympathetic ophthalmia has decreased with improvements in microsurgical technique and antibiotic use.[15]

Sympathetic ophthalmia may appear similar both clinically and pathologically to Vogt-Koyanagi-Harada syndrome (VKH). VKH is a systemic disorder involving many organs including the eye, ear, skin, and meninges. Also similar to sympathetic ophthalmia, a specific immune response is felt to be pathogenic. Researchers have shown that peripheral blood lymphocytes from patients with VKH are stimulated by uveal extracts or pigment.[17] Later studies by Maezawa and colleagues showed that cytotoxic T-cells from 6 patients with VKH demonstrated specific killing against a P-36 melanoma cell line which bore cross-reactive antigens with normal melanocytes, and that a monoclonal antibody against Leu-2a could block this response.[18]

Although autoimmunity appears to play a pathogenic role in human uveitis, an antigen-specific response has been difficult to demonstrate by studies of peripheral blood from patients. Nussenblatt and coworkers showed an increased cellular immune response against retinal S-antigen in patients with uveitis,[19] and Chan and colleagues demonstrated antiretinal autoantibodies in patients with VKH, Behçet's disease, and sympathetic ophthalmia.[20] Recent studies have shown that uveitis patients may have a specific cellular immune response to certain fragments of retinal S-antigen.[21] But antibodies against retinal antigens are also found in the sera of normal controls,[22] and although patients with uveitis appear to have increased levels of activated T-cells in their peripheral blood, these lymphocytes do not seem to be antigen specific.[23,24] However, few antigen-specific cells are probably needed to induce disease, and they may be more localized in the eye, explaining the confusing findings based on studies of peripheral circulation.

CORTICOSTEROID THERAPY

Although the autoimmune pathogenesis for human uveitis has not been definitively proven, therapy for ocular inflammatory disease has been based on suppressing a presumed autoimmune response. Corticosteroids have remained the mainstay of therapy for uveitis since their first use in the early 1950s. One of the major causes of visual loss from uveitis is cystoid macular edema. Cystoid macular edema results from a breakdown of the blood-retinal barrier with leakage of protein and fluid into the macula, the area of the retina serving central vision. Cook and MacDonald demonstrated that cortisone could restore normal permeability to capillaries in the eye,[25] and Gordon reported on the beneficial effects of corticosteroid therapy in the treatment of ocular inflammatory disease.[26,27]

Synthetic glucocorticoids can have both antiinflammatory and immunosuppressive effects depending on dosage and route of administration.[28] Topical application of corticosteroids is an effective way to treat uveitis limited to the anterior segment of the eye. Corneal penetration of the topical steroid preparations is high enough to allow therapeutic levels in the aqueous humor, especially in an inflamed eye. Topical corticosteroids avoid many of the systemic side effects of steroids, however, cataract and steroid-induced glaucoma are two of the possible local adverse effects of steroid eye drops. Unfortunately, in the phakic eye, therapeutic levels of corticosteroids cannot be obtained in the vitreous with topical administration. So for the treatment of uveitis affecting the posterior segment of the eye other routes of administration are needed.

Corticosteroids can be injected periocularly. Long-acting steroid injections are especially useful for treating uniocular disease, and result in therapeutic drug levels in the posterior segment of the eye. Adverse effects of periocular injections of corticosteroids include glaucoma, penetration of the eye, fibrosis, and a melting of the sclera secondary to inhibited collagen synthesis in an eye with scleral inflammation. Systemic corticosteroids remain the initial treatment of choice for most patients with bilateral sight-threatening autoimmune uveitis. Oral prednisone at an initial dose of 1 to 1.5 mg/kg has been effective in treating many forms of uveitis. In addition, we have successfully used short courses of pulse intravenous methylprednisolone for patients with severe disease activity (unpublished data). Nevertheless, many patients remain resistant or become intolerant of corticosteroid therapy. Based on the understanding that autoimmunity may play a pathogenic role in many forms of uveitis, researchers began investigating the use of immunosuppressive drugs for the treatment of ocular inflammatory disease.

IMMUNOSUPPRESSIVE THERAPY FOR UVEITIS

Almost all the currently available immunosuppressive agents have been tried for the treatment of uveitis, but the most commonly used drugs are azathioprine, cyclophosphamide, and cyclosporine. Azathioprine (Imuran) was one of the first immunosuppressive agents used in the treatment of autoimmune uveitis. Initially developed as a therapy for rheumatoid arthritis and other systemic autoimmune diseases in the mid-1960s, azathioprine was soon tried for the treatment of steroid-resistant uveitis.[29] Azathioprine is an antimetabolite that alters purine metabolism after conversion to the active agent, 6-mercaptopurine. The drug is administered orally at a dose of 1–2.5 mg/kg and has been associated with bone marrow suppression, gastrointestinal symptoms, and secondary infections. Newell and Krill reported that some patients with uveitis could be successfully treated with azathioprine.[30] Andrasch and colleagues showed that about half the patients with uveitis treated with azathioprine and low dose corticosteroids had a favorable response.[31] A single case report stated the successful use of azathioprine for the treatment of sympathetic ophthalmia,[32] however, other researchers give conflicting results.[30]

Some researchers have reported good results treating Behçet's disease with azathioprine. The disease is characterized by oral and mucosal ulcerations and a recurrent uveitis that is usually resistant to corticosteroids.[33] Azathioprine at a dose of 2.5 mg/kg per day was shown to prevent the development of new ocular disease and to decrease rates of recurrent ocular disease in patients with Behçet's disease.[34] Aoki and Sugiura reported that greater than 50% of Behçet's patients had improvement in their ocular disease with azathioprine,[35] but again, others have reported less success.[36]

Cyclophosphamide (Cytoxan) is a nitrogen mustard derivative alkylating agent that supresses humoral and cellular immunity. This drug has been used extensively for the treatment of Wegener's granulomatosis, significantly reducing disease morbidity and improving survival.[37,38] Cyclophosphamide has also been effectively used in the treatment of rheumatoid arthritis and its ocular complications.[39,40] Cyclophosphamide at doses of 1–2 mg/kg per day has now been used to treat a number of forms of uveitis including Behçet's disease and sympathetic ophthalmia.[41–43] However, the benefits of cyclophosphamide for autoimmune uveitis have not been well documented in large, prospective, randomized clinical trials.

Other cytotoxic agents have been used in the treatment of autoimmune uveitis. Chlorambucil (leukoran) has been effectively used in the treatment of the ocular complications of Behçet's disease by a number of investigators,[44–46] although not all reports are uniformly enthusiastic.[47] Data also suggest that chlorambucil may be effective in the treatment of sympathetic ophthalmia,[45,48] and the ocular inflammatory disease associated with juvenile rheumatoid arthritis.[49,50] Similarly, methotrexate has been successfully used in the treatment of some patients with corticosteroid-resistant ocular inflammation including sympathetic ophthalmia and scleritis.[51,52]

The development of animal models of autoimmune uveitis has been extremely useful for developing and testing the safety and efficacy of immunosuppressive drugs for uveitis. The use of cyclosporine was first evaluated for ocular autoimmune disease using the S-antigen-induced model of experimental autoimmune uveitis. Experiments clearly demonstrated the efficacy of cyclosporine in preventing the development of disease in rats.[53,54] At a dose of 10 mg/kg per day, disease was prevented in 100% of Lewis rats immunized with retinal S-antigen. Cyclosporine was effective, even when therapy was started 1 week after immunization, when immunocompetent cells capable of inducing disease are already present.

Based on these data in experimental animals, cyclosporine at a dose of 10 mg/kg per day was used to treat patients with uveitis resistant to corticosteroids and immunosuppressive agents. In an initial clinical study, 7 of 8 patients with bilateral sight-threatening posterior uveitis responded with improved visual acuity and disappearance of ocular inflammatory activity.[55] In a second study, 15 of 16 patients demonstrated improvement in visual acuity or intraocular inflammation after two to 18 months follow-up (FIGURE 3).[56] Other studies also demonstrated the efficacy of cyclosporine in the treatment of autoimmune uveitis. In a controlled, randomized clinical trial, Masuda and Nakajima showed that cyclosporine was more effective than colchicine for the treatment of Behçet's disease.[57]

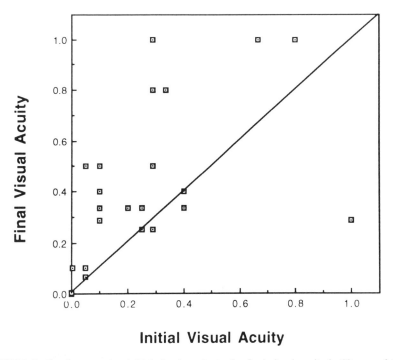

Initial Visual Acuity

FIGURE 3. Graph comparing initial visual acuity to the final visual acuity in 32 eyes of 16 patients after two to 18 months of follow-up. Visual acuity is represented as a fraction; 20/20 is 1, 20/200 is 0.1, no light perception is 0. Points above the diagonal line indicate improvement in visual acuity after cyclosporine therapy.

Clinical studies showed that renal toxicity limited the therapeutic success of cyclosporine as the sole drug for treating uveitis. Renal biopsies from 17 uveitis patients treated with cyclosporine for at least one year demonstrated definitive signs of cyclosporine toxicity when compared to age-matched controls.[58] In an attempt to decrease cyclosporine-induced renal toxicity, lower doses of cyclosporine (5 mg/kg per day) were combined with low doses of prednisone (10–20 mg/day). Studies using the combination of lower doses of cyclosporine with low dose prednisone have been effective in treating patients with uveitis.[59,60] With time, corticosteroids may be tapered and discontinued, and some patients have been successfully maintained on cyclosporine alone at doses of less than 2 mg/kg per day.[61] In a randomized, double-masked trial, cyclosporine was found to be equally effective as prednisone for the treatment of endogenous uveitis. However, patients who failed therapy with both drugs alone, showed additional improvement when both drugs were used together.[62]

Recently we reviewed the treatment of 19 patients with ocular Behçet's syndrome with combined cyclosporine A and prednisone therapy.[63] All patients had previously failed treatment with corticosteroids alone. Mean follow-up on combined therapy was 51 months with initial doses of cyclosporine ranging from 2.7 to 10.9 mg/kg. Visual acuity remained stable or improved in 28 of 37 eyes (76%) during the course of therapy. Visual acuity was significantly improved after 3 months of treatment ($p < 0.001$), but then tended to diminish with time despite continued therapy. Cyclosporine was discontinued because of adverse effects in only 3 of the 19 patients. In this study, the addition of small to moderate doses of prednisone appeared to allow effective use of smaller dosages of cyclosporine, thereby limiting the adverse effects of cyclosporine therapy.

The addition of azathioprine to therapeutic regimens of cyclosporine and prednisone have been shown superior to therapy with cyclosporine and prednisone alone in the prevention of graft rejection.[64,65] However, this "triple therapy" has only been used sporadically in the treatment of autoimmune uveitis,[66] and may warrant further investigation. A recent study showed that much lower doses of cyclosporine could be effectively used in the treatment of uveitis when combined with ketaconazole, a P-450 microsomal enzyme inhibitor.[67]

Animal models of autoimmune uveitis have also been useful in testing three new immunosuppressive agents for the treatment of uveitis: FK 506, rapamycin, and mycophenolate mofetil. FK 506 was first found in a soil sample obtained from Tsukuba, Japan in 1984.[68] Like cyclosporine, FK 506 inhibits expression of early T-cell activation genes, encoding IL-2, IL-3, IL-4, interferon-gamma, GM-CSF, and C-myc.[69,70] FK 506 has been shown to suppress the proliferative response in murine and human mixed lymphocyte responses at about 100 times lower concentration than cyclosporine,[68,71] and is effective in inhibiting transplant rejection in experimental animals and humans. FK 506 is also being tried for the treatment of various autoimmune diseases. Kawashima and colleagues first demonstrated that FK 506 could inhibit the development of EAU in rats.[72] Ming and coworkers in our laboratory later showed that FK 506 not only inhibited the development of EAU, but also decreased MHC class II antigen expression on ocular resident cells and IL-2 receptor expression on T lymphocytes in the eye.[73] Fujino and others showed that FK 506 at a dose of 0.5 mg/kg per day could prevent the development of EAU in primates,[74] and later experiments demonstrated that FK 506 could suppress ongoing ocular inflammation in animals, suggesting a role for the treatment of patients.[75] A multicenter clinical open trial of FK 506 has been started in refractory uveitis patients; mostly patients with Behçet's disease.[76] Initial data showed that 18 of 30 (62%) patients improved with FK 506 therapy at initial doses of 0.05 to 0.2 mg/kg per day; however, follow-up was less than 3 months for all dosage groups. Adverse effects of therapy included renal impairment in 4 patients, tremor in 3 cases, nausea in 2 cases, hyperglycemia in 1 case, hyperkalemia in 1 case, and chest discomfort in 1 case. Further studies of FK 506 for the treatment of corticosteroid-resistant uveitis are ongoing.

The macrolide rapamycin also inhibits T lymphocyte proliferation by interfering with IL-2 and IL-4 signal transduction that cannot be overcome by the addition of these cytokines.[77–80] Rapamycin has also been shown to prolong survival of allografts in a number of rejection models. Roberge and colleagues have shown that rapamycin at doses as low as 0.1 mg/kg per day effectively inhibited the development of EAU in Lewis rats.[81] This was true whether rapamycin therapy was initiated at the time of immunization or 7 days after immunization. Rats treated with rapamycin had an average 9% weight reduction during the first week of therapy; however, the initial weight lost was regained during the second week of therapy.

Mycophenolate mofetil is another new immunosuppressive compound and inhibits proliferative responses of human and rodent T and B lymphocytes to mitogens.[82] Researchers have shown that doses of mycophenolate mofetil sufficient to prevent allograft rejection in mice inhibited the incorporation of labeled thymidine into DNA in the lymph nodes and spleen of mice but not in the germinal cells of the testis or in the basal epithelial cells of the jejunum.[83] In addition, mycophenolate mofetil did not produce neutropenia, anemia, or thrombocytopenia, suggesting that this drug has lymphocyte-selective antiproliferative effects *in vivo* and can inhibit both cell-mediated and humoral immune responses without major side effects. Recently, Gery and coworkers showed that orally administered mycophenolate mofetil completely prevented the development of EAU in 10 of 12 animals at 2 weeks following immunization with retinal S-Antigen.[84] The drug also inhibited adoptively transferred EAU, and delayed disease onset and reduced disease severity when administered on days 7–20 after immunization. The authors concluded that mycophenolate mofetil affects both the afferent and efferent processes of EAU without weight loss or other adverse effects, suggesting that the drug may be useful for the treatment of uveitis in humans.

NEW THERAPEUTIC APPROACHES

Although immunosuppressive agents have been effective in treating patients with autoimmune uveitis, serious side effects have limited their use and fostered a search for new therapeutic approaches. The route of antigen administration partly determines the type of immune response that is induced, and oral administration of antigen can induce a state of immunologic tolerance to the fed antigens.[85] Oral tolerance has been demonstrated in several animal models of autoimmune disease including experimental allergic encephalomyelitis.[86] Nussenblatt and coworkers showed that oral administration of the S-antigen molecule prevented or markedly diminished the clinical appearance of S-antigen-induced uveitis,[87] and subsequent studies showed that oral administration of a uveitogenic peptide could diminish the severity of EAU induced by the whole S-antigen molecule.[88]

Recently Weiner and colleagues presented the results of a 1-year, double-masked, randomized clinical trial of 30 patients with relapsing-remitting multiple sclerosis. Fifteen patients received daily capsules of bovine myelin protein and 15 received a control protein. Six of the 15 patients in the myelin-treated group had at least one major exacerbation while 12 of 15 had an attack in the control group ($p = 0.06$). Subgroup analysis showed that males and HLA-DR2- individuals benefitted most from myelin therapy. In addition, T-cells reactive with myelin basic protein were reduced in the myelin-treated group.[89] Importantly, no important side effects of the treatment have been reported. A similar prospective, randomized, double-masked clinical trial is under way at the National Eye Institute, where patients with uveitis are treated with capsules of bovine retinal antigens or control proteins.

Researchers are also attempting to inhibit inflammation by interfering with cell adhesion. In both human and experimental uveitis, ocular tissues are infiltrated with mononuclear and polymorphonuclear cells recruited from the circulation. Cell adhesion is mediated by surface proteins, and increased expression of these cell adhesion molecules appears to promote the migration of leukocytes to areas of inflammation including the eye.[90] Intercellular adhesion molecule-1 (ICAM-1) is a member of the immunoglobulin supergene family,[91] and binds to two members of the β2 integrin family of cell adhesion molecules, lymphocyte function-associated antigen-1 (LFA-1) and Mac-1. In contrast to LFA-1 and Mac-1, which are predominantly expressed on leukocytes, ICAM-1 is mostly expressed on nonhematopoietic cells. ICAM-1 can be expressed on the human cornea, retinal pigment epithelium (RPE), capillary endothelium of the iris, ciliary body, choroid, and retina, and on glial cells in the retina.[90,92-95] We have previously shown that ICAM-1 is expressed on the RPE, vascular endothelium, and retinal glial cells in human eyes with posterior uveitis.[90]

More recently, we have demonstrated that ICAM-1 is expressed in the eyes of mice immunized with retinal antigens before histologic evidence of inflammation, and that monoclonal antibodies against both ICAM-1 and LFA-1 inhibited the development of EAU in these animals.[96] Proliferative responses to lipopolysaccharide, PPD, and IRBP of lymphocytes obtained from the draining lymph nodes were also decreased in mice treated with these antibodies. These data suggest that drugs to block cell adhesion molecules may be useful for the treatment of uveitis in humans. In fact, part of the antiinflammatory effect of immunosuppressive agents may be secondary to the inhibition of cell adhesion molecules.[97] In the eye, researchers have shown that FK 506 inhibits the expression of ICAM-1 on retinal pigment epithelial cells,[98] and a number of antiinflammatory agents have been shown to down regulate adhesion molecule expression in eyes with EAU.[99]

SUMMARY

The number of effective drugs for the treatment of autoimmune uveitis has greatly increased over the past 40 years. Many patients previously condemned to blindness can now be successfully treated with new immunosuppressive agents. New targets of the immune system, such as cell adhesion molecules, may offer novel therapeutic approaches for the treatment of inflammatory disease. However, since the catholicon for uveitis is not yet available, the search for new antiinflammatory therapy continues.

REFERENCES

1. UHLENHUTH, P. T. 1903. Zur lehre von der unterscheidung verschiedener eiweissarten mit hilfe spezifixher sera, in Fetschrift zum 60 geburstag von Robert Koch: 49–74. Fischer. Jena, Germany.
2. ELSCHNIG, A. 1910. Albrecht von Graefes Arch. Ophthalmol. 76: 509–46.
3. WACKER, W. B. & M. M. LIPTON. 1965. Nature 206: 253–258.
4. WACKER, W. B., C. M. KASLOW, J. A. YANKEELOV & D. T. ORGANISCIACK. 1977. J. Immunol. 119: 1949–1958.
5. CASPI, R. R., F. G. ROBERGE, C. C. CHAN, B. WIGGERT, G. J. CHADER, L. A. ROZENSZAJN, Z. LANDO & R. B. NUSSENBLATT. 1988. J. Immunol. 140: 1490–1495.
6. CHAN, C. C., M. MOCHIZUKI, R. B. NUSSENBLATT, A. G. PALESTINE, C. MCALLISTER, I. GERY & D. BENEZRA. 1985. Clin. Immunol. Immunopathol. 35: 103–110.
7. CHAN, C. C., M. MOCHIZUKI, A. G. PALESTINE, D. BENEZRA, I. GERY & R. B. NUSSENBLATT. 1985. Cell. Immunol. 96: 430–434.
8. CHAN, C. C., R. R. CASPI, M. NI, W. C. LEAKE, B. WIGGERT, G. J. CHADER & R. B. NUSSENBLATT. 1990. J. Autoimmunity 3: 247–255.
9. MOCHIZUKI, M., T. KUWABARA, C. C. CHAN, R. B. NUSSENBLATT, D. C. DETCALFE & I. GERY. 1984. J. Immunol. 133: 1699–1701.

10. Hirose, S., T. Kuwabara, R. B. Nussenblatt, B. Wiggert, T. M. Redmond & I. Gery. 1986. Arch. Ophthalmol. **104:** 1698–1702.
11. Schalken, J. J., A. H. M. van Vugt, H. J. Sinkens, P. H. M. Bovee-Geurts, W. J. DeGrip & R. M. Broekhuyse. 1988. Graefe's Arch. Clin. Exp. Ophthalmol. **226:** 255–261.
12. Broekhuyse, R. M., E. D. Kuhlmann, H. J. Winkens & A. H. Van Vugt. 1991. Exp. Eye Res. **52:** 465–474.
13. Marak, G. E., Jr. 1979. Surv. Ophthalmol. **24:** 141–156.
14. Chan, C. C., D. BenEzra, S. M. Hsu, A. G. Palestine & R. B. Nussenblatt. 1985. Arch. Ophthalmol. **103:** 198–202.
15. Lubin, J. R., D. M. Albert & M. Weinstein. 1980. Ophthalmology **87:** 109–121.
16. Chan, C. C., D. BenEzra, M. M. Rodrigues, A. G. Palestine, S. M. Hsu & R. B. Nussenblatt. 1985. Ophthalmology **92:** 580–590.
17. Momoeda, S. 1976. Acta Soc. Ophthalmol. Jpn **80:** 491–495.
18. Maezawa, H., A. Yano, M. Taniguchi & S. Kojima. 1982. Ophthalmologica **185:** 179–186.
19. Nussenblatt, R. B., I. Gery, E. J. Ballentine & W. B. Wacker. 1980. Am. J. Ophthalmol. **89:** 173–179.
20. Chan, C. C., R. B. Nussenblatt, A. G. Palestine, F. Roberge & D. BenEzra. 1985. Ophthalmology **92:** 1025–1028.
21. de Smet, M. D., M. Mochizuki, I. Gery, V. J. Singh, T. Shinohara, B. Wiggert, G. J. Chader & R. B. Nussenblatt. 1991. Am. J. Ophthalmol. **110:** 135–142.
22. Forrester, J. V. 1992. Eye **6:** 433–446.
23. Dick, A., Y. F. Cheng, A. T. Purdie, J. M. Liversidge & J. V. Forrester. 1992. Eye **6:** 643–647.
24. Deschennes, J., D. H. Char, S. Kaliter. 1988. Br. J. Ophthalmol. **72:** 83–87.
25. Cook, C. & R. K. MacDonald. 1951. Br. J. Ophthalmol. **35:** 730–735.
26. Gordon, D. M. 1954. Am. J. Ophthalmol. **37:** 533–538.
27. Gordon, D. M. 1956. Am. J. Ophthalmol. **41:** 593–600.
28. Drews, J. 1990. Immunosuppression. *In* Immunopharmacology. Principles and Perspectives: 141–145. Springer-Verlag. New York, N.Y.
29. Corley, C. C., S. E. Lessner & W. E. Larsen. 1966. Am. J. Med. **41:** 404–412.
30. Newell, F. W. & A. E. Krill. 1967. Trans. Ophthalmol. Soc. UK **87:** 499–511.
31. Andrasch, R. H., B. Pirofsky & R. P. Burns. 1978. Arch. Ophthalmol. **96:** 247–251.
32. Moore, C. E. 1968. Br. J. Ophthalmol. **52:** 688–690.
33. Behçet, H. 1937. Dermatol. Wochenshr. **46:** 414–419.
34. Yazici, H., H. Pazarli, C. G. Barnes, Y. Tüzün, Y. Öyazgan, A. Silman, S. Serdaroglus, V. Oguz, S. Yurdakul, G. E. Lovatt, B. Yazichi, S. Somani & A. Müftüoglu. 1990. N. Engl. J. Med. **322:** 281–285.
35. Aoki, K. & S. Sugiura. 1976. Mod. Probl. Ophthalmol. **16:** 309–313.
36. Baer, J. C., C. S. Foster & M. B. Raizman. 1989. Ophthalmology **96** (Suppl.): 128.
37. Fauci, A. S., B. F. Haynes, P. Katz & S. M. Wolff. 1983. Ann. Intern. Med. **98:** 76–85.
38. Hoffman, G. S., G. S. Kerr, R. Y. Leavitt, C. W. Hallahan, R. S. Lebovics, E. D. Travis, M. Rottem & A. S. Fauci. 1992. Ann. Intern. Med. **116:** 488–498.
39. Foster, C. S., S. L. Forstot & L. A. Wilson. 1984. Ophthalmology **91:** 1253–1263.
40. Hurd, E. R., W. B. Snyder & M. Ziff. 1970. Am. J. Med. **48:** 273–278.
41. Oniki, S., K. Kurakazu & K. Kawata. 1976. Jpn J. Ophthalmol. **20:** 32–40.
42. Buckley, C. E. III & J. P. Gills, Jr. 1969. Arch. Intern. Med. **124:** 29–35.
43. Martenet, A. C. 1976. Ophthalmologica (Basel) **172:** 106–115.
44. O'Duffy, J. D., D. M. Robertson & N. P. Goldstein. 1984. Am. J. Med. **76:** 75–84.
45. Godfrey, W. A., W. V. Epstein, G. R. O'Connor, S. J. Kumura, M. J. Hogan & R. A. Nozik. 1974. Am. J. Ophthalmol. **78:** 415–428.
46. Tricoulis, D. 1976. Br. J. Ophthalmol. **60:** 55–57.
47. Tabbara, K. F. 1983. Ophthalmology **90:** 906–908.
48. Jennings, T. & H. H. Tessler. 1989. Br. J. Ophthalmol. **73:** 140–145.
49. Kanski, J. J. 1977. Arch. Ophthalmol. **95:** 1794–1797.
50. Foster, C. S., L. P. Fong & G. Singh. 1989. Ophthalmology **96:** 281–288.

51. LAZAR, M., M. J. WEINER & I. H. LEOPOLD. 1969. Am. J. Ophthalmol. **67:** 383–387.
52. HOANG-XUAN, T., C. S. FOSTER & B. A. RICE. 1990. Ophthalmology: 892–898.
53. NUSSENBLATT, R. B., M. M. RODRIGUES, W. B. WACKER, S. J. CEVARIO, M. SALINAS-CARMONA & I. GERY. 1981. J. Clin. Invest. **67:** 1228–1231.
54. NUSSENBLATT, R. B., M. M. RODRIGUES, M. C. SALINAS-CARMONA, I. GERY, S. CEVARIO & W. WACKER. 1982. Arch. Ophthalmol. **100:** 1146–1149.
55. NUSSENBLATT, R. B., A. G. PALESTINE, A. H. ROOK & I. SCHER. 1983. Lancet **2:** 235–238.
56. NUSSENBLATT, R. B., A. G. PALESTINE & C. C. CHAN. 1983. Am. J. Ophthalmol. **96:** 275–282.
57. MASUDA, K. & A. NAKAJIMA. 1985. A double-masked study of cyclosporine in Behçet's diseases. *In* Cyclosporin Treatment in Behçet's disease. R. Schindler, Ed.: 162–164. Springer-Verlag. Berlin, Germany.
58. PALESTINE, A. G., H. A. AUSTIN, J. E. BALOW, T. T. ANTONOVYCH, G. SABNISS, H. G. PREUSS & R. B. NUSSENBLATT. 1986. N. Engl. J. Med. **314:** 1293–1298.
59. DIAZ-LLOPIS, M., M. CERVERA & J. L. MENETO. 1990. Curr. Eye Res. **9**(Suppl.): 17–23.
60. TOWLER, H. M. A., P. H. WHITING & J. V. FORRESTER. 1990. Eye **4:** 514–520.
61. BIELORY, L., C. HOLLAND, P. GASCON & L. FROHMAN. 1988. Transplant. Proc. **20**(Suppl. 4): 144–148.
62. NUSSENBLATT, R. B., A. G. PALESTINE, C. C. CHAN, G. STEVENS, JR., S. D. MELLOW & S. B. GREEN. 1991. Am. J. Ophthalmol. **112:** 138–146.
63. WHITCUP, S. M., E. C. SALVO, JR., M. D. DE SMET & R. B. NUSSENBLATT. 1992. Ophthalmology **99**(Suppl.): 138.
64. PERKINS, J. D., S. STERIOFF, R. H. WIESNER, K. P. OFFORD, J. RAKELA, E. R. DICKSON & R. A. F. KROM. 1987. Transplant. Proc. **19:** 2434–2436.
65. WIESSNER, R. H., J. LUDWIG, R. A. F. DROM, J. E. HAY & B. VAN HOEK. 1993. Mayo Clin. Proc. **93**(68): 69–79.
66. HOOPER, P. L. & H. J. KAPLAN. 1991. Ophthalmology **98:** 944–951.
67. DE SMET, M. D., R. I. RUBIN, S. M. WHITCUP, J. S. LOPEZ, H. A. AUSTIN & R. B. NUSSENBLATT. 1992. Am. J. Ophthalmol. **113:** 687–690.
68. GOTO, T., H. HATANAKA, M. OKUHARA, M. KOHSAKA, H. AOKI & H. IMANAKA. 1991. Transplant Proc. **23:** 2713–2717.
69. DI PADOVA, F. D. 1989. Pharmacology of cyclosporine. Pharmacol. Rev. **41:** 373–405.
70. TOCCI, M. J., D. A. MATKOVICH, K. A. COLLIER, P. KWOK, F. DUMONT, S. LIN, S. DEGUDICIBUS, J. J. SIEKIERKA, J. CHIN & N. I. HUTCHINSON. 1989. J. Immunol. **143:** 718–726.
71. ZEEVI, A., M. WOAN, G-Z. YAO, R. VENKATARAMANAN, S. TODO, T. E. STARZL & R. J. DUQUESNOY. 1991. Transplant. Proc. **23:** 2928–2930.
72. KAWASHIMA, H., Y. FUJINO & M. MOCHIZUKI. 1988. Invest. Ophthalmol. Vis. Sci. **29:** 1265–1271.
73. MING, N., C. C. CHAN, R. B. NUSSENBLATT & M. MOCHIZUKI. 1990. Autoimmunity **8:** 43–51.
74. FUJINO, Y., M. MOCHIZUKI, C. C. CHAN, J. RABER, S. KOTAKE, I. GERY & R. B. NUSSENBLATT. 1991. Curr. Eye Res. **10:** 679–690.
75. KAWASHIMA, H. & M. MOCHIZUKI. 1990. Exp. Eye Res. **51:** 565.
76. MOCHIZUKI, M., K. MASUDA, T. SAKANE, G. INABA, K. ITO, M. KOGURE, N. SUGINO, M. USUI, Y. MIZUSHIMA, S. OHNO, Y. MIYANAGA, S. HAYASAKA & K. OHIZUMI. 1991. Transplant. Proc. **23:** 3343–2246.
77. DUMONT, F. J., M. J. STARUCH, S. L. KOPRAK, M. R. MELINO & N. H. SIGAL. 1991. J. Immunol. **144:** 251–258.
78. BIERER, B. E., P. S. MATTILA, R. F. STANDAERT, L. A. HERZENBERG, S. J. BURAKOFF, G. CRABTREE & S. L. SCHREIBER. 1990. Proc. Natl. Acad. Sci. USA **87:** 9231–9235.
79. BIERER, B. E., S. L. SCHREIBER & S. J. BURAKOFF. 1991. Eur. J. Immunol. **21:** 439–445.
80. HENDERSON, D. J., I. NAYA, R. V. BUNDICK, G. M. SMITH & J. A. SCHMIDT. 1991. Immunology **73:** 316–321.
81. ROBERGE, F. G., D. XU, C. C. CHAN, M. D. DE SMET, R. B. NUSSENBLATT & H. CHEN. 1993. Curr. Eye Res. **12:** 197–203.

82. EUGUI, E. M., S. J. ALMQUIST, C. D. MULLER & A. C. ALLISON. 1991. Scand. J. Immunol. **33:** 161–174.
83. EUGUI, E. M., A. MIRKOVICH & A. C. ALLISON. 1991. Scand. J. Immunol. **33:** 175–183.
84. GERY, I., A. C. ALLISON, N. MILLER-RIVERO, B. P. VISTICA, N. P. CHANAUD III & R. B. NUSSENBLATT. 1993. Invest. Ophthalmol. Vis. Sci. **34:** 1480.
85. WELLS, H. 1911. J. Infect. Dis. **9:** 147–171.
86. BITAR, D. M. & C. C. WHITACRE. 1988. Cell. Immunol. **112:** 364–370.
87. NUSSENBLATT, R. B., R. R. CASPI, R. MAHDI, C. C. CHAN, F. ROBERGE, O. LIDER & H. L. WEINER. 1990. J. Immunol. **144:** 1689–1695.
88. THURAU, S. R., C. C. CHAN, E. SUH & R. B. NUSSENBLATT. 1991. J. Autoimmun. **4:** 507–516.
89. WEINER, H. L., G. A. MACKIN, M. MATSUI, E. J. ORAV, S. J. KHOURY, D. M. DAWSON & D. A. HAFLER. 1993. Science **259:** 1321–1324.
90. WHITCUP, S. M., C. C. CHAN, Q. LI & R. B. NUSSENBLATT. 1992. Arch. Ophthalmol. **110:** 662–666.
91. STAUNTON, E. D., S. D. MARLIN, C. STRATOWA, M. L. DUSTIN & T. A. SPRINGER. 1988. Cell **52:** 925–933.
92. ELNER, V. M., S. G. ELNER, M. A. PAVILACK, R. F. TODD III, B. Y. J. T. JUE & A. R. HUBER. 1991. Am. J. Pathol. **138:** 525–536.
93. FORRESTER, J. V., J. LIVERSIDGE & H. S. DUA. 1990. Curr. Eye Res. **9**(Suppl.): 183–191.
94. KAMINSKA, G. M., J. Y. NIEDERKORN & J. P. McCULLEY. 1991. Invest. Ophthalmol. Vis. Sci. **32**(Suppl.): 677.
95. WAKEFIELD, D., P. McCLUSKEY & P. PALLADINETTI. 1992. Arch. Ophthalmol. **110:** 121–125.
96. WHITCUP, S. M., L. R. DEBARGE, R. R. CASPI, R. HARNING, R. B. NUSSENBLATT & C. C. CHAN. Clini. Immunol. Immunopathol. (In press.)
97. PETZELBAUER, P., G. STINGL, K. WOLFF & B. VOLC-PLATZER. 1991. J. Invest. Dermatol. **96:** 362–369.
98. LIVERSIDGE, J., A. W. THOMSON & J. V. FORRESTER. 1991. Transplant. Proc. **23:** 3339–3342.
99. LAI, J., C. C. CHAN, Q. LI & S. M. WHITCUP. 1993. Invest. Ophthalmol. Vis. Sci. **34:** 1206.

Immunosuppressive Treatment of Chronic Liver Disease

E. ANTHONY JONES[a] AND NORA VALERIA BERGASA[b,c]

[a]Department of Medicine
Royal Free Hospital
London, United Kingdom

[b]Liver Diseases Section
National Institutes of Health
Bethesda, Maryland

Several chronic liver diseases have been classified as having an autoimmune basis, notably idiopathic (autoimmune) chronic active hepatitis, primary biliary cirrhosis (PBC), primary sclerosing cholangitis (PSC), and immunocholangitis.

AUTOIMMUNE CHRONIC ACTIVE HEPATITIS

Idiopathic chronic active hepatitis, which is characterized histologically by piecemeal necrosis of periportal hepatocytes,[1] was the first liver disease for which an autoimmune pathogenesis was postulated, and this hypothesis is supported by experimental findings.[2] It is much less common than chronic viral hepatitis. The rationale for treating this disease with immunosuppressive drugs, principally corticosteroids, is considered to have been established, and is based on the results of three controlled clinical trials.[3-5] These trials appear to show that corticosteroid therapy is associated with improved survival,[3-5] although progression of the disease to cirrhosis does not seem to be prevented by this therapy.[6] Differences of opinon remain concerning the magnitude of the desirable initial dose of corticosteroids (e.g., in the range of 30 to 60 mg of prednisolone daily) for treatment of this disease and how soon a minimal maintenance dose can be achieved (usually a few weeks). The serum level of alanine aminotransferase is regarded as an important marker of disease activity and hepatocellular necrosis during immunosuppressive therapy, although periodic needle biopsies of the liver provide more definitive information on the activity and progression of the disease. The desirable maintenance dose of corticosteroid is the lowest dose that appears to adequately control the activity of the disease (usually 5 to 20 mg of prednisolone daily). Alternate-day corticosteroid therapy has not been convincingly shown to improve the therapeutic index of this class of drugs. In some patients, the disease process appears to burn itself out, usually after several years, and, if this happens, it may be possible to wean the patients off corticosteroids altogether. However, most patients require immunosuppressive treatment indefinitely and any attempt to slowly withdraw corticosteroids typically precipitates serum biochemical and histological relapses of disease activity.[7,8] Azathioprine (usually 50 to 100 mg daily) is often given in addition, as reduction of corticosteroids is possible

[c]Author to whom correspondence should be addressed. Present affiliation: Laboratory of the Biology of Addictive Diseases, The Rockefeller University, 1230 York Avenue, New York, New York 10021-6399.

without precipitating a relapse of desease activity.[9] It is generally agreed that asymptomatic patients with substantial disease activity should be treated with immunosuppression, although asymptomatic patients were not included in the original trials.[10,11] Immunosuppressive drugs, other than corticosteroids and azathioprine, have not been systematically assessed in the management of this disease.

OTHER AUTOIMMUNE CHRONIC LIVER DISEASES

More recently PBC, which is characterized by a chronic nonsuppurative destructive cholangitis affecting septal and the larger interlobular intrahepatic bile ducts,[12] has also been classified as an autoimmune disease.[13] PBC has been regarded as a rare disease, but it is being increasingly recognized, particularly in asymptomatic patients.[14] A fair body of evidence is consistent with PBC having an autoimmune pathophysiological basis, but this evidence is not conclusive and the interesting possibility that an infectious agent may be involved in the pathogenesis of the disease cannot be excluded at the time of writing.[15-18] The first controlled trial of an immunosuppressive drug for PBC was the azathioprine trial conducted by Heathcote and her colleagues in the 1970s.[19] Several trials of other immunosuppressive drugs for this disease have subsequently been conducted and published.[20-25]

Primary sclerosing cholangitis is characterized by a chronic fibrosing cholangitis affecting larger (intrahepatic and/or extrahepatic) bile ducts than those involved in PBC.[26] Available information on this disease suggests that it may have an autoimmune basis.[27] However, primary sclerosing cholangitis is even rarer than PBC, and immunosuppressive therapies for PBC tend to be used as models for the treatment of primary sclerosing cholangitis.[26] Recently, a form of cholangitis very similar to PBC has been described, and it has been termed immunocholangitis.[28] This condition may well have an autoimmune basis, but its treatment with immunosuppressive drugs is currently empiric. Thus, current interest in immunosuppressive treatment for autoimmune chronic liver disease is focused largely on PBC.

IMMUNOSUPPRESSIVE DRUGS AND PBC

The rationale for trials of immunosuppressive drugs in PBC is based on evidence that suggests that autoimmune phenomena contribute to the pathogenesis of this disease.[13] As PBC is chronic and slowly progressive, a necessary property of treatment for this disease is that it be suitable for long-term use. Because of the toxicities associated with the administration of classical immunosuppressive drugs, it has seemed prudent to select for treatment patients with symptomatic disease and reduced life expentancy.[23] However, there appears to be a general consensus that by the time a major complication of chronic liver disease has developed, there is little room for immunosuppressive drugs to be effective. Furthermore, whether to treat the asymptomatic patients is a major issue. The prognosis of asymptomatic PBC is uncertain,[29] but recent data dependent on patient selection criteria have suggested that mean live expectancy in a population of patients with asymptomatic PBC is significantly reduced.[30] Thus, it may be appropriate to evaluate an immunosuppressive drug for the treatment of patients with asymptomatic PBC, providing administration of the drug is sufficiently free from serious side effects. The properties of mycophenolate mofetil suggest that it might be a suitable drug for administration in such a trial.[31]

During the past 7 years, the results of 5 clinical trials of immunosuppressive drug in patients with PBC have been published. The drugs studied were azathioprine,[20,21] chlorambucil,[22] prednisolone,[23] cyclosporine,[24] and methotrexate.[25] The doses of these drugs given to patients with PBC in the trials tended to be low, presumably because of apprehension over the potential for serious short-term and long-term side effects if high doses of these drugs are administered. Four of the trials were controlled. The MTX trial was uncontrolled. Only in one of the trials, the multi-center trial of azathioprine, were a substantial number of patients studied.

A major issue in trials of immunosuppressive drugs in PBC is the problem of what to monitor during immunosuppressive therapy. It is routine to record symptoms, serum biochemistry, and hepatic histologic findings. Fatigue and pruritus are usually assessed using subjective scores. Attempts are being made to make the criteria used in such scores more consistent and meaningful by making scores more dependent on questions that require less subjective answers. Pruritus may also be assessed by quantitating its behavioral consequence, scratching activity. Recently this approach has been facilitated by developing a monitoring system that records the total amount of scratching activity carried out by the middle fingernail of the dominant hand independent of body movements.[32] The device developed is well tolerated by patients and can be used to quantitate scratching activity throughout the day and night. It has been applied successfully to assess the effect of a drug on scratching activity in patients with pruritus due to PBC[33] and appears to have considerable potential for the objective evaluation of antipruritic medications. However, caution is necessary in applying this approach to assess progression of PBC, as pruritus may regress spontaneously with the development of hepatocellular failure.[34] It is not clear whether a decrease in ALT or alkaline phosphatase associated with immunosuppressive therapy may reflect a slowing of progression of the disease, providing the immunosuppressive drug does not have a direct effect on bilirubin metabolism. Serum bilirubin appears to be an important index of prognosis in PBC, and serum bilirubin[35] is a major component of prognostic scores that have been developed for PBC.[21,36] Serum albumin, which appears to depend on both the rate of albumin synthesis[37] and the plasma volume in chronic liver disease,[38] may also be a useful marker in assessing the effects of an immunosuppressive drug on PBC. However, appreciable changes in either serum bilirubin or serum albumin do not occur until the disease process of PBC has undergone appreciable progression.[35] There is clearly a need for serum biochemical markers of PBC that would be useful if applied in the early stages of the disease, including the asymptomatic phase. The limitation of routine serum biochemistry in monitoring progress in patients with PBC is illustrated by the occurrence of florid bile duct lesions characteristic of the disease in liver biopsies from some untreated patients who have normal values for serum bilirubin, ALT, and alkaline phosphatase.[39] In therapeutic trials in PBC, a liver biopsy is usually obtained at the outset and at one or two yearly intervals thereafter. The value of serial liver biopsies in assessing progression in an individual patient is severely limited by sampling error. However, this problem is much less important in a clinical trial in which mean scores for histological changes (such as inflammation, fibrosis, and stage of disease) are determined from examination of coded slides from control and treated groups. Such comparisons probably provide meaningful data on the efficacy of a drug, providing the design of the trial is satisfactory and the numbers of patients in each group are adequate.

Effects of Immunosuppressives on Symptoms in PBC

In an open label trial of MTX (15 mg/week orally) conducted at the National Institutes of Health (NIH), appreciable improvement in scores for both fatigue and pruritus were apparent after 12 months of therapy.[40] Analogous findings in another open label trial of MTX were similar.[25] In some patients, in whom scratching activity was quantitated serially, an improvement in puritus score correlated with a decrease in scratching activity. Fatigue and pruritus also appeared to be less in patients treated with chlorambucil,[22] prednisolone,[23] or cyclosporine[24] than in patients in corresponding control groups.

Effects of Immunosuppressives on Serum Biochemistry in PBC

In the second year of the NIH trial, mean values for serum bilirubin, ALT, and alkaline phosphatase were lower than before treatment. A frequent observation in this trial was an increase in serum ALT above the initial baseline value 4–8 months after starting therapy. No new symptoms or signs have been observed when patients on MTX develop a further increase in their ALT level. Without altering the dose of MTX, increased ALT levels during the first few months of therapy subsequently decreased so that at one year they were similar to or less than baseline values.[40] These findings are in broad agreement with analogous findings observed by Kaplan.[25] At NIH, liver biopsies have not been obtained when serum ALT values have been high during the first year of therapy. Particularly striking were data on serum bilirubin in the chlorambucil trial.[22] In the treated group, the mean bilirubin remained unchanged over the four-year period of the trial, whereas in the control group it increased progressively. Values for mean serum bilirubin tended to decrease on MTX therapy[25] and tended to be less in patients receiving prednisolone[23] or cyclosporine[24] than in patients in corresponding control groups. In addition, values for serum ALT and alkaline phosphatase also tended to be lower in patients treated with prednisolone or cyclosporine than in respective controls. Furthermore, values for serum albumin tended to be higher in patients treated with chlorambucil, prednisolone, or cyclosporine than in those in corresponding controls groups.

It would seem logical to obtain in a trial of a new therapy in PBC serial biochemical measurements that, in contrast to routine serum biochemical data, constitute a quantitative test of biliary (or hepatocellular) function. However, such tests (e.g., galactose elimination capacity, the MEGX test, and fasting and postprandial serum bile acid levels) constitute extra work and expense and there is a strong impression that some centers, who might otherwise participate in a trial, would not be motivated to do additional tests. In the NIH, fasting and two-hour postprandial serum bile acid levels tended to be lower after 12 months on MTX than before therapy.[40]

Effects of Immunosuppressives on Histology in PBC

In the NIH trial, the mean score for hepatic inflammation was less after 12 months on MTX than before therapy.[41] A similar observation was made in the other MTX trial.[25] In addition, hepatic inflammation appeared to be less in patients receiving chlorambucil,[22] prednisolone,[23] or cyclosporine[24] than in respective controls. So far there has been no convincing evidence that therapy with any immunosuppressive drug retards hepatic fibrogenesis or progression of histologic stage of disease. Indeed, in the NIH trial, MTX therapy appeared to be associated with an increase in the mean score of hepatic fibrosis. Furthermore, in one patient, there was an increase of ballooning of hepatocytes which was interpreted as MTX toxicity and led to discontinuation of the drug in that patient.[40]

Effects of Immunosuppressives on Immune Markers in PBC

It is conceivable that immune markers that reflect an autoimmune process contributing to the pathogenesis of PBC may be of value in assessing the effects of an immunosuppressive drug on this disease. In patients with PBC, IgM is not only present in increased concentrations in most sera[41] but the IgM present has abnormal immunoreactive properties that may potentially contribute to the pathogenesis of the disease, such as the ability to activate complement.[42] In the chlorambucil trial, the mean serum IgM level remained elevated in the control group, whereas in the treated group it had become normal by one year and remained normal.[22] Similar data have been obtained in some patients treated with MTX in the NIH trial.[40] In both of these trials, treatment tended to be associated with a lowering of the IgM serum levels, although this phenomenon may represent a nonspecific effect of immunosuppression. Serum levels of the intercellular adhesion molecules ICAM1, VCAM-1, and E-selectin have been shown to be elevated in patients with PBC.[43,44] A lowering of the serum levels of these immune markers or of other immune markers, such as Tac peptide,[45] in association with the administration of an immunosuppressive drug may reflect a beneficial effect of the disease process of PBC, although in the NIH pilot study with MTX, serum levels of these soluble adhesion molecules did not decrease after one year of treatment in spite of the reduction of serum levels of liver associated enzymes and the decreased intensity of the inflammatory infiltrate associated with MTX treatment.[40,44]

Effects of Corticosteroids on PBC

As corticosteroids have excellent immunosuppressive properties,[46] it is unfortunate that their use in PBC is not recommended because of their apparent tendency to precipitate or exacerbate severe metabolic bone disease.[47] Perhaps for this reason, there has been only one controlled trial of corticosteroids in PBC. This trial clearly showed that apparent beneficial effects induced by 12 months of prednisolone therapy were associated with increased loss of trabecular bone volume and a reduction in the bone resorption surface. The positive effects of prednisolone in this trial were sufficiently encouraging that the authors did not conclude that corticosteroids have no place in the treatment of PBC. Instead, they raised three important issues. First, it may be possible to prevent corticosteroid-induced accelerated bone loss, perhaps with estrogens. Second, it may be possible to identify patients at particular risk of accelerated bone loss (e.g., by measuring calcium absorption) and to avoid corticosteroids in this subgroup. Finally, careful monitoring of bone loss may facilitate the safe administration of corticosteroids in PBC.

Immunosuppression-Related Tumors and PBC

In the trials in which the numbers of patients studied were small, no malignancies have been reported, and in the azathioprine trial, the incidence of malignancies was higher in the placebo-treated group.[21] Nevertheless, the principal potential long-term side effect of classical immunosuppressive drugs is an increased risk of developing malignancies. This potential risk remains a major factor limiting the more widespread assessment of immunosuppressive drugs in the management of PBC.[48]

Effects of Immunosuppressives on Survival in PBC

The authors of the multicenter azathioprine trial developed a prognostic index to facilitate analysis of their data. Components of this index are bilirubin, age, albumin, and the presence histologically of cirrhosis and central cholestasis.[21] A prognostic index for PBC has also been developed at the Mayo Clinic.[36] An important difference between the two indices is that the Mayo score does not include histology. A common feature of both is that they are highly dependent on late features of the disease, such as an elevated serum bilirubin. Thus, both are probably of limited value in assessing the effects of immunosuppressive drugs in patients with early PBC. Currently, neither of these indices is widely accepted in studies designed to evaluate the effects of immunosuppressive drugs on PBC.

In contrast, death and referral for liver transplantation constitute definitive end points for studies of the effects of immunosuppressive drugs on PBC. The percentage of patients that underwent liver transplantation or died in the azathioprine trial was slightly less in the treated group than in the placebo group. The numbers in the other controlled trials were too small to make any comments on the effects of treatment on survival.[22–24] When the survival data in the azathioprine trial were analyzed by the use of the Kaplan Meier method, the difference between treated and control groups was not significant. However, when the Cox regression model was applied the difference between the two groups was highly significant. During the 120 months period of the trial, the main survival was 20 months longer in the azathioprine group than in the placebo group. The main limitation of this trial was the high attrition rate (38%). The authors advocated azathioprine for the routine treatment of PBC, but this recommendation has not been generally accepted.[21]

FUTURE FOR TREATMENT OF AUTOIMMUNE LIVER DISEASE

Clearly, there is room for more effective and safer immunosuppressive therapy for chronic autoimmune liver diseases. Potentially useful approaches for the future include the design of drugs with selective immunosuppressive actions (such as mycophenolate mofetil), the administration of theapeutic antibodies (e.g., anti-Tac or anti-ICAM1), and the use of cytokine antagonists. If an ongoing infection as the etiology of PBC remains uncorfirmed and further evidence for an autoimmune contribution to the pathogenesis of PBC accumulates, the rationale for administering a potent immunosuppressive agent to patients with PBC will be enhanced. In this context, drugs that do not fulfill classical criteria of immunosuppressive agents may not adequately suppress autoimmune manifestations of the disease and consequently may not have the potential of significantly increasing survival. Of the nonimmunosuppressive drugs that have been used in the treatment of PBC, ursodeoxycholic acid (UDCA) is currently receiving considerable attention and is being increasingly used for the routine treatment of PBC. The popularity of this agent is based on its very low toxicity and the results of a multicenter European trial which appeared to show that the administration of UDCA was associated with a favorable trend in symptoms, serum biochemistry, histology, and even survival.[49] These findings are not universally accepted and have not been confirmed by other groups.[50] However, while UDCA is not a classical immunosuppressive, this agent has been shown to mediate immunomodulatory effects.[51,52] These effects may include suppression of increased expression of HLA antigens on biliary epithelial cells.[52] Such an action of UDCA, if confirmed, may imply that this agent might augment suppression of a component of an immunological reaction contributing to tissue injury in PBC. This line of reasoning may be used as a rationale to justify trials to assess the effects of UDCA in combination with a classical immunosuppressive, such MTX, in the management of PBC. Of greater potential interest would appear to be the development of drugs with potent immunosuppressive properties, but that lack the undesirable myelosuppressive and carcinogenic properties of the classical immunosuppressive drugs. In this context, mycophenolate mofetil shows considerable promise and merits evaluation for its possible efficacy in the treatment of PBC. A particularly intriguing therapeutic trial would be an assessment of the effects of a combination of mycophenolate mofetil and anti-Tac on PBC. Mycophenolate mofetil does not inhibit early stages of lymphocyte activation, including expression of IL-2R.[31] By inhibiting clonal proliferation of T and B cells, mycophenolate mofetil may freeze activated cells for elimination or inactivation by anti-Tac. Hypothetically, such potentially synergistic effects of two potent immunosuppressive therapeutic agents could substantially suppress the disease process of PBC.

REFERENCES

1. DE GROOTE, J., V. J. DESMET, P. GEDOGK, G. KORB, H. POPPER, H. POULSEN, P. J. SCHEUER, M. SCHMID, H. THALER, E. UEHLINGERAND & W. WEPLER. 1968. A classification of chronic hepatitis. Lancet **ii:** 626–628.
2. LOHSE, A. W. 1991. Experimental models of autoimmune hepatitis. Semin. Liver Dis. **11**(3): 241–247.
3. COOK, G. C., R. MULLIGANAND & S. SHERLOCK. 1971. Controlled trial of corticosteroid therapy in active chronic hepatitis. Q. J. Med. **158:** 159–185.
4. SOLAWAY, R. D., W. H. J. SUMMERSKILL, A. H. BAGGENSTOSS, M. G. GEALL, G. L. GITNICK, L. R. ELVEBACKAND & L. J. SCHOENFIELD. 1972. Clinical, biochemical, and histological remission of severe chronic active liver disease: a controlled study of treatments and early prognosis. Gastroenterology **63**(5): 820–833.
5. MURRAY-LYON, I. M., R. B. STERNAND & R. WILLIAMS. 1973. Controlled trial of prednisolone and azathioprine in active chronic hepatitis. Lancet **i:** 735–737.
6. CZAJA, A. J., G. L. DAVIS, J. LUDWIG & H. TASWELL. 1984. Complete resolution of inflammatory activity following corticosteroid treatment of HBsAg-negative chronic active hepatitis. Hepatology **4**(4): 622–627.
7. CZAJA, A. J., J. LUDWIG & A. H. BAGGENSTOSS. 1981. Corticosteroid-treated chronic active hepatitis in remission. N. Engl. J. Med. **304:** 5–9.
8. HEGARTY, J. E., K. T. NOURI AURI, B. PORTMANN, A. L. W. F. EDDLESTON & R. WILLIAMS. 1983. Relapse following treatment withdrawal in patients with autoimmune chronic active hepatitis. Hepatology. **3:** 685–689.
9. STELLON, A. J., J. J. KEATING, P. J. JOHNSON, I. G. MCFARLANE & R. WILLIAMS. 1988. Maintenance of remission in autoimmune chronic active hepatitis with azathioprine after corticosteroid withdrawal. Hepatology **8:** 781–784.
10. BERK, P. D., E. A. JONES, P. H. PLOTZ, L. B. SEEF & E. C. WRIGHT. 1976. Corticosteroid therapy for chronic active hepatitis. Ann. Intern. Med. **85**(4): 523–525.
11. WRIGHT, E. C., L. B. SEEF, P. D. BERK, E. A. JONES & P. H. PLOTZ. 1977. Treatment of chronic active hepatitis: an analysis of three controlled trials. Gastroenterology **73:** 1422–1430.
12. SCHEUER, P. 1967. Primary biliary cirrhosis. Proc. R. Soc. Med. **60:** 1257–1260.
13. JAMES, S. P., J. H. HOOFNAGLE, W. STROBER & E. A. JONES. 1983. NIH conference: primary biliary cirrhosis: a model autoimmune disease. Ann. Intern. Med. **99**(4): 500–512.
14. KAPLAN, M. 1987. Primary biliary cirrhosis. N. Engl. J. Med. **316:** 521–528.
15. STEMEROWICZ, R., B. MOLLER, A. RODLOFF, M. FREUDENBERG, U. HOPF, C. WITTENBRINK, R. REINHARDT & C. GALANOS. 1988. Are mitochondrial antibodies in primary biliary cirrhosis induced by R (rough)-mutants of enterobacteriaceae? Lancet: 1166–1169.

16. HOPF, U., R. STEMEROWICZ, A. RODLOFF, C. GALANOS, B. MOLLER, H. LOBECK, M. FREUDENBERG & D. HUHN. 1989. Relation between *Escherichia coli* R (rough)-forms in gut, lipid and in liver, and primary biliary cirrhosis. Lancet: 1419–1422.

17. HOPF, U. & R. STEMEROWICZ. 1991. Recent developments in primary biliary cirrhosis: etiology and treatment. Immunol. Res. **10**(3–4): 508–517.

18. BURROUGHS, A. K., P. BUTLER, M. J. E. STERNBERG & H. BAUM. Molecular mimicry in liver disease. Nature **358**: 377–378.

19. HEATHCOTE, J., A. ROSSAND & S. SHERLOCK. 1976. A prospective controlled trial of azathioprine in primary biliary cirrhosis. Gastroenterology **70**: 656–660.

20. CROWE, J., E. CHRISTENSEN, M. SMITH, M. COCHRANE, L. RANEK, G. WATKINSON, D. DONIACH, H. POPPER, N. TYGSTRUP & R. WILLIAMS. 1980. Azathioprine in primary biliary cirrhosis: a preliminary report of an international trial. Gastroenterology **78**: 1005–1010.

21. CHRISTENSEN, E. 1989. Prognostication in primary biliary cirrhosis: relevance to the individual patient. Hepatology **10**(1): 111–113.

22. HOOFNAGLE, J., G. DAVIS, D. SCHAFER, M. PETERS, M. AVIGAN, S. PAPPAS, R. HANSON, G. MINUCK, G. DUSHEIKO, G. CAMPBELL, R. MACSWEEN & E. A. JONES. 1986. Randomized trial of chlorambucil for primary biliary cirrhosis. Gastroenterology **91**: 1327–1334.

23. MITCHINSON, H. C., M. F. BASSENDINE, A. J. MALCOLM, E. J. WATSON, C. O. RECORD & O. F. W. JAMES. 1989. A pilot, double-blind, controlled 1-year trial of prednisolone treatment in primary biliary cirrhosis: hepatic improvement but greater bone loss. Hepatology **10**: 420–429.

24. WIESNER, R. H., E. R. DICKSON, K. D. LINDOR, R. JORGENSEN, N. F. LARUSSO & W. BALDUS. 1990. A controlled clinical trial of cyclosporine in the treatment of primary biliary cirrhosis. N. Engl. J. Med. **322**(22): 1419–14245.

25. KAPLAN, M. M. & T. A. KNOX. 1991. Treatment of primary biliary cirrhosis with low-dose weekly methotrexate. Gastroenterology **101**(5): 1332–1338.

26. LARUSSO, N., R. H. WIESNER, J. LUDWIG & R. L. MACCARTHY. 1984. Primary sclerosing cholangitis. N. Engl. J. Med. **310**(14): 899–903.

27. BODENHIMER, H. C., JR. N. F. LARUSSO, W. R. THAYER JR., C. CHARLAND, P. STAPLES & J. LUDWIG. 1983. Elevated circulating immune complexes in primary sclerosing cholangitis. Hepatology **3**: 150–154.

28. BRUNNER, G. & O. KLINGE. 1987. A cholangitis with antinuclear antibodies (immunocholangitis) resembling chronic destructive nonsuppurative cholangitis. Dtsch. Med. Wochenschr. **112**(38): 1454–1458.

29. ROLL, J., J. L. BOYER, D. BARRY & G. KLATSKIN. 1983. The prognostic importance of clinical and histologic features in asymptomatic and symptomatic primary biliary cirrhosis. N. Engl. J. Med. **308**: 1–7.

30. BALASUBRAMANIAM, K., P. M. GRAMBSCH, R. H. WIESNER, K. D. LINDOR & E. R. DICKSON. 1990. Diminished survival in asymptomatic primary biliary cirrhosis. A prospective study. Gastroenterology **98**(6): 1567–1571.

31. ALLISON, A. C. 1991. Approaches to the design of immunosuppressive agents. *In* Molecular Biology of Immunosuppression. A. Thompson, Ed. Open University Press. Buckingham, England.

32. TALBOT, T., J. SCHMITT, N. V. BERGASA, E. A. JONES & E. WALKER. 1991. Application of piezo film technology for the quantitative assessment of pruritus. Biomed. Instrum. Technol. **25**: 400–403.

33. BERGASA, N. V., T. L. TALBOT, D. W. ALLING, J. M. SCHMITT, E. C. WALKER, B. L. BAKER, J. C. KORENMAN, Y. PARK, J. H. HOOFNAGLE & E. A. JONES. 1992. A controlled trial of naloxone infusions for the pruritus of chronic cholestasis. Gastroenterology **102**(2): 544–549.

34. LLOYD-THOMAS, H. G. L. & S. SHERLOCK. 1952. Testosterone therapy for the pruritus of obstructive jaundice. Br. Med. J. **2**: 1289–1291.

35. SHAPIRO, J. M., H. SMITH & F. SCHAFFNER. 1979. Serum bilirubin: prognostic factor in primary biliary cirrhosis. Gut **20**: 137–140.

36. DICKSON, E. R., P. M. GRAMBSCH, T. R. FLEMING, L. D. FISHER & A. LANGWHORTHY. 1989. Prognosis in primary biliary cirrhosis: a model for decision making. Hepatology **10:** 1–7.

37. TAVILL, A. S., A. GRAIGIE & V. M. ROSENOER. 1968. The measurement of the synthetic rate of albumin in man. Clin. Sci. **34:** 1–28.

38. ROTHSCHILD, M. A., M. ORATZ, D. ZIMMON, S. S. SCHREIBER, I. WEINER & A. VAN CANEGHEM. 1969. Albumin synthesis in cirrhotic subjects with ascites studied with carbonate-^{14}C. J. Clin. Invest. **48:** 340–350.

39. MITCHINSON, H. C., M. F. BASSENDINE, A. HENDRICK, M. K. BENNETT, G. BIRD, A. J. WATSON & O. F. W. JAMES. 1986. Positive antimitochondrial antibody but normal alkaline phosphatase: is this primary biliary cirrhosis? Hepatology **6**(6): 1279–1284.

40. BERGASA, N. V., J. H. HOOFNAGLE, D. KLEINER, Y. PARK & E. A. JONES. 1992. Methotrexate (MTX) for primary biliary cirrhosis (PBC): interim analysis of an open label study. Hepatology **16:** 516 (Abstr.).

41. FEIZI, T. 1968. Immunoglobulins in chronic liver disease. Gut **9:** 193–198.

42. LINGREN, S. & S. ERIKSSON. 1982. IgM in primary biliary cirrhosis. Gut **99:** 636–645.

43. ADAMS, D. H., E. MAINOLFI, P. BURRA, J. M. NEUBERGER, R. AYERS, E. ELIAS & R. ROTHLEIN. 1992. Detection of circulating intercellular adhesion molecule-1 in chronic liver diseases. Hepatology **16:** 810–814.

44. BERGASA, N. V., W. NEWMAN, R. ROTHLEIN, E. A. JONES & D. H. ADAMS. 1993. Serum levels of soluble adhesion molecules (I-CAM-1, V-CAM1 and E-selectin) are markedly elevated in primary biliary cirrhosis (PBC) and unaffected by low oral methotrexate therapy. Gastroenterology **104**(4): A877.

45. WALDMAN, T. A. 1986. The structure, function, and expression of interleukin-2 receptors on normal and malignant lymphocytes. Science **232:** 727–732.

46. FAUCI, A. S. & D. C. DALE. 1974. The effect of in vivo hydrocortisone on subpopulations of human lymphocytes. J. Clin. Invest. **53:** 240–246.

47. HOWAT, H. T., A. J. RALSTON, H. VARLEY & A. J. WILSON. 1966. The late results of long term treatment of primary biliary cirrhosis by corticosteroids. Rev. Intern. Hepatol. **16:** 227–238.

48. WANG, K. K., A. J. CZAJA, S. J. BEAVER & V. L. W. GO. 1989. Extrahepatic malignancy following long-term immunosuppressive therapy of severe hepatitis B surface antigen–negative chronic active hepatitis. Hepatology **10:** 39–43.

49. POUPON, R. E., B. BALKAU, E. ESCHWEGE & R. POUPON. 1991. A multicenter, controlled trial of ursodiol for the treatment of primary biliary cirrhosis. UDCA-PBC Study Group. N. Engl. J. Med. **324**(22): 1548–1554.

50. HEATHCOTE, E. J. L., K. CAUCH, V. WALKER, R. J. BAILEY, L. M. BLENDIS, C. N. GHENT, G. Y. MINUK, S. C. PAPPAS, L. SCULLY, U. P. STEINBRECHER, L. SUTHERLAND, C. N. WILLIAMS, L. WOROBETZ, R. A. MILNER, I. R. WANLESS & H. WITT-SULLIVAN. 1992. The Canadian multi-centre double blind randomized controlled trial of ursodeoxycholic acid in primary biliary cirrhosis. Hepatology **16**(4): 91 A.

51. YOSHIKAWAS, M., T. TSUJII, K. MATSUMURA, J. YAMAO, Y. MATSUMURA, R. KUBO, H. FUKUI & S. ISHIZAKA. 1992. Immunomodulatory effects of ursodeoxycholic acid on immune responses. Hepatology. **16**(2): 358–364.

52. CALMUS, Y., P. GANE, P. ROUGER & R. POUPON. 1990. Hepatic expression of class I and class II major histocompatibility complex molecules in primary biliary cirrhosis: effect of ursodeoxycholic acid. Hepatology **11:** 12–15.

Mycophenolate Mofetil Can Prevent the Development of Diabetes in BB Rats[a]

LIMING HAO, SIU-MEI CHAN, AND KEVIN J. LAFFERTY[b]

The Barbara Davis Center for Childhood Diabetes
University of Colorado Health Sciences Center
4200 East 9th Avenue
Denver, Colorado 80262

INTRODUCTION

The new immunosuppressive agent mycophenolic mofetil (MM) is an enzyme inhibitor acting on the pathway of purine nucleotide synthesis.[1,2] This drug can block lymphocyte proliferation and has been reported to facilitate long-term allograft survival.[3–6] Our previous work shows that MM facilitates islet allografting and induces donor-specific tolerance in recipient animals.[3] However, MM treatment failed to prevent islet graft destruction following transplantation to spontaneously diabetic recipients.[7] In this study, we have examined the capacity of MM treatment of diabetes-prone BB rats, from an early age, to prevent the activation and expansion of autoreactive T cells and, thus, prevent the spontaneous development of diabetes.

MATERIALS AND METHODS

Animals

Bio-Breeding (BB) rats (RTI[u]) were bred at the Barbara Davis Center animal care unit from a breeding nucleus kindly provided by Drs. A. Naji and C. F. Barker of the University of Pennsylvania, Philadelphia, Pa. The incidence of diabetes in our BB colony is about 60% both in males and in females; clinical disease develops between the ages of 60 and 130 days.

MM Preparation and Administration

MM was kindly supplied by Syntex Research (Palo Alto, Calif.) and prepared as described previously.[1–3] In order to test the capacity of MM to inhibit the development of diabetes in the BB rat, animals were treated with either MM or vehicle only. The animals were dosed orally with MM, at 20 mg/kg per day. Control animals were dosed with equal amounts of vehicle alone. The blood glucose levels of all the animals were followed for up to 200 days.

Blood Glucose Determination

Blood samples (10 μl) were collected from the tail of the rats. The blood glucose concentration was read by using an ExacTech TM blood glucose meter (MediSense, Inc., Abington, United Kingdom).

[a] Supported in part by a grant from National Institutes of Health DK33470.
[b] Author to whom correspondence should be addressed.

Histological Examination

The pancreases of all BB rats were removed and fixed in formal saline for 24 hours. The tissue was then transferred to 75% alcohol. Paraffin sections were stained with hematoxylin-eosin and aldehyde fuchsin. Tissues were examined histologically to determine the degree of tissue damage and mononuclear cell infiltration.

RESULTS

MM Prevents the Development of Diabetes in BB Rats

BB rats develop diabetes that in many respects resembles human type I diabetes.[8] It has been reported that the diabetic syndrome in BB rats results from the

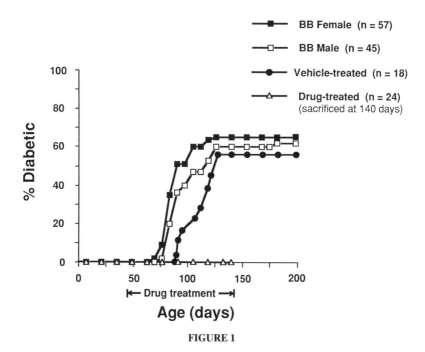

FIGURE 1

destruction of pancreatic β cells by cell-mediated immune response which is characterized by mononuclear cell infiltration of pancreatic islets.[9,10]

Data from FIGURE 1 show that the incidence of diabetes in our BB colony is approximately 60% both in males and in females. In the vehicle-treated control group, 10/18 (55%) BB rats became diabetic over the same time period as our colony. However, when 24 BB rats were treated with MM (20 mg/kg per day, from 40–140 days of age), none developed diabetes. Fourteen of the 24 animals were sacrificed for histological examination at the cessation of drug treatment (140 days). Thirteen of these animals showed no evidence of insulitis, and one had some lymphocyte infiltration in some islets. These data demonstrate that MM can prevent the development of spontaneous diabetes in BB rats as long as the treatment is maintained.

Short-Term Treatment with MM Does Not Prevent the Development of Diabetes in BB Rats

The above data show that MM can prevent the spontaneous development of diabetes in the BB rats, and the development of lymphocytic infiltration around islets during the period of drug treatment. However, this effect is dependent on the

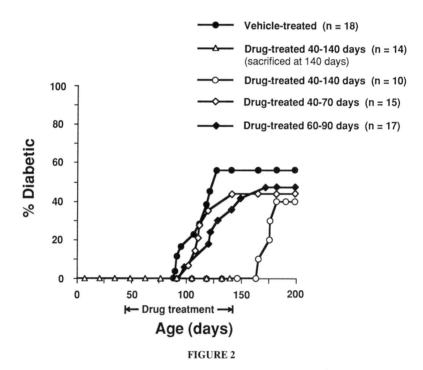

FIGURE 2

continuous presence of the drug. We next set out to determine the effect of drug treatment on the subsequent development of disease following drug withdrawal. FIGURE 2 shows results obtained when BB rats were treated with MM for 30 days at different ages (from 40–70 days of age and from 60–90 days of age, respectively). No significant difference in the development of diabetes was observed between these short-term treated groups and the vehicle control group. FIGURE 2 also demonstrated that MM can only block disease during the period of therapy. Ten animals treated with MM from 40–140 days of age were followed to 200 days of age. When drug treatment was terminated at 140 days, 4/10 (40%) of animals went on to develop diabetes at approximately 160–180 days.

DISCUSSION

Prevention of diabetes at an early age is an ideal way to control this disease and its subsequent complications. It has been reported that anti-CD4 treatment given to NOD mice and BB rats can prevent both the development of diabetes and the formation of insulitis.[11,12] Immunosuppressive agents, such as CsA, can also reduce the incidence of diabetes in BB rats when the drug is given at 60–70 days of age. However, insulitis remains present in this case,[13] which indicates that CsA may affect the effector stage of the inflammation.[14]

We have shown in this paper that brief treatment with MM (30 days) during the prediabetic phase had little effect on the development of diabetes. Continuous treatment of disease-prone BB rats with MM prevents both insulitis and diabetes. However, animals became diabetic after the withdrawal of the drug treatment. These data suggest that MM is affecting the early stage of the disease development, presumably the expansion of lymphocytes responsible for the destruction of islet β cells. Interestingly, MM can induce a specific immune tolerance to alloantigens when adult animals are transplanted with allograft.[3] However, when MM is given at the early age of the spontaneous diabetic animals, at the time when lymphocytes responsible for the destruction of islet β cells are thought to be activated, no specific tolerance to the autoantigens developed. This phenomenon may indicate that the mechanism of T cell activation and the function of the activated T cells may differ between autoimmune diabetes and the development of islet allograft rejection.

ACKNOWLEDGMENTS

The authors thank Drs. Anthony Allison and Elsie Eugui at Syntex Research for providing the agent. The authors also thank Anthony Valentine for his technical assistance.

REFERENCES

1. EUGUI, E. M., A. M. MIRKOVICH & A. C. ALLISON. 1991. Lymphocyte-selective anti-proliferative and immunosuppressive effects of mycophenolic acid in mice. Scand. J. Immunol. **33:** 161.
2. EUGUI, E. M., S. J. ALMQUIST, C. D. MULLER, et al. 1991. Lymphocyte-selective sytostatic and immunosuppressive effects of mycophenolic acid in vitro: role of deoxyguanosine nucleotide depletion. Scand. J. Immunol. **33:** 175.
3. HAO, L., F. CALCINARO, R. G. GILL, et al. 1992. Facilitation of specific tolerance induction in adult mice by RS-61443. Transplantation **53:** 590–595.
4. MORRIS, R. E., E. C. HOYT, M. P. MURPHY, et al. 1990. Mycophenolic acid morpholinoeth-ylester (RS-61443) is a new immunosuppressant that prevents and halts heart allograft rejection by selective inhibition of T and B cell purine synthesis. Transplant. Proc. **22:** 1659.
5. MORRIS, R. E., J. WANG, J. R. BLUM, et al. 1991. Immunosuppressive effect of morpho-linoethyl ester of mycophenolic acid (RS-61443) in rats and nonhuman primate recipients of heart allografts. Transpl. Proc. **23:** 14.
6. PLATZ, K. P., H. W. SOLLINGER, D. A. HULLETT, et al. 1991. RS-61443—a new potent immunosuppressive agent. Transplantation **51:** 27.
7. HAO, L., Y. WANG, S. M. CHAN & K. J. LAFFERTY. 1992. Effect of mycophenolate mofetil on islet allografting to chemically induced or spontaneously diabetic animals. Transplant. Proc. **24:** 2843.

8. MARLISS, E. B., A. F. NAKHOODA, P. POUSSIER, *et al.* 1982. The diabetic syndrome of the "bb" Wistar rat: possible relevance to type I (insulin dependent) diabetes in man. Diabetologia **22:** 225.

9. LOGOTHETOPOULOS, J., N. VALIQUETTE, E. MADURA, *et al.* 1984. The onset and progression of pancreatic insulitis in the overt, spontaneously diabetic, young adult BB rat studied by pancreatic biopsy. Diabetes **33:** 33.

10. WANG, Y., O. PONTESILLI, R. G. GILL, *et al.* 1991. The role of CD4+ and CD8+ T cells in the destruction of islet grafts by spontaneously diabetic mice. Proc. Natl. Acad. Sci. USA **88:** 527.

11. SHIZURU, J., E. C. TAYLOR, B. A. BANKS, *et al.* 1988. Immunotherapy of nonobese diabetic mouse: treatment with an antibody to T helper lymphocytes. Science **240:** 659.

12. LIKE, A. A., C. A. BIRON, E. J. WERINGER, *et al.* 1986. Prevention of diabetes in Biobreeding/Worcester rats with monoclonal antibodies that recognize T lymphocytes or natural killer cells. J. Exp. Med. **164:** 1145.

13. LIKE, A. A., V. DIRODI, S. THOMAS, *et al.* 1984. Prevention of diabetes mellitus in the BB/W rat with cyclosporin-A. AJP **117:** 92.

14. WANG, Y., M. McDUFFIE, I. N. NOMIKOS, *et al.* 1988. Effect of cyclosporine on immunologically mediated diabetes in nonobese diabetic mice. Transplantation **46:** 101s.

The Use of Nicotinamide in the Prevention of Type 1 Diabetes

R. B. ELLIOTT, C. C. PILCHER, A. STEWART,[a]
D. FERGUSSON,[b] AND M. A. McGREGOR

Department of Pediatrics
School of Medicine
University of Auckland
Private Bag 92019
Auckland, New Zealand

[a]*Biostatistics Unit*
Department of Community Health
School of Medicine
Auckland, New Zealand

[b]*Department of Psychological Medicine*
School of Medicine
University of Otago
Christchurch, New Zealand

INTRODUCTION

Type 1 diabetes is characterized by the slow destruction of the β cells of the islets of Langerhans, which is accompanied by an intra islet chronic inflammatory process. The cellular component of this process involves the whole congeries of chronic inflammatory immune cells, and is signaled by the appearance of antibodies to a variety of β cell components. Some of these antibodies may appear by the age of 2 years,[1] and exist for many decades before eventual severe β cell depletion and clinical symptoms of the disease.[2] Thus, there is a time window for therapeutic intervention to prevent the disease, commencing with the first appearance of these antibodies.

The chronic inflammatory islet process is distinguishable from other autoimmune diseases only in the specificity of the target tissue—and even this is not monospecific, as the islet disease may be accompanied by multiple organ inflammations (e.g., thyroid, gastric mucosa, adrenals).

The practical possibilities for designing therapeutic interventions in humans are limited by our current knowledge (TABLE 1) and by safety. While in rodent models of Type 1 diabetes (BB rat, NOD mouse), a large number of interventions have been shown to prevent the subsequent onset of diabetes, many of these are unsafe in humans, e.g., intraperitoneal silica, immunosuppression.

The humoral antibody predictors of the disease in humans are not foolproof. The addition of a metabolic marker of β cell disease (first phase insulin release) is only predictive very close to the clinical onset of diabetes.[3] The ideal intervention in humans is therefore the one with the maximum safety, as inevitably some subjects may be treated unnecessarily if very early intervention is attempted. Accordingly we have selected nicotinamide as a possible preventive agent. It has been shown to prevent diabetes in the NOD mouse[4] (but not the BB rat) and to exhibit β cell cytoprotective effects in the presence of cytolytic macrophages[5] or β cytolytic concentrations of NO·[6] or IL1β.[7,8] The available information on acute toxicity of nicotinamide is reassuring, and it has been used in large doses for long periods for other diseases without apparent long-term ill effects.

IN VIVO EXPERIMENTAL EVIDENCE THAT NICOTINAMIDE MAY PREVENT TYPE 1 DIABETES

The NOD Mouse

The spontaneously diabetic insulin-dependent albino mouse (NOD) provides a reasonable model of the human disease. In our colony, 30–40% of females develop diabetes between 115 and 250 days. There is evidence of macrophage and lympho-cytic infiltration in and just outside the islets. Islet and insulin autoantibodies appear from about day 40, and eventual major β cell loss occurs.

TABLE 1. Possibilities for Therapeutic Intervention in the Islet Inflammatory Process

Component	Proposed Mechanisms	Intervention
1. Etiopathogenesis	Genetic + unknown environmental	? Diet ? Viral vaccine ? Peptide vaccination
2. Initiating macrophage invasion	Release of cytokines release of NO· or other radicals	Anticytokine therapy, NO·, or other radical scavengers or inhibitors, antimacrophage agents[a]
3. T cell invasion	Release of cytokines ? Release of NO· or other radicals	Anticytokine therapy, NO· or other radical scavengers or inhibitors, anti CD4 CD8 therapy[a]

[a]This may be specific (e.g., monoclonal antibodies) or nonspecific (e.g., immunosuppression).

Effects of Nicotinamide on Diabetes Incidence in the NOD Mouse

Litters are separated at 20 days, and only the females studied for the evolution of diabetes, in groups of 19–24. Animals were fed nicotinamide (1% w/w in chow or 1% w/v in their drinking water from weaning).

The protective effect of both is shown in FIGURE 1. The major protective effect is apparent up to 250 days, but wanes somewhat in older animals. A smaller dose (0.1%) is not effective, and giving the nicotinamide after 60 days is ineffective, i.e., there is a critical dose and a critical time of introduction to produce protection. Nicotinamide reduces the degree of islet inflammation (TABLE 2).

First-Degree Relatives of Insulin-Dependent Diabetics

First-degree relatives (3,600) of all ages were screened for islet cell antibodies by a sensitive indirect immunofluorescent technique,[9] with 5.6% showing islet cell antibodies ≥ 10 international units. Glycated hemoglobin (GHb) and first phase

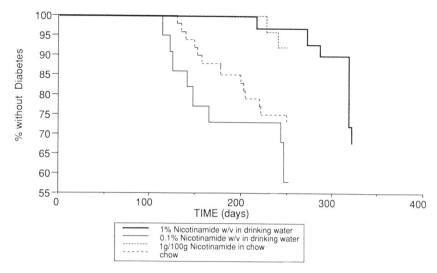

FIGURE 1. Comparison of diabetes rates in NOD mice given nicotinamide.

insulin release (FPIR − 1' + 3' levels, conducted according to an internationally accepted protocol)[10] were measured in the antibody "positive" group.

We selected from these antibody-positive relatives groups with criteria used in other studies of the natural history of the disease.

a. Age < 16 years, ICA ≥ 80 units, FPIR < 67 mmol/l,[10] and normal initial GHb. These were the criteria used by Chase *et al.*[11] in a natural history study.

b. Age < 10 years, ICA ≥ 10 units, with no overt evidence of diabetes initially. These were the criteria used by Riley *et al.*[12]

c. All ages, ICA ≥ 20 units, with no evidence of overt diabetes. These were the criteria used in a combined study from the Barts-Windsor-Oxford[13] Gainesville[12] groups. We only treated these individuals with nicotinamide when their FPIR fell below 80 mmol/l initially or subsequently.

TABLE 2. Insulitis in Female NOD Mice Given 1% W/V Nicotinamide in Drinking Water from Weaning (Day 20)

	No. Mice	Prevalence of Insulitis	Insulitis Score	Number with Intense Insulitis +ICA[a] + IAA[b]
Day 40				
Nicotinamide	22	24%	2.9 ± 1.4	1
Control	21	57%	9.6 ± 2.6	4
Day 250				
Nicotinamide	14	86%	21.3 ± 6.4	1
Control	14	100%	60.9 ± 8.5	4

[a]Islet cell antibodies.
[b]Insulin autoantibodies.

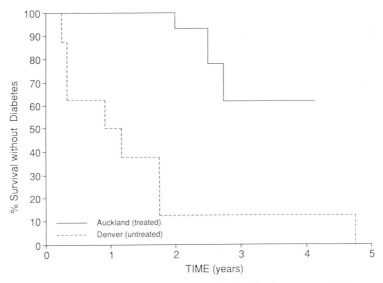

FIGURE 2. Effect of nicotinamide on diabetes rates in Auckland vs. untreated Denver cases. Criteria: ICA ≥ 80 units; age < 16 years; FPIR < 67; initial glycated Hb normal.

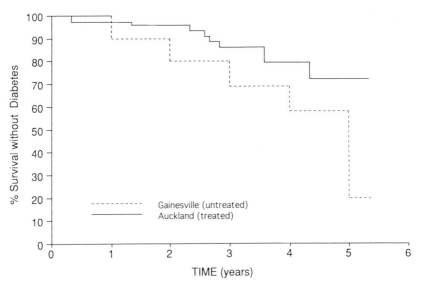

FIGURE 3. Effect of nicotinamide on diabetes rates in Auckland vs. untreated Gainesville cases. Criteria: ICA ≥ 10 units; age < 10 years.

The results of these comparisons are shown in FIGURES 2, 3, and 4. In each instance the diabetes incidence is less in the treated groups than in the historical international controls—by at least 50%. Nevertheless, many biases may have contributed to these comparisons, although there is remarkable agreement in the historical control results between the three centers (Denver, Gainesville, Barts) when age and level of ICA are taken into consideration.

Diabetes Unrelated 5–7 Year Old School Children

In this study, 33,658 children aged 5.0–7.9 years and resident in Auckland were randomly selected (by school) from a total population of 81,993 who were of that age

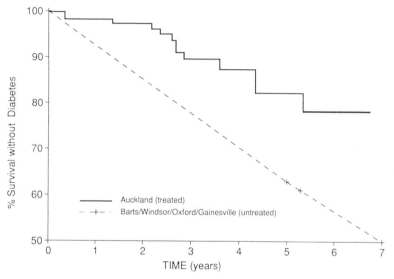

FIGURE 4. Effect of nicotinamide on diabetes rates in Auckland vs. untreated Barts/Windsor/ Oxford/Gainesville cases. Criteria: ICA ≥ 20 units; any age.

in a three-year sampling frame 1988–91. Those with ICA ≥ 20 units and those with ICA = 10 units + FPIR < 100 mmol/l and who further consented, were treated with nicotinamide. Treatment continued until either ICA disappeared or diabetes developed. Of this 33,658, a total of 20,195 consented to testing for ICA over the three-year period. The subject years exposure to diabetes risk was calculated for the three groups—in the (random) control group, the 20,195 consenting children and the 13,463 who were approached for testing and declined. The incidence of diabetes in the three groups has been studied in the 1.7–4.7 years of follow-up to date (TABLE 3).

These results demonstrate a high degree of protection from diabetes in the tested/intended to treat group ($8.1/10^5$ per yr) compared with the untested controls ($20.1/10^5$ per yr). This cannot be attributed to a bias introduced by consent to testing. The 4 tested children who have developed diabetes to date in the tested group, all

TABLE 3. Population Prevention Strategy

	Number	Exposure Years	No. Diabetics	Rate (10^5/yr)	Mean Age (yr)
Controls	48,335	322,000	48	20.1[a]	9.6
Accepted Testing	20,195	49,000	4	8.1[a]	8.9
"Refused" Testing	13,463	33,000	5	15.1	9.0

[a]Difference (proportional hazards estimate) $p = 0.03$.

had some unusual features (TABLE 4). Considering the efficacy of nicotinamide treatment alone (i.e., eliminating case 2 from both the observed and expected numbers of diabetics), the protection afforded is about 70% to date.

DISCUSSION

In humans, a protective effect of nicotinamide similar to that found in the NOD mouse is apparent, although of a lesser degree. This lesser effect is not surprising given the variable age at which nicotinamide was given, compared with that in the mouse experiments and the lesser dose/kg used in humans. We do not know as yet whether the protective effect wanes with advancing age, as in the NOD mouse. Nicotinamide given to children recently diagnosed as diabetic is without effect.[14]

The vitamin amide protects β cells against the cytolytic activity of streptozotocin *in vivo,* and is thought to do so by the rapid increase in intracellular levels of NAD following administration.[15] It is agreed that these high levels of NAD arise from inhibition of one of the pathways of metabolism of NAD—poly adenyl ribose polymerase (PARP).[16] *De novo* synthesis of NAD from nicotinamide is thought to be less important at high concentrations of nicotinamide. There is some evidence of very rapid incorporation of an analogue, 6 amino nicotinamide, into the corresponding 6 amino NAD, at very low concentrations (see FIGURE 5). It is thus probable that nicotinamide may contribute to the intracellular pool of NAD via either mechanism, depending on the dose given and whether the DNA repair enzyme has been markedly induced by DNA fragmentation.

In *in vitro* experiments, interleukin 1β can cause impairment of β cell function or β cell death,[7] and this can be prevented by exposure of the cells to nicotinamide in concentrations of ≥ 10 mmolar (see TABLE 5). Syngeneic activated macrophages added to rat islets in culture can kill β cells, but similar additions to other cell lines do not result in cell death.[5] Such macrophages produce cytokines capable of killing β cells, but specific antisera to these cytokines do not inhibit the cell killing. Nicotinamide can prevent this β cell toxic effect of the macrophages, and it is thought that it may do so by inhibiting the action of cytokine generated NO· radicals in β cells or the macrophages themselves.[6] 3-Amino benzamide is somewhat less effective in these *in*

TABLE 4. Possible Modifying Circumstances in the Four Failures of the Preventive Strategy

Case 1.	Impaired glucose tolerance before treatment started.
Case 2.	No islet cell antibodies on screening or at time of diagnosis, i.e., never treated.
Case 3.	Not compliant with treatment.
Case 4.	Accompanying persistent IgA deficiency.

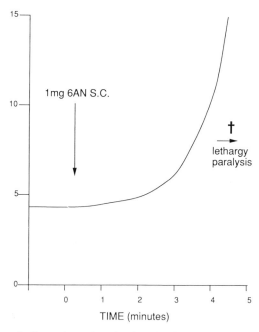

FIGURE 5. Temporal effects of 6-amino nicotinamide (6AN) on blood glucose 6 AN → 6A NAD (inhibition of glycolysis) in Swiss mice.

vitro systems, although an equally effective PARP inhibitor.[6] It is not an NAD precursor.

Nicotinamide is an O· radical scavenger, and may also inhibit free radical (e.g., NO·, O·, HCLO·) generation. The susceptibility of the β cell to such toxic agents may relate to its curiously ineffectual free radical scavenging systems.

Most of the proposed mechanisms of action of nicotinamide require levels of ≥ 10 mmolar *in vitro*. *In vivo* doses of about 500 mg/kg per day (i.e., 1–3 mmolar at most if distributed uniformly in body water) are effective in rodents in both preventing diabetes caused by the β cell toxin streptozotocin, or in the spontaneous diabetes of the NOD mouse. Protective effects in humans seem to be attained with

TABLE 5. Effect of Nicotinamide on Interleukin 1β Inhibition of Glucose-Stimulated Insulin Release from Islets In Vitro[a]

	Basal	Glucose Stimulated
Control	183 ± 32	2037 ± 363
IL-1β (10 U-ml)	191 ± 28	1025 ± 126
IL-1β (50 U-ml)	176 ± 39	185 ± 41
IL-1β (10) + Nic (10 mM)	179 ± 33	1993 ± 284[b]
IL-1β (50) + Nic (10 mM)	187 ± 37	1007 ± 123[b]

[a]Data from Reference 8.
[b]$p < 0.001$ with respect to the group treated with IL-1β alone.

serum levels of nicotinamide an order less. It is thus possible that mechanisms other than PARP inhibition may account for part of the *in vivo* protective effect, or this may reflect the difficulty of translating from cell biology experiments on rodent cells to the human *in vivo*.

SAFETY

Nicotinamide has a reassuring toxicity record in doses of less than 3 g/day in adults. No liver enzyme changes are seen in children with doses of 1.2 g/m^2/day of a slow-release preparation.

Doses of 10 g/day in humans cause acute heptocellular changes, which disappear after treatment is stopped.

Chronic adverse effects have been postulated but not observed in humans. Nicotinamide given to rats concurrently with streptozotocin—a known carcinogen—induces β cell adenomas,[17] but nicotinamide alone given long term to rats does not cause cancer. DNA repair is significantly delayed by tissue levels of ≥ 10 mmolar nicotinamide, and this may increase susceptibility to mutagenesis. Maximum plasma levels of nicotinamide attained with 2 g of slow release nicotinamide given to adult humans is < 1 mmol/l, and thus doses in excess of 10 g/dose would be needed to cause significant PARP inhibition—a dose that causes acute jaundice.

Nicotinamide given in food to rats (1% w.w.) causes poor weight gain associated with reduced food intake; 1% in drinking water does not cause either of these effects in mice. Sixty-four of the 5–7 year old school children enrolled in the study described above, given 1 g/day of a slow release formulation and confirmed as compliant, showed no significant change in their weight or height standard deviation score over two years. Nicotinamide, unlike nicotinic acid, does not appear to cause insulin resistance. Its effects on the developing fetus are unknown.

SUMMARY

Nicotinamide can protect the NOD mouse from diabetes if given early enough and in sufficient dose. The effect partly wanes with time. There is reduced islet inflammation. Similar protective effects can be demonstrated in quasi-experimental interventions in humans—both diabetes related and unrelated deemed at risk of developing diabetes by reason of having islet cell antibodies.

Nicotinamide protects isolated islets *in vitro* from the toxicity of a number of agents, but only in doses that produce significant PARP inhibition, and increased intracellular levels of NAD.

It is unlikely that the protective effect demonstrated in humans is due to significant PARP inhibition, as the levels of nicotinamide achieved with the doses used are too low. Other effects of the vitamin are more likely, e.g., increase in NAD pool size by *de novo* synthesis, or inhibition of free radical generation.

The drug appears to be safe in the doses employed in humans.

REFERENCES

1.   PILCHER, C. C., K. DICKENS & R. B. ELLIOTT. 1991. ICA only develop in early childhood. Proceedings 11th International Immunology and Diabetes Workshop. Diabetes Res. Clin. Pract. **14:** S82.

2. GORSUCH, A. N., J. LISTER, B. M. DEAN, *et al.* 1981. Evidence for a long prediabetic period in type 1 (insulin dependent) diabetes mellitus. Lancet **2:** 1363–1365.
3. CHASE, H. P., M. A. VOSS, N. BUTLER-SIMON, S. HOOPS, D. O'BRIEN & M. J. DOBERSEN. 1987. Diagnosis of pre-type 1 diabetes. J. Pediatr. **111:** 807–812.
4. YAMADA, K., K. NONAKA, T. HANAFUSA, A. MIYAZAKI, H. TOYOSHIMA & S. TARUI. 1982. Preventive and therapeutic effects of large-dose nicotinamide injections on diabetes associated with insulitis. Diabetes **31:** 749–753.
5. KRÖNCKE, K-D., J. FUNDA, B. BERSCHICK, H. KOLB & V. KOLB-BACHOFEN. 1991. Macrophage cytotoxicity towards isolated rat islet cells: neither lysis nor its protection by nicotinamide are beta-cell specific. Diabetologia **34:** 232–238.
6. KALLMAN, B., V. BURKART, K-D. KRÖNCKE, V. KOLB BACHOFEN & H. KOLB. 1992. Toxicity of chemically generated nitric oxide towards pancreatic islet cells can be prevented by nicotinamide. Life Sci. **51:** 671–678.
7. MANDRUP-POULSEN, T., K. BENDTZEN, J. NERUP, C. A. DINARELLO, M. SVENSON & J. H. NIELSON. 1986. Affinity-purified human interleukin 1 is cytotoxic to isolated islets of Langerhans. Diabetologia **29:** 63–67.
8. BUSCEMA, M., C. VINCI, C. GATTA, M. A. RABUAZZO, R. VIGNEN & F. PURRELLO. 1992. Nicotinamide partially reverses the interleukin-1β inhibition of glucose-induced insulin release in pancreatic islets. Metabolism **41:** 296–300.
9. PILCHER, C. C. & R. B. ELLIOTT. 1990. A sensitive and reproducible method for the assay of human islet cell antibodies. J. Immunol. Methods **129:** 111–117.
10. SMITH, C. P., A. J. K. WILLIAMS, J. M. THOMAS, R. ARCHIBALD, V. D. ALGAR, G. F. BOTTAZZO, E. A. M. GALE & M. O. SAVAGE. 1988. The pattern of basal and stimulated insulin responses to intravenous glucose in first degree relatives of type 1 (insulin dependent) diabetic children and unrelated adults aged 5–50 years. Diabetologia **31:** 430–434.
11. ELLIOTT, R. B. & H. P. CHASE. 1991. Prevention or delay of type 1 (insulin dependent) diabetes mellitus in children using nicotinamide. Diabetologia **34:** 362–365.
12. RILEY, W. J., N. K. MACLAREN, J. KRISCHER, *et al.* 1990. A prospective study of the development of diabetes in relatives of patients with insulin-dependent diabetes. N. Engl. J. Med. **323:** 1167–1172.
13. BONIFACIO, E., P. J. BINGLEY, M. SHATTOCK, B. M. DEAN, D. DUNGER, E. A. M. GALE & G. F. BOTTAZZO. 1990. Quantification of islet cell antibodies and prediction of insulin-dependent diabetes. Lancet **335:** 147–149.
14. CHASE, H. P., N. BUTLER-SIMON, S. GARG, M. MCDUFFIE, S. L. HOOPS & D. O'BRIEN. 1990. A trial of nicotinamide in newly diagnosed patients with type 1 (insulin-dependent) diabetes mellitus. Diabetologia **33:** 444–446.
15. LEDOUX, S. P., C. R. HALL, P. M. FORBES, N. J. PATTON & G. L. WILSON. 1988. Mechanisms of nicotinamide and thymidine protection from alloxan and streptozocin toxicity. Diabetes **37:** 1015–1019.
16. OKAMOTO, H., H. YAMAMO, S. TAKASAWA, C. INQUE, K. TERAZONO, K. SHIGA & M. KITAGAWA. 1988. Molecular mechanism of degeneration, oncogenesis and regeneration of pancreatic B-cells of islets of Langerhans. *In* Frontiers in Diabetes Research. Lessons from animal diabetes II. E. Shafrir & A. E. Renold, Eds.: 149–157. John Libby and Co. London, England.
17. YAMAGAMI, T., A. MIWA, S. TAKASAWA, H. YAMAMOTO & H. OKOMOTO. 1985. Induction of rat pancreatic beta-cell tumors by the combined administration of streptozotocin or alloxan and poly (adenosine diphosphate ribose) synthetase inhibitors. Cancer Res. **45:** 1845–1849.

Early Diagnosis and Specific Treatment of Insulin-Dependent Diabetes[a]

NOEL MACLAREN,[b] ANDREW MUIR,
JANET SILVERSTEIN, YAO-HUA SONG,
JIN XIONG SHE, JEFFREY KRISCHER, MARK ATKINSON,
AND DESMOND SCHATZ

Departments of Pathology and Laboratory Medicine, and Pediatrics
University of Florida College of Medicine
Gainesville, Florida 32610

THE PROBLEM WITH INSULIN-DEPENDENT DIABETES

Insulin-dependent diabetes (IDD) remains a serious, incurable autoimmune disease[1,2] in which a number of characteristic complications are seen increasingly with time following diagnosis. Blindness, renal failure, heart disease, peripheral vascular disease, stroke, and peripheral and sympathetic neuropathies are some of the common outcomes. The therapeutic problem of IDD is that there is no practical way of delivering replacement doses of insulin that closely mimic normal endogenous secretion. As a result of giving relatively large, intermittent boluses of insulin into the subcutaneous tissues—the currently available means of delivery—excessive glycemic excursions follow food intake, exercise, fasting, sleep, and a variety of stresses. Prolonged hyperglycemia leads to nonenzymatic glycosylation of a variety of bodily proteins and to the formation of advanced glycosylation end products. These include families of glucose-derived imidazole and pyrrole based, cross-linked, extracellular proteins.[3] Basement membranes of blood vessels so affected thicken, they lose their charge and become porous to macromolecules, with resultant microvascular diseases including those of the retinae and kidneys. Once established, these lesions become irreversible irrespective of subsequent improvements in glycemic control.[4–8] Clearly, a better clinical approach to IDD is needed. Indeed, one might argue that investigative diabetologists should feel obligated to try to find solutions to this problem for their patients. Their goals should include the amelioration of the pathogenic processes and the delay of the progression to complete insulin dependence. The following addresses progress in the prediction of IDD, as well as intervention strategies that should be closely related to the stage of the natural history of pathogenic events.

NATURAL HISTORY OF IDD

As shown in FIGURE 1, an individual destined to develop IDD has a number of inherited susceptibilities. The disease is polygenic and incompletely penetrant. One

[a]The findings reported here were supported by grants RO1 HD19469 and POI DK 39079 from National Institutes of Health, and 1921523 from the Juvenile Diabetes Foundation.

[b]Address correspondence to: Department of Pathology and Laboratory Medicine, Box 100275, J. Hillis Miller Health Center, University of Florida College of Medicine, Gainesville, Florida 32610.

third of identical twins affected by IDD become concordant for the disease, as do some 6% of nonidentical siblings. The risk of IDD in HLA identical siblings of affected probands rises to 1 in 7 but is as high as 1 in 4 when siblings share HLA haplotypes that contain both DR3 and DR4 alleles. Among caucasians without close relatives affected by IDD, the HLA-DQ alleles which have arginine at residue 52 of their alpha chains and a non–aspartic acid residue at position 57 of their beta chains encode the greatest risk.[9–11] Another gene has been located near the insulin and IGF-2 genes on chromosome 11,[12,13] and more are likely to be identified soon.[14]

At present, it remains unclear whether the beta cell mass of the person at genetic risk is normal or not. In any event, it is believed that the pathogenic sequence of

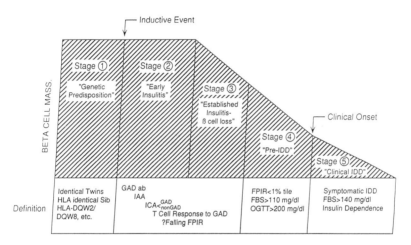

FIGURE 1. The proposed pathogenic stages of IDD. Putative preventive treatments of IDD will have variable effectiveness for patients at different stages of the disease. Those that have a genetic predisposition, but no active autoimmunity, are at stage 1. After an as yet unknown disease-inducing event, autoimmunity to islet cell antigens (GAD$_{65}$, IAA, ICA) begins and early insulitis appears (stage 2). As the inflammatory lesion progresses, β-cell toxicity leads to clinically undetectable decreases in islet function (stage 3). As clinical IDD becomes more imminent, diminished insulin responses to secretagogues and mild elevations of fasting blood glucose occur (stage 4). When most of the β-cell mass has been destroyed, overt IDD is diagnosed (stage 5). GAD, glutamic acid decarboxylase; IAA, insulin autoantibody; ICA, islet cell autoantibody; FPIR, first-phase insulin release; FBS, fasting blood sugar; OGTT, oral glucose tolerance test.

events must be induced by a chance environmental encounter.[1,2] Strong candidates for induction are immunizations against infectious agents such as viruses or food antigens that have molecular homologies with islet autoantigens. Putative examples are the P-2 protein of Coxsackie B viruses and glutamic acid decarboxylase (GAD),[15] or bovine serum albumin and an islet cell protein of 69 kDa.[16]

The process once induced can be marked by the appearance of antiislet autoantibodies in the peripheral blood. Previous studies have indicated that autoantibodies to insulin or to an islet cell protein of 64 kDa appear first.[17] The 64 kDa antigen, reported to be the lower molecular isoform of GAD (GAD$_{65}$),[18] has had its gene cloned and expressed in a variety of recombinant expression vectors.[15] Another autoantibody that may occur relatively early is that against an islet cell protein of 38 kDa.[19,20] Since these autoantibodies immunoprecipitate labeled islet cell proteins in their native configurations, they are likely to recognize conformational epitopes. The 2 antigens (38 kDa and GAD_{65}) can also induce the proliferative responses of peripheral blood T cells as presented by autologous macrophages.[19,20]

As beta cells become damaged by the autoimmune process, additional antibodies to many islet cell autoantigens arise (TABLE 1). Those of greatest clinical importance

TABLE 1. Islet Cell Autoantigens of Insulin-Dependent Diabetes[a]

Autoantigen	Characteristics
Sialoglycolipid	Target of ICA in humans, GM2-1, non–beta cell specific
Glutamate decarboxylase	Target of 64KA/GADAb in humans and animal models of IDD, two forms (GAD 65 and 67), cellular immune antigen, synaptic-like microvesicle protein, disease modifying antigen
Insulin	Target of IAA in humans and NOD mice, cellular immune antigen, disease modifying antigen
Insulin receptor	Target of autoantibodies in humans, determined by bioassay
38 kDa	Target of 38KA in humans, induced by cytomegalo virus, localized to insulin secretory granules, cellular immune antigen, multiple antigens of this M_r?
Bovine serum albumin	Target of BSA Ab, antigen in humans and animal models of IDD, contains ABBOS peptide, has molecular mimic in beta cell p69 protein (PM-1), disease modifying antigen
Glucose transporter	Target of autoantibodies in humans, inhibits glucose stimulation, Glut-2 directed?
Heat shock protein 65	Target of autoantibodies and cellular immunity in NOD mice, disease modifying antigen, contains p277 peptide
Carboxypeptidase H	Target of autoantibodies in humans, identified by immunoscreening of islet cDNA, insulin secretory granule protein
52 kDa	Target of autoantibodies in humans and NOD mice, molecular mimic with Rubella virus
ICA12/ICA512	Target of autoantibodies in humans, identified by immunoscreening of islet cDNA, 512 homology to CD45
150 kDa	Target of autoantibodies in humans, beta cell specific, membrane associated
RIN polar	Target of autoantibodies in humans and NOD mice, present on insulinoma cells

[a]The effect of daily prophylactic NPH insulin replacement therapy in NOD mice from 4 weeks to 180 days. The histology score represents only nondiabetic animals and was coded as fractions up to a maximum of 3.[26]

are islet cell autoantibodies (ICA) detectable through indirect immunofluorescence of cryosectioned pancreas. Some, but not all, ICA are attributable to antiislet GAD reactivity.[21] In association with the appearance of these markers of the autoimmunological process underlying IDD, there is a progressive loss of beta cells. This is reflected initially by a loss of the first phase of plasma insulin responses (FPIR) to a 0.5 g dose of intravenous glucose (IVGTT). Eventually, the FPIR falls below the first percentile of normal controls. At this point in the process, the risk of IDD within the next 5 years exceeds at least 50%. Later still, the ability of the beta cell to respond to other secretogogues such as arginine or tolbutamide also become impaired, followed by the appearance of hyperglycemia to oral glucose (glucose intolerance) or food.[22] At this point, proximity of the onset of symptomatic diabetes can be variable dependent upon the patient's age. After diagnosis of symptomatic IDD and initiation of replacement therapy, some recovery of insulin secretory capacity for a few months is common. This may result from beta cell rest induced by the exogenous insulin. In this quiescent state, the functions of surviving beta cells may recover, and the expression of autoimmunizing beta cell autoantigens may be reduced.

PREDICTABILITY OF INSULIN-DEPENDENT DIABETES

It follows from the foregoing that IDD is relatively predictable through the detection of autoimmune markers of the disease among high-risk relatives coupled with specific tests of beta cell functions. The risk is best expressed through the device of life table analyses.[23] We and at least one other group have been able to show that ICA are associated with an increased risk of IDD dependent upon their titer.[24,25] End point titers of ICA are expressed in Juvenile Diabetes Foundation units through comparison with an international standard accepted by the Immunology of Diabetes Workshops. The higher the titer, the greater the risk for future disease. Insulin autoantibodies (IAA) are clinically reliable only when detected by radioimmunoassay. When found by themselves, they weakly predict IDD. IAA however are highly associated with ICA, and when these autoantibodies occur together, the risks of IDD are more than additive.[23,26] Using data developed by us, the risk of IDD over 5 years approximates 10% for IAA alone, 25% for ICA alone, 50% for IAA plus ICA, and as much as 65% for high titered ICA plus impaired FPIR to IVGTT. These risks appear to be greater for young infants and children than for older adults with identical laboratory findings.

These data are sufficiently robust to provide the basis for intervention trials. It needs to be emphasized that most patients who develop IDD know of no similarly affected close relative. Thus it will be important to document the ability to predict IDD in the general population through antibody screening tests. Although not yet confirmed by others, we have found that age-matched, normal school children can be predicted to progress to IDD on the basis of ICA screening just as well as relatives can (FIGURE 2). These preliminary results need to become firm before interventions can be proposed in prediabetic persons ascertained from ICA/IAA screening of the normal population.

INTERVENTION STRATEGIES TO PREVENT DIABETES

By the time of clinical diagnosis, the majority of the beta cells have already been destroyed.[27] Thus, considerable recovery of function at this stage of the disease would not be expected. General immunosuppression through the use of cyclosporin or Imuran, however, does promote preservation of C-peptide secretion which unfortunately does not persist indefinitely, despite continued immunosuppression.[28] Our own studies have been with Imuran, a purine antagonist with a spectrum of immunosuppression that is relatively restricted to NK and Ts cells. A short course of glucocorticoids was given initially to all patients. Therapeutic benefits were confined to those with a lymphopenic response to the drug. By the end of the first year, 15% of controls versus 50% of the Imuran-treated patients were judged to be in remission as based upon a near normal hemoglobin A1c and peak C-peptide responses to

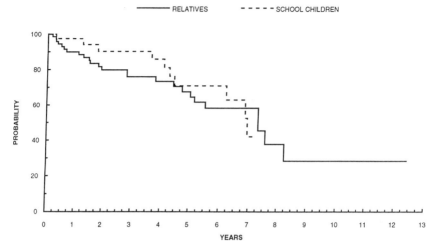

FIGURE 2. Kaplan-Meier life table estimates the chance of remaining IDD free for unaffected first-degree relatives and U.S. school children ages 5–17 years with islet autoantibodies (ICA) of 10 or more JDFu. The probability of developing IDD is not statistically significantly different ($p = 0.7$) between the two groups.

Sustacal challenge of over 0.5 pmol/L.[29] As shown in FIGURE 3, the benefits were more apparent in those patients that had the best initial plasma C-peptide responses to oral Sustacal.

Just as the institution of insulin replacement therapy often promotes a "honeymoon" remission, so has intensive insulin replacement through the first year or so after diagnosis enhanced the patient's capacity to secrete insulin.[30] In the stage

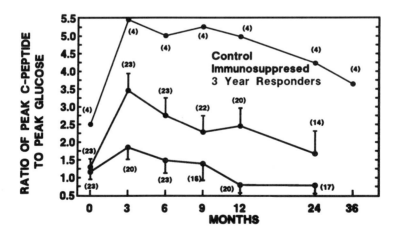

FIGURE 3. The figure shows that those 4 of 14 newly diagnosed patients treated by long term azathioprine, who responded best after 2 years of treatment, were the same ones that had least metabolic impairment at diagnosis as determined by the peak plasma C-peptide to blood glucose ratio following a standard oral Sustacal (7 ml/kg) challenge.

of the disease just prior to diagnosis, we have had apparent success with Imuran in several patients. Such benefits, however, in the long term need to be balanced against the potential risks of viral-associated neoplasias such as B cell lymphoma.

There is current interest in the possibility that superoxides or nitric oxide, generated within the islet inflammatory lesion (insulitis), may damage beta cells as part of the pathogenic process leading to IDD. Accordingly, there may be potential for the use of antioxidant drugs such as probucol or the poly-ADP ribose polymerase inhibitor nicotinamide to protect the beta cell from the damage that results from depletion of intracellular NAD during the DNA repair that follows oxidant DNA induced damage. Further, inducible nitric oxide can be inhibited in rodents by aminoguanidine, and while this drug needs to be assessed for its possible value to prevent diabetes, it should be noted that the inducible form of nitric oxide synthase has not yet been clearly identified in humans.

In our own studies in NOD mice, daily subcutaneous injections of NPH insulin dramatically reduced both the frequency of diabetes and the severity of insulitis (TABLE 2).[31] The effect may be due to (1) induced beta cell rest, as discussed earlier, (2) a direct stimulatory effect of insulin on T lymphocytes enabling tolerance to be restored, or (3) insulin immunization which in some way could inhibit the autoimmune attack on beta cells. Based upon these NOD studies, we have begun a study of high-risk relatives who have ICA of 20 JDF units or greater as well as loss of FPIR to

TABLE 2. Effects of Prophylactic Insulin Therapy in NOD Mice

	Diabetes	Insulitis
Insulin	3/34 (9%)[a]	0.5 ± 0.7[b]
Placebo	17/26 (65%)	2.7 ± 0.8

[a] $p < 0.0001$.
[b] $p < 0.001$.

iv glucose. Twice daily insulin prophylactic therapy will be given in an open, randomized trial. Based upon our findings that the risk of IDD in such relatives approximates 60% over 5 years, we estimate that we will need approximately 110 patients to demonstrate a fall to 40% in the diabetes rate (80% power; $p < 0.5$ one-tail test). To get this number, we will have to screen as many as 20,000 relatives. Obviously, this can only be achieved through cooperative multicenter trials. In preliminary studies of 10 patients enrolled in the studies to date, we find that an NPH insulin dose of 0.2 U/kg per day divided twice daily is well tolerated and suitable for our studies. No subjects have yet developed IDD.

We have two other intervention methods in NOD mice that may have applicability to human trials. The first exploits the old observation that oral ingestions of large amounts of an antigen can diminish the degree of immune responsiveness resulting from subsequent immunization by the antigen. Thus, ingestion of self-antigens targeted by autoimmunological diseases might diminish the severity of the pathogenic process. We began studies in NOD mice that involved giving them intermittent 1 mg doses of porcine insulin from early life and found that onset of hyperglycemia was delayed, an effect that was more common in females and not accompanied by obvious declines in the severity of the insulitis lesions. We have also been able to show a similar protective effect using partially purified oral recombinant GAD$_{65}$; however, bacterial lysate fed controls showed protective effects also. Weiner and colleagues have reported similar findings to ours with oral insulin, and could transfer the protection to untreated mice using splenocytes from treated animals in cotransfer experiments.[32] This documents that the protective process is active and probably involves regulatory T cells. Further, the group reports that orally fed glucagon is also effective in delaying IDD. Since glucagon has never been incriminated as an antigen targeted in IDD,[33] it is possible that oral ingestion of islet antigens generates regulatory T cells which traffic to the islets and release inhibitory cytokines such as TGF-beta and IL-10 upon contact with their antigen. The insulitis lesion thus becomes suppressed through paracrine actions that inhibit other ongoing autoimmune responses (i.e., bystander effect). Since no appreciable side effects would be expected, oral insulin/GAD therapy would seem worthy of a clinical trial in early human IDD.

Finally, in consideration of the possible mechanisms involved in prophylactic insulin therapy, we have begun a series of studies in the NOD mouse to attempt to bolster its immunological tolerance to islet antigens. We immunized the mice with monthly doses of porcine insulin suspended in incomplete Freund's adjuvant. The result was striking protection from diabetes. We found no preventive effect after immunizing against BSA and its ABBOS peptide, both of which have been recently implicated in human IDD.[34] When insulin was fractionated into its A and B chains, only immunization by B chain was effective and the therapeutic response was successfully transferred to untreated recipients by the splenocytes isolated from B-chain-immunized, but not A-chain-immunized, donors. These findings suggest that there may be a dominant epitope on B chain insulin that conveys immunoprotection.

These findings argue that daily prophylactic insulin therapy is ready for multicenter human trials, but should only be advocated in high-risk relatives. The therapy is sufficiently invasive that it should not be offered to those with only modest risks for the disease. Further human studies of oral insulin/GAD/glucagon should be soon undertaken in ICA-positive relatives who do not yet have impaired FPIR. Finally, we suspect that the future in IDD prevention may lie in islet antigen vaccination strategies, which could be applied even to those with only a low risk of IDD.

REFERENCES

1. ATKINSON, M. A. & N. K. MACLAREN. 1990. What causes diabetes? Sci. Am. **262**(7): 61–71.
2. MACLAREN, N. K., D. SCHATZ, A. DRASH & G. GRAVE. 1989. The initial pathogenic events in insulin-dependent diabetes. Diabetes **38:** 534–539.
3. BROWNLEE, M., H. VLASSARA, T. KOONEY, P. ULRICH & A. CERAMI. 1986. Aminoguanidine prevents diabetes induced arterial wall protein cross-linking. Science **232:** 1629–1632.
4. 1991. Diabetes Epidemiology Research International Mortality Study Group. Major cross-country differences in risk of dying for people with IDDM. Diabetes Care **14:** 49–54.
5. 1987. The DCCT Research group results of feasibility study. Diabetes Care **10:** 1–19.
6. FORD, E. S. & F. DESTEFANO. 1991. Risk factors for mortality from all causes and from coronary heart disease among persons with diabetes. Findings from the National Health and Nutrition Examination Survey I epidemiologic follow-up study. Am. J. Epidemiol. **133:** 1220–1230.
7. BROWNLEE, M., H. VLASSARA & A. CERAMI. 1984. Nonenzymatic glycosylation and the pathogenesis of diabetic complications. Ann. Intern. Med. **101:** 527–537.
8. VIBERTI, G. 1988. Etiology and prognostic significance of albuminuria in diabetes. Diabetes Care **11:** 840–845.

9. TODD, J. A., J. I. BELL & H. O. MCDEVITT. 1987. HLA-DQ beta gene contributes to susceptibility and resistance to insulin-dependent diabetes mellitus. Nature **329:** 599–604.
10. WINTER, W. E., M. OBATA, A. MUIR & N. K. MACLAREN. 1991. Heritable origins of type 1 (insulin-dependent) diabetes mellitus: immunogenetic update. Growth Genet. Horm. **7:**(2): 1–6.
11. TODD, J. A. 1990. Genetic control of autoimmunity type I diabetes. Immunol. Today **11:** 122–129.
12. JULIER, C., R. N. HYER, J. DAVIES, F. MERLIN, P. SOULARUE, L. BRIANT, G. CATHELINEAU, I. DESCHAMPS, J. I. ROTTER, P. FROGUEL, *et al.* 1991. Insulin-IGF2 region on chromosome 11p encodes a gene implicated in HLA-DR4-dependent diabetes susceptibility. Nature **354:** 155–159.
13. BAIN, S., J. PRINS, C. HEARNE, N. RODRIGUES, B. ROWE, L. PRITCHARD, R. RITCHIE, J. HALL, D. UNDLIEN, K. RONNINGEN, D. DUNGER, A. BARNETT & J. TODD. 1992. Insulin gene region-encoded susceptibility to type 1 diabetes is not restricted to HLA-DR4 positive individuals. Nature/Genetics **2:** 212–215.
14. TODD, J. A. & S. C. BAIN. 1992. A practical approach to identification of susceptibility genes for IDDM. Diabetes **41:** 1029–1034.
15. KAUFMAN, D., M. ERLANDER, M. CLARE-SALZLER, M. ATKINSON, N. MACLAREN & A. TOBIN. 1992. Autoimmunity to two forms of glutamate decarboxylase in insulin-dependent mellitus. J. Clin. Invest. **89:** 283–292.
16. KARJALAINEN, J., J. M. MARTIN, M. KNIP, J. ILONEN, B. ROBINSON, E. SAVILAHTI, H. K. AKERBLOM & H.-M. DOSCH. 1992. A bovine albumin peptide as a possible trigger of insulin-dependent diabetes mellitus. N. Engl. J. Med. **327**(5): 302–327.
17. ATKINSON, M. A., N. K. MACLAREN, D. SCHARP, P. LACY & W. J. RILEY. 1990. 64,000 M_r autoantibodies as predictors of insulin-dependent diabetes. Lancet **335:** 1357–1360.
18. BAEKKESKOV, S., H. J. ANASTOOT, S. CHRISTGAUN, A. REETZ, M. SOLIMENA, M. CASCALHO, F. FOLLI, H. RICHTER-OLESEN & P. DE CAMILLI. 1990. Identification of the 64K autoantigen in insulin-dependent diabetes as the GABA-synthesizing enzyme glutamic acid decarboxylase. Nature **347:** 151–156.
19. ATKINSON, M., D. KAUFMAN, L. CAMPBELL, K. GIBBS, S. SCHAH, D-F. BU, M. ERLANDER, A. TOBIN & N. MACLAREN. 1992. Response of peripheral blood mononuclear cells to glutamate decarboxylase in insulin dependent diabetes. Lancet **339:** 458–459.
20. ROEP, B. O., S. D. ARDEN, R. R. DE VRIES & J. C. HUTTON. 1990. T-cell clones from a type 1 diabetes patient respond to insulin secretory granule proteins. Nature **345:** 632–634.
21. ATKINSON, M. A., D. L. KAUFMAN, D. NEWMAN, A. J. TOBIN & N. K. MACLAREN. 1993. Islet cell cytoplasmic autoantibody reactivity to glutamate decarboxylase in insulin-dependent diabetes. J. Clin. Invest. **91:** 350–356.
22. MACLAREN, N. K. 1988. Perspectives in diabetes: how, when, and why to predict IDDM. Diabetes **37**(12): 1591–1994.
23. KRISCHER, J., N. MACLAREN, W. RILEY, D. SCHATZ, R. P. SPILLAR, S. SCHWARTZ, J. MALONE, S. SHAH, C. VADHEIM, J. ROTTER & J. SILVERSTEIN. Insulin and islet cell autoantibodies in the development of diabetes in relatives of patients with insulin dependent diabetes: a prospective study. J. Clin. Endocrinol. Metab. (In press.)
24. BONIFACIO, E., P. J. BINGLEY, M. SHATTOCK, B. M. DEAN, D. DUNGER, E. A. GALE & G. F. BOTTAZZO. 1990. Quantification of islet-cell antibodies and prediction of insulin-dependent diabetes. Lancet **335:** 147–149.
25. RILEY, W. J., N. K. MACLAREN, J. KRISCHER, R. SPILLAR, J. SILVERSTEIN, D. SCHATZ, S. SHAH, C. VADHEIM & J. ROTTER. 1990. A prospective study of the development of diabetes in relatives of patients with insulin dependent diabetes. N. Engl. J. Med. **323:** 1167–1172.
26. ATKINSON, M. A., N. K. MACLAREN, W. J. RILEY, W. E. WINTER, D. D. FISK & R. P. SPILLAR. 1986. Are insulin autoantibodies markers for insulin-dependent diabetes mellitus? Diabetes **35:** 894–898.
27. GEPTS, W. 1965. Pathologic anatomy of the pancreas in juvenile diabetes mellitus. Diabetes **14:** 619–633.
28. MARTIN, S., G. SCHERNTHANER, J. NERUP, F. A. GRIES, V. A. KAIVISTO, J. DUPRE, E.

STANDL, P. HAMET, R. MCARTHUR, M. H. TAN, *et al.* 1991. Follow-up of cyclosporin A treatment in type 1 insulin dependent diabetes mellitus: lack of long-term effects. Diabetologia **34:** 429–434.

29. SILVERSTEIN, J., N. MACLAREN, W. RILEY, R. SPILLAR, D. RADJENOVIC & S. JOHNSON. 1988. Immunosuppression with azathioprine and prednisone in recent-onset insulin-dependent diabetes mellitus. N. Engl. J. Med. **319**(10): 599–604.

30. ATKINSON, M., N. MACLAREN, R. LUCHETTA & I. BURR. 1990. Insulitis and diabetes in NOD mice reduced by prophylactic insulin therapy. Diabetes **39**(8): 933–937.

31. ZHANG, I., L. DAVIDSON, G. EISENBARTH & H. L. WEINER. 1991. Suppression of diabetes in non-obese diabetic mice by oral administration of porcine insulin. Proc. Natl. Acad. Sci. USA **88:** 10252–10256.

Lessons Learned from Use of Cyclosporine for Insulin-Dependent Diabetes Mellitus

The Case for Immunotherapy for Insulin-Dependent Diabetics Having Residual Insulin Secretion

JEFFREY L. MAHON, JOHN DUPRE,
AND CALVIN R. STILLER[a]

Department of Medicine
University of Western Ontario
London, Ontario, Canada

INTRODUCTION

Insulin-dependent diabetes mellitus (IDDM) is marked by selective loss of the beta-cells of the pancreas, hyperglycemia, and a tendency to ketosis. For 70 years, the mainstay of therapy has been lifelong, daily insulin injections following symptomatic beta-cell failure. Despite this, IDDM has conveyed an immense societal and personal burden of suffering through premature mortality,[1] structural complications,[1,2] and the direct and indirect costs attending these problems.[3] This poor outcome, and laboratory and clinical observations that suggested that beta-cell loss was immune mediated in IDDM,[4] led to trials of cyclosporine for newly diagnosed IDDM in the 1980s.[5-14] Long-term use of cyclosporine has not emerged as a viable treatment for IDDM largely because of the drug's potential for irreversible nephrotoxicity.[15,16] However, these trials yielded insights that may eventually lead to a substantive reduction in the burden of IDDM. In this paper, we will first summarize the experience with cyclosporine for IDDM with emphasis on the randomized trials. We will then outline some lessons from this experience. Finally, using these lessons and the findings of the recently completed Diabetes Control and Complications Trial, we will develop an argument for further, careful testing of immunotherapy in insulin-dependent diabetics having residual insulin secretion.

TRIALS OF CYCLOSPORINE FOR IDDM

The Open Trials

The assessment of cyclosporine for newly diagnosed IDDM proceeded through the usual sequence of open, nonrandomized trials[5-11] to double-blind, placebo-controlled, randomized trials.[12-14] The largest open trials were conducted in Canada[6] and France.[10,11] The randomized trials were undertaken in France,[12] and Northern

---

[a]Author to whom correspondence should be addressed at: University Hospital, P.O. Box 5339, London, Ontario, Canada, N6A 5A5.

Europe and Canada.[13] A third, smaller randomized trial was completed in Miami but has not been fully reported[14] and will not be considered here.

The open trials were not undertaken with the aim of definitively establishing the efficacy of cyclosporine for IDDM, but were essential in justifying the randomized trials. Several observations in the open trials were confirmed in the randomized trials and bear reiteration:

1. Unprecedently high rates of "clinical remission," where this was defined as a non–insulin-receiving state with non-diabetic-range fasting blood glucose levels, were seen within the first year of diagnosis.[6,8,10,11] These remissions were associated with similarly unprecedented preservation of endogenous insulin secretion as determined by insulin connecting-peptide (C-peptide) levels in the peripheral blood.[6,11]
2. Clinical remissions were associated with the time of introduction of cyclosporine relative to the duration of symptomatic hyperglycemia. Specifically, the earlier the drug was started, the greater the chance of a remission.[6,9] If cyclosporine was started after more than two months of overt IDDM, remissions were very unlikely.[6] As well, remissions were virtually always lost within a few weeks of stopping cyclosporine.[6]
3. Endogenous insulin secretion appeared to be maintained for as long as cyclosporine was given.[6,11] Despite this, clinical remissions were usually lost by the second year.[6,10,11] This paradox was directly confirmed in a randomized trial,[13] but remains incompletely explained. Limited observations in the open trials have suggested that declining insulin sensitivity contributed to the loss of glycemic control.[10,17]

The assessment of efficacy in the open trials used insulin dosage, glycemic control, and C-peptide levels. Because all three were subject to patient, physician, and disease-process factors other than cyclosporine, confirmation of the findings required trials with randomization, placebo controls, and double blinding.

The French Multicenter Randomized Trial

The first such trial to be reported was a multicenter study from France.[12] One hundred and twenty-two patients, with a mean age of 25 years (range 15 to 40 years) and a mean duration of symptomatic hyperglycemia of 10 weeks, were randomized. Insulin dosage was minimized as consistent with maintenance of blood glucose levels < 7.8 mM before meals and < 11.1 mM after meals. A "complete remission" required these blood glucose levels and a glycated hemoglobin (GHb) level $\leq 7.5\%$ (upper limit of normal 5.8%) in the absence of insulin injections. "Partial remissions" required the same glycemic parameters and an insulin dosage of < 0.25 units/ kilogram per day. The rates of complete remission at 9 months were 24% in the cyclosporine group and 6% in the placebo group ($p < 0.01$). Statistically significant increases in the combined rate of complete and partial remissions were also seen in the cyclosporine group at 6 (cyclosporine 46% vs. placebo 29%, $p = 0.05$) and 9 months (cyclosporine 37% vs. placebo 14%, $p < 0.01$). By post hoc analysis, complete remissions in both treatment groups were associated with symptoms of shorter duration and greater body weight at entry. However, formal statistical assessment of an interaction between these variables, cyclosporine or placebo treatment, and remissions was not done. Comparison of beta-cell function between the two groups was also not done, although in a follow-up report C-peptide levels from the cyclosporine group were found to be maintained in comparison to non-cyclosporine-treated, historical controls.[11]

The Canadian-European Randomized Trial

The second double-blind, placebo-controlled, randomized trial of cyclosporine for IDDM to be reported was a multicenter Canadian-European trial.[13] One hundred and eighty-eight patients were randomized within 14 weeks of onset of symptoms and within no more than 6 weeks of starting insulin therapy. The mean age was 22 years. Most (86%) patients were at least 16 years old. The study was designed to assess the effects of cyclosporine through one year on clinical remissions and beta-cell function in terms of glucagon-stimulated C-peptide secretion. Insulin therapy was given to maintain capillary blood glucose levels < 7.8 mM before meals and the dose was minimized as far as possible without exceeding this target. Two end points were defined in advance. A non-insulin-receiving (NIR) remission required these glycemic targets without insulin therapy for at least 2 weeks. A second, compound end point required either an NIR remission or a glucagon-stimulated C-peptide level of at least 0.6 nM (a value attained in > 90% of normal subjects).

Glycemic control by GHb level was not different between the groups at 3, 6, and 12 months.[13] At the same time, NIR remissions were significantly more frequent in the cyclosporine group at 6 months (cyclosporine 39% vs. placebo 19%, $p = 0.003$) and 12 months (cyclosporine 24% vs. placebo 10%, $p = 0.009$). Regarding beta-cell function, a higher mean glucagon-stimulated C-peptide level in the cyclosporine group was present at 90 days and was maintained to one year, whereas the mean values in the placebo group showed the expected pattern of a peak at 3 months followed by progressive decline. By 12 months, the mean glucagon-stimulated C-peptide level was significantly higher in the cyclosporine group (cyclosporine 0.46 nM vs. placebo 0.35 nM, $p < 0.002$). This difference occurred despite a statistically significant converse difference between the groups at entry.

A striking interaction between cyclosporine treatment, duration of disease, and NIR remissions was seen in the Canadian-European trial.[13] The NIR remission rate at 12 months among patients with short duration disease, where the definition of short duration was not data driven and was ≤ 6 weeks of symptoms before entry with ≤ 2 weeks of insulin therapy, was highly significantly different (cyclosporine 32% vs. placebo 3%, $p = 0.001$). No difference was observed in NIR remissions at 12 months among patients with long-duration disease (cyclosporine 19% vs. placebo 15%, $p = 0.55$). An interaction between early treatment and response to cyclosporine was also suggested in respect to endogenous insulin secretion. The rate of remission at 12 months by the compound end point among patients with short duration disease was 40% for the cyclosporine group and 16% for the placebo group ($p = 0.02$), whereas the respective rates among patients with long-duration disease were 28% and 24% ($p = 0.58$).

These interactions were assessed by multiple logistic regression analysis controlling for other baseline variables (sex, age, body mass index, and C-peptide level).[13] Only duration of disease continued to show an interaction between treatment and remissions. The difference in efficacy of cyclosporine between short- and long-duration patients for both end points was statistically significant at 6 months (NIR remission, $p = 0.003$; compound end point, $p = 0.02$) and showed a clear trend at 12 months (NIR remission, $p = 0.06$; compound end point, $p = 0.15$).

LESSONS FROM THE CYCLOSPORINE TRIALS FOR IDDM

The lessons from the randomized trials of cyclosporine for IDDM address the biology of the disease and have important implications for future clinical trials of immunotherapy for IDDM.

The Biology of Beta-Cell Loss

The most important conclusion from the experience with cyclosporine therapy for IDDM is that an immune-mediated process causes beta-cell loss in human IDDM. With Hill's observations on causation in mind,[18] the randomized trials of cyclosporine remain the only definitive proof to date for this cause and effect sequence. All other laboratory and clinical observations before and since the cyclosporine randomized trials have provided strong, but circumstantial, evidence for such a relationship. The use of double blinding in the cyclosporine trials brought additional rigor to this causal inference—a rigor that was not present for unavoidable reasons in the only other large randomized, but open, trial of immunosuppression (prednisone and azathioprine) for IDDM in which a similar effect on the natural history of the disease was seen.[19] Thus, the randomized trials of cyclosporine for IDDM remain the strongest available data in support of further efforts to identify effective, safe immunotherapy for the disease.

A second biological lesson from the cyclosporine trials concerns the immunological mechanism of beta-cell loss. In view of the drug's action,[20] it is reasonable to conclude that a T-lymphocyte directed, lymphokine-mediated process governs beta-cell loss at the time of onset of symptomatic IDDM. While this conclusion may not bear upon earlier immunopathological events in IDDM, it has established the efficacy of at least one mechanism of action that should be considered when choosing immunotherapy for future studies.

A third biological lesson from the cyclosporine trials addresses the tempo of beta-cell loss, which had been hypothesized to follow an unremitting, steady course.[21] The Canadian-European randomized trial demonstrated a large difference in remission rates in association with a difference in duration of symptomatic disease of only six weeks.[13] That such a short time is important relative to the known period of beta-cell autoimmunity of several years[22] suggests that beta-cell loss is greatly accelerated at onset of overt disease. This differential response was unlikely to have arisen through glucose toxicity because glycemic control was not different between the two groups.[13] Furthermore, while the interaction was demonstrated by a *post hoc* subgroup analysis, its validity was strengthened by the consistency of similar associations seen in the open trials,[6,9] the fact that the subgroup analysis was not data driven, and the high level of statistical significance associated with the difference in remission rates between short- and long-duration patients.[13] The importance of this observation is that it supports the hypothesis that beta-cell loss at other times in the disease, including the pre-IDDM period, may pass through active and quiescent phases. This observation is consistent with findings in identical twins who are discordant for IDDM for a period of time beyond which it is extremely unlikely that the second twin will develop IDDM, but in which the nondiabetic twin shows evidence of beta-cell autoimmunity.[23] If this hypothesis is true, then it raises the possibility that less toxic, intermittent immunotherapy during active periods of autoimmunity in the pre-IDDM phase may be sufficient to prevent further beta-cell loss.

End Points and Strategies for Future Clinical Trials

While the above biological lessons have obvious importance to future clinical trials of immunotherapy for IDDM, there were other lessons from the cyclosporine trials that carry direct implications for the design of such trials, including preventative trials that are soon starting for nondiabetic individuals at high risk for IDDM because of their family history and the presence of markers of beta-cell autoimmunity such as islet cell antibodies.[24,25]

First, such trials will probably always include outcome measures of efficacy based upon blood glucose level and endogenous insulin secretion,[26] as these are the cardinal pathophysiological features of IDDM. However, the discrepancy between loss of glycemic control and preservation of endogenous insulin secretion seen in the cyclosporine trials calls for concurrent assessment of insulin action. Studies of insulin sensitivity are labor intensive and are particularly difficult in children. It is hoped that simpler, valid measures of insulin sensitivity will be forthcoming that will make assessment of insulin sensitivity feasible for most subjects enrolled in these trials. Meantime, the experience from the cyclosporine trials suggests, at the least, that a representative sample of adult subjects within these trials should also have prospective, serial insulin sensitivity studies.

A second observation from the cyclosporine trials having a bearing on future clinical trials of immunotherapy for IDDM is that a cause and effect relationship has been established between improved endogenous insulin secretion and improved glycemic control. Several large studies had previously shown an association between higher C-peptide levels and more normal glycemic control.[27–30] However, the observational nature of those data did not yield conclusive evidence for cause and effect. The Canadian-European randomized trial provided the proof: under randomized, double-blind, placebo-controlled conditions, insulin-dependent diabetics given a treatment that maintained endogenous insulin secretion for one year were less likely to be receiving insulin as compared with those not receiving the treatment.[13] This difference in insulin use did not occur at the cost of worse glycemic control[13] and is not explained by other metabolic effects of cyclosporine.[31]

A third lesson from the cyclosporine trials relates to the potential for recovery of insulin secretion present at onset of overt IDDM. The Canadian-European trial[13] and open observations from the Canadian[6] and French study groups[11] showed that maximal beta-cell secretory capacity, once IDDM is diagnosed, approached normal in a substantive proportion of patients. Furthermore, such levels of beta-cell function appeared to be maintained for as long as immunosuppression was given.[6,11] That this recovery in insulin secretion may be clinically important is supported by two observations. First, in the Canadian-European randomized trial, it was associated with improved glycemic control, at least to one year.[13] Second, in a large cross-sectional study of long-standing insulin-dependent diabetics, stimulated C-peptide levels of at least 0.2 nM were associated with lower GHb levels and lower daily doses of insulin.[30]

These observations on the recovery and maintenance of beta-cell function after diagnosis of IDDM, and the effect it has on glycemic control, have become very important in light of the recent findings of the Diabetes Control and Complications Trial (DCCT).[32] In the DCCT, approximately 1400 insulin-dependent diabetics were randomized to receive a program of intensive management—including multiple daily insulin injections or a continuous subcutaneous insulin infusion, frequent home capillary blood glucose monitoring, and weekly follow-up by health care personnel—or standard management. The intensive program was designed to attain a GHb as close to normal as safely possible. Standard management was designed to keep the patient free of symptomatic hyper- and hypoglycemia and accepted a higher GHb level. Through a mean follow-up of approximately 7 years, the relative risks for each of retinopathy, nephropathy, and peripheral neuropathy were reduced by approximately 50% in intensively treated patients. At the same time, there was about a threefold increase in severe hypoglycemia among intensively treated subjects.[32] Moreover, the ability to safely transfer the experience with the intensive program necessary to obtain near-normal GHb levels in the highly motivated group of patients in the DCCT to the much larger and less compliant constituency of diabetics in the community remains a major practical problem. Thus, the DCCT has conclusively established a cause and effect relationship between glycemic control and diabetic microvasculopathy and neuropathy. In doing so, it has also provided strong justification for further clinical trials in which identification of safe, practicable, and cost-effective strategies of improving glycemic control in established IDDM is a major clinical goal.

Taken together, the cyclosporine trials and DCCT have proven an important chain of cause and effect. From the cyclosporine trials, the chain begins with enhancement of endogenous insulin secretion by immunotherapy at the time of diagnosis of IDDM causing, in turn, more normal glycemic control. From the DCCT, more normal glycemic control reduces the risk for microvascular complications and neuropathy.

The inference that more normal endogenous insulin secretion causes fewer structural diabetic complications is not weakened by studies that have assessed the relationship between endogenous insulin secretion and complications.[33-41] An inverse association between urine or blood C-peptide levels and microvascular complications or neuropathy has been seen in some studies,[33-35] but not in others.[36-41] However, all of these data were cross-sectional and studied insulin-dependent diabetics that were insulinopenic. The observational nature of the data makes it impossible to adequately address confounding variables, the most obvious of which is disease duration. An analysis that assesses the association between C-peptide levels and complications while controlling for disease duration may not be sufficient to control for confounding because of the high inverse correlation between duration of diabetes and C-peptide levels.[36] This problem of collinearity can only be fully addressed by a randomized trial having endogenous insulin secretion as the experimental variable. Furthermore, it is plausible that an association between insulin secretion and long-term complications would consistently emerge if insulin-dependent diabetics with more normal insulin secretion were studied. Such levels of secretion are evidently not possible in "untreated" IDDM after 5 to 10 years but may be obtained with immunotherapy shortly after onset of IDDM, where the potential for recovery and maintenance of beta-cell function is at its greatest for any time after onset of disease.

The rationale for two experimental initiatives in clinical IDDM is greatly strengthened with the recognition of a causal sequence between enhanced endogenous insulin secretion and fewer structural diabetic complications. First, evolving efforts to identify effective means of preserving beta-cell secretion prior to onset of overt IDDM receive major justification. Second, the question of the potential clinical benefit of immunotherapy for insulin-dependent diabetics who retain endogenous insulin secretion can be reopened.[16]

THE CASE FOR FURTHER TESTING OF IMMUNOTHERAPY FOR INSULIN-DEPENDENT DIABETICS WITH RESIDUAL INSULIN SECRETION

At present, there are three experimental strategies of prevention of beta-cell loss that may eventually reduce the burden of IDDM. Immunotherapy at onset of overt

IDDM can be considered "tertiary prevention," where the pathological event being prevented is complete beta-cell loss. The aim of "secondary prevention" is to identify nondiabetic individuals with active, subclinical beta-cell loss by genetic, immune, and metabolic markers and then prevent IDDM with immunotherapy. Testing of two secondary preventions (exogenous insulin[24] and nicotinamide[25]) will soon start. In "primary prevention," the putative environmental factors responsible for initiating beta-cell autoimmunity are identified and eliminated.[42] Removal of cow's milk protein from the diet in the first year of life will probably be the first such environmental manipulation to be assessed.[43]

It is unarguable that secondary and primary prevention hold greater promise than tertiary prevention for reducing the burden of IDDM. We strongly support continuing exploration of these alternatives. However, there is strong rationale for continuing to test tertiary prevention when the limitations and advantages of the three preventative approaches are compared.

The main advantage of secondary and primary prevention over tertiary prevention follows from preservation of greater beta-cell function. Effective primary or secondary prevention should eliminate the need for exogenous insulin therapy. This has generally not been possible with tertiary prevention but is an important clinical result given the major impact on quality of life attendent to daily insulin injections. Furthermore, enhanced beta-cell function through secondary prevention, and attaining normal beta-cell function through primary prevention, may completely prevent structural complications in the longer term. However, there are limitations to primary and secondary prevention that do not pertain to tertiary prevention.

Secondary Prevention

For secondary prevention, the assessment of risk for IDDM by markers of beta-cell autoimmunity and impaired beta-cell function has been almost entirely limited to those at increased risk for IDDM, specifically, first-degree relatives of insulin-dependent diabetics.[44] Even in this high-risk group the positive predictive value of current markers for IDDM remains less than 100%. This leads to two major clinical consequences, neither of which occurs in tertiary prevention, that follow from falsely identifying someone to be at increased risk for IDDM. First, the person will be unnecessarily exposed to potentially harmful immunotherapy. Second, a person who will never become diabetic will be needlessly "labeled" to be at high risk for a major, lifelong illness. In our view, the potential psychological, social, and economic effects of IDDM labeling are serious and remain inadequately assessed.[45]

The proportion of individuals misclassified in this way depends directly upon the positive predictive value of the test(s). At present, the best validated marker for IDDM is high levels (≥ 20 Juvenile Diabetes Foundation units) of serum islet-cell antibodies (ICA). About 35% of first-degree relatives with ICA at this level will require insulin within 5 years and, with considerably less precision because of limited follow-up to date, about 70% (95% confidence limits: 45%, 100%) will need insulin within a decade.[46] As well, it appears that a proportion of these individuals will never develop IDDM.[47] The positive predictive value for IDDM can be raised to levels that approximate 100% when other markers of beta-cell autoimmunity and beta-cell loss are included. In particular, lost first-phase insulin response in nondiabetic, ICA-positive persons with an immediate family history of IDDM signals a probability for insulin therapy of about 90% within 3 years.[44]

While such certainty for IDDM provides a strong basis for testing immunotherapy to prevent exogenous insulin therapy, it is debatable whether there is any benefit in terms of long-term reduction of diabetic complications by this strategy over tertiary prevention. There may be no important differences in metabolic function bearing upon risk of structural complications between individuals who have lost first-phase insulin response but who are maintained in a non-insulin-receiving state through secondary prevention versus those who are receiving insulin and who maintain endogenous insulin secretion under tertiary prevention.[48] Specifically, it is plausible that normal GHb levels can be sustained by exogenous insulin therapy with little difficulty for several years in most, if not all, patients receiving tertiary prevention. If so, the difference between secondary prevention using current risk markers and tertiary prevention is the respective risk-benefit ratios of (1) fewer patients needing exogenous insulin therapy but with the consequences arising from false-positive diagnostic errors, and (2) all patients needing exogenous insulin therapy but without the consequences of false-positive diagnostic errors. This comparison assumes that the same immunotherapeutic agent is used for secondary and tertiary prevention. Given the potential seriousness of false-positive errors in this setting, these risk-benefit ratios may be similar.

Prediction of risk for IDDM, including development of models that do not need profound beta-cell dysfunction for high positive predictive values, is likely to improve. However, other limitations to secondary prevention will remain that support an argument for tertiary prevention. First, the predictive markers have largely been assessed in subjects with an immediate family history of IDDM who are at higher risk for disease than the general population. These individuals account for 10% of cases of IDDM and contribute relatively little to the total disease burden. Because it is highly unlikely that a perfect predictive model will ever be obtained, and because the baseline risk for disease is much lower in the general population, the impact of false-positive labeling for IDDM in terms of the number of false-positive errors and undesirable effects they have in a general population screening program will necessarily be much larger than for screening in first-degree relatives. Furthermore, it is highly improbable that completely effective preventative immunotherapy will be identified for either population. Thus, it can be expected that a large number of newly diagnosed insulin-dependent diabetics will continue to enter the health care system for many years. Safe, effective tertiary prevention would be an important therapeutic option for these individuals.

Primary Prevention

A strategy of primary prevention for IDDM is based on the premise that environmental factors induce beta-cell autoimmunity and loss in genetically suscep-tible persons.[42] There are three advantages of primary prevention over secondary and tertiary prevention that make it, in theory, the most attractive strategy in the long term. First, it avoids the adverse effects of immunotherapy (unlike secondary and tertiary prevention). Second, it will yield completely normal beta-cell function (unlike secondary and tertiary prevention). Third, it will not "medicalize" healthy individuals (unlike secondary prevention). However, there are some important potential disadvantages to primary prevention that do not apply to secondary and tertiary prevention.

First, the process of definitively identifying the environmental factor or factors that cause beta-cell loss and IDDM is formidible and will probably take decades of study. It will require randomized trials in which experimental control of the sus-pected factor leads to a reduction in the incidence of IDDM. Even under the most efficient circumstances (in which enrollment is limited to subjects at high baseline risk for IDDM, that is, first-degree relatives of insulin-dependent diabetics), several thousand relatives will need to be randomized and followed for 5 to 10 years because the baseline incidence of disease is very low. The task becomes more daunting given the working hypothesis that several environmental factors including stress, recurrent nonspecific viral infections, and common dietary constituents may induce beta-cell autoimmunity over a series of "multiple hits."[49,50] In the meantime, the opportunity to improve the long-term prognosis of patients with subclinical or overt IDDM through secondary or tertiary prevention may be at hand.

Second, in view of the multiple hit hypothesis, it seems unlikely that environmental manipulation will prevent all cases of IDDM. Thus, it can be expected that individuals will continue to present for many years to come with subclinical or established IDDM for which secondary or tertiary prevention may be beneficial.

REQUIREMENTS FOR CLINICAL TRIALS OF IMMUNOTHERAPY FOR INSULIN-DEPENDENT DIABETICS WITH RESIDUAL INSULIN SECRETION

If one accepts the rationale for testing immunotherapy in insulin-dependent diabetics with residual beta-cell function, what are the key components of such a trial?

Above all, it is essential that the experimental intervention have a long record of use (we would suggest a minimum of 5 to 10 years) in a large number of patients, from which acceptably low risks of toxicity can be precisely defined and weighed against the benefit that the trial is designed to detect. At present, there is at least one candidate agent, nicotinamide,[25] but it is expected that others will emerge through further long-term experience with immunotherapy in transplantation and autoimmune diseases. Such a safety record notwithstanding, careful monitoring for toxicity, both expected and unexpected, would be necessary as would independent safety committees having authority to stop the trial in the event of serious adverse effects.

Second, there are some important inclusion criteria to consider. First, there must be no doubt that subjects have IDDM, with documentation of ketosis being preferred. Second, to maximize potential recovery of beta-cell function, the majority of subjects should have overt IDDM of no more than 3 months. However, consideration could be given to enroll subjects with IDDM of more than 3 months who continue to secrete insulin. If so, stimulated C-peptide levels above 0.2 nM would be an acceptable cut point, as this was the level that was clearly associated with better long-term glycemic control in a large, representative sample of patients with IDDM.[30] Third, children and adolescents should not be enrolled if the experience with the test therapy is not sufficient to precisely define its safety in younger patients.

Third, the primary end point upon which the sample size is based would be an improvement in GHb that is of sufficient magnitude and duration to cause a reduction in diabetic complications. While it would not be necessary to repeat the DCCT to an end point of changes in diabetic retinopathy, that trial has provided a direct measure of the difference (about 1.5%) and duration (about 5 years) in GHb levels that is clinically important. Prospective assessment of weight and insulin dose will also be required in view of the primary end point of GHb.

Fourth, given that the primary outcome measure is glycemic control, it would be essential that placebo controls and double blinding be used. Furthermore, the strategy of insulin therapy, home glucose monitoring, and advice on diet and exercise should be given with the aim of obtaining a GHb as close to normal as safely possible and would need to be explicitly outlined and identically applied in both groups. Discontinuation of insulin therapy would not be an outcome of interest in such a trial nor would systematic attempts be made to minimize insulin dosage. It would be necessary that GHb levels be regularly determined and given to the treating diabetologist. Provided that the test therapy has no side effects that lead to unblinding, this strategy of providing subjects and investigators with the primary outcome measure should not introduce bias.

Fifth, there are several other secondary outcomes that would need to be compared between the experimental and control groups. The most important of these is endogenous insulin secretion. Measurement of meal-stimulated C-peptide levels is probably the easiest and least noxious for patients. An interim comparison of C-peptide levels between the experimental and control group would be important from which a decision to stop the trial could be made. If the test therapy could not significantly enhance endogenous insulin secretion relatively early on, then there would be no point in finishing the trial. For reasons presented earlier, an additional measure of interest would be insulin sensitivity. The simplest, validated measure of insulin sensitivity in established IDDM at present applies the minimal model technique to a frequently sampled, three-hour intravenous glucose tolerance test.[17] Finally, assessment of quality of life by a disease-specific, reliable, and responsive instrument such as the Diabetes Quality of Life measure[51] and prospective collection of costing data serving a cost-utility analysis would be desirable.

CONCLUSIONS

The randomized trials of cyclosporine for IDDM have definitively proven that beta-cell loss in human IDDM is immune mediated. They have also shown that a T-lymphocyte-directed, lymphokine-mediated mechanism governs at least some beta-cell loss, that the intensity of beta-cell autoimmunity fluctuates over time, and have established a cause-effect relationship between enhanced beta-cell function and more normal glycemic control in IDDM. Combined with the results of the DCCT, the cyclosporine trials have defined a sequence of cause and effect that moves from enhancement of endogenous insulin secretion by immunotherapy to more normal glycemic control to reduction in microvascular complications and neuropathy. We expect that further clinical trials will follow from these insights and hope that these efforts will lead to a major reduction in the disease's burden of suffering.

REFERENCES

1. BORCH-JOHNSEN, K. 1989. The prognosis of insulin dependent diabetes mellitus: an epidemiological approach. Dan. Med. Bull. **36:** 336–348.
2. ORCHARD, T. J., J. S. DORMAN, R. E. MASER, D. J. BECKER, A. L. DRASH, D. ELLIS, R. E. LAPORTE & L. H. KULLER. 1990. Prevalence of complications of IDDM by sex and duration. Diabetes **39:** 1116–1124.
3. THE CARTER CENTER OF EMORY UNIVERSITY. 1985. Closing the gap: the problem of diabetes mellitus in the United States. Diabetes Care **8:** 391–406.
4. CAHILL, G. F. & H. O. MCDEVITT. 1981. Insulin dependent diabetes mellitus: the initial lesion. N. Engl. J. Med. **304:** 1454–1465.
5. STILLER, C. R., J. DUPRE, M. GENT, M. R. JENNER, P. A. KEOWN, A. LAUPACIS, R. MARTELL, N. W. RODGER, B. VON GRAFFENRIED & B. M. J. WOLFE. 1984. Effects of cyclosporine immunosuppression in insulin-dependent diabetes mellitus of recent onset. Science **223:** 1362–1367.
6. DUPRE, J., C. R. STILLER, M. GENT, DONNER A., B. VON GRAFFENREID, G. MURPHY, D. HEINRICHS, M. R. JENNER, P. A. KEOWN, A. LAUPACIS, J. MAHON, R. MARTELL, N. W.

RODGER & B. M. J. WOLFE. 1988. Effects of immunosuppression with cyclosporine in insulin-dependent diabetes mellitus of recent onset: the Canadian open study at 44 months. Transplant. Proc. **20:** 184–192.

7. ASSAN, R., G. FEUTREN, M. DEBRAY-SACHS, M. C. QUINIOU-DEBRIE, C. LABORIE, G. THOMAS, L. CHATENOUD & J. F. BACH. 1985. Metabolic and immunological effects of cyclosporin in recently diagnosed type 1 diabetes mellitus. Lancet **i:** 67–71.

8. LEVY-MARCHAL, C. & P. CZERNICHOW. 1986. Effect of different doses of cyclosporine A (CsA) on the early phase of overt insulin-dependent diabetes mellitus (IDDM) in children. Transplant. Proc. **28:** 1543–1544.

9. BOUGNERES, P. F., J. C. CAREL, L. CASTANO, C. BOITARD, J. P. GARDIN, P. LANDAIS, J. HORS, M. J. MIHATSCH, M. PAILLARD, J. L. CHAUSSAIN & J. F. BACH. 1988. Factors associated with early remission of type 1 diabetes in children treated with cyclosporine. N. Engl. J. Med. **318:** 663–670.

10. BOUGNERES, P. F., P. LANDAIS, C. BOISSON, J. C. CAREL, N. FRAMENT, C. BOITARD, J. L. CHAUSSAIN & J. F. BACH. 1990. Limited duration of remission of insulin dependency in children with recent overt type 1 diabetes treated with low-dose cyclosporin. Diabetes **39:** 1264–1272.

11. ASSAN, R., G. FEUTREN, J. SIRMAI, C. LABORIE, C. BOITARD, P. VEXIAU, H. DU ROSTU, M. RODIER, M. FIGONI, P. VAGUE, J. HORS & J. F. BACH. 1990. Plasma C-peptide levels and clinical remissions in recent-onset type 1 diabetic patients treated with cyclosporin A and insulin. Diabetes **39:** 768–774.

12. FEUTREN, G., L. PAPOZ, R. ASSAN, B. VIALETTES, G. KARSENTY, P. VEXXIAU, H. DU ROSTU, M. RODIER, J. SIRMAI, A. LALLEMAND & J. F. BACH. 1986. Cyclosporin increases the rate and length of remissions in insulin-dependent diabetes of recent onset. Lancet **ii:** 119–123.

13. THE CANADIAN-EUROPEAN RANDOMIZED CONTROL TRIAL GROUP. 1988. Cyclosporin-induced remission of IDDM after early intervention. Diabetes **37:** 1574–1582.

14. SKYLER, J. S. 1987. Immune intervention studies in insulin-dependent diabetes mellitus. Diabetes Metab. Rev. **3:** 1017–1035.

15. FEUTREN, G. & M. MIHATSCH. 1992. Risk factors for cyclosporine-induced nephropathy in patients with autoimmune diseases. N. Engl. J. Med. **326:** 1654–1660.

16. FATHMAN, C. G. & B. D. MYERS. 1992. Cyclosporine therapy for autoimmune disease. N. Engl. J. Med. **326:** 1693–1695.

17. HRAMIAK, I. M., J. DUPRE & D. T. FINEGOOD. 1993. Determinants of clinical remission in recent-onset IDDM. Diabetes Care **16:** 125–132.

18. HILL, A. B. 1984. A Short Textbook of Medical Statistics. 11th Edit. Hodder and Stoughton. London, England.

19. SILVERSTEIN, J., N. MACLAREN, W. RILEY, R. SPILLAR, D. RADJENOVIC & S. JOHNSON. 1988. Immunosuppression with azathioprine and prednisone in recent-onset insulin-dependent diabetes mellitus. N. Engl. J. Med. **319:** 599–604.

20. VAN BUREN, C. T. 1986. Cyclosporine: progress, problems, and perspectives. Surg. Clin. North Am. **66:** 435–449.

21. EISENBARTH, G. S. 1986. Type 1 diabetes mellitus. A chronic autoimmune disease. N. Engl. J. Med. **314:** 1360–1368.

22. GORSUCH, A. N., K. M. SPENCER, J. LISTER, J. M. MCNALLY, B. M. DEAN, G. F. BOTTAZZO & A. G. CUDWORTH. 1981. Evidence for a long prediabetic period in type 1 (insulin dependent) diabetes mellitus. Lancet **ii:** 1363–1365.

23. MILLWARD, B. A., L. ALVIGGI, P. J. HOSKINS, C. JOHNSTON, D. HEATON, G. F. BOTTAZZO, D. VERGANI, R. D. G. LESLIE & D. PYKE. 1986. Immune changes associated with insulin dependent diabetes may remit without causing the disease: a study in identical twins. Br. Med. J. **292:** 793–796.

24. KELLER, R. J., G. S. EISENBARTH & R. A. JACKSON. 1993. Insulin prophylaxis in individuals at high risk of type 1 diabetes. Lancet **341:** 927–928.

25. CHASE, P., J. DUPRE, J. MAHON, R. EHRLICH, E. GALE, H. KOLB, E. LAMPETER & J. NERUP. 1992. Nicotinamide and prevention of diabetes. Lancet **339:** 1051.

26. AMERICAN DIABETES ASSOCIATION: POSITION STATEMENT. 1990. Prevention of type 1 diabetes. Diabetes **39:** 1151–1152.

27. DAHLQVIST, G., L. BLOM, P. BOLME, L. HAGENFELDT, F. LINDGREN, B. PERSSON, B. THALME, M. THOERELL, & S. WESTIN. 1982. Factors influencing the magnitude, duration, and rate of fall of B-cell function in type 1 diabetic children followed for two years from their clinical diagnosis. Diabetologia **31:** 664–669.
28. AGNER, T., P. DAMM & C. BINDER. 1987. Remission in IDDM: prospective study of basal C-peptide and insulin dose in 268 consecutively studied patients. Diabetes Care **10:** 164–169.
29. CLARSON, C., D. DANEMAN, A. L. DRASH, D. J. BECKER & R. M. EHRLICH. 1987. Residual beta-cell function in children with IDDM: reproducibility of testing and factors influencing insulin secretory capacity. Diabetes Care **10:** 33–38.
30. THE DCCT RESEARCH GROUP. 1987. Effects of age, duration and treatment of insulin-dependent diabetes mellitus on residual beta-cell function: observations during eligibility testing for the Diabetes Control and Complications Trial (DCCT). J. Clin. Endocrinol. Metab. **65:** 30–36.
31. ROBERTSON, P., G. FRANKLIN & L. NELSON. 1989. Intravenous glucose tolerance and pancreatic islet B cell function in patients with multiple sclerosis during two years' treatment with cyclosporine. Diabetes **38:** 58–64.
32. THE DCCT RESEARCH GROUP. N. Engl. J. Med. (In press.)
33. EFF, C., O. FABER & T. DECKERT. 1979. Persistent insulin secretion assessed by plasma C-peptide estimation in long-term juvenile diabetics with a low insulin requirement. Diabetologia **15:** 169–172.
34. SJOBERG, S., R. GUNNARSSON, M. GJOTTERBERG, A. K. LEFVERY, A. PERSSON & J. OSTMAN. 1987. Residual insulin production, glycemic control and prevalence of microvascular lesions and polyneuropathy in long-term type 1 diabetes mellitus. Diabetologia **30:** 208–213.
35. THE DCCT RESEARCH GROUP. 1988. Factors in the development of diabetic neuropathy. Diabetes **37:** 476–481.
36. MADSBAD, S., E. LAURITZEN, O. K. FABER & C. BINDER. 1986. The effect of residual beta-cell function on the development of diabetic retinopathy. Diabetes Med. **3:** 42–45.
37. BODANSKY, H. J., S. MEDBAK, P. L. DRURY & A. G. CUDWORTH. 1981. Plasma C-peptide in long-standing type 1 diabetics with and without microvascular complications. Diabetes Med. **7:** 265–269.
38. SBERNA, P., U. VALENTINI, A. CIMINO, M. SABATTI, A. ROTONDI, M. CRISTIQ & S. SPANDRIO. 1986. Residual B-cell function in insulin dependent (type 1) diabetics with and without retinopathy. Acta Diabetol Lat. **23:** 339–344.
39. BIRES, B., W. FOLLANSBEE & T. ORCHARD. 1989. Does residual beta-cell function relate to the complications of IDDM? (abstract) Diabetes **38**(Suppl. 1): 91A.
40. SMITH, R. B. W., D. A. PYKE, P. J. WATKINS, C. BINDER & O. K. FABER. 1979. C-peptide response to glucagon in diabetics with and without complications. N. Zealand Med. J. **89:** 304–306.
41. HAUMONT, D., H. BORCHY, D. TOUSSAINT & M. DESPONTIN. 1982. Exogenous insulin needs. Relationship with duration of diabetes, C-peptidemia, insulin antibodies, and retinopathy. Helv. Paediatr. Acta **37:** 143–150.
42. DIABETES EPIDEMIOLOGY RESEARCH INTERNATIONAL. 1987. Preventing insulin dependent diabetes mellitus: the environmental challenge. Br. Med. J. **295:** 479–481.
43. SAVILAHTI, E., J. TUOMILEHTO, T. T. SAUKKONEN, H. K. AKERBLOM & E. T. VIRTALA. 1993. Increased levels of cow's milk and beta-lactoglobulin antibodies in young children with newly diagnosed IDDM. Diabetes Care **16:** 984–989.
44. BINGLEY, P. J., E. BONIFACIO & E. A. M. GALE. 1993. Can we really predict IDDM? Diabetes **42:** 213–220.
45. JOHNSON, S. B., W. J. RILEY, C. A. HANSEN & M. A. NURICK. 1990. Psychological impact of islet-cell antibody screening. Diabetes Care **13:** 93–97.
46. BONIFACIO, E., P. J. BINGLEY, B. M. DEAN, M. SHATTUCK, D. DDUNGER, E. A. M. GALE & G. F. BOTTAZO. 1990. Quantification of islet-cell antibodies and prediction of insulin-dependent diabetes. Lancet **335:** 147–149.
47. MCCULLOCH, D. K., L. J. KLAFF, S. E. KAHN, S. L. SCHOENFIELD, C. J. GREENBAUM, R. S. MAUSETH, E. A. BENSON, G. T. NEPOM, L. SHEWAY & J. P. PALMER. 1990. A prospective

study of subclinical beta-cell dysfunction among first-degree relatives of IDDM patients: 5 yr follow-up of the Seattle family study. Diabetes **39:** 549–556.

48. DUPRE, J., I. HRAMIAK, J. L. MAHON & C. R. STILLER. 1990. Induction and pathophysiology of remission of insulin-dependent diabetes mellitus during administration of cyclosporin. Horm. Res. **33:** 152–158.

49. PATRICK, S. L., C. S. MOY & R. E. LAPORTE. 1989. The world of insulin-dependent diabetes mellitus: what international epidemiologic studies reveal about the etiology and natural history of IDDM. Diabetes Metab. Rev. **5:** 571–578.

50. NERUP, J., T. MANDRUP-POULSEN, J. MOLVIG, S. HELQVIST, L. WOGENSEN & J. EGEBERG. 1988. Mechanisms of pancreatic beta-cell destruction in type 1 diabetes. Diabetes Care. **11**(Suppl. 1): 16–23.

51. THE DCCT RESEARCH GROUP. 1988. Reliability and validity of a diabetes quality-of-life measure for the diabetes control and complications trial (DCCT). Diabetes Care **11:** 275–32.

Strategies in Immunotherapy of Insulin-Dependent Diabetes Mellitus

JEAN-FRANÇOIS BACH

Hopital Necker
Immunologie Clinique
161 rue de Sevres
75743 Paris Cedex 15, France

INTRODUCTION: NEED FOR ALTERNATIVE TREATMENT TO INSULIN

Insulin therapy is a good treatment of insulin-dependent diabetes mellitus (IDDM). When adequately applied, it avoids the occurrence of the severe manifestations of ketoacidosis and delays the onset of degenerative complications. However, insulin therapy is unsatisfactory in several regards.

In the first place, due to its discontinuous administration, it does not allow the diabetic patient to respond to physiological variations in glucose levels, leading to long periods of hyperglycemia. It is generally assumed that the longer these periods, the higher the risk of degenerative complications. In fact, these degenerative complications do occur in a high percentage of cases after a few decades.

Additionally, insulin therapy exposes patients to the discomfort and (potentially lethal) risks of hypoglycemia and imposes a number of constraints, linked to the requirement for daily monitoring of glucose metabolism and repeated subcutaneous injections. Lastly, insulin therapy is particularly difficult to adapt for use in adolescents.

The question has been raised as to the relative weight of these difficulties compared to the potential risks of immunointervention. This is a difficult problem, particularly since risks associated with immunological treatment are very variable, depending on the methods used, and to some extent they are not fully appreciated as far as the long-term outcome is concerned. One would ideally like to be able to stop insulin in a complete and definitive fashion while keeping satisfactory metabolic control. If this goal is not achievable, it is also important to consider the possibility of delaying for a few years the onset of insulin therapy, particularly in childhood, or to ensure optimal metabolic control, when it is not accessible by insulin therapy.

IMMUNOPREVENTION OF IDDM IN ANIMAL MODELS

A wide array of immunosuppressive agents have been shown capable of preventing the onset of IDDM in the NOD mouse and in the BB rat. These agents are listed in TABLE 1. Most of these agents have been used in this context prophylactically, before the appearance of overt diabetes and even often before insulitis. The list of agents shown to still be active once diabetes is clinically apparent or to prevent the transfer of diabetes afforded by spleen cells derived from diabetic mice is much shorter. It would be interesting to determine the correspondence between the stages at which immunosuppression is still efficacious in experimental models and the corresponding stages of the human disease, as defined below.

364

TABLE 1. Immunotherapy of Diabetes in NOD Mice

Agent	References	Prevention Treatment Started ≤3 Months of Age	Prevention of Diabetes Transfer	Prevention of Cytoxan Induced IDDM	Treatment of Overt Diabetes
Immunosuppressive agents					
Cyclosporin	15	+			±
FK506	16, 18, 59	+		+	
Rapamycin	19	+			−
ALS	13		+		
Monoclonal antibodies					
αCD3	8, 20	+			+
αTCR	21	+		+	+
αVβ8	22			+	
αCD4	9, 13, 23–25	+	+	+	+
αCD8	13, 26 Our unpublished data	+	+	+	+
αclass II	27	+	+ (neonate)	+	
αclass I	28			+	
αIL-2R	29	+			
αCD45RA	30	+			
αγIFN	31, 32		+	+	
αIL-6	32		+	+	
Cytokines					
IL-1	33, 34	+	+		
IL-4	75	+			
TNFα	33, 35	+	+		
DAB 486 IL-2	10		+		
Immunomodulations					
Ciamexone	36	+??			
LZ8	37	+			
THI tetra OH butyl imidazole	38		+		+
OK432	39, 40	+			
CFA	41–43	+			
BCG	44	+		+	
Miscellaneous					
Antioxydants	45	+ (with steroids)			
Vitamin D3	46				
Gangliosides	47	+			
Con A	48	+			
Hsp65/peptide	49	+			
Insulin (parenteral)	50, 51	+	+		
Insuline (oral)	52	+			
Diets	53	+			±−
Nicotinamide	54	+			
Immunoglobulins	55	+			
Silica	56	+		+	

REMISSIONS OF HUMAN DIABETES INDUCED BY
IMMUNOSUPPRESSIVE AGENTS

A number of agents have been used to induce remission of human IDDM. Only a limited number of these studies were controlled in an adequate way. In fact, only three studies using cyclosporin were randomized with a placebo group.[1–7] Another study using azathioprine and steroids was also performed with a randomized protocol but without a placebo group (impossible to introduce for practical reasons).[63] All other studies were essentially pilot nonrandomized studies, the interpretation of which is made difficult because of the common spontaneous evolution of IDDM towards remission in the year following the first requirement for insulin (honeymoon). TABLE 2 presents the main studies reported so far. It is important to mention that all patients enrolled in these studies were treated by insulin for less than two months. Importantly, the remission rate was strictly dependent upon the duration of disease at onset of immunosuppressive treatment and on initial C peptide levels.[1–4]

It could be shown in the most recent cyclosporin studies that remissions could be obtained with minimal immediate toxicity (notably nephrotoxicity, as proven by renal biopsy) and without opportunistic infections. The metabolic control was at least as good as that achieved with conventional insulin therapy (HbA1c < 6.5%).

Few immunotherapy studies have been performed in prediabetic subjects (subjects at risk of diabetes presenting no sign of carbohydrate metabolism disturbance). None of these studies was randomized against placebo, which is absolutely mandatory in this setting in view of the imperfect reliability of the prediction of the definition of the prediabetic state.

LIMITATIONS OF CONVENTIONAL IMMUNOSUPPRESSION IN
RECENTLY DIAGNOSED DIABETICS

The induction of human IDDM remissions by cyclosporin and azathioprine has had the important merit of confirming that human IDDM, like NOD mouse or BB

TABLE 2. Therapeutic Trials in Human IDDM

	Reference
Immunosuppressive agents	
Cyclosporine	1–7
+ nicotinamide	57
+ bromocriptine	58
FK 506	59
Corticosteroids	60
Azathioprine	61, 62
+ corticosteroids	63
+ thymostimulin	64
Miscellaneous	
Nicotinamide	65, 66, 67, 68, 69
Insulin	70
iv immunoglobulins	71
Lymphocyte transfusion	72
Pancreatic irradiation	73
Thymopoietin	74

TABLE 3. Cyclosporine in IDDM: Results of Placebo-Controlled Trials

	Complete Remission Rate (%)		
	6 Months	9 Months	12 Months
CDF study (n = 122)[2]			
CyA (all patients)	25.4	22.4	17.5
(CyA > 300 ng/ml,			
trough blood level)	(37.5)	(37.0)	(32.3)
placebo	18.6	5.8	0
Can-Eur study[3]			
CyA	38.7	—	24.2
(CyA, sympt < 6 weeks)	(55.3)	—	(31.6)
placebo	19.1	—	9.8

rat IDDM, is of autoimmune origin and that the remarkable results obtained with various forms of immunointervention in these animal models should be applicable to the human disease.

It remains true, however, that it is hard to envisage their generalized application at the present time because of three areas of difficulty:

- An insufficient rate of response.
- The relapses that occur rapidly when stopping the immunosuppressive treatment, less rapidly but also consistently when continuing the treatment.
- Side effects essentially linked to the direct drug toxicity (no manifestation of overimmunosuppression has so far been observed).

Insufficient Remission Rate

The rate of cyclosporin-induced remission was overall 27% at one year and 17.5% at two years[5] when considering complete remissions from insulin dependency. Figures were higher when considering optimizing patient selection conditions (early therapy as assessed by C peptide values) and cyclosporin administration (blood trough levels > 300 ng/ml) (TABLE 3). These results were confirmed in studies performed in Paris since the completion of the CDF study.

However, a significant percentage of patients still do not respond to cyclosporin even when considering these optimal conditions. In addition, such conditions are difficult to meet in individual cases inasmuch as many patients are not referred to the specialized center in due time.

The absence of predictive factors of remission, other than high remaining β cell mass (or related parameters such as weight loss or duration of disease symptoms), or even of genetic (HLA) or immunologic (autoantibodies) factors, indicates that most patients, like NOD mice and BB rats, should be sensitive to immunointervention if the treatment were applied earlier.

Solutions

Improving the remission rate involves earlier intervention (at the prediabetes stage) as well as more immediate and complete damping of the islet-specific autoimmune response than that afforded by cyclosporin.

Relapses of Diabetes

As also shown in animal models, diabetes reappears soon after cessation of immunosuppressive therapy (1–3 months), a problem seen with all autoimmune diseases treated with any chemical immunosuppressive agent. This observation indicates that immunosuppression does not induce any state of tolerance but rather acts by allowing transient "freezing" of the autoimmune response.

More disappointingly, diabetes relapses also appear when the immunosuppressive treatment is continued.[6] The onset of relapses is then delayed (1–4 years), but all patients finally relapse. The longest remissions so far reported were 3–4 years. In fact, the appearance of these relapses could have been predicted in view of previous data showing that partial pancreatectomy (80%) in normal rats ultimately leads to chronic hyperglycemia. One assumes that reduced β cell mass leads to transient hyperglycemia which in turn induces insulin resistance and glucotoxicity. It has indeed been shown, both in children and in adults, that relapses occurring under cyclosporin were essentially of the metabolic type, due to insulin resistance (within good persisting C peptide levels).

Solutions

Prevention of immunologic relapses requires induction of tolerance to islet autoantigen. Avoiding metabolic relapses requires earlier intervention.

Hazards of Immunosuppressive Treatment

Immunosuppressive treatments are associated with a number of side effects. One must distinguish those related to direct drug toxicity and those that are the consequence of overimmunosuppression. It should be realized, however, that these complications are not observed at a similar rate as in organ transplantation, due to the lower intensity of immunosuppression used and to the shorter treatment duration.

Concern for drug-induced toxicity has essentially focussed so far around the problem of cyclosporin-induced nephrotoxicity. Some nephrotoxicity was indeed demontrated in the initial studies,[2–3] although it was always moderate. None of the patients treated in Paris, even the first few that showed moderate nephrotoxicity on renal biopsies, have today any sign of renal failure (as studied by creatinine clearance).[7] Monitoring drug dosage according to creatininemia and drug blood levels has permitted the avoidance of the occurrence of harmful toxicity. It remains that this potential risk complicates the drug handling, and one would fear a higher toxicity if the drug usage were generalized to nonspecialized centers.

Overimmunosuppression-associated side effects (opportunistic infections, malignancies) have not been a significant problem so far (TABLE 4), but one cannot claim that this would still be the case for longer duration treatments.

Solutions

One can hope to reduce direct drug toxicity by using less toxic drugs. Unfortunately, no drug has been convincingly shown so far to be as efficient as cyclosporin with less toxicity (including cyclosporin analogues, azathioprine, FK506 and mycophenolic acid).

Drug combinations, as used in organ transplantation, are an alternative possibility, but one is reluctant to expose diabetic patients to the risks of overimmunosuppression that this may potentially involve.

The alternative solution is obviously to reduce the duration of immunosuppressive treatment by inducing tolerance.

IMMEDIATE AND COMPLETE "FREEZING" OF THE ANTIISLET AUTOIMMUNE RESPONSE

Experience in organ transplantation has fully demontrated that cyclosporin A and azathioprine are essentially active in prophylaxis of immune responses. They may show some effect on established response as long as the response is not too intense, but in this case the effect is not immediate (1–2 weeks). These limitations explain why these agents are not used in the treatment of acute rejection episodes. One prefers in this setting to use antilymphocyte antibodies (ALG, anti–T cell

TABLE 4. Absence of Overimmunosuppression in Cyclosporin-Treated Diabetics (CDF Study)

	Cyclosporine	Placebo
Infections		
Benign	37/61	26/54
Severe	0	0
Lymphomas	0/657	0/150
Ig abnormality (IEF)[a]	0/59	0/38

[a]IEF: isoelectrofocussing of serum.

monoclonals) or high-dose steroids. One may tentatively interpret this insufficient effect of these drugs in this hyperimmune status by assuming that the drug effects are then overwhelmed by the intensity of cytokine production and expression of their receptors.

These comments probably apply to recent onset IDDM where the islet specific T cell response is at its highest level at the time of emergence of insulin dependency. In this context one should rather use agents whose action is not limited by T cell hyperactivity. Monoclonal antibodies reacting with antigens whose expression on T cell membrane is not affected by cell activation (e.g., CD3, CD4) can be used. There are even agents whose action may be increased during T cell activation, such as IL-2 toxin conjugates whose binding to T cell IL-2 receptors is favored by activation.

Studies in the NOD mouse indicate that anti-CD3,[8] anti-CD4,[9] and IL-2 toxin[10] still show a strong immunosuppressive effect when applied in this context (diabetes transfer, overt diabetes). Conversely, cyclosporin rapidly loses its efficacy after mice have become diabetic.[11]

We were ourselves interested in two approaches of this type. Four patients were treated with OKT3, an anti-CD3 monoclonal antibody. Unfortunately, the study had to be stopped because of the intensity of the symptoms associated with the first injection of the antibody (chills, fever, headache, prostration, diarrhea, vomiting). In

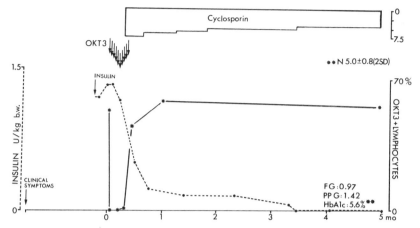

FIGURE 1. Treatment of a recently diagnosed diabetic patient with OKT3 (5 mg) followed by cyclosporin (abbreviations: FG, fasting glycemia; PPG, postprandial glycemia).

the only patient who received 5 injections, a decrease in insulin need was observed (FIGURE 1). In the same vein, more recently, we undertook an open label trial with DAB486 IL-2, a DNA recombinant manifactured conjugate of human IL-2 and diphtheria toxin fragment B. Cyclosporin treatment was started 45 days after the 2-week IL-2 toxin treatment but at a dosage (5 mg/kg per d) known not to induce remission of IDDM, particularly when started as late as 2–3 months after initiation of insulin therapy. Results shown in FIGURE 2 are very much in favor of a therapeutic effect when compared to the latest historical consecutive series of patients treated with cyclosporin alone (at 7.5 mg/kg per d). The frequency of remission was at least as high as with cyclosporin. The effect was paradoxically better with the lowest IL-2 toxin dose, suggesting that the highest dose induced some β cell toxicity or inhibited

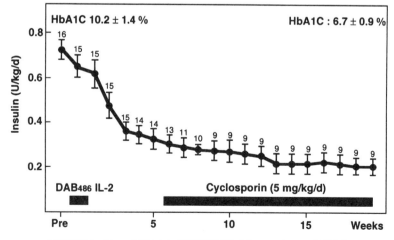

FIGURE 2. Phase I/II trial of DAB486 IL-2 in recent onset IDDM.

some IL-2 receptor positive suppressor cells. There was no significant cyclosporin-induced nephrotoxicity. One may assume that IL-2 toxin treatment induced a rapid clearance of intraislet IL-2 receptor bearing activated T cells, that cannot be achieved by cyclosporin alone.

SEARCH FOR TOLERANCE

The autoantigen(s) triggering the anti-islet T cell response at the origin of IDDM is not determined, making the search for tolerance induction protocols difficult. Some experimental studies in the NOD mouse suggest that tolerance can be induced by administration of recombinant glutamic acid decarboxylase (GAD), but these data need confirmation with adequate controls and extension to include treatment of mice with established insulitis and disease.

Another approach consists of using the β cell autoantigens present in the few persisting β cells by targeting the other components of the antigen recognition complex: MHC molecules, the TCR/CD3 complex, or other transduction associated molecules (CD4).

We have obtained results in the NOD mouse that indicate the feasibility of this approach. Anti-H-2 class II monoclonal antibodies prevent the onset of IDDM when applied before two months of age.[12] The prevention is complete and definitive without further treatment. It is resistant to cyclophosphamide. However, the treatment is no longer effective if applied after two months of age.

Conversely, anti-CD3 monoclonal antibody therapy begun shortly after the mice have become diabetic induces long-term remission of diabetes.[8] The remission is not immediate, taking 4–6 weeks to be complete. It is then usually permanent, at least over the four months of follow-up. Interestingly, the remissions are not associated with the clearing of insulitis which is still prevalent with both CD4 and CD8 T cells.

Similar results have been reported for antilyphocyte serum and mixtures of depleting anti-CD4 and anti-CD8 monoclonal antibodies.[13]

It will be interesting to assess the capacity of other methods (parenteral GAD, oral GAD, or insulin) to achieve similar tolerance states when applied as late as was performed with the anti-CD3 antibody.

EARLY TREATMENT

Most of the approaches discussed above would clearly be improved if immunotherapy could be applied earlier, when more β cells persist, at a time when hopefully the autoimmune response is more sensitive to immunointervention. The large number of treatments active at this stage in the NOD mouse (TABLE 1) is self-explanatory. In fact, one could even hope at the earliest stages to successfully apply relatively nonspecific therapies such as those based on favorable environmental factors (diets, nonspecific immunostimulation such as that generated by viral or bacterial infections), or β cell protection (the concept behind the use of nicotinamide). Preferably, one could think of using the tolerance-inducing procedures discussed in the preceding section.

Early therapy is dependent on precocious and reliable prediction. The improved knowledge of IDDM-predisposing genes (HLA, TAP 2),[14] and non-HLA genes (essentially known so far only in the mouse) allows at least for the present time improved focussing on subjects at risk, in diabetics' families. The emergence of new autoantibody assays (GAD, BSA) complementing the already very highly predictive ICAs gives hope that the prediction rate should progressively reach values over 90%, a mandatory condition to propose preventive methods on a large scale.

SUMMARY AND CONCLUSIONS

Complete and definitive prevention of diabetes obtained in animal models by using a number of diversified maneuvers has elicited major hope for immunoprevention of the disease in man. Therapeutic trials of immunosuppressive drugs in human IDDM have opened the way towards prevention or cure of the disease. Difficulties encountered, including requirement for chronic immunosuppression and risk of metabolic relapses, suggest two complementary approaches: precocious intervention based on early and reliable disease prediction, and tolerance-inducing regimens, hopefully using shorter and innocuous therapy. Animal data suggest that this is indeed an achievable goal.

REFERENCES

1. ASSAN, R., G. FEUTREN, J. SIRMAI, C. LABORIE, C. BOITARD, P. VEXIAU, H. DU ROSTU, M. RODIER, M. FIGONI, P. VAGUE, J. HORS & J. F. BACH. 1990. Plasma C-peptide levels and clinical remissions in recent-onset type 1 diabetic patients treated with cyclosporin A and insulin. Diabetes **39:** 768–774.
2. FEUTREN, G., L. PAPOZ, R. ASSAN, B. VIALETTES, G. KARSENTY, P. VEXIAU, H. DU ROSTU, M. RODIER, J. SIRMAI, A. LALLEMAND & J. F. BACH. 1986. Cyclosporin increases the rate and length of remissions in insulin-dependent diabetes of recent onset. Lancet **2:** 119–124.
3. CANADIAN-EUROPEAN RANDOMIZED CONTROL TRIAL GROUP. 1988. Cyclosporin-induced remission of IDDM after early intervention. Association of 1 yr of cyclosporin treatment with enhanced insulin secretion. Diabetes, **37:** 1574–1582.
4. BOUGNÈRES, P. F., J. C. CAREL, L. CASTANO, C. BOITARD, J. P. GARDIN, P. LANDAIS, J. HORS, M. J. MIHATSCH, M. PAILLARD, J. L. CHAUSSAIN & J. F. BACH. 1988. Factors associated with early remission of type I diabetes in children treated with cyclosporine. N. Engl. J. Med. **318:** 663–670.
5. ASSAN, R., G. FEUTREN & J. SIRMAI. 1988. Cyclosporin trials in diabetes: updated results of the French experience. Transplant Proc. **20:** 178–183.
6. BOUGNÈRES, P. F., P. LANDAIS, C. BOISSON, J. C. CAREL, N. FRAMENT, C. BOITARD, J. L. CHAUSSAIN & J. F. BACH. 1990. Limited duration of remission of insulin dependency in children with recent overt type I diabetes treated with low-dose cyclosporin. Diabetes **39:** 1264–1272.
7. ASSAN, R., J. TIMSIT, G. FEUTREN, P. BOUGNÈRES, P. CZERNICHOW, T. HANNEDOUCHE, C. BOITARD, L. H. NOEL, M. J. MIHATSCH & J. F. BACH. The kidney of cyclosporine-treated diabetic patients: a long-term clinico-pathologic study. Clin. Nephrol. (In press.)
8. CHATENOUD, L., E. THERVET, J. PRIMO & J. F. BACH. 1992. Remission of established diabetes in diabetic NOD mice using anti-CD3 monoclonal antibody. C. R. Acad. Sci. Paris **315:** 225–228.
9. HUTCHINGS, P., L. O'REILLY, N. M. PARISH, H. WALDMANN & A. COOKE. 1992. The use of a non-depleting anti-CD4 monoclonal antibody to re-establish tolerance to β cells in NOD mice. Eur. J. Immunol. **22:** 1913–1918.
10. PACHECO-SILVA, A., M. G. BASTOS, R. A. MUGGIA, O. PANKEWYCZ, J. NICHOLS, J. R. MURPHY, T. B. STROM & V. E. RUBIN-KELLEY. 1992. Interleukin 2 receptor targeted fusion toxin (DAB486-IL-2) treatment blocks diabetogenic autoimmunity in non-obese diabetic mice. Eur. J. Immunol. **22:** 697–702.

11. WANG, Y., M. MCDUFFIE, I. N. NOMIKOS, L. HAO & K. J. LAFFERTY. 1988. Effect of cyclosporine on immunologically mediated diabetes in nonobese diabetic mice. Transplantation 46(Suppl. 2): 101–106.

12. TIMSIT, J., W. SAVINO, C. BOITARD & J. F. BACH. 1989. The role of class II major histocompatibility complex antigens in autoimmune diabetes: animal models. J. Autoimmun. 2 (Suppl.): 115–129.

13. MAKI, T., T. ICHIKAWA, R. BLANCO & J. PORTER. 1992. Long-term abrogation of autoimmune diabetes in nonobese diabetic mice by immunotherapy with anti-lymphocyte serum. Proc. Natl. Acad. Sci. USA 89: 3434–3438.

14. CAILLAT-ZUCMAN, S., E. BERTIN, J. TIMSIT, C. BOITARD, R. ASSAN & J. F. BACH. 1992. TAP1 and TAP2 transporter genes and predisposition to insulin dependent diabetes mellitus. C. R. Acad. Sci. Paris 315: 535–539.

15. MORI, Y., M. SUKO, H. OKUDAIRA, I. MATSUBA, A. TSURUOKA, A. SASAKI, H. YOKOYAMA, T. TANASE, T. SHIDA, M. NISHIMURA, E. TERADA & Y. IKEDA. 1986. Preventive effects of cyclosporin on diabetes in NOD mice. Diabetologia 29: 244–247.

16. MIYAGAWA, J., K. YAMAMOTO, T. HANAFUSA, N. ITOH, C. NAKAGAWA, A. OTSUKA, H. KATSURA, K. YAMAGATA, A. MIYAZAKI, N. KONO & S. TARUI. 1990. Preventive effect of a new immunosuppressant FK-506 on insulitis and diabetes in nonobese diabetic mice. Diabetologia 33: 503–505.

17. CARROLL, P. B., A. G. TZAKIS, C. RICORDI, H. R. RILO, K. ABU-EL-MAGD, N. MURASE, Y. J. ZENG, R. ALEJANDRO, D. MINTZ & T. E. STARZL. 1991. The use of FK 506 in new-onset type I diabetes in man. Transplant. Proc. 23: 3351–3353.

18. STRASSER, S., J. CEARNS-SPIELMAN, P. CARROLL & R. ALEJANDRO. 1992. Effect of FK 506 on cyclophosphamide-induced diabetes in NOD mice. Diabetes Nutr. Metab. 5: 61–63.

19. BAEDER, W. L., J. SREDY, S. N. SEHGAL, J. Y. CHANG & L. M. ADAMS. 1992. Rapamycin prevents the onset of insulin-dependent diabetes mellitus (IDDM) in NOD mice. Clin. Exp. Immunol. 89: 174–178.

20. HAYWARD, A. R. & M. SHRIBER. 1992. Reduced incidence of insulitis in NOD mice following anti-CD3 injection: requirement for neonatal injection. J. Autoimmun. 5: 59–67.

21. SEMPÉ, P., P. BÉDOSSA, M. F. RICHARD, M. C. VILLA, J. F. BACH & C. BOITARD. 1991. Anti-α/β T cell receptor monoclonal antibody provides an efficient therapy for autoimmune diabetes in nonobese diabetic (NOD) mice. Eur. J. Immunol. 21: 1163–1169.

22. BACELJ, A., B. CHARLTON & T. E. MANDEL. 1989. Prevention of cyclophosphamide-induced diabetes by anti-Vβ8 T-lymphocyte-receptor monoclonal antibody therapy in NOD/Wehi mice. Diabetes 38: 1492–1495.

23. WANG, Y., L. HAO, R. G. GILL & K. J. LAFFERTY. 1987. Autoimmune diabetes in NOD mouse is L3T4 T-lymphocyte dependent. Diabetes 36: 535–538.

24. KOIKE, T., Y. ITOH, T. ISHII, I. ITO, K. TAKABAYASHI, N. MARUYAMA, H. TOMIOKA & S. YOSHIDA. 1987. Preventive effect of monoclonal anti-L3T4 antibody on development of diabetes in NOD mice. Diabetes 36: 539–541.

25. SHIZURU, J. A., C. TAYLOR-EDWARDS, B. A. BANKS, A. K. GREGORY & C. G. FATHMAN. 1988. Immunotherapy of the nonobese diabetic mouse: treatment with an antibody to T-helper lymphocytes. Science 240: 659–662.

26. HUTCHINGS, P. R., E. SIMPSON, L. A. O'REILLY, T. LUND, H. WALDMANN & A. COOKE. 1990. The involvement of Ly2+ T cells in beta cell destruction. J. Autoimmun. 3: 101–109.

27. BOITARD, C., A. BENDELAC, M. F. RICHARD, C. CARNAUD & J. F. BACH. 1988. Prevention of diabetes in nonobese diabetic mice by anti-I-A monoclonal antibodies. Transfer of protection by splenic T cells. Proc. Natl. Acad. Sci. USA 85: 9719–9723.

28. TAKI, T., M. NAGATA, W. OGAWA, N. HATAMORI, M. HAYAKAWA, J. HARI, K. SHII, S. BABA & K. YOKONO. 1991. Prevention of cyclophosphamide-induced and spontaneous diabetes in NOD/Shi/Kbe mice by anti-MHC class-I Kd monoclonal antibody. Diabetes 40: 1203–1209.

29. KELLEY, V. E., G. N. GAULTON, M. HATTORI, H. IKEGAMI, G. EISENBARTH & T. B. STROM. 1988. Anti-interleukin 2 receptor antibody suppresses murine diabetic insulitis and lupus nephritis. J. Immunol. 140: 59–61.

30. SEMPÉ, P., S. EZINE, J. MARVEL, P. BÉDOSSA, M. F. RICHARD, J. F. BACH & C. BOITARD. Role of CD4+CD45TA+ T cells in the development of autoimmune diabetes in the non-obese diabetic (NOD) mouse. Int. Immunol. (In press.)

31. DEBRAY-SACHS, M., C. CARNAUD, C. BOITARD, H. COHEN, I. GRESSER, P. BEDOSSA & J. F. BACH. 1991. Prevention of diabetes in NOD mice treated with antibody to murine IFNγ. J. Autoimmun. **4:** 237–248.

32. CAMPBELL, I. L., T. W. H. KAY, L. OXBROW & L. C. HARRISON. 1991. Essential role for interferon gamma and interleukin-6 in autoimmune insulin-dependent diabetes in NOD/WEHI mice. J. Clin. Invest. **87:** 739–742.

33. JACOB, C. O., S. AISO, S. A. MICHIE, H. O. MCDEVITT & H. ACHA-ORBEA. 1990. Prevention of diabetes in nonobese diabetic mice by tumor necrosis factor (TNF): similarities between TNF-alpha and interleukin 1. Proc. Natl. Acad. Sci. USA **87:** 968–972.

34. FORMBY, B., C. JACOBS, P. DUBUC & T. SHAO. 1992. Exogenous administration of IL-1 α inhibits active and adoptive transfer autoimmune diabetes in NOD mice. Autoimmunity **12:** 21–27.

35. SATOH, J., H. SEINO, T. ABO, S. TANAKA, S. SHINTANI, S. OHTA, K. TAMURA, T. SAWAI, T. NOBUNAGA, T. OTEKI, K. KUMAGAI & T. TOYOTA. 1989. Recombinant human tumor necrosis factor α suppresses autoimmune diabetes in nonobese diabetic mice. J. Clin. Invest. **84:** 1345–1348.

36. KRUG, J., E. F. LAMPETER, A. J. K. WILLIAMS, E. PROCACCINI, C. CARTLEDGE, A. SIGNORE, P. E. BEALES & P. POZZILLI. 1992. Immunotherapy with ciamexon in the non obese diabetic (NOD) mouse. Horm. Metab. Res. **24:** 1–4.

37. KINO, K., K. MIZUMOTO, T. SONE, T. YAMAJI, J. WATANABE, A. YAMASHITA, K. YAMAOKA, K. SHIMIZU, K. KO & H. TSUNOO. 1990. An immunomodulating protein Ling Zhi-8 (LZ-8) prevents insulitis in non-obese diabetic mice. Diabetologia **33:** 713–718.

38. MANDEL, T. E., M. KOULMANDA & I. R. MACKAY. 1992. Prevention of spontaneous and cyclophosphamide-induced diabetes in non-obese diabetic (NOD) mice with oral 2-acetyl-4-tetrahydroxybutylimidazole (THI), a component of caramel colouring III. Clin. Exp. Immunol. **88:** 414–419.

39. TOYOTA, T., J. SATOH, K. OYA, S. SHINTANI & T. OKANO. 1986. Streptococcal preparation (OK-432) inhibits development of type I diabetes in NOD mice. Diabetes **35:** 496–499.

40. SHINTANI, S., J. SATOH, H. SEINO, Y. GOTO & T. TOYOTA. 1990. Mechanism of action of a streptococcal preparation (OK-432) in prevention of autoimmune diabetes in NOD mice. Suppression of generation of effector cells for pancreatic B cell destruction. J. Immunol. **144:** 136–141.

41. SADELAIN, M. W. J., H. Y. QIN, J. LAUZON & B. SINGH. 1990. Prevention of type I diabetes in NOD mice by adjuvant immunotherapy. Diabetes **39:** 583–589.

42. MCINERNEY, M. F., S. B. PEK & D. W. THOMAS. 1991. Prevention of insulitis and diabetes onset by treatment with complete Freund's adjuvant in NOD mice. Diabetes **40:** 715–725.

43. ULAETO, D., P. E. LACY, D. M. KIPNIS, O. KANAGAWA & E. R. UNANUE. 1992. A T-cell dormant state in the autoimmune process of nonobese diabetic mice treated with complete Freund's adjuvant. Proc. Natl. Acad. Sci. USA **89:** 3927–3931.

44. HARADA, M., Y. KISHIMOTO & S. MAKINO. 1990. Prevention of overt diabetes and insulitis in NOD mice by a single BCG vaccination. Diabetes Res. Clin. Pract. **8:** 85–89.

45. RABINOVITCH, A., W. L. SUAREZ & R. F. POWER. 1992. Combination therapy with an antioxidant and a cordicosteroid prevents autoimmune diabetes in NOD mice. Life Sci. **51:** 1937–1943.

46. MATHIEU, C., J. LAUREYS, H. SOBIS, M. VANDEPUTTE, M. WAER & R. BOUILLON. 1992. 1,25-Dihydroxyvitamin D3 prevents insulitis in NOD mice. Diabetes **41:** 1491–1495.

47. WILBERZ, S., L. HERBERG & A. E. RENOLD. 1988. Gangliosides in vivo reduce diabetes incidence in non-obese diabetic mice. Diabetologia **31:** 855–857.

48. PEARCE, R. B. & C. M. PETERSON. 1991. Studies of concanavalin A in nonobese diabetic mice. I. Prevention of insulin-dependent diabetes. J. Pharmacol. Exp. Ther. **258:** 710–715.

49. ELIAS, D., D. MARKOVITS, T. RESHEF, R. VAN DER ZEE & I. R. COHEN. 1990. Induction and therapy of autoimmune diabetes in the non-obese diabetic (NOD/LT) mouse by a 65-kDa heat shock protein. Proc. Natl. Acad. Sci USA 87: 1576–1580.

50. ATKINSON, M. A., N. K. MACLAREN & R. LUCHETTA. 1990. Insulitis and diabetes in NOD mice reduced by prophylactic insulin therapy. Diabetes 39: 933–937.

51. THIVOLET, C. H., E. GOILLOT, P. BEDOSSA, A. DURAND, M. BONNARD & J. ORGIAZZI. 1991. Insulin prevents adoptive cell transfer of diabetes in the autoimmune non-obese diabetic mouse. Diabetologia 34: 314–319.

52. ZHANG, Z. J., L. DAVIDSON, G. EISENBARTH & H. L. WEINER. 1991. Suppression of diabetes in nonobese diabetic mice by oral administration of porcine insulin. Proc. Natl. Acad. Sci. USA 88: 10252–10256.

53. ELLIOTT, R. B., S. N. REDDY, N. J. BIBBY & K. KIDA. 1988. Dietary prevention of diabetes in the non-obese diabetic mouse. Diabetologia 31: 62–64.

54. YAMADA, K., K. NONAKA, T. HANAFUSA, A. MIYAZAKI, H. TOYOSHIMA & S. TARUI. 1982. Preventive and therapeutic effects of large-dose nicotinamide injections on diabetes associated with insulitis. An observation in nonobese diabetic (NOD) mice. Diabetes 31: 749–753.

55. FORSGREN, S., A. ANDERSSON, V. HILLÖRN, A. SÖDERSTRÖM & D. HOLMBERG. 1991. Immunoglobulin-mediated prevention of autoimmune diabetes in the non-obese diabetic (NOD) mouse. Scand. J. Immunol. 34: 445–451.

56. CHARLTON, B., A. BACELJ & T. E. MANDEL. 1988. Administration of silica particles or anti-Lyt2 antibody prevents beta-cell destruction in NOD mice given cyclophosphamide. Diabetes 37: 930–935.

57. VIALETTES, B., R. PICQ, M. DU ROSTU, B. CHARBONNEL, M. RODIER, J. MIROUZE, P. VEXIAU, P. PASSA, M. PEHUET & F. ELGRABLY. 1990. A preliminary multicentre study of the treatment of recently diagnosed type 1 diabetes by combination nicotinamide-cyclosporin therapy. Diabet. Med. 7: 731–735.

58. ATKISON, P. R., J. L. MAHON, J. DUPRE, C. R. STILLER, M. R. JENNER, T. L. PAUL & C. I. MOMAH. 1990. Interaction of bromocriptine and cyclosporine in insulin dependent diabetes mellitus: results from the Canadian open study. J. Autoimmun. 3: 793–799.

59. CARROLL, P. B., S. STRASSER & R. ALEJANDRO. 1991. The effect of FK-506 on cyclophosphamide-induced diabetes in the NOD mouse model. Transplant. Proc. 23: 3348–3350.

60. SECCHI, A., M. R. PASTORE, A. SERGI, A. E. PONTIROLI & G. POZZA. 1990. Prednisone administration in recent onset type I diabetes. J. Autoimmun. 3: 593–600.

61. HARRISON, L. C., P. G. COLMAN, B. DEAN, R. BAXTER & F. I. MARTIN. 1985. Increase in remission rate in newly diagnosed type I diabetic subjects treated with azathioprine. Diabetes 34: 1306–1308.

62. COOK, J. J., I. HUDSON, L. C. HARRISON, B. DEAN, P. G. COLMAN, G. A. WERTHER, G. L. WARNE & J. M. COURT. 1989. Double-blind controlled trial of azathioprine in children with newly diagnosed type I diabetes. Diabetes 38: 779–783.

63. SILVERSTEIN, J., N. MACLAREN, W. RILEY, R. SPILLAR, D. RADJENOVIC & S. JOHNSON. 1988. Immunosuppression with azathioprine and prednisone in recent-onset insulin-dependent diabetes mellitus. N. Engl. J. Med. 319: 599–604.

64. MONCADA, E., M. L. SRUBIRA, A. OLEAGA, F. GONI, A. SANCHEZ-IBARROLA, M. MONREAL, M. SEVILLA, M. J. GONI, A. YOLDI, D. TERAN & I. LLORENTE. 1990. Insulin requirements and residual beta-cell function 12 months after concluding immunotherapy in type I diabetic patients treated with combined azathioprine and thymostimulin administration for one year. J. Autoimmun. 3: 625–638.

65. LEWIS, C. M., D. M. CANAFAX, J. M. SPRAFKA & J. J. BARBOSA. 1992. Double-blind randomized trial of nicotinamide on early-onset diabetes. Diabetes Care 15: 121–123.

66. VAGUE, P., R. PICQ, M. BERNAL, V. LASSMANN-VAGUE & B. VIALETTES. 1989. Effect of nicotinamide treatment on the residual insulin secretion in type 1 (insulin-dependent) diabetic patients. Diabetologia 32: 316–321.

67. VAGUE, P., B. VIALETTES, V. LASSMANN-VAGUE & J. J. VALLO. 1987. Nicotinamide may extend remission phase in insulin-dependent diabetes. Lancet 1: 619–620.

68. POZZILLI, P., N. VISALLI, G. GHIRLANDA, R. MANNA & D. ANDREANI. 1989. Nicotinamide increases C-peptide secretion in patients with recent onset type 1 diabetes. Diabet. Med. **6:** 568–572.

69. MENDOLA, G., R. CASAMITJANA & R. GOMIS. 1989. Effect of nicotinamide therapy upon B-cell function in newly diagnosed type 1 (insulin-dependent) diabetic patients. Diabetologia **32:** 160–162.

70. KELLER, R. J., G. S. EISENBARTH & R. A. JACKSON. 1993. Insulin prophylaxis in individuals at high risk of type I diabetes. Lancet **341:** 927–928.

71. PANTO, F., C. GIORDANO, M. P. AMATO, A. PUGLIESE, M. DONATELLI, G. D'ACQUISTO & A. GALLUZZO. 1990. The influence of high dose intravenous immunoglobulins on immunological and metabolic pattern in newly diagnosed type I diabetic patients. J. Autoimmun. **3:** 587–592.

72. KRUG, J., H. I. VERLOHREN, B. BIERWOLF, E. LAMPETER, M. BORTE, U. NIETZSCHMANN, B. HAUSTEIN & D. LOHMANN. 1990. Lymphocyte transfusion in recent onset type I diabetes mellitus—a one-year follow-up of cell-mediated anti-islet cytotoxicity and C-peptide secretion. J. Autoimmun. **3:** 601–609.

73. DEMPE, A., W. BAASKE, R. VON BAEHR, S. KUTTNER, G. NEUBERT & K. NEUMEISTER. 1988. Remission of the newly diagnosed type 1 diabetes by radiation of the pancreas. Exp. Clin. Endocrinol. **92:** 123–125.

74. GIORDANO, C., F. PANTO, M. P. AMATO, N. SAPIENZA, A. PUGLIESE & A. GALLUZZO. 1990. Early administration of an immunomodulator and induction of remission in insulin-dependent diabetes mellitus. J. Autoimmun. **3:** 611–617.

75. RAPOPORT, M. J., A. JARAMILLO, D. ZIPRIS, A. H. LAZARUS, D. V. SERREZE, E. H. LEITER, P. CYOPICK, J. S. DANSKA & T. L. DELOVITCH. 1993. Interleukin 4 reverses T cell proliferative unresponsiveness and prevents the onset of diabetes in nonobese diabetic mice. J. Exp. Med. **178:** 87–99.

New Strategies for Clinical Islet Transplantation

The Role of Purified Grafts and Immunosuppressive Therapy

PAUL F. GORES,[a,c] DIXON B. KAUFMAN,[b]
AND DAVID E. R. SUTHERLAND[a]

[a]Department of Surgery
University of Minnesota Medical School
Minneapolis, Minnesota

[b]Department of Surgery
Northwestern University School of Medicine
Chicago, Illinois

The effectiveness of islet transplantation for the treatment of diabetes was first demonstrated in rodent models more than 20 years ago.[1,2] However, successful application of this approach to diabetic man remains problematic. Much of the blame for the failure of clinical islet transplantation has been ascribed to the nature of the islet preparation obtainable from the human pancreas, and a great deal of effort has focused on the development of more efficient methods of extracting islets in purified form. The dogma has been that avoidance of exocrine contamination is required lest the islets be destroyed by local release of proteolytic enzymes or by the heightened nature of the immune response to the accompanying acinar tissue. The recent demonstration that an insulin-independent state can be achieved by intraportal injection of unpurified preparations of autologous dispersed pancreatic tissue after duodenopancreatectomy invalidates the former,[3] and it is unclear to what degree immunogenicity is increased by the use of impure preparations of pancreatic islet tissue.

The most contaminated islet preparation possible, a whole pancreas, can be transplanted with a rejection rate not substantially different from other organs. It is our contention that innovative antirejection strategies designed to mitigate immune-mediated damage of allogeneic islet tissue, while simultaneously minimizing drug-induced diabetogenic toxicity, will enable islet transplantation to replace pancreas transplantation as the preferred mode of endocrine replacement therapy in uremic diabetic patients receiving a concomitant renal allograft. In this paper, we will review the evidence, such as it exists, regarding the influence contaminating exocrine tissue has on the fate of islet allografts both in respect to engraftment and immunogenicity. The characteristics of the immune response to islets in the form of a non–immediately vascularized graft will be examined and a rationale provided for the design of new immunosuppressive strategies to circumvent this immune response while at the same time minimizing diabetogenic effects of the immunosuppressive agents themselves.

[c]Address correspondence to: Box 277 UMHC, 420 Delaware Street S.E., Minneapolis, MN 55455.

NATURE OF THE ISLET PREPARATION

The initial successes with islet transplantation occurred in rodent models. The pancreas of these animals is flimsy in comparison to the more fibrous human pancreas. If one injects the duct of a rodent pancreas with collagenase solution and raises the temperature to 37°C, the gland readily dissociates, leaving the islets relatively free of contaminating exocrine tissue. It is then a practical matter to hand pick the 500 murine or 1000 rat islets required to reproducibly achieve normoglycemia in these allograft models. The purity of the preparations, in terms of islet tissue, is in excess of 95%. In their original report, Ballinger and Lacy showed that by injecting hand-picked islet preparations into the peritoneal cavity of chemically induced diabetic rats, glycosuria was reduced. However, a simple intraperitoneal injection of totally unpurified dispersed pancreatic tissue did not ameliorate diabetes in the three rats in whom it was tried.[2] In the two decades since these pioneering reports, numerous protocols utilizing purified preparations have been developed that lead to long-term survival of islet allografts in rodent models.[4,5]

In large animals, a minimum of 4000 islet/kg recipient body weight are necessary to restore euglycemia in autograft experiments[6,7] and probably something in excess of 8000 islets/kg are required in the setting of allogeneic islet transplantation.[8] Obviously, hand picking such numbers of islets is not practical. Furthermore, collagenase digestion is somewhat less effective in these large animal models and islets are often not completely separated from their acinar bed. Automated procedures have been developed,[9] but the yield in man is still marginal (3500–7000 islets/kg), with 50–75% of the original islet mass being lost during the final step of gradient centrifugation. Furthermore, the degree of purity (60–90%) is less than what can be obtained by hand picking. In order to obtain an adequate islet mass, most groups have resorted to pooling islets from multiple donors for transplantation to single individuals.

Although the preponderance of evidence suggests that exocrine contamination interferes with engraftment *in rodent models,*[10] the experience in large animals, including man, has been different. The original experiments by Mirkovitch *et al.,* in which autologous unpurified dispersed pancreatic tissue was shown to engraft within the spleen and prevent pancreatectomy-induced diabetes in dogs, suggested that purification would not be necessary in the clinical situation.[11] Other groups confirmed these findings in dogs and observed similar results in subhuman primate models.[12–15] Of more direct relevance to the problem of clinical islet allotransplantation is the experience with intraportal autotransplantation of dispersed pancreatic tissue garnered at the University of Minnesota over the past 15 years.[3] Since 1977, 28 patients have undergone total or near-total pancreatectomy as treatment for intractable chronic pancreatitis. Although the small remnant (less than 5%) of pancreas remaining after near-total pancreatectomy makes interpretation of the fate of the autograft problematic, since 1987 pylorus-saving total duodenopancreatectomy has been performed in eight patients. These pancreases are often fibrotic and have been subjected to previous surgical procedures, making the islet yield less than that attainable from the average cadaver donor pancreas. Nevertheless, since 1987 all five patients who received greater than 100,000 islets (3100 islets/kg recipient body weight) remain insulin independent. This series unequivocally demonstrates that gross exocrine contamination does not prevent islets from engrafting and functioning to maintain euglycemia when the dispersed tissue preparation is injected into the portal circulation. If proteolytic enzymes released by contaminating exocrine tissue in fact are deleterious, their effect is apparently mitigated by the dilution achieved by injection into a large, well-vascularized space.

The theoretical basis for the belief that immunogenicity is heightened by exocrine contamination of islet allografts is embodied in the passenger leukocyte concept.[16,17] Sensitization to alloantigen requires the presence of antigen-presenting cells. The hope has been that by developing procedures that provide very pure islet preparations, and thereby avoiding contamination by passenger leukocytes residing in the exocrine pancreas, immunogenicity will be reduced sufficiently to allow for successful allotransplantation. But a technique for the complete elimination of contaminating elements from the islet preparation has not, as of yet, been devised. Even the purest islet preparations contain significant numbers of lymphoid and dendritic cells capable of antigen presentation.[18] In fact, islets themselves contain an array of tissue types including endothelial and dendritic cells as well as passenger leukocytes. Unfortunately, even their elimination does not ensure success although the data in this regard are conflicting.[19,20]

However, it is clear that even rigorously purified beta cells, obtained by flow cytometric selection after tryptic dissociation of islets, are immunogenic.[21,22] *In vitro,* stimulator-type antigen-presenting cells may directly present class I MHC antigens to responder cells or class I alloantigens may be processed by responder antigen presenting cells for indirect presentation.[23] Thus, it is not surprising that the elimination of passenger leukocytes from a graft does not abolish the capacity of the tissue to immunize. Tissue immunogenicity is abrogated *in vitro* only when both stimulator and responder antigen-presenting cells are eliminated from the system.[21,23]

Thus, with regard to clinical application, it is apparent that the development of methods yielding increasingly pure populations of endocrine cells are not necessary for engraftment to take place or sufficient to allow for transplantation without the requirement for host immunosuppression.

The need for purification has been overemphasized. Impure preparations will engraft as long as the site of implantation can accommodate the large amount of tissue to be injected. For clinical success to occur, more effective regimens of immunosuppression need to be developed. This will require the introduction of new agents that lack the diabetogenic toxicities associated with current drugs, particularly corticosteroids and cyclosporine. A fundamental understanding of the immune response to a graft of dispersed tissue is required for rational protocol design.

IMMUNE RESPONSE TO NON–IMMEDIATELY VASCULARIZED GRAFTS

The achievement, even transiently, of a euglycemic, insulin-independent state after islet allotransplantation in man has occurred only rarely.[8] This may be due to transplantation of an inadequate mass of functional islets. The successes, which are essentially anecdotal in nature, have occurred only when excessive amounts of islets have been infused (>8000 IE/kg). This contrasts with the experience of islet autotransplantation after total pancreatectomy for benign disease where as few as 3100 IE/kg are sufficient to prevent the onset of diabetes.[3] This suggests that an immune mechanism may be responsible for the early failure of human islet allografts or that the drugs given to prevent rejection inhibit function.

A similar phenomenon occurs in rodent models of allotransplantation. Chemically induced diabetic recipients usually revert to normoglycemia within 1 to 5 days following transplantation. In the absence of immunosuppression, hyperglycemia commonly ensues 1 to 3 weeks later. Biopsy at that time reveals disruption of islet architecture with an intense lymphocytic infiltrate, and classic rejection is said to have occurred. The infiltrating cell population is comprised predominantly of

T lymphocytes with a paucity of macrophages present and no evidence of immuno-globulin deposition.[24]

Another form of immune-mediated dysfunction of islet allografts also occurs. Depending on the strain combination used, a variable percentage of recipients do not revert, even transiently, to a normoglycemic state following transplantation. This immediate failure of the allograft, termed primary nonfunction, varies in incidence from < 10% to > 40% depending on the strain combinations involved.

Immunohistochemical analysis of grafts manifesting primary nonfunction show apparently viable islets with insulin-containing cells against a background of a moderate inflammatory cell infiltrate. The infiltrate in these animals is more intense and contains more macrophages than infiltrates observed in normoglycemic allograft recipients or in recipients of isografts.[24] Immunoglobulin or complement deposition does not occur. These findings suggest that primary nonfunction of islet allografts is a manifestation of the host alloimmune response. We hypothesized that macrophages or macrophage byproducts either directly injure islets or inhibit their function until classic T-cell-mediated destruction supervenes. Injury of allogeneic islets might be caused by any of a variety of molecules synthesized and secreted by macrophages such as interleukin-1, tumor necrosis factor, or nitric oxide.

A central role for macrophages is also supported by the impact of various immunosuppressive agents on the functional outcome after islet transplantation. Immunodepletion of CD4 or CD8 T lymphocytes delays the onset of graft loss due to rejection but does not alter its incidence or that of primary nonfunction. However, intraperitoneal administration of the antimacrophage agent silica, which effectively depletes the recipient's macrophage population as documented by FACS analysis of peritoneal exudate cells, completely abolishes primary nonfunction.[24] Splenic T cell activity measured by the cell-mediated lympholysis assay is unaffected, and as one would expect, long-term graft survival is not enhanced by silica with the majority of grafts succumbing to classic rejection.

These data are consistent with the hypothesis that primary nonfunction results from an early cell-mediated response, involving primarily macrophages or their products, that either injures islets or inhibits their function until ultimate destruction by mediators of more delayed onset, CD4+ and CD8+ T cells, occurs.

These findings have clinical implications as well. Most clinical attempts of islet allotransplantation have not succeeded. Although it is difficult to accurately assign the cause of failure in the clinical setting, it is likely that some human islet allografts have failed because of macrophage-mediated primary nonfunction as well as classic T-cell-mediated rejection. The success of human islet transplantation should be enhanced by the development of agents with activity directed at macrophages as well as T lymphocytes that do not possess the diabetogenic toxicities associated with corticosteroids.

15-DEOXYSPERGUALIN

15-Deoxyspergualin (DSG), a synthetic derivative of spergualin, effectively prolongs graft survival in a variety of small and large animal models of allotransplantation.[25-27] It also has been used to reverse established rejection[28] and has been shown to be an effective immunosuppressant for autoimmune diseases.[29]

DSG's mechanism of action is unknown, although it appears to differ from that of other available immunosuppressive agents. It binds to a member of the heat shock protein 70 family and does not compete with the immunophilins cyclophilin or FK binding protein.[30] The drug appears to be a poor inhibitor of lymphocyte proliferation and may interfere at a later point in the activation process leading to the generation of antigen-specific cytotoxic T lymphocytes.[31] DSG has also been shown to inhibit several macrophage functions. It inhibits lysosomal enzyme release and superoxide production by macrophages[32] and inhibits class II MHC antigen induction in response to immunologic stimuli.[33] DSG has also been shown to block induction of ornithine decarboxylase activity, inhibition of which impairs macrophage function.[34,35]

Given our current understanding of the immunologic mediators responsible for primary nonfunction, DSG's antimacrophage activity makes it an interesting agent to test in experimental models of islet transplantation. However, effectiveness in preventing immune-mediated beta cell damage is only one characteristic required of an agent that will be useful in models of islet allotransplantation.

Posttransplant hyperglycemia is a well-recognized complication of immunosuppression with standard drugs. The newer agents, FK506 and rapamycin, appear to be diabetogenic as well.[36,37] For a new drug to make a substantial contribution toward increasing the effectiveness of islet transplantation, it must not only be an effective immunosuppressant but must be lacking in significant diabetogenic toxicity as well.

In order to assess its impact on beta cell function, we examined the short-term effects of DSG on glucose-induced insulin secretion in islets isolated from rat and human pancreases.[38] Insulin secretory capacity was unaffected by 24-hour incubation in the presence of concentrations of DSG that bracketed the levels achieved *in vivo*. In addition, we treated normal rats with DSG (1, 4, or 10 mg/kg per d intraperitoneally) for 1 week and found that glucose disposal and insulin secretion were unaffected. These results, along with the fact that hyperglycemia has not been reported either in experimental animals or in human cancer patients participating in phase I studies receiving doses 10-fold in excess of the dose used for transplant immunosuppression, indicate that DSG does not possess appreciable diabetogenic toxicity.

We evaluated the ability of DSG to enhance islet allograft survival in a murine model.[39] B10.BR Sg/SnJ (H − 2^k) islets were isolated by collagenase digestion, dextran gradient separation, and hand picking and transplanted beneath the renal capsule of streptozotocin-induced diabetic C57BL/6J (H − 2^b) recipients. Although a generous islet mass was used for each transplant (700–900 islets), 27% of nonimmunosuppressed recipients remained permanently hyperglycemic after transplantation (TABLE 1). Another 48% were rendered temporarily normoglycemic before allograft rejection occurred, while 25% remained normoglycemic indefinitely. The daily administration of DSG (0.625 mg/kg per d ip for 50–100 days) completely abrogated the phenomenon of primary nonfunction as well as that of classic rejection with all grafts surviving indefinitely (> 100 days). Furthermore, once DSG was stopped, graft function continued unabated although rejection could be induced with donor strain splenocyte injections.

Experiments using a syngeneic split transplant model have demonstrated that as few as 50 islets are capable of maintaining a normoglycemic state.[40] Therefore, the 700–900 islets used in our initial experiments with DSG represent a relatively excessive beta cell mass. More than 90% of the islets transplanted could be destroyed by mediators accompanying the nonspecific inflammation at the transplant site, yet enough beta cell mass would still be present to maintain euglycemia.

In order to more rigorously assess the effectiveness with which DSG inhibits the events responsible for primary nonfunction of islet grafts, we utilized a marginal islet mass (150 islets/recipient) transplant model.[41] A dose-response study of islet isografts (C57BL/6J) revealed that transplantation of 150 islets/recipient resulted in a 75% incidence (12 of 16 animals) of euglycemia at a mean of 39 ± 6 days posttransplant. The rate of cure was not increased by the administration of DSG

TABLE 1. Outcome of B10.BR Islet Allografts Transplanted to Normal and to DSG-Treated C57BL/6 Mice[a]

Immuno-suppression	n	Duration of Function (mean day ± SD)	Islet Survival (d)	No. with Primary Nonfunction (%)	No. Rejecting (n) (mean d ± SD)	No. Surviving Long Term (%)
None	48	33.2 ± 5.8[b]	0 × 13, 5, 6, 11, 12, 13 × 3, 14 × 3, 15 × 2, 16, 17, 18, 20 × 3, 21, 22, 23, 30, 39, >100 × 12	13 (27)	23 (48%)[c] (17.0 ± 1.5)	12 (25)[d]
DSG 0.625 mg/kg/d	8	100.0 ± 0.0[b]	100 × 8	0 (0)	0 (0%)[c]	8 (100)[d]

[a]Reprinted by permission of Appleton & Lange, Inc. Kaufman, D.B., M.J. Field, S.A. Gruber, A.C. Farney, E. Stephanian, P.F. Gores & D.E.R. Sutherland. 1992. Extended functional survival of murine islet allografts with 15-deoxyspergualin. Transplant. Proc. 24(3): 1045–1047.
[b]$p < 0.001$ (Student's t-test).
[c]$p < 0.05$ (Student's t-test).
[d]$p < 0.06$ (Student's t-test).

(0.625 mg/kg per d ip). However, the mean duration of hyperglycemia prior to cure was significantly reduced (18 ± 3 vs. 39 ± 6 days), suggesting that mediators of nonspecific inflammation inhibit freshly transplanted isologous beta cells as well.

Early beta cell dysfunction is more pronounced in the allogeneic setting with only 22% (2 of 9) of untreated recipients attaining euglycemia. Administration of DSG (0.625 mg/kg per d ip) increased the cure rate to 75% (6 of 8). Furthermore, the duration of temporary hyperglycemia posttransplant (23 ± 5 days) was significantly less than that seen in untreated isograft controls.

These results are consistent with the hypothesis that islet allografts are vulnerable to injury by macrophage-mediated mechanisms at the time of engraftment and suggest that DSG may be a valuable agent to employ in immunosuppressive protocols for clinical islet transplantation. However, quite often protocols capable of dramatically extending the survival of islet grafts in rodent models have little or no impact on graft survival in the more clinically relevant large animal models. Therefore, we examined the effect of adding DSG to a regimen consisting of conventional immunosuppressive agents, used at clinically tolerable doses, in the outbred canine islet allograft model.[42] In this model, prolonged allograft function can be achieved with the use of cyclosporine monotherapy.[43,44] However, the blood levels required (whole-blood HPLC trough levels of 600–1000 ng/ml), although well-tolerated by canines, cannot be maintained in humans because of the attendant nephrotoxicity. When cyclosporine is administered at clinically relevant doses, islet allograft function is not prolonged vis-a-vis a nonimmunosuppressed control group.[44] The addition of azathioprine to cyclosporine has no measurable effect, but a 14-day course of goat anti–dog antilymphoblast globulin together with cyclosporine and azathioprine does increase allograft survival marginally.[45] Regimens including the diabetogenic agent prednisone are less successful.

Therefore, we examined the effect of adding DSG to cyclosporine/azathioprine/ antilymphoblast globulin in this model. Experience with DSG in canine models of renal transplantation have been hampered by the species-specific gastrointestinal toxicity associated with this drug at doses readily tolerated by humans.[46] In order to avoid problems with gastrointestinal mucositis and bleeding, we added how lose DSG (0.5 mg/kg per d intravenously for 10 days) to a regimen of CSA/AZA/ALG. This dose of DSG contrasts to the well-tolerated clinical dose of 4 mg/kg per day.

Animals underwent total pancreatectomy after an overnight fast, and purified islet preparations were obtained by collagenase digestion and Ficoll density gradient centrifugation. An average of 7100 islets/kg recipient body weight were transplanted intraportally after the animals had been divided into three groups. Group I received CSA 20 mg/kg per d peroral, AZA 2.5 mg/kg per d po, and ALG 20 mg/kg per d iv for 14 days. Group II received CSA, AZA, and ALG at the same doses with the addition of DSG at 0.5 mg/kg per d for 10 days. Group III animals received islet autografts and were not immunosuppressed.

Trough blood levels of cyclosporine as determined by HPLC were in the clinically acceptable range of 150–250 ng/ml in these pancreatectomized animals. There was no evidence of gastrointestinal toxicity with this dose of DSG, although several of the dogs became transiently leukopenic. Importantly, the functional survival of islet allografts was significantly prolonged in the group of dogs receiving DSG compared to those who did not (TABLE 2).

Pilot Study of 15-Deoxyspergualin in Human Islet Transplantation

In light of the encouraging experimental work summarized above, we have embarked on a clinical trial of DSG in recipients of simultaneous islet/kidney transplants.[47] All patients were type I insulin-dependent diabetics with end stage nephropathy awaiting cadaveric transplantation. In each instance, islets for transplantation were obtained from a single donor (same as the kidney). Between February 1992 and April 1993, six patients were enrolled. One patient experienced a splenic capsular tear (requiring splenectomy) and is excluded from further analysis. In order to maximize yield, all patients received unpurified islets (dispersed pancreatic tissue) prepared by the automated method of collagenase digestion. Density gradient separation techniques were not employed.

We used DSG (4 mg/kg per d for 10 days beginning at the time of transplantation) along with ALG or antithymocyte globulin (20 mg/kg per d for 7 days) for induction and azathioprine (1.5 mg/kg per d), prednisone (1 mg/kg per d taper), and cyclosporine (8 mg/kg per d beginning on the fifth postoperative day) for maintenance immunosuppression.

In all patients, C-peptides were absent or barely detectable and did not rise following a mixed meal challenge (Ensure; Ross Laboratories).

TABLE 2. Functional Survival of Canine Islet Transplants According to Immunosuppressive Regimen

Group	n	Immunosuppression	Days of Function	Mean	Median
I	11	CSA, AZA, ALG	$0 \times 2, 2, 3, 4 \times 3,$ $6 \times 2, 22, 68$	10.8	4[a]
II	10	CSA, AZA, ALG, DSG	3, 11, 12×2, 19, 25, 34, 42, 67, 99	32.4	22[a]
III	3	None (autografts)	$> 90, > 90, > 90$	> 90	> 90

[a]$p = 0.01$.

A sustained period of insulin independence was achieved in each of the first two patients. The results of the subsequent three patients have not been as good. However, only the fourth patient, who received 520,000 150 μm islet equivalents (7027/kg body wt.), was a clear failure of immunosuppressive therapy. In this patient, some engraftment of insulin producing tissue occurred, as evidenced by a rise in C-peptide levels into the normal range (0.34 pm/ml basal, 0.42 pm/ml stimulated) at last follow-up 8 months posttransplantation, but this is far below the level of insulin secretion required to maintain normoglycemia in nondiabetic patients on mainte-nance immunosuppression after renal transplantation with CSA/AZA/prednisone (1.0 pm/ml basal, 2.3 pm/ml stimulated).[48,49] The third patient received an islet/ kidney transplant from a 9-year old donor, and only 189,000 IE (2242 IE/kg body wt.) were recovered. This is below the threshold of 3000–4000 IE/kg body wt. known to be required for the achievement of normoglycemia in nonimmunosuppressed canine or human islet autograft recipients. Although significant engraftment occurred (with basal C-peptide levels rising to 0.70–0.90 pm/ml), the islets were not capable of significantly increasing their rate of insulin secretion in response to a mixed meal challenge, and his glycemic control posttransplant was unaffected. The fifth patient received 515,000 IE (6321 IE/kg body wt.) and achieved excellent engraftment with basal C-peptide levels rising to 1.78 pm/ml 10 days posttransplant in the face of normal renal allograft function. Unfortunately, upon discharge from the hospital, he was noncompliant and was lost to follow-up for two weeks. When he returned, his serum creatinine had risen to 6.7 mg/dl and a biopsy-proven severe renal allograft rejection was diagnosed. Renal function was not salvaged with a course of increased steroids and OKT3. Some islet tissue has survived (basal C-peptide levels of 0.35–0.50 pm/ml) but is not sufficient to significantly impact upon his glycemic control.

The first two patients achieved a sustained period of insulin independence and will be described in some detail.

Patient 1

This 42-year-old male with retinopathy and end-stage nephropathy had a 25-year history of insulin dependence and was taking 38 units of insulin daily. On February 20, 1992 he received a simultaneous islet/kidney transplant from a 26-year-old cadaver donor matched for two HLA antigens (1A, 1B, O DR). The kidney transplant was performed while the pancreas, which had been preserved for 5½ hours in University of Wisconsin solution, was digested by the automated method. The resulting 18 ml of tissue containing 536,000 IE was suspended in 300 ml of Hanks solution and slowly injected into a branch of the superior mesenteric vein. The portal pressure rose from a baseline of 6 cm of water to 19 cm of water immediately following the injection. Liver function tests remained within normal limits, and no adverse long-term impact on hepatic function was noted.

The kidney and islets functioned immediately with serum creatinine falling to 1.0 mg/dl by the end of the first posttransplant week and C-peptide levels rising (FIGURE 1). In an effort to reduce metabolic demand on the islets and promote engraftment, exogenous insulin administration was continued.

One month posttransplant, although serum C-peptide levels were stable, serum creatinine rose to 1.9 mg/dl and a biopsy-proven moderate acute tubulointerstitial renal allograft rejection episode was diagnosed. This was successfully treated by increasing his prednisone dose to 2 mg/kg per day followed by a slow taper and administering a 7-day course of OKT3 (5 mg/day) with serum creatinine stabilizing in the 1.4–1.6 mg/dl range. From 3 months posttransplant until 11 months posttransplant, his insulin dose varied between 15 and 28 units daily. The islets continued to function with C-peptide levels 11 months posttransplant of 0.72 pm/ml (basal) and 1.70 pm/ml (stimulated). Glycemic control was excellent with Hgb A1c ranging between 5.7 and 6.1% (nl 4.3–6.0%). At this point, exogenous insulin administration was discontinued. He remained off insulin therapy for the next 5 months and although islet function, as reflected by C-peptide levels, remained stable, his glycemic control gradually deteriorated (Hgb A1c 6.7–6.9%). Sixteen months posttransplant, he resumed insulin therapy at a dose of 10 units/day, renal function remains stable, and Hgb A1c has returned to the normal range.

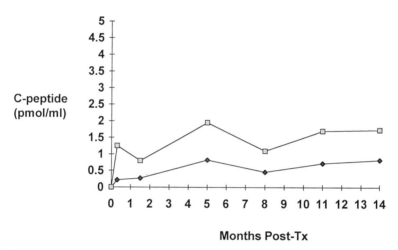

Months Post-Tx

FIGURE 1. Serum C-peptide levels in patient 1 as a function of time following simultaneous islet/kidney transplantation. Values are plotted as basal (diamonds) and after ingestion of 360 ml of Ensure, a liquid mixed meal containing 51 g carbohydrate, 13 g protein, and 13 g fat (squares).

Patient 2

This 32-year-old female with retinopathy and end-stage nephropathy had a 29-year history of insulin dependence and was taking 31 units of insulin daily. On March 19, 1992 she received a simultaneous islet/kidney transplant from a 29-year-old cadaver donor matched for two HLA antigens (O A, 1B, 1DR). Prior to processing, the pancreas was preserved for 2½ hours in University of Wisconsin solution. Tissue (41 ml) containing 626,000 IE was injected into the portal circulation with portal pressure transiently rising from 8 to 44 cm of water. Posttransplant, liver function tests remained in the normal range and again no adverse long-term sequelae were noted.

The kidney functioned immediately, with serum creatinine falling to 1.2 mg/dl. Islet engraftment was excellent as evidenced by high C-peptide levels measured 1 week posttransplant (basal 1.73 pm/ml, stimulated 4.80 pm/ml). A biopsy-proven kidney allograft rejection episode kidney allograft rejection episode occurring 3 weeks posttransplant was successfully treated with a 2 mg/kg per day prednisone taper and a 10 day course of ALG (20 mg/kg per day). Insulin therapy continued for the first 3 months posttransplant, and islet function remained stable (FIGURE 2). During the fourth posttransplant month, insulin administration was discontinued. Over the ensuing 7 months, the islets continued to function well and glycemic control remained good in the absence of exogenous insulin administration with Hgb A1c averaging 6.6%. A second biopsy-proven kidney allograft rejection episode occurred 11 months posttransplant, which was successfully reversed with increased steroids and OKT3. Insulin therapy was resumed around the time of her antirejection therapy, and although C-peptide levels remained high (FIGURE 2) glycemic control was suboptimal while on her steroid taper. Currently, 17 months posttransplantation, she is taking 10 mg Prednisone daily and is once again insulin independent.

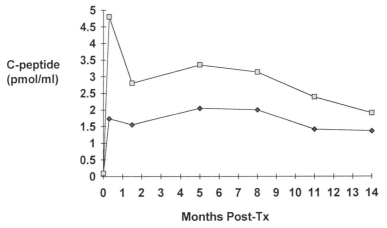

FIGURE 2. Serum C-peptide levels in patient 2 as a function of time following simultaneous islet/kidney transplantation. Values are plotted as basal (diamonds) and after ingestion of 360 ml of Ensure, a liquid mixed meal containing 51 g carbohydrate, 13 g protein, and 13 g fat (squares).

This series demonstrates unequivocally that elimination of contaminating exocrine tissue is not essential for engraftment and function of allogeneic islet tissue. The elimination of purification steps increases islet yield and avoids the necessity of resorting to multiple donors to obtain sufficient islet mass.

Unfortunately, the inclusion of corticosteroids in the immunosuppressive protocol with the attendant side effects of heightened resistance to the action of insulin, places excessive demands on islet function. 15-Deoxyspergualin is a promising agent for use in human islet transplantation. In this series its use was confined to the 10 days following transplantation, thus any beneficial effect it may have probably is related to its ability to blunt the nonspecific macrophage-driven inflammatory reaction surrounding freshly transplanted allogeneic tissue. As currently formulated, long-term therapy with DSG is impractical because it may only be given intravenously. Further progress awaits the elimination of corticosteroids from maintenance immunosuppressive protocols by substituting newer agents with similar therapeutic efficacy but lacking in the diabetogenic toxicity associated with steroid therapy.

REFERENCES

1. YOUNOSZAI, R., R. L. SORENSON & A. W. LINDALL. 1970. Homotransplantation of isolated pancreatic islets (abstract). Diabetes **19**(Suppl.): 406.
2. BALLINGER, W. F. & P. E. LACY. 1972. Transplantation of intact pancreatic islets in rats. Surgery **72**: 175–186.
3. FARNEY, A. C., J. S. NAJARIAN, R. E. NAKHLEH, G. LLOVERAS, M. J. FIELD, P. F. GORES & D. E. R. SUTHERLAND. 1991. Autotransplantation of dispersed pancreatic islet tissue combined with total or near-total pancreatectomy for treatment of chronic pancreatitis. Surgery **110**: 427–439.
4. SUTHERLAND, D. E. R. 1981. Pancreas and islet transplantation. I. Experimental studies. Diabetologia **20**: 161–185.
5. LACY, P. E. 1990. Islet transplantation. *In* The Diabetes Annual/5. K. G. M. M. Alberti & L. P. Krall, Eds.: 245–253. Elsevier. Amsterdam, the Netherlands.
6. WARNOCK, G. L. & R. V. RAJOTTE. 1988. Critical mass of purified islets that induce normoglycemia after implantation into dogs. Diabetes **37**: 467–470.
7. MUNN, S. R., D. B. KAUFMAN, R. M. MELOCHE, M. J. FIELD & D. E. R. SUTHERLAND. 1988. Weight-corrected islet counts are predictive of outcome in the canine intrahepatic islet autograft model. Diabetes Res. **9**: 121–124.
8. HERING, B. J., C. C. BROWATZKI, A. SCHULTZ, R. G. BRETZEL & K. F. FEDERLIN. 1993. Clinical islet transplantation—registry report, accomplishments in the past and future research needs. Cell Transplant. **2**: 269–282.
9. RICORDI, C., P. E. LACY, E. H. FINKE, B. J. OLACK & D. W. SCHARP. 1988. Automated method for isolation of human pancreatic islets. Diabetes **37**: 413–420.
10. GRAY, D. W. R., R. SUTTON, P. MCSHANE, M. PETERS & P. J. MORRIS. 1988. Exocrine contamination impairs implantation of pancreatic islets transplanted beneath the kidney capsule. J. Surg. Res. **45**: 432–442.
11. MIRKOVITCH, V. & M. CAMPICHE. 1977. Intrasplenic autotransplantation of canine pancreatic tissue: maintenance of normoglycemia after total pancreatectomy. Eur. Surg. Res. **9**: 173–190.
12. KRETSCHMER, G. J., D. E. R. SUTHERLAND, A. J. MATAS, T. L. CAIN & J. S. NAJARIAN. 1977. The dispersed pancreas: transplantation without islet purification in totally pancreatectomized dogs. Diabetologia **13**: 495–502.
13. KOLB, E., R. RUCHERT & F. LARGIADER. 1977. Intraportal and intrasplenic autotransplantation of pancreatic islets in the dog. Eur. Surg. Res. **9**: 419–426.
14. MIENY, C. J. & J. A. SMIT. 1978. Autotransplantation of pancreatic tissue in totally pancreatectomized baboons. S. Afr. J. Surg. **16**: 19–21.
15. GRAY, D. W. R., G. L. WARNOCK, R. SUTTON, M. PETERS, P. MCSHANE & P. J. MORRIS. 1986. Successful autotransplantation of isolated islets of Langerhans in the cynomologous monkey. Br. J. Surg. **73**: 850–853.
16. SNELL, G. D. 1957. The homograft reaction. Annu. Rev. Microbiol. **11**: 439–458.
17. LAFFERTY, K. J., S. J. PROWSE, C. J. SIMEONOVIC & M. S. WARREN. 1983. Immunobiology of tissue transplantation: a return to the passenger leukocyte concept. Annu. Rev. Immunol. **1**: 143–173.
18. SEVER, C. E., A. J. DEMETRIS, J. ZENG, P. CARROLL, A. TZAKIS, J. J. FUNG, T. E. STARZL & C. RICORDI. 1992. Composition of human islet cell preparations for transplantation. Acta Diabetol. **28**: 233–238.
19. FAUSTMAN, D., V. HAUPTFELD, P. LACY & J. DAVIE. 1981. Prolongation of murine islet allograft survival by pretreatment of islets with antibody directed to Ia determinants. Proc. Natl. Acad. Sci. USA **78**: 5156–5159.
20. GORES, P. F., D. E. R. SUTHERLAND, J. L. PLATT & F. H. BACH. 1986. Depletion of donor Ia+ cells prior to transplantation does not prolong islet allograft survival. J. Immunol. **137**: 1482–1485.

21. STOCK, P. G., N. L. ASCHER, S. CHEN, J. FIELD, F. H. BACH & D. E. R. SUTHERLAND. 1991. Evidence for direct and indirect pathways in the generation of the alloimmune response against pancreatic islets. Transplantation **52:** 704–709.

22. PIPELEERS, D. G., M. PIPELEERS-MARICHAL, B. VANBRABANDT & S. DUYS. 1991. Transplantation of purified islet cells in diabetic rats. II. Immunogenicity of allografted islet β-cells. Diabetes **40:** 920–930.

23. MIZOUCHI, T., H. GOLDING, A. S. ROSENBERG, L. H. GLIMCHER, T. R. MALEK & A. SINGER. 1985. Both L3T4+ and Lyt-2+ helper T cells initiate cytotoxic T lymphocyte responses against allogenic major histocompatibility antigens but not against trinitrophenyl-modified self. J. Exp. Med. **162:** 427–443.

24. KAUFMAN, D. B., J. L. PLATT, F. L. RABE, D. L. DUNN, F. H. BACH & D. E. R. SUTHERLAND. 1990. Differential roles of Mac-1+ cells, and CD4+ and CD8+ T lymphocytes in primary nonfunction and classic rejection of islet allografts. J. Exp. Med. **172:** 291–302.

25. NEMOTO, K., M. HAYASHI & F. ABE. 1987. Immunosuppressive activities of 15-deoxyspergualin in animals. J. Antibiot. **40:** 561–562.

26. SUZUKI, S., M. KANASHIRO & H. AMEMIYA. 1987. Effect of a new immunosuppressant, 15-deoxyspergualin, on heterotopic rat heart transplantation, in comparison with cyclosporine. Transplantation **44:** 483–487.

27. REICHENSPURNER, H., A. HILDEBRANT, P. HUMAN, D. H. BOEHM, A. G. ROSE, J. A. O'DELL, B. REICHARD & H. U. SCHORLEMMER. 1990. 15-Deoxyspergualin for induction of graft nonreactivity after cardiac and renal allotransplantation in primates. Transplantation **50:** 181–185.

28. AMEMIYA, H., S. SUZUKI, K. OTA, K. TAKAHASHI, T. SONODA, M. ISHIBASHI, R. OMOTO, I. KAYAMA, K. DOHI, Y. FUKUDA & K. FUKAO. 1990. A novel rescue drug, 15-deoxyspergualin. Transplantation **49:** 337–343.

29. MAKINO, M., M. FUJIWARA, T. AOYAGI & H. UMEZAWA. 1987. Immunosuppressive activities of deoxyspergualin. I. Effect of the long-term administration of the drug on the development of murine lupus. Immunopharmacology **14:** 107–114.

30. NADLER, S. G., M. A. TEPPER, B. SCHACTER & C. E. MAZZUCCO. 1992. Interaction of the immunosuppressant deoxyspergualin with a member of the HSP 70 family of heat shock proteins. Science **258:** 484–486.

31. YUH, D. D. & R. E. MORRIS. 1993. The immunopharmacology of immunosuppression by 15-deoxyspergualin. Transplantation **55:** 578–591.

32. DICKNEITE, C., H. U. SCHORLEMMER, E. WEINMANN, R. R. BARLETT & H. H. SEDLACEK. 1987. Skin transplantation in rats and monkeys: evaluation of efficient treatment with 15-deoxyspergualin. Transplant. Proc. **19:** 4244–4247.

33. DICKNEITE, G., H. U. SCHORLEMMER, P. WALTER, J. THIES & H. J. SEDLACEK. 1986. The influence of deoxyspergualin on experimental transplantation and its immunopharmacological mode of action. Behring Inst. Mitt. **80:** 93–102.

34. HIBASAMI, H., T. TSUKADA, R. SUZUKI, K. TAKANO, S. TAKAJI, T. TAKEUCHI, S. SHIRAKAWA, T. MURATA & K. NAKASHIMA. 1991. 15-Deoxyspergualin, an antiproliferative agent for human and mouse leukemia cells, shows inhibitory effects on the synthetic pathway of polyamines. Anticancer Res. **11:** 325–330.

35. KIERSZENBAUM, F., J. J. WIRTH, P. P. McCANN & A. SJOERDSMA. 1987. Impairment of macrophage function by inhibitors of ornithine decarboxylase activity. Infect. Immun. **55:** 2461–2464.

36. RICORDI, C., Y. ZENG, R. ALEJANDRO, A. TZAKIS, R. VENKATANAMANAN, J. FUNG, D. BEREITER, D. H. MINTZ & T. E. STARZL. 1991. In vivo effect of FK506 on human pancreatic islets. Transplantation **52:** 519–522.

37. WHITING, P. H., J. WOO, B. J. ADAM, N. U. HASAN, R. J. L. DAVIDSON & A. W. THOMSON. 1991. Toxicity of rapamycin—a comparison and combination study with cyclosporine at immunotherapeutic dosage in the rat. Transplantation **52:** 203–208.

38. XENOS, E. S., D. CASANOVA, D. E. R. SUTHERLAND, A. C. FARNEY, J. J. LLOVERAS & P. F. GORES. 1993. In vivo and in vitro effect of 15-deoxyspergualin on pancreatic islet function. Transplantation **56:** 144–147.

39. KAUFMAN, D. B., M. J. FIELD, S. A. GRUBER, A. FARNEY, E. STEPHANIAN, P. F. GORES & D. E. R. SUTHERLAND. 1992. Extended functional survival of murine islet allografts with 15-deoxyspergualin. Transplant. Proc. **24:** 1045–1047.
40. OHZATO, H., J. PORTER, A. P. MONACO & T. MAKI. 1993. Fifty islets maintain euglycemia and survive longer than 200 islets in allogeneic and xenogeneic diabetic hosts. Transplant. Proc. **25:** 953–954.
41. KAUFMAN, D. B., A. C. FARNEY, M. J. FIELD, E. STEPHANIAN, P. F. GORES & D. E. R. SUTHERLAND. Effect of 15-deoxyspergualin on immediate function and long-term survival on transplanted islets in recipients of a marginal islet mass. (Submitted)
42. STEPHANIAN, E., J. J. LLOVERAS, D. E. R. SUTHERLAND, A. C. FARNEY, M. J. FIELD, D. B. KAUFMAN, B. D. MATTESON & P. F. GORES. 1992. Prolongation of canine islet allograft survival by 15-deoxyspergualin. J. Surg. Res. **52:** 621–624.
43. ALEJANDRO, R., R. CUTFIELD, F. L. SHIENVOLD, Z. LATIF & D. M. MINTZ. 1985. Successful long-term survival of pancreatic islet allografts in spontaneous or pancreatectomy-induced diabetes in dogs. Diabetes **34:** 825–828.
44. KNETEMAN, N. M., D. ALDERSON & D. W. SCHARP. 1987. Long-term normoglycemia in pancreatectomized dogs following pancreatic islet allotransplantation and cyclosporine. Transplantation **44:** 595–599.
45. KAUFMAN, D. B., P. MOREL, R. CONDIE, M. J. FIELD, M. ROONEY, P. TZARDIS, P. STOCK & D. E. R. SUTHERLAND. 1991. Beneficial and detrimental effects of RBC-absorbed antilymphocyte globulin and prednisone on purified canine islet autograft and allograft function. Transplantation **51:** 37–42.
46. TODO, S., N. MURASE, D. KAHN, C. E. PAN, K. OKUDA, S. CEMEJ, A. CASAVILLA, V. MAZZAFERRO, A. GHALAB, B. S. RHOE, M. YANG, K. TNAIGUCHI, M. NALESNIK, L. MAKOWKA & T. E. STARZL. 1988. Effect of 15-deoxyspergualin on experimental organ transplantation. Transplant. Proc. **20**(S1): 233–236.
47. GORES, P. F., J. S. NAJARIAN, E. STEPHANIAN, J. J. LLOVERAS, S. L. KELLEY & D. E. R. SUTHERLAND. 1993. Insulin independence in type I diabetes after transplantation of unpurified islets from single donor with 15-deoxyspergualin. Lancet **341:** 19–21.
48. SCHARP, D. W., P. E. LACY, J. V. SANTIAGO, C. S. McCULLOUGH, L. G. WEIDE, P. J. BOYLE, L. FALQUI, P. MARCHETTI, C. RICORDI, R. L. GINGERICH, A. S. JAFFE, P. E. CRYER, D. W. HANTO, C. B. ANDERSON & M. W. FLYE. 1991. Results of our first nine intraportal islet allografts in type 1, insulin-dependent diabetic patients. Transplantation **51:** 76–85.
49. KATZ, H., M. HOMAN, J. VELOSA, P. ROBERTSON & R. RIZZA. 1991. Effects of pancreas transplantation on postprandial glucose metabolism. N. Engl. J. Med. **325:** 1278–1283.

A Powerful Antiinflammatory Therapy Is Effective in the Treatment of Idiopathic Thrombocytopenia

ADRIANA MENICHELLI AND
DOMENICO DEL PRINCIPE[a]

Department of Public Health and Cellular Biology
University "Tor Vergata"
Via O. Raimundo
00173 Rome, Italy

Since 1984, we have treated 50 children affected with immune thrombocytopenic purpura (ITP) with a single intravenous injection of 15 mg/kg methylprednisolone (MP), which was repeated only for three consecutive days[1] according to the schedule proposed in our preliminary paper.[2] In all patients, a rapid cessation of bleeding, starting a few hours following the first injection of MP, before the increase of platelet number, was observed. The rate of response to steroid bolus was comparable to that obtained by treatment with high doses of immunoglobulins.[3] At the end of the therapy, in fact, 80% of the patients showed a platelet count above the danger zone ($> 50 \times 10^9/l$). The remission lasted 1 month in 50% and 4 months in 30% of patients. No side effects were observed. A few single doses of MP, in fact, even if very high, do not produce harmful effects because kinetics and metabolism of this steroid are dose dependent.[4]

ITP of childhood is usually a self-limited disorder, and the majority of children will have a complete remission without therapy within a few weeks to months. Serious, life-threatening bleeding can occur, however, if platelet counts are persistently below 20,000/μl. Intravenous injections of high doses of MP given in pulses represent a useful and economic tool to manage ITP of childhood, which rapidly restores the platelet count to safe levels. This therapeutic approach, now employed in many clinical institutions, increases the steroid pharmacologic effects minimizing, in the meantime, either the toxic effects of a long-term therapy or those resulting from its abrupt cessation.[5] Symptoms of chronic steroid toxicity and withdrawal syndromes have never been reported in patients treated with MP pulses. Significant suppression of the hypothalamus-pituitary-adrenal system, in fact, has not been observed even after prolonged and repeated steroid pulse therapy.[6]

The most interesting finding emerging from our study is, in our opinion, that thrombocytopenia may be cured in a high percentage of patients with a powerful antiinflammatory therapy. The effects of glucocorticoids on inflammatory and immunologic systems are very complex. These hormones profoundly affect kinetics and functional properties of inflammatory cells. In particular, they interfere with the production of tumor necrosis factor-alpha from macrophages and of interleukin-1 (IL-1) from monocytes at different levels, and inhibit the release of IL-1 into the extracellular fluids. Another mechanism of the antiinflammatory action is mediated by the action of second messengers. Very important among these is lipocortin, a member of a family of proteins that inhibits phospholipase A_2 activity, thereby

[a] Author to whom correspondence should be addressed.

decreasing the production of potent mediators of inflammation.[7] With the intermittent administration of glucocorticoids there is only a limited, short-lasting interference with the immunologic system. The immune suppressive effects last, in fact, only the first 12 hours when steroids are given in pulses, and increasing the dosage does not increase the duration or the degree of immune suppression. A sustained immune suppression is obtained, in fact, only when the hormone is given at least twice a day and for a long period of time.[4]

On the basis of the observation that most patients who were previously refractory to immune suppressive treatments, including the standard steroid therapy, are responsive to MP pulses, it may be inferred that inflammatory processes play an important role in the pathophysiology of ITP, at least in some cases. We have yet to understand which mechanism sustains the prolonged remission showed by some patients treated with only three MP pulses.

REFERENCES

1. DEL PRINCIPE, D., A. MENICHELLI, P. G. MORI, D. DE MATTIA, G. MANCUSO, V. CARNELLI, L. ZANESCO, M. JANKOVIC, M. CALMASINI, A. AMICI, C. MIANO, D. ROSATI, G. CIAVARELLA, G. ODDO, P. GIULOTTO, G. MASERA & T. LANZA. 1987. Acta Haematol. **77:** 226–230.
2. MENICHELLI, A., D. DEL PRINCIPE & E. REZZA. 1984. Arch. Dis. Child. **59:** 777–779.
3. MORI, P. G., G. MANCUSO, D. DEL PRINCIPE, M. DUSE, R. MINIERO, R. TOVO, M. BARDARE, V. CARNELLI & D. DE MATTIA. 1983. Arch. Dis. Child. **58:** 851–855.
4. FREY, F. J. 1987. Kinetics and dynamics of prednisolone. Endocr. Rev. **8:** 453–473.
5. DEL PRINCIPE, D. & A. MENICHELLI. 1988. Acta Haematol. **79:** 224–226.
6. MILLER, J. J., III. 1980. Pediatrics **65:** 989–994.
7. SAEZ-LLORENS, X., O. RAMILO, M. M. MUSTAFA, J. MERTSOLA & G. H. MCCRACKEN. 1990. J. Pediatr. **116:** 671–684.

Interaction of Diltiazem and Rapamycin on Survival of Rat Cardiac Allografts

LOUIS DUMONT, HUIFANG CHEN, DASHENG XU, AND
PIERRE DALOZE

Département de Pharmacologie et de Chirurgie
Faculté de Médecine
Université de Montréal

Laboratoire de Chirurgie Expérimentale
Centre de Recherche
Hôpital Notre-Dame
Montréal, Quebec, Canada H3C 3J7

INTRODUCTION

Diltiazem, a benzothiazepine-like Ca^{2+} antagonist, possesses significant immuno-modulator properties as demonstrated with *in vivo* and *in vitro* models, and these experimental data translated into clinical benefits.[1,2] The molecular targets of Ca^{2+} antagonist immunomodulation are at the level of lymphocyte activation and include inhibition of IL-2 encoding mRNA, IL-2 receptor expression, and IL-2 production.[3,4] Rapamycin, a macrolide antibiotic, was found to be a potent immunosuppressor, and its mechanism of action is believed to be related to inhibition of lymphokine signal transduction.[5] Since both diltiazem and rapamycin interact at different levels of lymphocyte activation, we investigated their possible synergistic effects on rat cardiac allograft survival.

MATERIALS AND METHODS

Heterotopic heart transplants were placed intraabdominally by a modification of the method of Ono and Lindsey.[6] Donor (Wistar-Furth) and recipient (Lewis) rats were anesthetized with pentobarbital (40 mg/kg) intraperitoneally (ip) and supple-mented with chloral hydrate (160 mg/kg) as necessary. Donor hearts were perfused through the thoracic inferior vena cava with heparinized saline to chill them to 4°C prior to ligation of the vena cava and pulmonary veins. The grafts were kept in 4°C saline less than 30 minutes. After exposing the infrarenal vena cava and aorta of the recipient, anastomoses of the donor pulmonary artery to recipient vena cava, and the donor aorta to recipient aorta, were carried out using 10–0 nylon sutures. Cardiac activity was assessed daily through abdominal palpation. The time of rejection was defined as the last day of palpable cardiac contraction and confirmed histologically after laparotomy.

Following the surgical procedures, 4 groups of allograft recipients were studied. Untreated allografts were used as the control group. One group received a 14-day continuous intravenous therapy with rapamycin, 0.02 mg/kg per day. Another group received diltiazem alone at a dose of 2.50 mg/kg per day by gavage. Five recipients were treated with both rapamycin 0.02 mg/kg per day and diltiazem 2.50 mg/kg per day.

Rapamycin (Wyeth-Ayerst) was diluted in a vehicle (10% Tween 80, 20% NN-N-dimethylacetamide and 70% polyethylene glycol 400) and administered intravenously (iv) for 14 days using a 2002 osmotic pump (Alzet®) via a lumbar vein. The rapamycin-filled pumps were primed for 2–3 hours in saline at 37°C. Diltiazem (Nordic Merrell Dow Research) was diluted in sterile water, and the concentrated solution (10 mM) was kept refrigerated. A diluted solution was prepared and administered daily by gavage. Untreated isograft recipients (Lewis-Lewis) were included in the follow-up studies and sacrificed on the 60th day posttransplantation to allow histopathological studies.

Following sacrifice of recipients, a complete morphological examination was carried out and a sample of the left ventricle was used for histopathology (eosin, hematoxylin). All data are expressed as mean ± standard error of the mean (SEM). Statistical analysis was performed using the ANOVA and the Student's t-test for unpaired data, and the statistical significance was set at $p < 0.05$.

TABLE 1. Mean Survival Time of Cardiac Allografts

Group	Treatment	Dose (mg/kg per day)	Survival (days)
1	Control	—	6.4 ± 0.2^a
2	Rapamycin	0.02	27.2 ± 8.3^b
3	Diltiazem	2.50	12.0 ± 1.2^b
4	Rapamycin	0.02	35.2 ± 9.7^b
	+ diltiazem	2.50	

[a]Mean ± SEM (n = 5–6 per group).
[b]Significantly different from untreated allografts.

RESULTS

All recipients had a successful implantation of the donor heart. Isografts (Lewis-Lewis) had an uneventful posttransplantation follow-up, and they were sacrificed 60 days later. In untreated or vehicle-infused allograft recipients, the survival time was 6 to 7 days (TABLE 1). Experiments carried out with rapamycin alone resulted in significant prolongation of mean graft survival time (27.2 ± 8.3 days, $p < 0.001$). Allograft recipients treated with diltiazem also had a significant increase in mean survival time (12.0 ± 1.2 days, $p < 0.01$) but to a lesser degree than rapamycin alone (FIGURE 1). When rapamycin, 0.02 mg/kg per day, and diltiazem, 2.50 mg/kg per day, were combined, the mean survival time was increased to 35.2 ± 9.7 days ($p < 0.001$).

In all groups studied, daily measurement of body weight was carried out. No statistically significant difference in body weight was found between control and treated recipients. None of the animals treated with rapamycin, diltiazem, or their combinaison showed any sign of drug toxicity.

DISCUSSION

The present experiments examined the efficacy of the benzothiazepine-like Ca^{2+} antagonist diltiazem and the macrolide antibiotic rapamycin upon cardiac allograft survival in rats. Although most *in vitro* studies suggested that calcium antagonists possess immunosuppressive properties, animal studies failed to demonstrate either in the presence of nifedipine (dihydropyridine) or verapamil (phenylalkylamine) any significant prolongation of graft survival except when high supratherapeutic doses were utilized.[3,7,8] On the contrary, the present report as well as data collected from previous studies suggested that diltiazem and clentiazem, two benzothiazepine-like Ca^{2+} antagonists, were able to prolong significantly rat cardiac allograft survival when they were administered alone and at clinically relevant concentrations.[1] These results and the fact that a beneficial pharmacokinetic interaction has been reported between diltiazem and cyclosporine let us to consider these compounds (diltiazem, clentiazem) as the drugs of choice when Ca^{2+} antagonists have to be administered in transplanted patients.

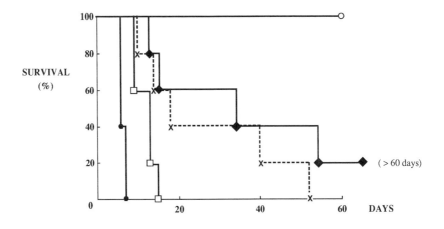

Data are expressed as % of allografts that survived at a given time.

o   = isografts.
●   = control allografts.
x   = allografts treated with rapamycin, 0.02 mg/kg/day.
□   = allografts treated with diltiazem, 2.50 mg/kg/day.
◆   = allografts treated with both rapamycin and diltiazem.

FIGURE 1. Effects of diltiazem and rapamycin on survival rate of rat cardiac allografts.

The new immunosuppressive agent rapamycin, after convincing experimental studies,[9] has entered the clinical trial phase. Previous studies have demonstrated that its safety and efficacy were improved when combined with other pharmacologic agents.[10,11] In the present study, we could not demonstrate significant synergistic or additive immunosuppressive properties when diltiazem and rapamycin were combined, although the mean survival time of cardiac allografts was slightly increased. Further studies should evaluate the benefits of a reduced rapamicin toxicity with this combination therapy since deleterious rapamycin–vessel wall interaction (vasculitis) has been reported and diltiazem has been shown to provide significant vascular protective effects.

REFERENCES

1. DUMONT, L., H. CHEN, P. DALOZE, D. XU & D. GARCEAU. 1993. Immunosuppressive properties of the benzothiazepine calcium antagonists, diltiazem and clentiazem, with and without cyclosporine in heterotopic rat heart transplantation. Transplantation 56: 181–184.

2. WAGNER, K. & H-H. NEUMAYER. 1987. Influence of the calcium antagonist diltiazem on delayed graft function in cadaveric kidney transplantation: results of a 6-month follow-up. Transplant. Proc. 19: 1353.

3. GRIER, G. A. & A. M. MASTRO. 1985. Mitogen and co-mitogen stimulation of lymphocytes inhibited by three Ca^{++} antagonists. J Cell. Phys. 124: 131.

4. WEIR, M. R., R. PEPPLER, D. GOMOLKA & B. S. HANDWERGER. 1991. Additive inhibition of afferent and efferent immunological responses of human peripheral blood mononuclear cells by verapamil and cyclosporine. Transplantation 51: 851.

5. KAHAN, B. D., J. Y. CHANG & S. N. SEHGAL. 1991. Preclinical evaluation of a new potent immunosuppressive agent, rapamycin. Transplantation 52: 185.

6. ONO, K. & E. S. LINDSEY. 1969. Improved technique of heart transplantation in rats. J. Thorac. Cardiovasc. Surg. 57: 225.

7. FOEGH, M. L., B. S. KHIRIBADI & P. W. RAMWELL. 1985. Prolongation of rat cardiac allograft survival by Ca^{++} blockers. Transplantation 40: 211.

8. TESI, R. J., J. HONG, K. M. H. BULL, B. M. JAFFE & M. A. MCMILLEN. 1987. In vivo potentiation of cyclosporine immunosuppression by calcium antagonists. Transplant. Proc. 19: 1382.

9. MORRIS, R. E. 1992. Rapamycins: antifungal, antitumor, antiproliferative, and immunosuppressive macrolides. Transplant. Rev. 6: 39.

10. KIMBALL, P. M., R. H. KERMAN & B. D. KAHAN. 1991. Production of synergistic but nonidentical mechanisms of immunosuppression by cyclosporine and rapamycin. Transplantation 51: 486.

11. STEPKOWSKI, S. M., H. CHEN, P. DALOZE & B. D. KAHAN. 1991. Prolongation by rapamycin of heart, kidney, pancreas, and small bowel allograft survival in rats. Transplant Proc. 23: 507.

Antioxidants Inhibit Activation of Transcription Factors and Cytokine Gene Transcription in Monocytes

MARIOLA ILNICKA, SIMON W. LEE,
AND ELSIE M. EUGUI

Syntex Research
3401 Hillview Avenue
Palo Alto, California 94303

INTRODUCTION

We have established that oxidants such as hydrogen peroxide, in concentrations that do not affect cell viability, prime human monocytic lineage cells (U937) so that LPS induces the formation of IL-1β mRNA and protein.[1] Activation of transcription factors such as AP-1 may be involved in this process. Antioxidants that prevent the activation of transcription factors may inhibit IL-1β gene transcription. To test this hypothesis, we analyzed the mechanism by which some antioxidants inhibit the production of IL-1 and IL-6 by human peripheral blood mononuclear cells (PBM) stimulated with LPS.

RESULTS

Human PBM were purified by Ficoll-Paque gradient and adherence to plastic petri dishes. LPS treatment of these cells induced the production of IL-1α, IL-1β, TNFα, and IL-6 mRNAs and proteins. Immunoassay of human PBM culture supernatants showed that the antioxidant tetrahydropapaveroline (THP, RS 78414) inhibited LPS-induced cytokine production without affecting overall protein synthesis.[2] Northern blot analysis showed that within 3 hours of treatment, THP markedly decreased the steady-state levels of IL-1α, IL-1β, and IL-6 mRNAs but not of other reference mRNAs (FIGURE 1A and B). The IC_{50} of inhibition was about 1 to 2 μM. Nuclear run-on experiments showed that THP inhibited LPS-induced IL-1β gene transcription (FIGURE 1C), suggesting that the effect of THP is at the transcriptional level.

Transcription of genes is usually promoted by DNA-binding transcription factors. Gel mobility assays using nuclear extracts of PBM activated by LPS in the presence of THP showed NFκB (FIGURE 2A) and AP-1 (FIGURE 2B) to be markedly decreased 1 hour after drug addition. When THP was added to nuclear extracts from LPS-activated cells and incubated prior to analysis, THP did not affect binding of NFκB (FIGURE 2C) and AP-1 (FIGURE 2D) to cognate DNA sequences. These findings suggest that antioxidants inhibit the activation of transcription factors, including NFκB and AP-1, and the transcription of IL-1β gene. The mechanism(s) by which antioxidants decrease TNFα and IL-6 mRNAs have not been analyzed.

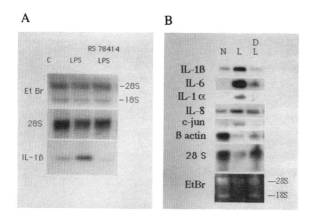

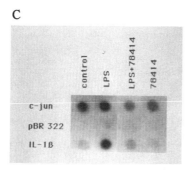

FIGURE 1. A: Northern blot analysis of monocyte mRNA following treatment with LPS and THP (RS 78414, 5 μM) for 3 h. Top panel, ethidium bromide staining of RNA gel (Et Br); middle and bottom panels, blots probed with labeled 28S oligonucleotides and IL-1β cDNA. c, control. **B:** Monocytes were cultured as described for A. Northern blots were probed successively. N, control; L, LPS; D, drug treatment (THP). **C:** Nuclear run-on assay of THP-treated and LPS-activated monocytes. Monocytes were cultured for 2 h, and nuclei were isolated. mRNA transcripts were labeled with radioactive UTP and hybridized to cDNA immobilized on nitrocellulose membranes. LPS stimulated IL-1β gene transcription and THP decreased LPS-induced IL-1β transcription but did not affect c-jun transcription. pBR 322, negative control.

A 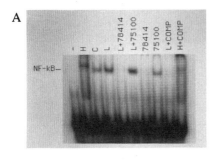 B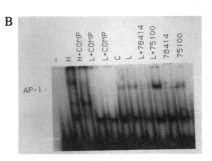

C 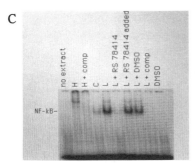 D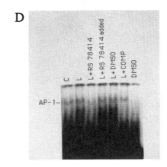

FIGURE 2. Gel mobility shift assays of monocyte nuclear extracts. **A** and **B:** Inhibition of NF-κB and AP-1 binding to DNA sequences following LPS treatment in the presence of THP. A gel mobility shift kit was purchased from Gibco/BRL, and assays were performed according to the manufacturer's procedures. LPS enhanced DNA-binding activities, which were significantly decreased by THP treatment. Legends: −, labeled oligo alone; H, positive control with HeLa nuclear extract; C, no treatment; L, LPS; COMP, oligo competitor; 75100, a control drug, which is not an antioxidant. Competition showed sequence specificity of the DNA binding. **C** and **D:** THP effect on NF-κB and AP-1 binding when added exogenously to isolated nuclear extracts. Nuclear extracts were prepared 1 h after treatment. As shown in A and B, THP inhibited NF-κB and AP-1 binding when added together with LPS. When THP was added to extracts derived from LPS-activated monocytes (L + RS 78414 added), no decrease of DNA binding activities was observed for either NF-κB or AP-1. Thus, THP decreased the activation of transcription factors but had no direct effect on DNA binding.

REFERENCES

1. LEE, S. W. & M. ILNICKA. Oxidant priming of human monocytic lineage cells to produce IL-1β. Ann. New York Acad. Sci. (This volume.)
2. EUGUI, E. M., B. DELUSTRO, S. ROUHAFZA, M. ILNICKA, S. LEE, R. WILHEIM & A. C. ALLISON. Some antioxidants inhibit, in a coordinate fashion, the production of TNFα, IL-1β, and IL-6 in LPS-activated monocytes. (Submitted for publication.)

Hydrogen Peroxide Primes Promonocytic U937 Cells to Produce IL-1β

SIMON W. LEE AND MARIOLA ILNICKA

Syntex Research
3401 Hillview Avenue
Palo Alto, California, 94304

INTRODUCTION

We have previously published that the LPS-stimulated promonocytic U937 cell line produces very little IL-1β mRNA and protein; addition of phorbol ester (PMA) increases their formation.[1] Committed monocytic precursors (THP-1) and peripheral blood monocytes produce high levels of IL-1β mRNA in response to LPS even in the presence of cycloheximide (unpublished data). Thus, the capacity to produce IL-1β is minimal in early monocytic precursors and increases as the cells differentiate into monocytes, which possess factors required for LPS signal transduction and IL-1β gene transcription. To investigate the factors involved in IL-1β gene transcription, we analyzed IL-1β mRNA following treatment of U937 cells with LPS and various reagents. We have now established that H_2O_2, in concentrations that do not affect viability, primes the U937 cells so that LPS induces the formation of IL-1β mRNA and protein. *De novo* synthesis of transcription factors such as AP-1 may be involved.

RESULTS

Simultaneous exposure of U937 cells to H_2O_2 and LPS induces detectable levels of IL-1β mRNA after 6 hours (FIGURE 1A). Pretreatment of U937 cells with H_2O_2 primes the U937 cells so that LPS induces the formation of IL-1β mRNA and protein (FIGURE 1B). The mechanism of H_2O_2 action is distinct from PMA induction because it is not sensitive to staurosporin A treatment (FIGURE 1C), which enhanced the steady-state concentration of IL-1β mRNA in the presence of hydrogen peroxide and LPS. Expression of IL-1β mRNA is down regulated by antioxidants such as mannitol (FIGURE 1D) and DMSO. Preliminary studies indicate that the action of H_2O_2 is dose dependently accompanied by calcium ion mobilization. Either EDTA or EGTA (1 mM) added at the time of stimulation reduced IL-1β mRNA expression by 70%. Preformed IL-1β mRNA induced by H_2O_2/LPS cotreatment was selectively destabilized by Dexamethasone in a manner similar to that described in PMA-induced U937 and LPS-treated peripheral blood monocytes.[2] IL-1β mRNA formation was diminished in the presence of cycloheximide, suggesting that mRNA expression is mediated by *de novo* synthesis of protein factors.

Gene transcription is mediated by activation of nuclear transcription factors that are DNA binding proteins. Gel shift mobility assays using nuclear extracts of U937 activated by H_2O_2/LPS showed that AP-1 was essentially unchanged at 0.5 hours but was markedly increased at 4 hours after stimulation (FIGURE 2). c-Fos mRNA was not elevated by H_2O_2/LPS treatment. Consistent with the earlier findings, staurosporin A treatment enhanced AP-1 activity in H_2O_2/LPS-activated cells. These findings suggest H_2O_2 priming induces changes in the cells, which leads to activation of transcription factor AP-1 at 4 hours and synthesis of detectable levels of IL-1β mRNA at 6 hours. Thus, in promonocytic cells, the absence of transcription factors such as AP-1 limits expression of the IL-1β gene in response to LPS. Oxidants such as H_2O_2 prime the cells for IL-1β production. The synthesis and activation of

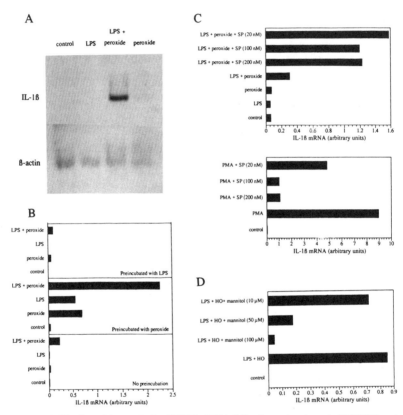

FIGURE 1. A: Northern blot analysis of U937 mRNA following cotreatment of LPS (10 μg/ml) and hydrogen peroxide (1 mM). RNA were isolated by the acidified guanidine thioisocyanate procedure.[2] **B:** Priming of U937 cells by hydrogen peroxide. U937 cells were incubated with LPS or hydrogen peroxide for 16 hours. Cells were washed with warmed RPMI medium, and media were replaced with media containing LPS, hydrogen peroxide, or both. RNA were isolated after 24 hours of incubation. **C:** Differential effect of staurosporin A on hydrogen peroxide/LPS and PMA-treated U937 cells. Cells were treated with hydrogen peroxide/LPS or PMA (100 nM) in the presence of 20 to 200 nM of staurosporin A for 16 hours. PMA, phorbol ester; SP, staurosporin A. Staurosporin A, a known inhibitor of PKC, inhibited IL-1β mRNA accumulation induced by PMA but enhanced the peroxide effect. **D:** Down regulation of IL-1β mRNA accumulation by antioxidant mannitol. IC_{50} of mannitol was about 30 μM. RNA quantification was performed by dot-blot analysis and densitometry.

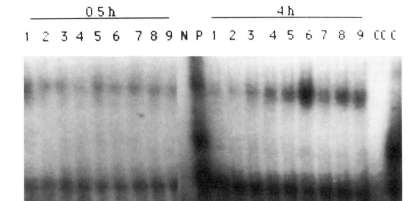

FIGURE 2. Enhancement of AP-1 activity by hydrogen peroxide and LPS in U937 cells. Treatments are described below. Nuclear extracts were prepared after 0.5 and 4 hours of treatment. Gel mobility assay was performed. 1, no treatment; 2, LPS; 3, hydrogen peroxide; 4, LPS and hydrogen peroxide; 5, PMA; 6, LPS, hydrogen peroxide and staurosporin A; 7, PMA and staurosporin A; 8, LPS, hydrogen peroxide, and okadaic acid; 9, PMA and okadaic acid; N, negative control (labeled oligo); P, positive control (Hela nuclear extract, Gibco/BRL); CC, competitor control; C, Hela nuclear extract and competitor.

transcription factors such as AP-1 may be involved in oxidant priming. Consequently, antioxidants that inhibit the stimulation of transcription factors down regulate the transcription of the IL-1β gene (Ilnicka *et al.,* this volume).

REFERENCES

1. LEE, S. W., A.-P. TSOU, H. CHAN, J. THOMAS, K. PETRI, E. M. EUGUI & A. C. ALLISON. 1988. Glucocorticoids selectively inhibit the transcription of the interleukin 1β gene and decrease the stability of interleukin 1β mRNA. Proc. Natl. Acad. Sci. USA **85:** 1204–1208.
2. AMANO, Y., S. W. LEE & A. C. ALLISON. 1992. Inhibition by glucocorticoids of the formation of interleukin-1a, interleukin-1β, and interleukin-6: mediation by decreased mRNA stability. Mol. Pharmacol. **43:** 176–182.

Structure-Function Analysis of Integrin-Mediated Cell Functions by Novel Nonpeptidic Conformational Mimetics of the Arg-Gly-Asp and Leu-Asp-Val Amino Acid Sequences

OFER LIDER,[a] RAMI HERSHKOVIZ,[a] RONEN ALON,[b]
AND NOAM GREENSPOON[c]

[a]Department of Cell Biology
[b]Department of Membrane Research and Biophysics
[c]Department of Organic Chemistry
The Weizmann Institute of Science
Rehovot 76100, Israel

The extravasation of cells from blood vessels and their ensuing tissue localization depend on receptor-mediated recognition of components of blood vessel walls and the extracellular matrix (ECM).[1] Fibronectin (FN), an ECM-derived cell-adhesive glycoprotein, is present in a variety of matrices and in the plasma.[2] FN is involved in processes that include wound healing, embryonic cell migration and differentiation, cell activation, proliferation, and adhesion.[3] Cell binding to immobilized FN is mediated primarily by surface integrins of the β_1 (CD29; VLA) subfamily of receptors.[4] The interaction of FN with these integrins relies on its central cell-binding domain and depends on the cell adhesion motif Arg-Gly-Asp (RGD), which is recognized primarily by the $\alpha_5\beta_1$ (VLA-5) integrin, and by the Leu-Asp-Val (LDV) sequence present on the alternative spliced sequences of the CS1 region of FN,[1] the binding of which is primarily mediated by the $\alpha_4\beta_1$ integrin (VLA-4).[5]

To study the structural parameters determining RGD and LDV specificity and affinity for their respective integrins, we prepared a series of novel nonpeptidic mimetics of the two sequences, as well as control compound mimetics of the Arg-Gly-Glu (RGE) and Leu-Glu-Val (LEV) sequences, and studied their interactions with various cell types.

ANALYSIS OF RGD MIMETICS

We have designed various structural mimetics of the tripeptide sequence, which consist of differentially spaced guanidinium and carboxylic groups. We have found that structures that contain guanidinium and carboxylic groups separated by an 11 carbon atom backbone mimic the distal configuration of functional RGD sequence. These compounds acquire a considerable affinity for the RGD-dependent platelet $\alpha_{IIb}\beta_3$ integrin and inhibited platelet aggregation with an IC_{50} at the sub-mM range. Furthermore, these compounds interfered with the binding of T-lymphocytes and metastatic tumor cells to immobilized FN. A structural mimetic of the RGE sequence, and structures with incorrect spacing between the functional groups, failed to inhibit these interactions. *In vivo,* an RGD surrogate effectively inhibited the elicitation of a delayed-type hypersensitivity reaction mediated by T cells.[6]

ANALYSIS OF LDV MIMETICS

To probe the structural requirements for LDV recognition by integrins and to examine the inhibition of LDV-dependent cell-FN interactions, we have designed and constructed a novel Ψ-S-CH$_2$ peptide bond surrogate that was employed in the formation of LDV surrogates. The synthesis of the Ψ-S-CH$_2$ surrogates is based on Michael addition of 4-methyl pentane thiol to an itaconic acid diester to form an S-CH$_2$ bond. We have found that the LDV surrogates comprised of 4-methyl pentanoate-Asp-i-Butyl amide and 8-methyl-3-(2-methylpropyl aminocarbonyl)-5-thia nonanoic acid interfered with CD4$^+$ human T cell adhesion to FN *in vitro,* with an ED$_{50}$ of 280 μg/ml. A control structural mimetic of the LEV peptide did not interfere with T cell–FN interaction. The specificity of the reaction was substantiated by the finding that the LDV mimetics did not interfere with T cell adhesion to laminin, another major cell-adhesive glycoprotein of the extracellular matrix. That the nonpeptidic mimetics of LDV interfered markedly with T cell–FN adhesive interactions indicate that the peptide bond and the amine and carboxyl end groups of the tripeptide make only a minor contribution to the integrin binding affinity (Greenspoon, N., *et al.,* in preparation).

Thus, such nonpeptidic constructs of short adhesion motifs of FN could provide novel insights into the fundamental mechanisms of receptor–ECM ligand interactions, and serve as competitive antagonists of potential therapeutic value.

REFERENCES

1. HYNES, R. O. 1992. Integrins: versatility, modulation, and signaling in cell adhesion. Cell **69:** 11–25.
2. YAMADA, K. M. 1991. Fibronectin and other cell interactive glycoproteins. *In* Cell Biology of Extracellular Matrix. E. D. Hay, Ed.: 111–148. Plenum Press. New York, N.Y.
3. PROCTOR, R. A. 1987. Fibronectin: a brief overview of its structure, function, and physiology. Rev. Infect. Dis. **9**(S4): 317–321.
4. SPRINGER, T. A. 1990. Adhesion receptors of the immune system. Nature **346:** 425–433.
5. SHIMIZU, Y. & S. SHAW. 1991. Lymphocyte interactions with extracellular matrix. FASEB J. **5:** 2292–2299.
6. GREENSPOON, N., R. HERSHKOVIZ, R. ALON, D. VARON, B. SHENKMAN, G. MARX, S. FEDERMAN, G. KAPUSTINA & O. LIDER. 1993. Structural analysis of integrin recognition and the inhibition of integrin-mediated cell functions by novel nonpeptidic surrogates of the Arg-Gly-Asp sequence. Biochemistry **32:** 1001–1008.

Effects of Cyclosporine-A and Cyclosporine-G on ADP-Stimulated Aggregation of Human Platelets

MARIANA S. MARKELL,[a,d] JULIO FERNANDEZ,[b]
ULHAS P. NAIK,[b] YIGAL EHRLICH,[c]
AND ELIZABETH KORNECKI[b]

[a] Departments of Medicine and Surgery
[b] Department of Cell Biology and Anatomy
SUNY Health Science Center at Brooklyn,
Brooklyn, New York

[c] CSI/IBR Center for Developmental Neuroscience
CUNY at Staten Island
Staten Island, New York

Use of cyclosporine-A (CSA) has been associated with a variety of clinical disorders that may be related to platelet dysfunction, including accelerated atherosclerosis, increased thrombotic episodes,[1] a hemolytic-uremic syndrome, and other sporadic reports of a vasculitic type picture in patients with cyclosporine nephrotoxicity.[1] Studies utilizing platelet-rich plasma (PRP) from CSA-treated renal transplant recipients suggest that these platelets are abnormally hyperaggregable when stimulated by ADP, collagen, and epinephrine.[2,3] In the present study, we compared dose- and time-response curves of CSA pretreatment in PRP to the curves of the norvaline substituted analogue, cyclosporine-G (CSG), which has less nephrotoxicity than CSA in animal models,[4] in order to determine if there was a difference in effect on platelet function.

MATERIALS AND METHODS

Whole blood (90 ml) was collected from healthy drug-free volunteers into the anticoagulant sodium citrate. Gel-filtered platelets (GFP) were prepared as previously described.[5] The final platelet count was 2×10^8/ml PRP and GFP were maintained at 37°C for all subsequent experiments. Platelet aggregations were carried out in a Lumi dual channel platelet aggregometer (Chronolog, Havertown, Pa.). Aggregations were plotted on a dual channel recorder as a change in optical transmission following the addition of the platelet agonist ADP (2.1 μM, final concentration) to 0.45 ml aliquots of the GFP suspension in the presence of added fibrinogen (0.41 mg/ml). The extent of aggregation was measured 3 minutes following the addition of ADP and was expressed as light transmission units (LTU). The initial velocity of aggregation was measured in light transmission units per minute (LTU/min).

[d] Address correspondence to: Division of Renal Disease, Box 52, SUNY Health Science Center at Brooklyn, 450 Clarkson Ave., Brooklyn, N.Y. 11203.

Purified cyclosporine-A (lot no. 88272.01) and cyclosporine-G [lot no. 90920 (56529)] were kindly supplied by the Sandoz Pharmaceuticals Corporation (East Hanover, N.J.). Cyclosporine vehicle solutions were prepared following the protocols supplied by Sandoz. CSA was dissolved in a minimum volume of 100% ethyl alcohol, mixed with Tween 20 (Fisher Scientific, Fair Lawn, N.J.) and diluted with 0.15 M NaCl. The final concentrations of Tween 20 and ethanol in the GFP suspensions were 0.001% and 0.006% respectively. Cyclosporine-G was dissolved in phosphate-buffered saline (PBS) containing 0.5% glucose and 3.5% BSA. Polyvinyl-pyrrolidone, molecular weight 40,000 (PVP-40), was used as a hydrophobic carrier.[6] Following solubilization in ethanol at 1 mg/ml concentration, the CSG solution was

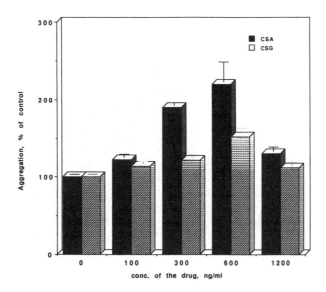

FIGURE 1. Effect of the concentration of CSA or CSG on hyperaggregation of platelets. PRP were incubated with various concentrations of CSA or CSG for 60 minutes at 37°C, and then 0.45 ml of PRP were added to the aggregometer. Platelet aggregation was induced by the addition of ADP (2 μM). The data represent the percent change in extent of ADP-induced platelet aggregation in CSA-treated platelets and CSG-treated platelets as compared to the vehicle-treated platelets. Values are the mean $\pm$ SEM for 6 experiments.

diluted 10-fold in PBS containing 35 mg/ml of PVP-40 at pH 7.40. The solution was then lyophilized and reconstituted in distilled water and the resulting stock solution stored at 4°C. All subsequent dilutions were made with 0.15 M saline. Control, vehicle solutions were prepared in an identical fashion to stock solutions except that addition of CSA or CSG was omitted. Dose-response studies were performed by incubation of 0.45 ml GFP with various concentrations of the drugs or vehicle in the aggregometer for 60 minutes under stirring conditions. Time course studies required incubations with the cyclosporines or vehicles with 6.0 ml GFP for up to 3 hours with gentle mixing. Aliquots of GFP (0.45 ml) were removed at various time intervals, supplemented with 0.41 mg/ml fibrinogen, and platelet aggregation was initiated by the addition of ADP as detailed above.

RESULTS

FIGURE 1 shows a dose-response curve comparing CSA- to CSG-treated platelets at 60 minutes incubation time. The peak effect is at approximately 600 ng/ml in this experiment for both drugs. However cyclosporine-A causes a greater than 200% increase in aggregation over control whereas, cyclosporine-G causes less than a 150% increase. FIGURE 2 shows a comparison of time-course curves, comparing CSA and CSG, using 1000 ng/ml solutions and reveals that a difference in the enhancement of ADP-stimulated platelet aggregation appears by 5 minutes and persists at as

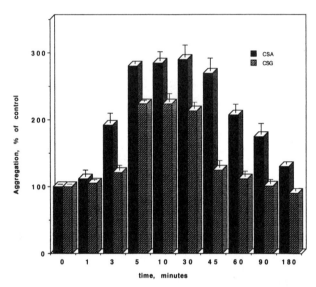

FIGURE 2. Effect of time of incubation of platelets with CSA vs. CSG on platelet hyperaggregability. CSA (1 μg/ml) or CSG (1 μg/ml) or respective vehicles were added to PRP. At various time points from 1 minute to 180 minutes, aliquots (0.45 ml) of PRP were added to the aggregometer and platelet aggregation was induced by the addition of ADP (2 μM). The data represent the percent change in the extent of aggregation between the CSA- or CSG-treated platelets and the vehicle-treated platelets. Values are mean ± standard error of the mean (SEM) for 6 experiments.

long as 60 minutes preincubation. The proaggregant effect with CSG is 40–100% less than the effect with CSA, depending on the preincubation time studied. In addition, the CSA effect appears to persist at longer incubation times, whereas, the CSG effect returns toward control value.

DISCUSSION

Platelet functional abnormalities play a role, not only in thrombotic events, but also in the generation of atherosclerosis, which is the leading cause of death in the long-term transplant recipient[7] and hypothetically in the genesis of chronic rejection.[8] Comparison of the dose response curves for CSG and CSA (FIGURE 1) reveals that CSG has less of a proaggregant effect on platelets at the peak concentration, which is within the range for peak cyclosporine concentrations. In addition, comparison of time-response curves (FIGURE 2) suggests that although the CSA proaggregant effect persists at longer preincubation time intervals up until 60 minutes, at which time platelets begin to lose viability, the CSG effect returns to near control values by 45 minutes. This finding suggests that the CSG effect may be transient. Although correlation with *in vivo* studies will be necessary, the relatively favorable profile of cyclosporine-G with regard to ADP-stimulated platelet aggregation *in vitro* suggests that CSG-treated patients may be expected to have fewer platelet-related complications, including early graft thrombosis, vasculitides and perhaps accelerated atherogenesis.

REFERENCES

1. REMUZZI, G. & T. BERTRANI. 1989. Renal vascular and thrombotic effects of cyclosporine. Am. J. Kid. Dis. **13**(4): 261–272.
2. COHEN, H., G. H. NEILD, R. PATEL, *et al.* 1988. Evidence for chronic platelet hyperaggregability and in vivo activation in cyclosporine-treated renal allograft recipients. Thromb. Res. **49**(1): 91–101.
3. GRACE, A. A., M. A. BARRADAS, D. P. MIKHAILIDIS, *et al.* 1987. Cyclosporine A enhances platelet aggregation Kid. Int. **32**: 889–895.
4. TEJANI, A., J. LANCMAN, A. POMERANZ, M. KHAWAR & C. CHEN. 1988. Nephrotoxicity of cyclosporine A and cyclosporine G in a rat model. Transplantation **45**(1): 184–187.
5. KORNECKI, E., Y. H. EHRLICH & R. H. LENOX. 1984. Platelet-activating factor–induced aggregation of human platelets specifically inhibited by triazobenzodiazepines. Science **226**: 1454–1456.
6. YONISH-ROUACH, M. SHINITZKY & M. RUBINSTEIN. 1990. A method for preparing biologically active aqueous cyclosporine A solutions avoiding the use of detergents or organic solvents. J. Immunol. Methods **135**: 147–153.
7. MAHONEY, J. F., R. I. CATERSON, C. A. POLLOCK, *et al.* 1990. Coronary artery disease is the major late complication of successful cadaveric renal transplantation. Clin. Trans. **4**: 129–132.
8. TILNEY, N. L., W. D. WHITLEY, J. R. DIAMONF, J. W. KUPIEC-WEGLINSKI & D. H. ADAMS. 1991. Chronic rejection—an undefined conundrum. Transplantation **52**: 389–398.

Relationship of Ionized Magnesium and Cyclosporine Level in Renal Transplant Recipients

MARIANA S. MARKELL,[a,b,e] BELLA T. ALTURA,[c]
YVONNE SARN,[a] RANDALL BARBOUR,[d]
ELI A. FRIEDMAN,[a] AND BURTON M. ALTURA[a,c]

[a]Department of Medicine
[b]Department of Surgery
[c]Department of Physiology
[d]Department of Pathology
SUNY Health Science Center at Brooklyn
Brooklyn, New York

Cyclosporine (CSA) use in transplantation has been reported to cause low serum total magnesium (TMg) values during the early posttransplant period, independent of the organ transplanted.[1] The pathogenesis of CSA-induced hypomagnesemia is believed to be a defect in renal tubular handling of magnesium.[2] Atherosclerotic cardiovascular disease is a leading cause of death in the long-term (>10 year) cyclosporine-treated renal transplant recipient,[3] and hypomagnesemia has been implicated as a factor in promotion of atherogenesis.[4] In humans, hypomagnesemia has been associated with increased incidence of hypertension,[2] insulin resistance,[5] and *in vitro,* CSA-treated mesangial cells, cultured in the absence of magnesium, demonstrate an enhanced contractile response to vasoconstrictor substances, which is diminished by the presence of magnesium in the incubation medium.[6] In this study, we utilized a novel ion selective electrode to measure the ionized, biologically active fraction of serum ionized magnesium (IMg^{2+}) in long-term cyclosporine-treated renal transplant recipients.

METHODS

Serum samples were collected from 27 random stable renal transplant recipients (RTRs) attending transplant clinic and 34 age- and sex-matched control (nontransplanted) subjects with normal renal function. Total cholesterol, total calcium and magnesium, and serum creatinine values were measured using a Kodak DT-60 Ektachem analyzer. Ionized calcium and magnesium values were drawn concomitantly with CSA level and analyzed in triplicate using an ion selective electrode and a NOVA Biomedical Stat Profile 8 Analyzer (NOVA Biomedical Corp., Waltham, Mass) as previously described. All values were repeated three times, and the average value used for statistical analyses. Insulin values were measured in triplicate using the INCSTAR radioimmunoassay kit (INCSTAR Sci. Tech. Research, Stillwater,

[e]Address correspondence to: Box 52, Division of Nephrology, SUNY Health Science Center at Brooklyn, 450 Clarkson Ave., Brooklyn, N.Y. 11203.

Minn.). Cyclosporine-A was measured by high-performance liquid chromatography (HPLC) before and 6 to 8 hours following ingestion of the daily dose. GFR was estimated by counting of 6 timed blood and urine samples following subcutaneous injection of I^{125}-iothalamate. Statistical analyses were performed using 2-tailed Student's t-test or Pearson correlation as appropriate. A p value of <0.05 was considered significant.

RESULTS

Compared with 34 age-matched control subjects, the 27 RTRs had pronounced deficits in mean IMg^{2+} (0.50 ± 0.02 vs. control 0.61 ± 0.06 mM/L, $p < 0.05$) but only slight deficits in mean total Mg (0.78 ± 0.02 vs. 0.84 ± 0.017 mM/L). Initial IMg^{2+} value varied inversely with concomitant CSA trough level ($r = 0.55$, $p < 0.005$). Following ingestion of CSA, coincident with the rise in CSA levels, mean IMg^{2+} fell to 0.45 ± 0.01 mM/L, $p = 0.05$. Sixteen (59%) of the CSA-treated RTRs were

TABLE 1. General Characteristics of Renal Transplant Recipients with Profound Hypomagnesemia and Those Remaining Normomagnesemic.

	Hypomagnesemic	Normomagnesemic
Number	16	11
Age (yrs)	43 ± 3.1	34.2 ± 3.1
Weight (kg)	71.2 ± 3.4	80.1 ± 6.2
Body surface area	1.75 ± 0.04	1.8 ± 0.05
Time posttransplant (mos)	29.2 ± 4.9	41.8 ± 8.26
Male/female	7/9	7/4
Race (B/W/H/A)	5/4/5/2	4/2/2/3
CSA dose (mg/kg)	5.14 ± 0.45	4.53 ± 0.7
Prednisone dose (mg)	9.67 ± 0.76	11.1 ± 1.08
Hypertension	16 (100%)	11 (100%)
Lasix dose (mg)	91.4 ± 15.4	83.6 ± 16.6

significantly hypomagnesemic ($IMg^{2+} < 0.52$ mM/L). General characteristics of the two groups are shown in TABLE 1. There were no significant differences between the groups when examined for race or sex, number of hypertensives, dose of immunosuppression or lasix, weight or body surface area. Patients with hypomagnesemia tended to be slightly older, and to have had their transplant more recently but these differences did not reach significance. Comparison of laboratory values is shown in TABLE 2. Hypomagnesemic patients had lower TMg values, higher CSA trough values, lower urinary magnesium excretion, and higher fasting insulin values than RTRs who remained normomagnesemic. They did not differ as regards GFR, measured by iothalamate clearance, ionized calcium values, or lipid profile.

DISCUSSION

We have demonstrated that a subset of CSA-treated renal transplant recipients have profound deficits in both ionized and total magnesium that cannot be explained simply on the basis of diuretic use. Ionized magnesium values were low in the presence of relatively normal total magnesium values. IMg^{2+} values measured in a concomitant blood sample varied inversely with the CSA trough level, and magnesium values fell in 100% of patients at the time of concomitant peak CSA level, suggesting that CSA may have an acute effect on ionized magnesium. Hypomagnesemia has been associated with abnormalities of glucose tolerance, specifically in insulin resistant states.[5] Hyperinsulinemia in the patients with magnesium deficiency may represent insulin resistance. Urinary magnesium values were lower in the hypomagnesemic renal transplant patients when compared with normomagnesemic renal transplant patients, suggesting that the hypomagnesemic patients, who were on average 2 years posttransplant, had total body magnesium depletion rather than an ongoing "urinary leak." Hypomagnesemia could contribute to CSA toxicity, both in an acute and chronic form, in that CSA toxicity is associated with hypertension and decreased GFR, which may reflect altered vascular smooth muscle or mesangial cell contractility secondary to decreased intracellular magnesium values.

Thus, it appears that in our population of CSA-treated patients, deficits of ionized magnesium are common and may have been underrecognized because total

TABLE 2. Comparison of Laboratory Values for CSA-Treated Renal Transplant Recipients with Hypomagensemia and Those Remaining Normomagnesemic.[a]

	Hypomagnesemic	Normomagnesemic
Number	16	11
GFR (ml/min)	49.9 ± 5.4	36.5 ± 5.2
Trough CSA level	169.3 ± 26.9	52.5 ± 15.1*
Fasting insulin (mIU/ml)	16.0 ± 1.6	10.8 ± 1.34*
Urinary Mg (mg/24 hr)	70.1 ± 8.5	104.5 ± 6.5*
Ionized calcium (mM/L)	1.19 ± 0.02	1.19 ± 0.03
Total Mg (mM/L)	0.71 ± 0.03	0.87 ± 0.06**
Ionized Mg^{2+} (mM/L)	0.43 ± 0.015	0.58 ± 0.01***
Total cholesterol (mg/dl)	248.7 ± 12.5	252 ± 18.2
Triglycerides (mg/dl)	189.5 ± 16.1	237.5 ± 40.4
High-density lipoproteins (mg/dl)	58.3 ± 6.0	41.2 ± 4.77
Low-density lipoproteins (mg/dl)	158.7 ± 12.7	172.1 ± 15.8

[a]All values expressed as mean ± SEM. *$p < 0.05$ by 2-tailed Student's t-test for between group comparisons, **$p < 0.005$, ***$p < 0.0001$, all other values not significant.

serum magnesium values fell in the low normal range. The rapid measurement of serum or plasma ionized magnesium using ion selective electrodes should aid in the management of cyclosporine-treated renal transplant recipients in whom magnesium deficits may contribute to hypertension, hyperinsulinemia, cyclosporine nephrotoxicity, and accelerated atherosclerosis, which are encountered in this population.

REFERENCES

1. BARTON, C. H., N. D. VAZIRI, D. C. MARTIN, S. CHOI & S. ALIKHANI. 1987. Hypomagnesemia and renal magnesium wasting in renal transplant recipients receiving cyclosporine. Am. J. Med. 83: 693–699.
2. ELIN, R. J. 1988. Magnesium metabolism in health and disease. Dis. Month 34: 161–218.
3. MARKELL, M. S. & E. A. FRIEDMAN. 1989. Hyperlipidemia after organ transplantation. Am. J. Med. 87: 5-61N–5-67N.

4. ALTURA, B. M. 1988. Ischemic heart disease and magnesium. Magnesium: Exp. Clin. Res. **7:** 57–67.
5. RESNICK, L. M. 1992. Cellular calcium and magnesium metabolism in the pathophysiology and treatment of hypertension and related metabolic disorders. Am. J. Med. **93**(2A): 11S–20S.
6. FANDREY, J., P. M. ROB & W. JELKMANN. 1991. Theophylline and magnesium inhibit the contraction elicited with cyclosporine and angiotensin II in mesangial cell cultures. Nephron **57:** 94–98.
7. ALTURA, B. T., T. L. SHIREY, C. C. YOUNG, J. HITI, K. DELL'ORFANO, S. M. HANDWERKER & B. M. ALTURA. 1992. A new method for the rapid determination of ionized Mg^{2+} in whole blood, serum and plasma. Methods Find. Exp. Clin. Pharmacol. **14:** 297–304.

Studies on the Interaction of the Immunosuppressant 15-Deoxyspergualin with Heat Shock Proteins

STEVEN G. NADLER,[a] JEFFREY CLEAVELAND,[a]
MARK A. TEPPER,[a] CHRISTOPHER WALSH,[b]
AND KARI NADEAU[b]

[a] Bristol-Myers Squibb Pharmaceutical Research Institute
3005 First Avenue
Seattle, Washington 98121

[b] Harvard Medical School
Boston, Massachusetts

Recently, we have shown that the immunosuppressant 15-deoxyspergualin (DSG) specifically interacts with a member of the Hsp70 family of heat shock proteins.[1] In order to determine the solution binding constant of DSG for Hsc70, we have utilized two independent techniques: stimulation of heat shock protein ATPase activity and affinity capillary zone electrophoresis.

Heat shock proteins have been shown to be involved in several intracellular processes.[2] For members of the Hsp70 family of heat shock proteins, these functions can be grouped into two main areas which include their ability to act as "molecular chaperones" and their role in protein folding and unfolding reactions. Each of these functions requires the heat shock protein to bind and release its protein or peptide substrate. The release of peptides and proteins has been shown to be an ATP-dependent process; hence, peptides and proteins can stimulate the basal ATPase activity of Hsp70.[2] Since DSG is structurally similar to a tripeptide, we determined whether it was able to stimulate the ATPase activity of various members of the Hsp70 family of proteins. As seen in FIGURE 1, DSG stimulated the ATPase activity of bovine Hsc70 approximately twofold yielding a K_m for DSG binding to bovine Hsc70 of approximately 600 nM, and an affinity of 3.0 μM to mouse Hsp70. Interestingly, DSG did not stimulate the ATPase activity of DnaK, the bacterial form of Hsp70, or Mtp70, the mitochondrial form. To confirm these findings we have also used the technique of affinity capillary zone electrophoresis (ACE).[3] Using ACE, DSG was shown to bind to mouse Hsp70 with an affinity of 4.0 μM, which agrees well with the binding constant determined by stimulation of ATPase activity. DSG did not bind to DnaK or to Mtp70. These results confirm our previously reported studies and show that DSG binds to the *cytosolic* members of the Hsp70 family of proteins in solution.

To address the question of whether DSG may be binding at the peptide binding site, we radiolabeled a peptide with a sequence derived from cytochrome C. This peptide had a binding constant of approximately 10 μM for bovine Hsc70. Since DSG binds slightly better to Hsc70 than this peptide, we would have expected DSG to compete for the binding of the radiolabeled peptide if they both bound to the same site on the protein. Surprisingly, DSG competed very poorly for the binding of the peptide to Hsc70. This suggested that DSG was binding at a distinct site from the peptide binding site. FIGURE 2 shows that 5 mM of a peptide with the sequence KRQIYTDLEMNRLGK was unable to elute Hsc70 from a methoxy-DSG affinity

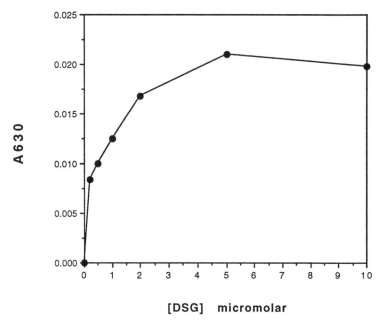

[DSG] micromolar

FIGURE 1. Stimulation of Hsc70 ATPase activity by 15-deoxyspergualin. Two μgrams of bovine Hsc70 was incubated with 500 μM ATP and varying amounts of deoxyspergualin for 60 minutes at 37°C. After the incubation, the amount of inorganic phosphate released was measured using a malachite green assay.

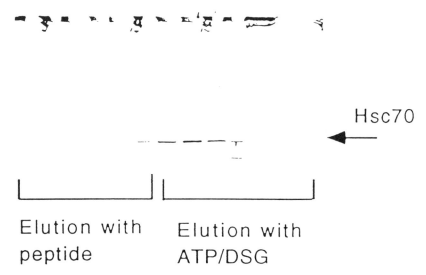

FIGURE 2. Methoxy-deoxyspergualin affinity chromatography of Jurkat cell lysates. Affinity chromatography was performed as previously described[1] with the following changes. After the high salt wash, protein was eluted with 5 mM of the peptide described above, followed by 5 mM of ATP plus DSG. A 12.5% gel was run, and proteins visualized by silver stain.

column providing additional evidence that DSG binds differently than peptides to Hsc70. These data would suggest that there are two distinct binding sites on Hsc70 in addition to the ATP binding site. As mentioned above, DSG can stimulate the ATPase activity of Hsc70. At concentrations above 200 μM, however, there was a dose-dependent decrease in ATPase activity, although based on ACE, DSG was still bound to the protein (data not shown). This lends additional support for our hypothesis that there are two binding sites on Hsc70 since it appears that the higher concentrations of DSG may be binding to an allosteric site and affecting the ATPase activity.

In conclusion, we have provided data that show that DSG binds to Hsc70 in solution. Since DSG reaches concentrations in lymphocytes greater than 50 μM (Nadler and Cleaveland, unpublished results) and the binding constant for Hsp70 is approximately 600 nM to 4 μM, clearly Hsp70 could be a target for the *in vivo* binding and immunosuppressive actions of DSG.

REFERENCES

1. NADLER, S. G., M. A. TEPPER, B. SCHACTER & C. E. MAZZUCCO. 1992. Science **258:** 484.
2. GETHING, M. J. & J. SAMBROOK. 1992. Nature **355:** 33.
3. AVILA, L. Z., Y. CHU, E. BLOSSEY & G. M. WHITESIDES. 1992. J. Med. Chem. **15:** 3040–3048.

4-Thiazolidinones, Potent Antioxidants, as Antiinflammatory Agents

J. A. PANETTA, J. K. SHADLE, M. L. PHILLIPS,
D. N. BENSLAY, AND P. P. K. HO

Lilly Research Laboratories
Lilly Corporate Center, 0444
Indianapolis, Indiana 46285

Oxygen-derived free radicals are important mediators of tissue injury associated with many disease states, inflammatory responses, and ischemic insults. For example, reactive oxygen species have been implicated in rheumatoid arthritis, myocardial infarction, muscular dystrophy, Parkinson's disease, stroke, and atherosclerosis. In inflammatory joint disease, many cells present in the inflamed joint (macrophages, neutrophils, endothelial cells) have the capacity when activated to produce large quantities of reactive oxygen metabolites such as superoxide anion (O_2^-), hydrogen peroxide (H_2O_2), and hydroxyl radical (OH·).[1,2] Iron plays a central role in both the generation and propagation of reactive oxygen species during an inflammatory event. These oxygen-derived radicals are capable of attacking the major classes of cellular components, such as lipids, proteins, and nucleic acids, thereby leading to tissue injury and cell death. Synovial fluid from knee joints of patients with rheumatoid arthritis contains increased levels of thiobarbituric acid–reactive (TBARS) substances, which correlates with clinical severity of the disease, suggesting an increase in oxidant-mediated membrane lipid peroxidation.[3]

We have developed a series of antioxidants that contain the backbone structure of butylated hydroxytoluene (BHT), a known antioxidant that is widely used in the food industry, and the thiazolidinone nucleus. The result of this approach is a series of potent inhibitors of iron-dependent lipid peroxidation. Several members of this series are extremely effective in animal models of arthritis (in particular, Freund's

	Dose mg/kg p.o.	% Inhibition of Bone Damage		% Inhibition of Paw Swelling Area Under Curve			Number of Rats
		Injected Paw	Uninjected Paw	A	B	C	
LY221068	50	76 ± 2*	78 ± 6*	29.4 ± 4.3	58.0 ± 2.9	72.4 ± 3.8	60
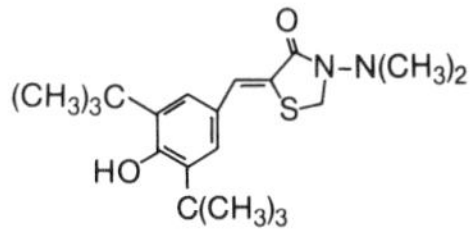	25	55 ± 7*	56 ± 9*	24.0 ± 7	41.0 ± 9	56.0 ± 12	15
	10	41 ± 9*	40 ± 5*	20.0 ± 14	24 ± 9	33 ± 9	15
	5	0	0	19 ± 7	14 ± 6	12 ± 6	10

*$p < 0.05$ as determined by two tailed Dunnett's t-test on raw data.

FIGURE 1. Dose response of LY221068 in the developing Freund's complete adjuvant induced arthritis in rats.

	Dose mg/kg p.o.	% Inhibition of Bone Damage		% Inhibition of Paw Swelling Area Under Curve			Number of Rats
		Injected Paw	Uninjected Paw	A	B	C	
LY269415	25	$81 \pm 2^*$	$86 \pm 1^*$	36 ± 5	56 ± 5	74 ± 8	20
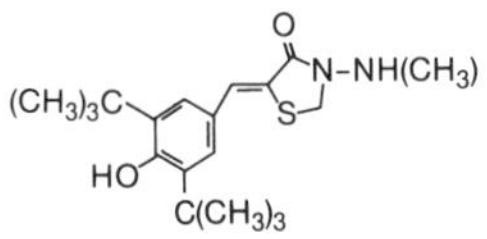	10	$58 \pm 5^*$	$80 \pm 6^*$	25 ± 5	37 ± 3	59 ± 6	15
	5	$36 \pm 5^*$	$52 \pm 12^*$	22 ± 10	21 ± 2	50 ± 8	15

$^*p < 0.05$ as determined by two tailed Dunnett's t-test on raw data.

FIGURE 2. Dose response of LY269415 in the developing Freund's complete adjuvant induced arthritis in rats.

complete adjuvant induced arthritis (FCA) model in rats). The compounds were administered orally, and inhibition of bone damage and soft tissue swelling of both the injected and uninjected paws was assessed for 28 days.

The A area under the paw volume curve represents the edematous reaction due to a nonimmune effect of injection of the adjuvant to the paw, while the B area under such a curve could result from a combination of the continuing presence of the irritant and immune-mediated inflammation. However, the C area is the paw volume curve of the uninjected paw, with the inflammatory response due to a systemic immune mediated reaction.

5-[3,5-bis(1,1 dimethylethyl)-4-hydroxy-phenyl]methylene]-3-(dimethyl-amino)-4- thiazolidinone, LY221068, and the monomethylamino analogue LY269415 are the most promising compounds with the minimum effective dose being 10 mg/kg per oral and 5 mg/kg po, respectively, and significantly inhibited the paw swelling under area C significantly more than either area A or B (FIGURES 1 and 2). The inhibition of bone damage for the injected and the uninjected paws paralleled the paw swelling inhibition. These results support the hypothesis that reactive oxygen species/lipid peroxidation may play an important role in the pathogenesis of rheumatoid arthritis.

REFERENCES

1. BABIOR, B. M. 1978. Oxygen dependent microbial killing by phagocytes. N. Engl. J. Med. **298:** 721–725.
2. FANTONE, J. C. & P. A. WARD. 1982. Role of oxygen derived free radicals and metabolites in leukocyte-dependent inflammatory reactions. Am. J. Pathol. **107:** 397.
3. ROWLEY, D. A., J. M. C. GUTTERIDGE, D. R. BLAKE, M. FARR & B. HALLIWELL. 1984. Lipid peroxidation in rheumatoid arthritis: thiobarbituric acid reactive material and catalytic iron salts in synovial fluid from rheumatoid patients. Clin. Sci. **66:** 691–695.

Effects of Methylprednisolone Administration on Lymphocyte LECAM-1, CD44, and LFA-1 Expression

Implications for Steroid-Induced Lymphopenia[a]

ROBERT SACKSTEIN

Bone Marrow Transplant Service
H. Lee Moffitt Cancer Center and
Research Institute
University of South Florida
College of Medicine
Tampa, Florida 33612

Corticosteroid therapy causes immunosuppression in part by depleting the bloodstream of the mature, recirculating pool of lymphocytes. This transient lymphopenia results from an inhibition of lymphocyte trafficking to peripheral lymph nodes, leading to a redistribution of circulating cells to other tissue compartments, such as bone marrow.[1-3] The first step in the migration ("homing") of lymphocytes to lymph node involves the specific attachment of the cells to lymph node high endothelial venules (HEV).[4] LECAM-1 (L-selectin), a 90,000 mw lymphocyte glycoprotein which mediates attachment to HEV, is the "lymph node homing receptor." In addition to this protein, two accessory HEV-binding molecules have also been identified: LFA-1 (CD11a/CD18) and CD44. Despite extensive knowledge of the biochemistry of these proteins and numerous physiologic studies of lymphocyte migration following corticosteroid therapy, our knowledge into the underlying molecular mechanisms for the steroid-induced decrease in lymphocyte migration to lymph nodes is incomplete. In rodents, there is evidence that steroids may decrease the capacity of HEV to bind lymphocytes.[5,6] In humans, this effect has not been demonstrated, and it may be hypothesized that steroids decrease expression of lymphocyte adhesion molecules specific for promoting entry into lymph node. The present study was undertaken to address this issue by analyzing the *in vivo* and *in vitro* effects of methylprednisolone on lymphocyte LECAM-1, CD44, and LFA-1 expression.

Flow cytometric analysis of peripheral blood lymphocytes isolated by density centrifugation was performed in tissue culture studies and following pulse methylprednisolone infusion *in vivo*. Six healthy volunteers underwent infusions of saline (placebo) and methylprednisolone (Solumedrol, 3 mg/kg in saline) over 15 minutes, and peripheral blood lymphocytes were isolated before, immediately after, and at 1, 2, 4, 8, 24, and 48 hours following infusions. Saline infusion (placebo) had no effect on lymphocyte counts or on the levels of expression of lymphocyte LECAM-1, CD44, or LFA-1 (both CD11a and CD18 chains). Following steroid infusion, lymphopenia

[a]This work was supported by a Veterans Affairs Career Development Award, V.A. Merit Grant 7687.03, National Institutes of Health General Clinical Research Center Grant M01-RR-05280, the Lou and Teresa Shinder CLL Research Fund, and the Stanley and Kathleen Glaser Research Foundation (University of Miami School of Medicine).

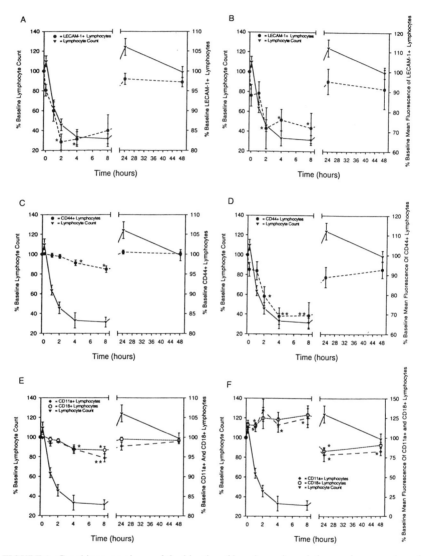

FIGURE 1. Graphic comparisons of the kinetics of lymphopenia and changes in expression of adhesion proteins following steroid infusion. Units shown are percentage relative to preinfusion values. Major changes are seen in the percentage of LECAM-1+ cells (graph A), and in the mean channel fluorescence levels of LECAM-1+ cells (graph B) and CD44+ cells (graph D). Results are mean ± standard error of the mean for percentage values. Compared to placebo, statistically significant ($p < 0.05$) decreases in lymphocyte counts were seen at 2, 4, and 8 hours; for adhesion proteins, statistical differences are as noted [$*p < 0.05$, $**p < 0.005$ by paired t-test (placebo vs. steroid)].

was observed within 1 hour and persisted for 8 hours but resolved by 24 hours. Concomitant with lymphopenia, there was a marked decrease in both the percentage and mean fluorescence intensity level of the LECAM-1+ lymphocytes, and the circulating cells did not adhere to HEV in an *in vitro* binding assay. There were minor changes in the percentage of CD44+ and LFA-1+ cells, while the mean fluorescence intensity level decreased for CD44+ cells and increased for LFA-1+ cells (FIGURE 1). All such changes in adhesion protein levels among circulating cells reversed with the resolution of lymphopenia. However, in tissue culture experiments, the expression of these adhesion proteins was not altered following incubation of lymphocytes for four hours utilizing either hydrocortisone (maximum dose 200 μg/ml) or methylprednisolone (maximum dose 40 μg/ml).

The results of this study provide an important insight into the mechanism of the lymphopenia of steroid therapy: the data support the notion that steroids inhibit lymphocyte migration to lymph node by decreasing expression of the major HEV-binding protein, LECAM-1, as well as the accessory protein CD44. Although *in vitro* studies indicate that lymphocyte expression of LECAM-1, CD44, or LFA-1 is not directly altered by steroids, the possibility that these agents may act indirectly *in vivo* by stimulating the release and/or promoting the activity of relevant biological mediators affecting lymphocyte adhesion protein expression needs further exploration.

ACKNOWLEDGMENTS

The author thanks Mr. Michael Borenstein and Mr. Rehan Naqui for expert technical assistance.

REFERENCES

1. FAUCI, A. S. & D. C. DALE. 1975. The effect of hydrocortisone on the kinetics of normal human lymphocytes. Blood **46:** 235–243.
2. FAUCI, A. S. & D. C. DALE. 1974. The effect of in-vivo hydrocortisone on subpopulations of human lymphocytes. J. Clin. Invest. **53:** 240–246.
3. HAYNES, B. F. & A. S. FAUCI. 1978. The differential effect of in-vivo hydrocortisone on the kinetics of subpopulations of human peripheral blood thymus-derived lymphocytes. J. Clin. Invest. **61:** 703–707.
4. CHIN, Y. H., R. SACKSTEIN & J. P. CAI. 1991. Lymphocyte homing receptors and preferential migration pathways. Proc. Soc. Exp. Biol. Med. **196:** 374–380.
5. COX, J. H. & W. L. FORD. 1982. The migration of lymphocytes across specialized vascular endothelium. Cell. Immunol. **66:** 407–422.
6. CHUNG, H. T., W. E. SAMLOWSKI & R. A. DAYNES. 1986. Modification of the murine immune system by glucocorticosteroids: alterations of the tissue localization properties of circulating lymphocytes. Cell. Immunol. **101:** 571–585.

CMT/NSAID Combination Increases Bone CMT Uptake and Inhibits Bone Resorption[a]

N. RAMAMURTHY,[b] M. LEUNG, S. MOAK,
R. GREENWALD, AND L. GOLUB

SUNY at Stony Brook

Old Westbury, Long Island Jewish Medical Center
New Hyde Park, New York

Collagenase and gelatinase belong to the matrix metalloproteinase (MMP) family, and these proteinases play a major role in collagen destruction in arthritic disorders, periodontal diseases, corneal ulcers, tumor invasion, etc. Extensive studies have confirmed that several tetracyclines (TCs), including the nonantimicrobial analogues known as the chemically modified tetracylines (CMTS), can inhibit collagenase and gelatinase activities and prevent pathologic tissue destruction.[1] Recently, Greenwald *et al.* described a synergism between nonsteroidal antiinflammatory drugs (NSAID) and CMT-1 in an adjuvant arthritis (AA) rat model.[2] Data reported in this study revealed that tetracyclines exhibit little antiinflammatory effect in AA rats in contrast to an NSAID such as flurbiprofen, which reduced joint swelling. Although each drug alone had only slight effects on joint bone loss, combining both compounds via daily oral gavage maximized the reduction of both inflammation and radiographic evidence of bone destruction. In addition, "combination" therapy completely inhibited MMP activity in the periarticular tissues. Tenidap (TD) is a novel oxindole NSAID that inhibits both lipoxygenase as well as cyclooxygenase. It has also been reported to inhibit the oxidative activation of neutrophil procollagenase. In the current study we examined the effect of TD on bone CMT uptake *in vivo* and the effect of both drugs on inflammatory bone destruction. Male Lewis rats were made arthritic by injecting Freund's adjuvant at the base of the tail. Arthritis became evident by 12–13 days. Treatment groups were as follows: normal, untreated AA, AA + TD (2 mg/rat), CMT (4 mg/rat), and AA + TD + CMT. All of the drugs were administered by oral gavage in 2% carboxymethyl cellulose for 23 days.

Joint scores and paw diameters were recorded weekly and at termination of the experiment. The whole legs were x-rayed on high resolution film and scored blindly by three readers from 0 (no damage) to 4 (maximal damage). Periarticular (PST) tissues were removed and extracted for collagenase and gelatinase. MMPs were assayed using radiolabeled collagen and gelatin and quantified by scintillation spectrometry or SDS-PAGE. The soft and hard tissues of the joints and serum were extracted with HPLC solvents, and the extracts analyzed for CMT levels using an HPLC technique.[3] Daily administration to AA rats of CMT in combination with TD markedly reduced ($p < 0.01$) MMP activities in PST and reduced bone destruction

[a]This study was supported by NIDR grant no. R37 DE-03987, ADAMH no. DA-47392, NIH no. GM-0818.

[b]Address correspondence to: Department of Oral Biology & Pathology. School of Dental Medicine, Health Sciences Center-South Campus, SUNY Stony Brook, Stony Brook, New York 11794-8702.

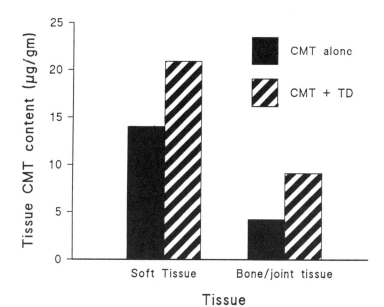

Tissue

FIGURE 1. Effect of Tenidap on CMT uptake in periarticular soft tissues (PST) and bones of tarsal joints. PST and bones were soaked in HPLC solvent (methanol:acetonitrile: 10 mM oxalic acid 1:1.5:2.5 pH 2.0) and homogenized by polytron for 30 seconds and extracted overnight. The supernatant was separated by centrifugation ($800 \times g$ 15 min) and passed through 0.3 μ acrodisc filter. Aliquots of the supernates were analyzed by HPLC using supelco LC-18-DB 5 μM C_{18} reversed-phase column. The eluant was monitored by UV-Vis detector at 360 nm. The area under the peaks was obtained by integration, and absolute quantity was obtained with a standard curve.

($p < 0.05$) more than either drug alone. "Combination" therapy increased CMT uptake in bone by 116% ($p < 0.05$) compared to the level seen in AA rats treated with CMT itself, but this effect was not seen in PST (FIGURE 1). In summary, these data indicate that severe inflammation reduces CMT uptake by AA bone. TD and other NSAIDs reduce inflammation, perhaps increasing blood delivery of CMT to the bone of the AA joints, thus promoting the ability of CMT to inhibit bone cell MMP activity. Past failures of MMP inhibitors to ameliorate radiologic severity in the AA rat may have been due to lack of concomitant antiinflammatory therapy.

REFERENCES

1. GOLUB, L. M., N. S. RAMAMURTHY, T. F. MCNAMARA, R. A. GREENWALD & B. R. RIFKIN. 1991. Tetracyclines inhibit connective tissue breakdown: new therapeutic implications for an old family of drugs. Crit. Rev. Oral Biol. Med. **2:** 297–322.
2. GREENWALD, R. A., S. A. MOAK, N. S. RAMAMURTHY & L. M. GOLUB. 1992. Tetracyclines suppress matrix metalloproteinase activity in adjuvant arthritis and in combination with flurbiprofen, ameliorate bone damage. J. Rheumatol. **19:** 927–938.
3. YU, Z., M. LEUNG, N. S. RAMAMURTHY, T. MCNAMARA & L. M. GOLUB. 1992. HPLC determination of a chemically modified non-antimicrobial tetracycline: biologic implications. Biochem. Med. Metab. Biol. **47:** 10–20.

Index of Contributors

423